T0292432

CURRENT CLINICAL PATHOLOGY

ANTONIO GIORDANO, MD, PHD
Philadelphia, PA, USA

SERIES EDITOR

More information about this series at http://www.springer.com/series/7632

Maria M. Picken • Guillermo A. Herrera
Ahmet Dogan

Editors

Amyloid and Related Disorders

Surgical Pathology and Clinical Correlations

Second Edition

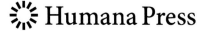 Humana Press

Editors
Maria M. Picken, MD, PhD
Professor of Pathology
Director of Surgical Pathology
Loyola University Medical Center
Department of Pathology
Maywood, IL, USA

Guillermo A. Herrera, MD
Albert G. And Harriet G. Smith
  Professor and Chair
LSU Health Shreveport
Department of Pathology
Shreveport, LA, USA

Ahmet Dogan, MD, PhD
Chief, Hematopathology Service
Memorial Sloan-Kettering Cancer Center
Department of Pathology and
  Laboratory Medicine
New York, NY, USA

ISSN 2197-781X   ISSN 2197-7828   (electronic)
Current Clinical Pathology
ISBN 978-3-319-19293-2   ISBN 978-3-319-19294-9   (eBook)
DOI 10.1007/978-3-319-19294-9

Library of Congress Control Number: 2015945563

Springer Cham Heidelberg New York Dordrecht London

Printed on acid-free paper

Humana Press is a brand of Springer
Springer International Publishing AG Switzerland is part of Springer Science+Business Media (www.springer.com)

This book is dedicated to our patients, past and present, with the hope that it will make a difference in the lives of future amyloidosis patients.

MMP, GAH, AD

Preface (Second Edition)

Amyloidosis, although known since the nineteenth century, retained for a long time the aura of a rare and obscure disease that was untreatable and mainly of purely academic interest. This state of affairs has, however, changed dramatically in recent years. With the new therapies that are now available, patients with systemic light chain amyloidosis (AL) may achieve a durable response and live for more than a decade from the time of their first diagnosis. Treatments for other types of systemic amyloidosis are also improving. Thus, in addition to liver transplantation, patients diagnosed with hereditary amyloidosis derived from a mutant transthyretin (ATTR) are currently being offered pharmacologic therapies that are in clinical trials. However, treatment outcomes are most successful when they are applied early in the disease process. Thus, now more than ever, early diagnosis is of the utmost importance. Although there are a number of excellent amyloidosis treatment centers around the world, early diagnosis of affected patients is reliant upon widespread and effective screening, and, despite advances in laboratory medicine, this still hinges upon the detection of deposits in tissues. Thus, the role of the pathologist in this process is critical. This book therefore has, as its primary focus, the diagnosis of amyloidosis in surgical pathology. Although written primarily for pathologists, it is hoped that this volume will also be helpful to those who would wish to gain insight into recent diagnostic and treatment options.

This second edition of "Amyloid and related disorders" has been expanded to include seven new chapters, while the prior content has been updated. The volume begins with a history of amyloid investigations and the latest nomenclature. Separate chapters are devoted to the mechanism of amyloidogenesis and an overview of AL, AA, ALECT2, hereditary, dialysis, and localized amyloidoses; a brief overview of cerebral amyloidoses is also included. In Part II, diseases that mimic amyloid and related disorders are discussed. Part III is entirely devoted to pathologic diagnosis, including the generic diagnosis of amyloid, and issues pertaining to amyloid typing that involve both antibody-based and proteomic methods. Part IV provides an overview of laboratory support for the diagnosis of amyloidosis, including serum, urine, bone marrow, and genetic studies. Part V provides an overview of amyloid pathologies in the genitourinary tract, cardiac, gastrointestinal/liver, and peripheral nervous systems; new chapters on lymph nodes and spleen, pulmonary, dermal, breast, and iatrogenic amyloidoses have been added.

Part VI discusses clinicopathologic issues and the role of solid organ transplantation, as well as recent advances in therapies for AL, hereditary, and AA amyloidosis. Brief chapters on relevant legal issues, and the patient's perspective, conclude Part VI.

Those who are interested in the amyloidoses are also encouraged to review the contents of "Amyloid: The Journal of Protein Folding Disorders" and contact the International Society of Amyloidosis (www.amyloidosis.nl). Resources available to patients include the Amyloidosis Foundation (http:// www.amyloidosis.org) and the Amyloidosis Support Group (http://www. amyloidosissupport.org).

It also behooves us to acknowledge that abnormal protein folding, the very essence of amyloid fibril formation, affects many more aspects of our lives than those covered by the chapters in this book. While amyloid formation represents a fundamental process in many diseases and aging, it also plays an important role in vertebrate and invertebrate biology, as functional amyloid; amyloid fibrils also have applications in the fields of nanotechnology and bioengineering. Therefore, understanding the driving forces behind both the regulated and unregulated formation of amyloid structures may help us to enlist that knowledge in the fight against disease and the aging process and may, unexpectedly, also lead to improvements in many other areas of our lives.

Maywood, IL, USA	Maria Mrozowicz Picken
Shreveport, LA, USA	Guillermo A. Herrera
New York, NY, USA	Ahmet Dogan

Acknowledgments

The editors would like to express their gratitude to the contributing authors and the publisher, Springer, and its Editors, Richard A. Hruska, Senior Editor, Clinical Medicine, and Michele Aiello, Developmental Editor, for editorial support during the publication process. Special thanks are due to Roger N. Picken for extensive editorial help.

Contents

Contributors

Ivona Aksentijevich, MD Inflammatory Disease Section, National Institutes of Health, National Human Genome Research Institute, Bethesda, MD, USA

Timothy Craig Allen, MD, JD Department of Pathology, The University of Texas Medical Branch, Galveston, TX, USA

Kevin Barton, MD Division of Hematology/Oncology, Loyola University Medical Center, Maywood, IL, USA

Merrill D. Benson, MD Department of Pathology and Laboratory Medicine, Indiana University School of Medicine, Van Nuys Medical Science Building, Indianapolis, IN, USA

Johan Bijzet, BSc Department of Rheumatology & Clinical Immunology, University Medical Center Groningen, University of Groningen, Groningen, The Netherlands

Francesca Brambilla, PhD Department of Proteomics and Metabolomics, Institute for Biomedical Technologies (ITB-CNR), Segrate (MI), Italy

Gian Luca Capello, BS Foundation IRCCS Policlinico San Matteo, Pavia, Italy

Department of Molecular Medicine, University of Pavia, Pavia, Italy

Lawreen H. Connors, PhD Departments of Pathology and Laboratory Medicine, Boston University School of Medicine, Boston, MA, USA

Amyloidosis Center, Boston University School of Medicine, Boston, MA, USA

Oscar W. Cummings, MD Department of Pathology, Indiana University Health, Indianapolis, IN, USA

Laura M. Dember, MD Renal, Electrolyte and Hypertension Division, Perelman School of Medicine, University of Pennsylvania, Philadelphia, PA, USA

Andrea Di Fonzo, PhD Department of Molecular Medicine and Amyloidosis Research and Treatment Center, Foundation IRCCS Policlinico San Matteo and University of Pavia, Pavia, Italy

Ahmet Dogan, MD, PhD Departments of Pathology and Laboratory Medicine, Memorial Sloan Kettering Cancer Center, New York, NY, USA

JaNean K. Engelstad, MS Peripheral Nerve Laboratory, Mayo Clinic, Rochester, MN, USA

Giovanni Ferraro, MSc Department of Molecular Medicine and Amyloidosis Research and Treatment Center, Foundation IRCCS Policlinico San Matteo and University of Pavia, Pavia, Italy

Muriel Finkel Amyloidosis Support Groups, Wood Dale, IL, USA

Janet A. Gilbertson, CSci, FIBMS UCL Division of Medicine, National Amyloidosis Centre, Royal Free Hospital, London, UK

Julian D. Gillmore, MBBS, MD, PhD, FRCP UCL Division of Medicine, National Amyloidosis Centre, Royal Free Hospital, London, UK

Karen L. Grogg, MD Department of Laboratory Medicine and Pathology, Mayo Clinic, Rochester, MN, USA

Philip N. Hawkins, PhD, FRCP, FRCPath, FMedSci UCL Division of Medicine, National Amyloidosis Centre, Royal Free Hospital, London, UK

Bouke P.C. Hazenberg, MD, PhD Department of Rheumatology & Clinical Immunology, University Medical Center Groningen, University of Groningen, Groningen, The Netherlands

Guillermo A. Herrera, MD Department of Pathology, Louisiana State University Health Sciences Center, Shreveport, LA, USA

W. Edward Highsmith Jr., PhD Department of Laboratory Medicine and Pathology, Mayo Clinic College of Medicine, Rochester, MN, USA

Alexander J. Howie, MD, FRCPath Department of Pathology, University College London, London, UK

Bertrand L. Jaber, MD, MS Division of Nephrology, Department of Medicine, St. Elizabeth's Medical Center, Tufts University School of Medicine, Boston, MA, USA

Alexandre Karras, MD Department of Nephrology, AP-HP, University Paris Descartes, Hôpital Européen Georges Pompidou, Paris, France

Jerry A. Katzmann, PhD Department of Laboratory Medicine and Pathology, Mayo Clinic, Rochester, MN, USA

Christopher J. Klein, MD Peripheral Nerve Laboratory, Mayo Clinic, Rochester, MN, USA

Chris P. Larsen, MD Nephropath, Little Rock, AR, USA

Francesca Lavatelli, MD, PhD Department of Molecular Medicine and Amyloidosis Research and Treatment Center, Foundation IRCCS Policlinico San Matteo and University of Pavia, Pavia, Italy

John C. Lee, MD Departments of Pathology and Laboratory Medicine, Boston University School of Medicine, Boston, MA, USA

John M. Lee, MD, PhD Department of Pathology and Laboratory Medicine, NorthShore University Health System, Evanston Hospital, Evanston, IL, USA

Reinhold P. Linke, MD, PhD Reference Center of Amyloid Diseases amYmed, Innovation Center of Biotechnology, Martinsried, Germany

Adam J. Loavenbruck, MD, MS Kennedy Laboratory, Department of Neurology, University of Minnesota, Minneapolis, MN, USA

Pierluigi Mauri, PhD Department of Proteomics and Metabolomics, Institute for Biomedical Technologies (ITB-CNR), Segrate (MI), Italy

Oana Madalina Mereuta, MD, PhD Department of Pathology, Memorial Sloan Kettering Cancer Center, New York, NY, USA

Giampaolo Merlini, MD Department of Molecular Medicine and Amyloidosis Research and Treatment Center, Foundation IRCCS Policlinico San Matteo and University of Pavia, Pavia, Italy

Patrizia Morbini, MD, PhD Pathology Unit, Department of Molecular Medicine, University of Pavia and Fondazione IRCCS Policlinico San Matteo, Pavia, Italy

David L. Murray, MD, PhD Department of Laboratory Medicine and Pathology, Mayo Clinic, Rochester, MN, USA

Mario Nuvolone, MD, PhD Institute of Neuropathology, University Hospital of Zurich, Zurich, Switzerland

Amyloidosis Research and Treatment Center, Foundation Scientific Institute Policlinico San Matteo, Department of Molecular Medicine, University of Pavia, Pavia, Italy

Laura Obici, MD Department of Molecular Medicine and Amyloidosis Research and Treatment Center, Foundation IRCCS Policlinico San Matteo and University of Pavia, Pavia, Italy

Carl J. O'Hara, MD Departments of Pathology and Laboratory Medicine, Boston University School of Medicine, Boston, MA, USA

Amyloidosis Center, Boston University School of Medicine, Boston, USA

Amanda K. Ombrello, MD Inflammatory Disease Section, National Human Genome Research Institute, National Institutes of Health, Bethesda, MD, USA

Giovanni Palladini, MD, PhD Department of Molecular Medicine and Amyloidosis Research and Treatment Center, Foundation IRCCS Policlinico San Matteo and University of Pavia, Pavia, Italy

Marco Paulli Foundation IRCCS Policlinico San Matteo, Pavia, Italy

Department of Molecular Medicine, University of Pavia, Pavia, Italy

Maria M. Picken, MD, PhD Department of Pathology, Loyola University Medical Center, Loyola University Chicago, Maywood, IL, USA

Emmanuelle Plaisier, MD, PhD Sorbonne Universités, UPMC Univ Paris 06, UMR_S 1155, Paris, France

Department of Nephrology and Dialysis, AP-HP, Hôpital Tenon, Paris, France

Anne Räisänen-Sokolowski, MD, PhD Transplantation Laboratory-HUSLAB, Helsinki University Central Hospital, Helsinki, HUS, Finland

Kimiyo M. Raymond, MD Department of Laboratory Medicine and Pathology, Mayo Clinic College of Medicine, Mayo Clinic, Rochester, MN, USA

E. Rene Rodriguez, MD Department of Pathology, Cleveland Clinic Lerner College of Medicine of Case Western Reserve University, Cleveland, OH, USA

Fausto J. Rodriguez, MD Department of Pathology, Division of Neuropathology, Johns Hopkins Hospital, Baltimore, MD, USA

Pierre Ronco, MD, PhD Sorbonne Universités, UPMC Univ Paris 06, UMR_S 1155, Paris, France

Department of Nephrology and Dialysis, AP-HP, Hôpital Tenon, Paris, France

UMR_S 1155, Batiment Recherche, Hôpital Tenon, Paris, France

Filiz Sen, MD Department of Pathology, Memorial Sloan Kettering Cancer Center, New York, NY, USA

S. Michelle Shiller, DO Department of Laboratory Medicine and Pathology, Mayo Clinic College of Medicine, Rochester, MN, USA

Department of Surgical Pathology, Baylor University Medical Center, Dallas, TX, USA

Paweena Susantitaphong, MD, PhD Division of Nephrology, Department of Medicine, St. Elizabeth's Medical Center, Tufts University School of Medicine, Boston, MA, USA

Extracorporeal Multiorgan Support Dialysis Center, Division of Nephrology, Department of Medicine, King Chulalongkorn Memorial Hospital, Chulalongkorn University, Bangkok, Thailand

Carmela D. Tan, MD Department of Pathology, Cleveland Clinic Lerner College of Medicine of Case Western Reserve University, Cleveland, OH, USA

Tom Törnroth, MD, PhD Transplantation Laboratory-HUSLAB, Helsinki University Central Hospital, Helsinki, HUS, Finland

Elba A. Turbat-Herrera, MD Departments of Pathology and Medicine, Louisiana State University, Shreveport, LA, USA

Ingrid I. van Gameren, MD, PhD Department of Rheumatology & Clinical Immunology, University Medical Center Groningen, University of Groningen, Groningen, The Netherlands

Laura Verga, DVM, PhD Pathology Unit, Department of Molecular Medicine, University of Pavia and Fondazione IRCCS Policlinico San Matteo, Pavia, Italy

Per Westermark, MD, PhD Department of Immunology, Genetics and Pathology, Rudbeck Laboratory, Uppsala University, Uppsala, Sweden

Part I

Introduction/General

Aspects of the History and Nomenclature of Amyloid and Amyloidosis

Per Westermark

A Short History of Amyloid

The longer you can look back
the further you can look forward
Winston Churchill

This chapter deals with some aspects of the history of amyloid and its evolving nomenclature. The history is interesting and contains some of the characteristics of human behavior, including envy and rigidity. Those with a particular interest are referred to a number of earlier publications [1–5]. In addition, some very interesting aspects of the modern history can be found in the proceedings from the international symposia on amyloidosis, particularly the first ones [6, 7].

The designation "amyloid" is actually a misnomer. As a human affliction, the term was coined by Rudolf Virchow when he used iodine to search for a cellulose- (or starch-) related substance. He found that corpora amylacea of the brain had some tinctorial properties that were reminiscent of starch and named the stained substance amyloid [8]. Corpora amylacea are not an example of what is now called amyloid, but Virchow expanded his studies to include tissues that contained (what we now understand must have been) systemic amyloidosis of the AA type and found similar staining properties. It should be emphasized that the condition was well known among pathologists before Virchow, but under other names. Amyloid means "starch-like" (amylon or amylum is starch in Greek and Latin, respectively), but only 5 years after the term amyloid had been coined, it was found that the deposited substance was mainly proteinaceous [9].

Thus, after the mistake with corpora amylacea, Virchow and others studied "real amyloid," most likely AA amyloidosis, the most prevalent systemic amyloidosis at that time. Although there are variations, in comparison to some other systemic amyloidoses, particularly AL amyloidosis, AA has a fairly constant tissue distribution pattern. Patients with a diverse amyloid distribution and symptoms that were most probably due to AL amyloidosis were described at an early date [10]. The term "senile amyloidosis" was coined by Soyka, who described a condition that was most likely senile systemic amyloidosis [11], today known to be derived from wild-type transthyretin (TTR) and therefore now called "wild-type ATTR (ATTRwt) amyloidosis" according to recommendations by the Nomenclature Committee of the International Society of Amyloidosis [12]. The term "primary generalized amyloidosis" was well described by Lubarsch in 1929 [13] although single cases probably had been reported earlier [14]. Localized,

P. Westermark, MD, PhD (✉)
Department of Immunology, Genetics and Pathology,
Rudbeck Laboratory, Uppsala University,
Uppsala SE 751 85, Sweden
e-mail: Per.Westermark@igp.uu.se

© Springer International Publishing Switzerland 2015
M.M. Picken et al. (eds.), *Amyloid and Related Disorders*, Current Clinical Pathology,
DOI 10.1007/978-3-319-19294-9_1

tumor-like amyloid had already been described in the nineteenth century and, similar to a large number of other medical conditions, careful and exact descriptions can be found in German literature from this period (e.g., see [15]). Cases of hereditary amyloidosis, which today is known to be a very heterogeneous group of disorders with varying biochemical nature and genetic background, and spread throughout the world, were also described [16]. An account of the most common form of hereditary amyloidosis, that is derived from TTR, was published in 1952, almost 100 years after the term amyloid was first coined [17]. The exact nature of this amyloid as derived from TTR was elucidated in 1978 [18]. This form of ATTR amyloidosis is found in many parts of the world and had been demonstrated to be due to a missense mutation [19]. Since then, a great number of different mutations in the TTR gene have been found, most of them associated with systemic amyloidosis and with varying phenotypes [20–22]. Later, several additional hereditary amyloidoses of various biochemical types were described, almost exclusively dominant hereditary, and due to missense mutations. Surprisingly, as late as 2008, a form of systemic amyloidosis that is not extremely rare was characterized [23].

Biochemical Nature of Amyloid

Even before the seminal discovery that amyloid has a distinctive fine fibrillar structure [24] in which the protein has adopted a high degree of β-sheet structure with the molecules regularly arranged and bound to each other by hydrogen bonds [25], an organized substructure for the hyaline amyloid had been proposed [26, 27]. Most important of all were the studies by Benditt and Eriksen, who showed that the deposits present in secondary systemic amyloidosis are characterized by one specific protein, which they called "protein A" (now protein AA) while the proteins in other types of amyloidosis were preliminarily called "protein B" [28]. They remarked, wisely, that there may be several B proteins. The techniques used to extract amyloid fibrils, dissolve them in chaotropic agents, and

purify the major proteins for characterization by Edman degradation revolutionized our comprehension of amyloid. Instead of being nonspecific degenerative materials, the amyloids were found to be polymers of highly specific proteins [29, 30]. At the end of the 1970s, four major amyloid fibril proteins had been described [18, 29–31]. Today, 31 different proteins have been accepted as major amyloid fibril proteins (Table 1.1).

Diagnosis of Amyloidosis

The introduction of the cotton dye Congo red was a great step forward in the identification of amyloid [32]. The dye was synthesized in 1883 for the textile industry, and there is evidence that its name has a firm connection with a political conference, held in Berlin in 1884–1885, where the colonial powers discussed Central Africa; thus, the name has nothing to do with the origin of the dye [33]. Congo red was introduced as an intravenous test for systemic amyloidosis in patients, since deposits in the tissues bound the dye, and enhanced plasma clearance was taken as a sign of disease [34]. A quite substantial amount of Congo red was injected, often more than 10 ml of a 1 % aqueous solution of the dye [35]. Although unreliable and potentially dangerous, this test seems to have continued in use until the 1970s [36, 37]. This can seem surprising to us now, when some laboratories hesitate to utilize Congo red in histopathology due to its potential to be carcinogenic [38]. As early as 1884, the dye was tested as a histological stain [39], but it was not until 1927 that its properties as an amyloid stain were described [26]. At that time, a very important property of amyloid stained with Congo red was identified: namely, the enhanced birefringence of amyloid in tissue sections viewed under polarized light [26]. In fact, this technique is still used in diagnostic work throughout the world. Diagnostic biopsies from organs showing symptoms had been used for some time (for examples and references, see [40]), but it was not until 1960 that the well-known rectal biopsy was introduced as a diagnostic tool for systemic amyloidosis [41]. This was a most important advance, since

Table 1.1 Amyloid fibril proteins and their precursors in human[a]

Fibril protein	Precursor protein	Systemic and/or localized	Acquired or hereditary	Target organs
AL	Immunoglobulin light chain	S, L	A, H[e]	All organs except CNS (Local AL amyloidosis may occur)
AH	Immunoglobulin heavy chain	S, L	A	All organs except CNS (Local AH amyloidosis may occur)
AA	(Apo) Serum amyloid A	S	A	All organs except CNS
ATTR	Transthyretin, wild type	S	A	Heart mainly in males, Ligaments, Tenosynovium
	Transthyretin, variants	S	H	PNS, ANS, heart, eye, leptomeninges
Aβ2M	β2-Microglobulin, wild type	L	A	Musculoskeletal system
	β2-Microglobulin, variant	S	H	ANS
AApoAI	Apolipoprotein A I, variants	S	H	Heart, liver, kidney, PNS, testis, larynx (C terminal variants), skin (C terminal variants)
AApoAII	Apolipoprotein A II, variants	S	H	Kidney
AApoAIV	Apolipoprotein A IV, wild type	S	A	Kidney medulla and systemic
AGel	Gelsolin, variants	S	H	PNS, cornea
ALys	Lysozyme, variants	S	H	Kidney
ALECT2	Leukocyte chemotactic factor-2	S	A	Kidney, primarily
AFib	Fibrinogen α, variants	S	H	Kidney, primarily
ACys	Cystatin C, variants	S	H	PNS, skin
ABri	ABriPP, variants	S	H	CNS
ADan[b]	ADanPP, variants	L	H	CNS
Aβ	Aβ protein precursor, wild type	L	A	CNS
	Aβ protein precursor, variant	L	H	CNS
APrP	Prion protein, wild type	L	A	CJD, Fatal insomnia
	Prion protein variants	L	H	CJD, GSS syndrome, Fatal insomnia
ACal	(Pro)calcitonin	L	A	C-cell thyroid tumors
AIAPP	Islet amyloid polypeptide[c]	L	A	Islets of langerhans, Insulinomas
AANF	Atrial natriuretic factor	L	A	Cardiac atria
APro	Prolactin	L	A	Pituitary prolactinomas, aging pituitary
AIns	Insulin	L	A	Iatrogenic, local injection
ASpc[d]	Lung surfactant protein	L	A	Lung
AGal7	Galectin 7	L	A	Skin
ACor	Corneodesmosin	L	A	Cornified epithelia, Hair follicles
AMed	Lactadherin	L	A	Senile aortic, Media

(continued)

Table 1.1 (continued)

Fibril protein	Precursor protein	Systemic and/ or localized	Acquired or hereditary	Target organs
AKer	Kerato-epithelin	L	A	Cornea, hereditary
ALac	Lactoferrin	L	A	Cornea
AOAAP	Odontogenic ameloblast-associated protein	L	A	Odontogenic tumors
ASem1	Semenogelin 1	L	A	Vesicula seminalis
AEnf	Enfurvitide	L	A	Iatrogenic, local injection

From Sipe et al. [12]
[a]Proteins are listed, when possible, according to relationship. Thus, apolipoproteins are grouped together, as are polypeptide hormones
[b]ADan is the product of the same gene as ABri
[c]Also called amylin
[d]Not proven by amino acid sequence analysis
[e]Benson et al. [46]

before 1950, only 7 % of patients were diagnosed before death [42]. The technique most commonly used today, biopsy from subcutaneous fat tissue, was developed a decade later in the 1970s [43]. Since then, biopsy techniques have been further expanded to include determination of the biochemical nature of an amyloid deposit; today, this is considered to be a necessary step in the clinical handling of patients with systemic amyloidosis. Although a biopsy with microscopic demonstration of amyloid is still the only way to obtain a diagnosis, a method for visualizing amyloid in vivo based on the ubiquitously present serum amyloid P (SAP) component has been successfully developed [44].

Nomenclature

What Is Amyloid?

Most of us working with amyloid believe that we know what amyloid is. However, when reading the modern scientific literature, one can begin to hesitate since the word is now used in different ways. In clinical pathological practice, amyloid is a homogenous extracellular deposit that stains specifically with Congo red, shows clear yellow to green birefringence in polarized light, and has a characteristic fine-fibrillar ultrastructure. It should be stressed that the Congo red staining should be performed under strictly controlled conditions; otherwise other tissue components may also be stained. Other staining methods may be used but are generally not regarded as being as specific. In addition to this "classical" amyloid, fibrils made in vitro that possess some amyloid properties are often called amyloid in the biochemical literature. Even inclusion bodies, which may or may not stain with Congo red, are often referred to as amyloid. Examples of such inclusions are the intranuclear aggregates in Huntington's disease and Lewy bodies in Parkinson's disease. In clinical pathology, it is wise to stay within the classical definition.

Older Nomenclatures

Over the decades, there have been a number of different nomenclatures. The most prevalent prior classification stems from 1935 and divides the amyloidoses into four groups: primary, secondary, tumor-forming, and the amyloidosis associated with multiple myeloma. Unfortunately, it is sometimes still in use, which creates unnecessary confusion (Table 1.2). For a long time, it was widely discussed whether the localized, often small, but dispersed deposits with amyloid staining properties are indeed "true" amyloid or not, and the designation "para-amyloid" was sometimes used to describe them [16, 45]. This name should be avoided.

Table 1.2 Terminology often used in the older literature which should now be abandoned

Designation to avoid	Reason for avoidance
Familial amyloidotic cardiomyopathy (FAC)	It is a systemic amyloidosis with deposits in other tissues as well
Familial amyloidotic polyneuropathy (FAP)	It is a systemic amyloidosis with deposits in other tissues as well
Primary amyloidosis	An old, inexact term. It was used for AL amyloidosis but also for hereditary amyloid forms
Secondary amyloidosis	An old, inexact term. It was used for AA amyloidosis but often also for amyloidosis with multiple myeloma and sometimes for localized amyloid in tumors
Senile cardiac amyloidosis	This term was used for wild type ATTR (senile systemic) amyloidosis. Although cardiac symptoms often predominate, it is a systemic disease
Senile systemic amyloidosis	This term was coined when the nature of the amyloid protein was unknown. Since the disease sometimes affects persons in their 50s, wild-type TTR amyloidosis is to be preferred

Modern Amyloid Nomenclature

At the international symposium on amyloidosis in 1974 in Helsinki, Finland, a committee was organized to oversee the nomenclature of the amyloid fibril proteins. Although only two amyloid proteins were known at the time (AA and AL), this decision proved prescient given the situation that pertains today, when at least 31 amyloid fibril proteins have been identified. The committee is now part of the International Society of Amyloidosis (ISA) and meets at each ISA symposium. On those occasions, the nomenclature committee updates the accepted amyloid fibril protein table and the updated nomenclature is published in the journal Amyloid. The latest nomenclature [12] is given in Table 1.1.

All amyloid proteins are designated as A plus a suffix, identifying the nature of the precursor.

Thus, immunoglobulin light chain amyloid protein is called AL (A+immunoglobulin light chain), transthyretin amyloid is ATTR, and so on. Any substitutions are indicated by a suffix, identifying the position in the mature protein flanked by the normal amino acid residue to the left and the variant to the right. If deemed important, the position based on the transcript may be given in parenthesis. Consequently, the most common transthyretin variant protein is designated ATTRVal30Met where valine is the normal residue and this is substituted by methionine and the translated gene product (p.TTRVal50Met) [12]. Amyloid deposits, and diseases, should be named after their main fibrillar protein and should also be identified as localized or systemic and whether they are sporadic or hereditary. Old designations, such as primary or secondary, typical or atypical, should be abandoned (Table 1.2). Familial amyloidotic polyneuropathy (FAP), which is very often used for hereditary ATTR amyloidosis, particularly with the Val30Met mutation, is also a designation that should be avoided although the name may be too well established to be replaced.

References

1. Kyle RA, Bayrd ED. Amyloidosis: review of 236 cases. Medicine. 1975;54:271–99.
2. Glenner GG. Amyloid deposits and amyloidosis. The β-fibrilloses. N Engl J Med. 1980;302:1283–92. 1333–43.
3. Cohen AS. General introduction and a brief history of amyloidosis. In: Marrink J, van Rijswijk MH, editors. Amyloidosis. Dordrecht: Martinus Nijhoff Publishers; 1986. p. 3–19.
4. Sipe JD, Cohen AS. Review: history of the amyloid fibril. J Struct Biol. 2000;130:88–98.
5. Westermark P. Amyloidosis and amyloid proteins: brief history and definitions. In: Sipe JD, editor. Amyloid proteins. The beta sheet conformation and disease. Weinheim: Wiley-VCH; 2005. p. 3–27.
6. Mandema E et al., editors. Amyloidosis. Amsterdam: Excerpta Medica; 1968.
7. Wegelius O, Pasternack A, editors. Amyloidosis. London: Academic; 1976.
8. Virchow R. Ueber eine im Gehirn und Ruckenmark des Menschen aufgefunde Substanz mit der chemishen Reaction der Cellulose. Virchows Arch Path Anat. 1854;6:135–8.
9. Friedreich N, Kekulé A. Zur Amyloidfrage. Virchows Arch Pathol Anat. 1859;16:50–65.

10. Wild C. Beitrag zur Kenntnis der amyloiden und der hyalinen Degeneration des Bindegewebes. Beitr Path Anat Physiol. 1886;1:175–200.
11. Soyka J. Ueber die amyloide Degeneration. Prag Med Wschr. 1876;1:165–71.
12. Sipe JD et al. Updated nomenclature 2014: amyloid fibril proteins and clinical classification of the amyloidoses. Amyloid. 2014;21:221–4.
13. Lubarsch O. Zur Kenntnis ungewöhnlicher Amyloidablagerungen. Virchows Arch Path Anat. 1929;271:867–89.
14. Herrera GA. The kidney in plasma cell dyscrasias: a current view and a look at the future. Contrib Nephrol. 2007;153:1–4.
15. Vossius A. Ueber amyloide Degeneration der Conjunctiva. Beitr Path Anat Allg Path. 1889;4:335–60.
16. Ostertag B. Demonstration einer eigenartigen familiären "Paramyloidose". Zentralbl Pathol. 1933;56:253–4.
17. Andrade C. A peculiar form of peripheral neuropathy: familial atypical generalized amylodosis with special involvement of the peripheral nerves. Brain. 1952;75:408–27.
18. Costa PP, Figueira AS, Bravo FR. Amyloid fibril protein related to prealbumin in familial amyloidotic polyneuropathy. Proc Natl Acad Sci USA. 1978;75:4499–503.
19. Tawara S et al. Identification of amyloid prealbumin variant in familial amyloidotic polyneuropathy (Japanese type). Biochem Biophys Res Commun. 1983;116:880–8.
20. Saraiva MJ. Hereditary transthyretin amyloidosis: molecular basis and therapeutical strategies. Expert Rev Mol Med. 2002;4(12):1–11.
21. Connors LH et al. Tabulation of human transthyretin (TTR) variants, 2003. Amyloid. 2003;10:160–84.
22. Rowczenio DM et al. Online registry for mutations in hereditary amyloidosis including nomenclature recommendations. Hum Mutat. 2014;35(9):E2403–12.
23. Benson MD et al. Leucocyte chemotactic factor 2: a novel renal amyloid protein. Kidney Int. 2008;74(2):218–22.
24. Cohen AS, Calkins E. Electron microscopic observations on a fibrous component in amyloid of diverse origins. Nature. 1959;183:1202–3.
25. Eanes ED, Glenner GG. X-ray diffraction studies on amyloid filaments. J Histochem Cytochem. 1968;16:673–7.
26. Divry P, Florkin M. Sur les propriétées optiques de l'amyloide. Comp Rend Soc Biol (Paris). 1927;97:1808–10.
27. Romhányi G. Uber die submikroskopische Struktur des Amyloid. Schweiz Z Path (Path Microbiol). 1949;12:253–62.
28. Benditt EP, Eriksen N. Chemical classes of amyloid substance. Am J Pathol. 1971;65:231–52.
29. Benditt EP et al. The major proteins of human and monkey amyloid substance: common properties including unusual N-terminal amino acid sequences. FEBS Lett. 1971;19:169–73.
30. Glenner GG et al. Amyloid fibril proteins: proof of homology with immunoglobulin light chains by sequence analysis. Science. 1971;172:1150–1.
31. Sletten K, Westermark P, Natvig JB. Characterization of amyloid fibril proteins from medullary carcinoma of the thyroid. J Exp Med. 1976;143:993–8.
32. Bennhold H. Eine specifische Amyloidfärbung mit Kongorot. Münch Med Wochenschr. 1922;69:1537–8.
33. Steensma DP. "Congo" red. Out of Africa? Arch Pathol Lab Med. 2001;125(2):250–2.
34. Bennhold H. Über die Asscheidung intravenös einverbleibten Kongorotes bei den verschiedensten Erkrankungen insbesondere bei Amyloidosis. Deutsch Arch Klin Med. 1923;142:32–46.
35. Morgan WKC, Mules JE. The intravenous Congo red test: a description of some unrecognized fallacies with suggested improvements. Am J Med Sci. 1960;239(1):61–70.
36. Ouchi E et al. Clinical significance of Congo red test. Tohoku J Exp Med. 1976;118(suppl):191–8.
37. Patra S, Jhala CI, Patra BS. Intravenous Congo red test in pulmonary tuberculosis for detection of amyloidosis, its value and limitations. J Assoc Physicians India. 1976;24(9):553–7.
38. Afkhami A, Moosavi A. Adsorptive removal of Congo red, a carcinogenic textile dye, from aqueous solutions by maghemite nanoparticles. J Hazard Mat. 2010;174:398–403.
39. Griesbach H. Weitere Untersuchungen über Azofarbstoffe behufs Tinction menchlischer und thierischer Gewebe. Zeitschr Wissenschaft Mikroskop Microskop Tech. 1886;3:358–85.
40. Symmers WSC. Primary amyloidosis: a review. J Clin Pathol. 1956;9:187–211.
41. Gafni J, Sohar E. Rectal biopsy for the diagnosis of amyloidosis. Am J Med Sci. 1960;240:332–6.
42. Editorial. Clinical diagnosis of amyloidosis. J Am Med Assoc. 1963;183(13):1104.
43. Westermark P, Stenkvist B. A new method for the diagnosis of systemic amyloidosis. Arch Intern Med. 1973;132:522–3.
44. Hawkins PN et al. Scintigraphic quantification and serial monitoring of human visceral amyloid deposits provide evidence for turnover and regression. Quart J Med. 1993;86:365–74.
45. Gellerstedt N. Die elektive, insuläre (Para-) Amyloidose der Bauchspeicheldrüse. Zugleich en Beitrag zur Kenntnis der "senilen Amyloidose". Beitr Path Anat. 1938;101:1–13.
46. Benson MD et al. Hereditary systemic immunoglobulin light-chain (AL) amyloidosis. XIVth International Symposium Amyloidosis, April 27–May 1, 2014, Indianapolis, IN.

Amyloid Diseases at the Molecular Level: General Overview and Focus on AL Amyloidosis

2

Mario Nuvolone, Giovanni Palladini, and Giampaolo Merlini

General Overview

In the vast and heterogeneous group of disorders collectively termed "amyloidoses", a protein or peptide loses, or fails to acquire, its physiologic, functional folding and, in its misfolded state, undergoes fibrillization and extracellular accumulation in the form of amyloid deposits [1]. These deposits display distinctive chemical, ultrastructural and tinctorial properties, which allow for their correct identification and help to distinguish amyloidoses from other pathologic conditions similarly characterized by abnormalities in protein conformation or metabolism [2, 3]. The process of amyloid formation and deposition ultimately results in tissue damage and organ dysfunction and is the pathological substrate of numerous clinical conditions, local or systemic, acquired or hereditary, extremely rare or rather frequent, which may represent a diagnostic challenge for pathologists and clinicians [1].

What Makes a Protein Amyloidogenic?

Based on extensive experimental evidence, any protein, either folded or natively unstructured, is predicted to form amyloid fibrils in vitro under appropriate circumstances [4]. However, only a limited number of proteins do so in vivo. The reason for this discrepancy is not fully understood, but it is assumed that the mild physico-chemical conditions of living systems and the existence of the orchestrated network of protein homeostasis (or proteostasis) contribute to preserve the folding state and function of the proteome [5, 6]. Nonetheless, there are situations where such constraints are no longer effective and, as a result, a protein or peptide aggregates and becomes toxic [1].

Decades of research and clinical observations have identified a few elements associated with the ability of a protein to form amyloid in vivo and give rise to disease (Fig. 2.1), and these include: (1) a pathologic and sustained increase in the concentration of a protein with increased propensity to

M. Nuvolone, MD, PhD
Institute of Neuropathology, University Hospital of Zurich, Schmelzbergstrasse 12, CH-8091 Zurich, Switzerland

Amyloidosis Research and Treatment Center, Foundation Scientific Institute Policlinico San Matteo, Department of Molecular Medicine, University of Pavia, Piazzale Golgi, 2, Pavia 27100, Italy
e-mail: mario.nuvolone@usz.ch

G. Palladini, MD, PhD • G. Merlini, MD (✉)
Department of Molecular Medicine and Amyloidosis Research and Treatment Center, Foundation IRCCS Policlinico San Matteo and University of Pavia, Piazzale Golgi, 2, 27100 Pavia, Italy
e-mail: giovanni.palladini@unipv.it; gmerlini@unipv.it

© Springer International Publishing Switzerland 2015
M.M. Picken et al. (eds.), *Amyloid and Related Disorders*, Current Clinical Pathology,
DOI 10.1007/978-3-319-19294-9_2

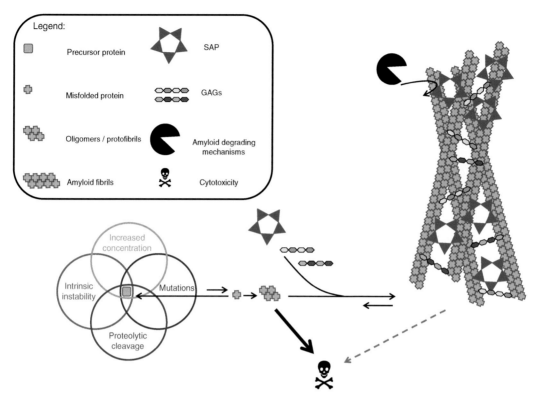

Fig. 2.1 Mechanisms of amyloid formation and toxicity. Intrinsic instability, increased concentration, mutations, proteolytic cleavage or a combination thereof can favour the conversion of the amyloidogenic precursor into its misfolded conformation. This process results in the formation of prefibrillar species and ultimately amyloid fibrils. Oligomers in equilibrium with amyloid fibrils are believed to exert a direct cytotoxic effect. Interactions with tissue factors, including glycosaminoglycans (*GAGs*) and serum amyloid P component (*SAP*), contribute to the formation and persistence of amyloid deposits, which contribute to the functional impairment of affected organs

aggregate; (2) an inherited modification of a protein primary sequence; (3) a proteolytic remodelling of a protein; (4) an intrinsic propensity to acquire a pathologic conformation [1].

More often, a combination of these factors actually determines the amyloidogenicity of an individual protein:

1. Increased concentration

    Some proteins can form amyloid only at persistently increased concentrations, as is the case for the acute phase reactant serum amyloid A (SAA) in chronic inflammations [7] and for wild-type β_2-microglobulin in patients with end-stage renal failure, where kidney-mediated clearance of this protein from the circulation is not efficiently replaced by dialysis [8].

2. Mutations

    Mutations, although frequently consisting of only a single amino acid substitution, can dramatically destabilize a protein and favour its aggregation and subsequent amyloid deposition—as demonstrated for cystatin C [9], transthyretin [10], lysozyme [11], gelsolin [12], apolipoprotein A-I [13] and β_2-microglobulin [14]. Such mutations (reported in a dedicated online registry [15], at www.amyloidosismutations.com) are the molecular substrate for a group of conditions that are collectively termed hereditary amyloidoses [16].

3. Proteolytic cleavage

    In the majority of cases, only a limited portion of the amyloidogenic precursor is actually found in amyloid deposits. The enzymes responsible for the proteolytic remodelling of the precursor are largely unknown. They are postulated to be extracellular and whether proteolysis occurs before or after the monomer has been incorporated within the amyloid fibrils is currently a matter of speculation [1]. There have been only a few cases where such enzymes have been unambiguously identified and the proteolysis has been shown to take place before amyloidogenesis: the enzyme furin, residing in the Golgi apparatus, cleaves ABri [17] and gelsolin [18] and the membrane proteases β- and γ-secretases release amyloid-β (Aβ) peptides from the amyloid precursor protein (APP) in Alzheimer's disease [19]. Remarkably, several mutations in genes encoding APP or presenilins, members of the γ-secretases, can strongly favour the amyloidogenic proteolytic cleavage of APP and are hence associated with familial forms of the disease [20].

4. Intrinsic instability

There are a few proteins that are believed to display an intrinsic propensity to adopt more than one conformation, a feature strongly influenced by hydrophobicity, electric charge and secondary structure [5] and which might—in the long term—lead to amyloid formation. Typical examples of this class of amyloidogenic proteins are transthyretin and apolipoprotein A-I, both associated, in their wild-type conformation, with ageing-related amyloid deposition [21–24]. The intrinsic instability of both proteins is further increased by pathogenic mutations associated with hereditary forms of the disease [25, 26]. Intriguingly, the propensity of wild-type transthyretin to form amyloid is also enhanced by exposure to a mutant disease-related form of the protein. In individuals heterozygous for one of the pathogenic mutation, both the mutated and the wild-type transthyretin are found in deposits [27–30], and this phenomenon explains why cardiac amyloid deposits can further progress in patients for whom liver transplantation has minimized the production of the mutant protein [27–29].

The inherent amyloidogenicity of a specific protein, per se, is not sufficient to explain the likelihood that amyloid deposition finally occurs in vivo. For example, only a minority of patients with long-lasting inflammation and subsequent elevation of SAA levels develop AA amyloidosis [31, 32]. Similarly, the disease-associated Val30Met mutation of transthyretin shows significant differences in penetrance and clinical presentation among different ethnic groups and geographic areas [33]. Other factors, both environmental and genetic, are probably involved and understanding their roles will certainly improve our current knowledge of amyloidogenesis and, hopefully, pave the way to the discovery of novel therapeutic approaches.

Common Constituents of Amyloid Deposits

Amyloid deposits are classified and named based on the chemical nature of the most abundant fibril protein, according to internationally adopted nomenclature guidelines [34]. However, additional components are regularly found in the deposits (Fig. 2.1), including proteoglycans [35], glycosaminoglycans [36], and the pentraxin family member, serum amyloid P component (SAP) [37]. Proteoglycans and glycosaminoglycans can contribute to the formation and stabilization of amyloid fibrils and, through their interaction with extracellular matrix elements, influence the localization of amyloid deposits [1]. The SAP component binds avidly and reversibly to all types of amyloid [38], a property which allows for the clinical use of a radiolabeled version of this protein for scintigraphic imaging of amyloid deposits [39, 40], and which renders amyloid resistant to degradation [41]. This latter feature, and the observation that mice genetically devoid of SAP show a delayed deposition of experimentally-induced amyloid [42], is the rationale for the development of therapeutic approaches aimed at reducing circulating and amyloid-associated SAP through small palindromic drugs and antibodies [43, 44], which have already started to enter into the clinical phase of testing [44].

Amyloid Structure

Electron microscopy and X-ray diffraction analysis have revealed that amyloid deposits are composed of rigid, non-branching fibrils with an average diameter of 7.5–10 nm and a cross-β super-secondary structure [45–47]. More recently, the application of solid-state nuclear magnetic resonance spectroscopy to large amyloid fibrils [48–50] and the successful preparation of microcrystals of small amyloid-like peptides which can be subjected to X-ray diffraction analysis [51, 52] have enabled refined structural studies of amyloids (reviewed in [3, 5, 53]), sometimes with atomic resolution [54, 55]. These results have corroborated the notion that, despite almost identical morphological and ultrastructural properties, amyloid fibrils do have a certain degree of variation [5], and this will hopefully deepen our understanding of the molecular basis of amyloid diseases.

Amyloid Formation: From Monomers to Fibrils

Self-intuitively, the transition from soluble monomeric and (usually) folded proteins to insoluble multimeric fibrillar aggregates with the above-mentioned structural properties requires drastic modifications of the protein's original conformation. This is believed to occur mainly through a partial unfolding of the native globular amyloidogenic precursor, or part of it, followed by aggregation of the unfolded moieties to finally form the amyloid fibrils [56, 57]. Said modifications are thermodynamically possible because the aggregation-prone unfolded state of the protein is separated from the native folded state—which corresponds to the minimum content of free energy and therefore to the most stable conformation—by a low energetic barrier which can be easily surmounted via naturally occurring thermal fluctuations [58].

However, alternative mechanisms can also play a role in amyloid fibrillogenesis. Under certain circumstances, globular proteins can oligomerize in a native-like state and only afterwards experience major conformational changes resulting in amyloid fibril formation [58]. This mechanism is reminiscent of the fibrillogenic pathway followed by naturally unfolded proteins and by protein fragments, which are unable to fold correctly when released from the protein of origin [58].

Irrespective of the pathway followed, amyloidogenesis entails the formation of expectedly heterogeneous intermediates, whose identity, biophysical properties and pathophysiological relevance are now the subject of extensive research [59–61].

Kinetics of Fibril Formation

In vitro studies have shown that amyloid fibril formation proceeds, in many instances, through a "nucleated growth" mechanism, which is reminiscent of the mechanism of crystallization [5]. Starting from a solution of monomeric proteins, there is an initial phase, termed lag phase, where aggregation does not occur. However, as soon as a critical nucleus has been generated, fibril formation begins and further proceeds with very fast kinetics: any amyloidogenic precursor in its aggregation-prone conformation is rapidly incorporated into the growing fibrils [1, 5, 62]. Moreover, fragmentation of growing fibrils and other nucleation events further accelerate amyloidogenesis [63].

The seeding mechanism may have clinical implications, since the process of amyloid resorption, following a positive response to therapy, usually leaves the seeds in tissues. In the case of a disease relapse, the seeds may trigger the rapid re-accumulation of amyloid deposits [64, 65].

Organ Tropism

In the localized forms of the disease, the site of amyloid deposition is determined by the cellular source of the amyloidogenic precursor: the pancreatic islets for the β-cell derived amylin in type two diabetes, the brain for the neuron-derived Aβ in Alzheimer's disease, the thyroid gland for the parafollicular cell-derived calcitonin in C-cell thyroid tumours, etc. Conversely, in systemic amyloidoses, the precursor protein circulates in the blood stream and has potential access to almost any organ or tissue in the body. Nonetheless, specific amyloidogenic proteins tend to deposit predominantly in defined organs, for example, the kidney for the fibrinogen Aα chain and leukocyte chemotactic factor 2, the joints for wild-type $β_2$-microglobulin, and the peripheral nerves for the transthyretin Met30 variant [1]. The reasons for the peculiar tropism of some amyloidogenic proteins are not fully known. Several factors could contribute to determining the site of amyloid deposition, including the presence of amyloid seeds, local protein concentration, pH, presence of proteolytic enzymes, interaction with collagen [66], glycosaminoglycans [67] or cellular receptors [1, 68].

Mechanisms of Tissue Damage

The process of amyloid formation and deposition usually results in tissue damage and organ dysfunction through mechanisms that have not been fully elucidated [1]. The presence of large amounts of amyloid material can subvert the tissue architecture and mechanically interfere with the physiologic function of affected organs (Fig. 2.1) [38].

However, compelling evidence now supports the idea that prefibrillar oligomeric species, and not fibrillar amyloid deposits, are the *bona fide* toxic species in amyloid diseases (Fig. 2.1) [1, 5]. Prefibrillar oligomers from transthyretin [69, 70], Aβ [71–73], immunoglobulin light chains [74–76] and the cellular prion protein [77] have been shown to be toxic in vitro and/or in vivo.

As a consequence of the conformational change underlying their formation, prefibrillar aggregates are expected to expose, at their surface, groups that are normally buried inside the folded proteins or dispersed in the natively unfolded proteins [5]. These structural properties of prefibrillar aggregates are regarded as potential effectors of amyloid toxicity [5] and recent in vitro studies support this hypothesis [78].

Immunoglobulin Light Chain Amyloidosis (AL)

With an overall incidence of 8.9 new cases per million person/year, immunoglobulin light chain (AL) amyloidosis is the most common form of systemic amyloidosis in Western countries [79, 80].

In this disease entity, a plasma cell clone is responsible for the production of monoclonal immunoglobulin light chains, which undergo aggregation and form amyloid deposits either systemically or, rarely, locally [81]. The latter condition is defined as localized AL amyloidosis and accounts for approximately 5 % of all AL cases.

The Amyloidogenic Clone

The plasma cell clone in systemic AL amyloidosis typically resides in the bone marrow, and the infiltrate is generally of modest size (median of bone marrow plasma cells: 9 %). The degree of plasma cell proliferation is usually low or undetectable [82], and less than 1 % of AL patients without multiple myeloma at diagnosis eventually progress to multiple myeloma over time [83]. Indeed, in AL amyloidosis the clinical manifestations are dominated by end-organ damage caused by the amyloidogenic light chains, rather than by the direct tumour burden of the plasma cell clone [81] (Fig. 2.2).

Exceptionally, AL amyloidosis can arise in association with Waldenström macroglobulinemia [84], light chain deposition disease [85], POEMS syndrome [86, 87], non-Hodgkin lymphoma [88, 89], and chronic lymphocytic leukemia [90].

Besides mature bone marrow plasma cells, the amyloidogenic clone also includes more undifferentiated bone marrow progenitors as well as mature B lymphocytes and plasma cells in peripheral blood [91–94]. Clonal plasma cell elements can also be found in the spleen and might serve as a source of amyloidogenic light chains [95].

Exposure to certain cytokines leads to in vitro differentiation of peripheral clonal elements into plasma cells that are very similar to their bone marrow counterparts [96]. These observations

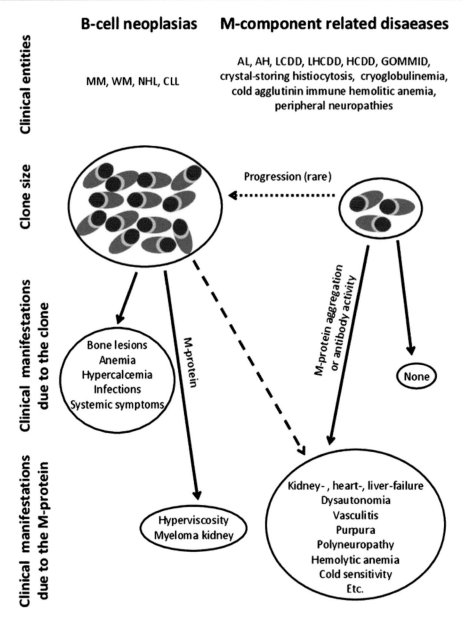

Fig. 2.2 B-cell neoplasia vs. M-component-related diseases. In B-cell neoplasias (*MM* multiple myeloma, *WM* Waldenström macroglobulinemia, *NHL* non-Hodgkin lymphoma and *CLL* chronic lymphocytic leukemia), the clinical pattern is usually dominated by systemic effects caused by expansion of the malignant clone, whereas the monoclonal protein may cause hyperviscosity syndrome or kidney damage. In less common disorders, termed M-component related disorders (*AL* immunoglobulin light chain amyloidosis, *AH* immunoglobulin heavy chain amyloidosis, *LCDD* light chain deposition disease, *LHCDD* light and heavy chain deposition disease, *HCDD* heavy chain deposition disease, *GOMMID* glomerulonephritis with organized microtubular monoclonal immunoglobulin deposits), the biological effects of the monoclonal protein may account for most of the clinical manifestations and determine the prognosis. There are overlaps between these two groups; for instance, the IgM of a patient with Waldenström macroglobulinemia may have a cold agglutinin activity and a myeloma clone can secrete an amyloidogenic light chain (*dashed line*). Rarely, M-component-related diseases can progress to an overt B-cell neoplasia (*dotted line*). (This is a modified version of a figure which was originally published in Blood. Merlini G, Stone MJ: Dangerous small B-cell clones. Blood 108:2520–30, 2006. © The American Society of Hematology)

suggest the existence of an intra-clonal differentiation process in AL: circulating elements would serve as precursors that are able to differentiate and sustain the accumulation of bone marrow plasma cells [97].

The degree of bone marrow infiltration and plasma cell clonality, with or without hypercalcemia, renal failure, anemia and lytic bone lesions attributable to clonal expansion of plasma cells (CRAB criteria) [98–100], the percentage of circulating peripheral blood plasma cells [101], serum levels of amyloidogenic free light chains [102–104] and other markers of plasma cell burden [104] are of prognostic value [105].

Clonotypic cells can contaminate apheretic stem cell harvests of AL patients and may contribute to relapse after high-dose chemotherapy followed by stem cell transplantation [93, 106].

The amyloidogenic clone has minimal but measurable kinetics of proliferation and replicating elements are represented by lymphoplasmacytoid cells within the bone marrow [91]. The percentage of bone marrow plasma cells in their DNA synthetic (S) phase of the cell cycle defines the so-called plasma cell labelling index and correlates with a poorer prognosis in AL patients [82].

Amyloidogenic plasma cells frequently display aneuploidy due to numerical chromosomal alterations [107]. Translocations affecting the 14q32 locus of immunoglobulin heavy chains are present in the majority of cases (>75 %) [108]. Particularly frequent are t(11;14)(q13;q32) [108] and t(4;14)(p16.3;q32) [109], present in 55 % and 14 % of cases, respectively. In contrast, hyperdiploidy is relatively uncommon with respect to other plasma cell disorders and is observed in only 11 % of AL cases [110]. Recently, gain of 1q21, which is present in approximately 20 % of AL cases, has been identified as an independent adverse prognostic factor in AL amyloidosis patients treated with standard chemotherapy [111].

Common single nucleotide polymorphisms representing risk alleles for MGUS [112] and multiple myeloma [113, 114] are also associated with AL amyloidosis, highlighting a common genetic susceptibility underlying these conditions [115]. Moreover, gene expression analysis has identi-

fied a set of 12 genes—including *CCND1*, the gene encoding cyclin D1—which can distinguish between AL amyloidosis and multiple myeloma with an accuracy of classification of 92 % [116]. According to this study, amyloidogenic plasma cells display an intermediate pattern of gene expression with respect to normal and myeloma plasma cells. The potential pathophysiological significance of cyclin D1 overexpression in amyloidogenic plasma cells has been the object of further investigations. In particular, cyclin D1 levels were found to be associated with preferential secretion of free light chains only and possibly with response to therapy and overall survival [117]. Moreover, amyloidogenic plasma cells were found to express CD32B [118] and, in a minority of cases, CD20 [119] and CD52 [120], which may be novel molecular targets for anti-AL immunotherapy.

Future studies will have to investigate to which extent chromosomal abnormalities, gene expression patterns or other genetic features of amyloidogenic plasma cells influence response to different chemotherapeutics or other aspects of the disease. The hope is that the increased mechanistic understanding of the biology of amyloidogenic plasma cells could guide therapeutic interventions against these small, yet detrimental clones [81].

Genetics of Amyloidogenic Light Chains

Only a small fraction of monoclonal light chains, believed to be less than 5 %, can form amyloid fibrils in vivo. In a clinical series of 1384 patients with a monoclonal gammopathy of undetermined significance, with an 11,009 person/years follow-up, only ten patients developed AL amyloidosis [121]. Analogously, only 1 % of patients with active multiple myeloma subsequently develop AL amyloidosis [122]. Therefore, the potential to form amyloid fibrils is believed to reside in specific structural features of immunoglobulin light chains. As opposed to other plasma cell disorders, the isotype of amyloidogenic light chains is, in most cases, λ (75 %). Moreover, germ-line gene usage for the variable region of λ light chains in

AL amyloidosis differ significantly from the germ-line gene usage observed in polyclonal bone marrow cells under normal conditions [123] due to the restricted usage of a small set of genes in AL [124, 125]. This phenomenon of gene restriction can be explained by the substantial over-representation of just three AL-associated gene segments, *IGLV2-14* (previously termed Vλ2), *IGLV3-1* (Vλ3r) and *IGLV6-57* (Vλ6a), which together encode 60 % of amyloid Vλ regions [123–125]. Of note, light chains belonging to the *IGLV6* family are almost invariably associated with AL amyloidosis [125]. On the other hand, germ-line gene usage in κ light chains is less well studied. It seems that a few gene segments (*IGKV1* and *IGKV3* families) are preferentially used in AL amyloidosis [125].

Recent results from a clinical series of 53 AL patients undergoing stem cell transplantation suggest that clonal variable light chain gene usage might influence global cardiac function and long-term mortality [126]. These preliminary observations, if confirmed, could shed new light on the mechanisms of amyloid toxicity and organ dysfunction.

In AL amyloidosis patients, immunoglobulin light chain variable regions were found to be hypermutated and mutations were not associated with intraclonal diversification within the bone marrow, indicating that amyloidogenic light chains undergo antigen-driven selection [127]. These data suggest that amyloidogenic clones may arise from a neoplastic transformation of differentiated B lymphoid elements selected during antibody response to a T-cell-dependent antigen [127, 128]. Recently, this type of analysis has also been extended to peripheral blood B cells, leading to the identification of some degree of intraclonal variation in circulating clones compared to bone marrow clones. Based on this finding, the existence of a common precursor that is subject to somatic mutation has been postulated [129].

Structural Features of Amyloidogenic Light Chains

Mutations in immunoglobulin light chains can exert a destabilizing effect on their structure [130–133], thus increasing their propensity to undergo misfolding and aggregation [134–138]. In this regard, crystallographic studies have been instrumental in analysing the similarities between amyloidogenic and non-amyloidogenic light chains [139, 140] and in determining the effect of specific mutations on the tertiary structure of the protein [141].

Compared to non-amyloidogenic light chains, the light chains associated with disease display a higher number of non-conservative mutations in specific structural regions, including the complementary determining regions 1 and 3, and some of these mutations are associated with serum free light chain levels in AL patients [142].

Post-translational modifications are believed to play a role in light chain amyloidogenicity, [143] and these include glycosylation, cysteinylation, tryptophan oxidation and truncation [144–148]. In general, data supporting the role of post-translational modifications in fibrillogenesis are scanty. The only exception is represented by truncation, whose role in amyloidogenesis has been extensively investigated based on the observation that AL deposits are mainly composed of the amino-terminal variable region and part of the constant region [143]. However, full-length light chains are found in the proteome of amyloid-laden tissue [149], and occasionally the constant region is the principal component of amyloid deposits [150]. The identity of the proteolytic enzymes responsible for this process remains obscure and, similarly, it is unknown whether proteolytic cleavage occurs before or after the monomeric light chain has been incorporated into higher-order aggregates. Biochemical studies based on a single recombinant light chain highlight a crucial role of the constant region at early stages of fibril formation [151] but whether this is a peculiar characteristic of the protein examined or a general feature of all amyloidogenic light chains is still to be determined.

Recently, proteomic studies on tissues from AL patients have supported the notion that peptides of the constant region of the amyloidogenic light chain are common constituents of amyloid deposits [149, 152–154]. Also, these analyses have been instrumental in identifying the hitherto-underestimated occurrence of cases–designated light + heavy chain amyloidosis or AHL amyloidosis—in which both the light and heavy chains of a monoclonal protein contribute to the formation amyloid deposits [155–157].

Mechanisms of Toxicity

As reported above, the exact mechanisms of tissue damage and organ dysfunction caused by the process of amyloid formation and deposition are not fully understood. Nonetheless, knowledge gained in the context of other forms of amyloidoses [71, 73, 158], as well as the growing body of evidence from experimental and clinical observations in AL, have contributed in recent years to significantly deepening our understanding of the pathophysiology of this disease. Key players in this process appear to be the immunoglobulin light chain fibril precursors. Indeed, exposure to physiologic levels of cardiotropic amyloidogenic light chains, in the absence of amyloid fibrils, can cause diastolic dysfunction in isolated mouse hearts [74] or inhibit pumping in the nematode—pharynx, which is evolutionary related to the vertebrate heart [159]. This leads to oxidative stress and impairs cell function [75], eventually resulting in apoptosis through the non-canonical p38α MAPK pathway [76, 160]. Whether this cellular response is elicited only in specific cell types or is a general event triggered by exposure to light chain oligomers needs to be determined.

Complementary evidence that prefibrillar species, rather than fibrillar deposits, are the culprit for most of the toxicity in AL amyloidosis comes from substantiated clinical findings. In particular, hematologic response to chemotherapy was shown to translate into significant improvement of organ function well before the resolution of amyloid deposits [161, 162]. These earlier observations have been subsequently corroborated by the discovery that chemotherapy-induced reduction of immunoglobulin free light chains, and presumably also of oligomers thereof, parallel the decrease of biochemical markers of cardiac dysfunction, despite an unchanged degree of myocardial amyloid deposits at echocardiography [163].

The cascade of events necessary for light chain oligomerization and the exact site where this process occurs are still enigmatic. Based on in vitro observations, immunoglobulin light chains can be internalized by cells through endocytosis [164, 165], and the existence of a putative cellular receptor mediating this process has been advocated [166]. Nonetheless, whether cellular internalization is a prerequisite for light chain toxicity or, alternatively, oligomers are built in the extracellular milieu and exert their detrimental effect through a different mechanism, remains to be elucidated.

Organ Tropism in AL Amyloidosis

With the exception of localized AL, where immunoglobulin light chain amyloid fibrils accumulate in proximity to the amyloidogenic plasma cell clone, amyloid deposits are mainly found at distal sites, in target organs, including the kidney, heart, liver and peripheral nervous system. Remarkably, any organ—excluding the central nervous system—can be potentially affected by this process (Fig. 2.3).

Laws governing the tissue tropisms of amyloidogenic light chains have not yet been elucidated. It has been hypothesized that the primary structure of the light chain plays a central role in determining tissue tropism, and this thinking is supported by the strong, albeit not absolute, association with *IGLV6-57* light chains and predominant, or exclusive, kidney involvement [123–125]. The peculiar tropism of *IGLV6-57* light chains for the kidney might be explained by a receptor-mediated interaction with mesangial cells [166, 167]. Recently, an association between soft tissue and bone involvement with *IGKV1* family [168], as well as an association between dominant cardiac involvement and the gene *IGLV1-44* [169] or *IGLV3* family [170], has been described. However, the germ-line gene alone is not sufficient to explain the phenomenon of tissue tropism of amyloidogenic light chains, as the pattern of amyloid deposition in individuals with the same germ-line gene origin can differ substantially [171]. Other factors, including somatic

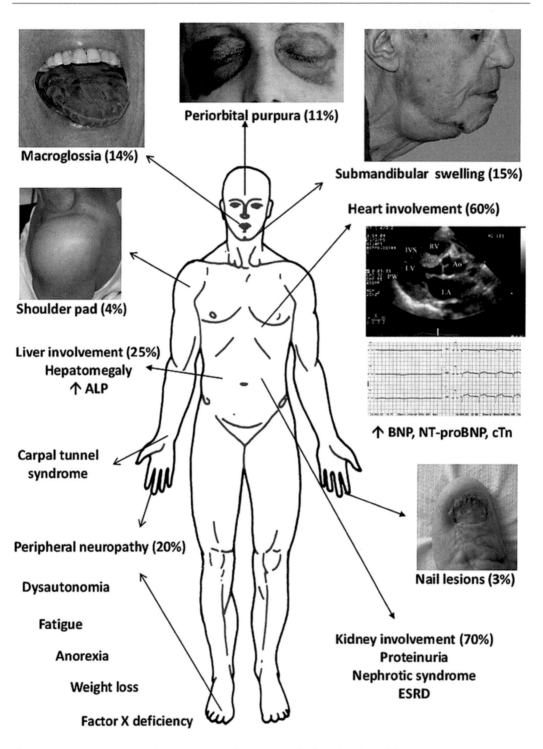

Fig. 2.3 The clinical spectrum of systemic AL amyloidosis. Clinical manifestations of systemic AL amyloidosis based on a clinical series of 1339 patients followed at our Center. Percentages refer to frequency at presentation.

BNP brain natriuretic peptide, *NT-proBNP* amino-terminal fragment of proBNP, *cTn* cardiac troponins, *ALP* alkaline phosphatase, *ESRD* end stage renal disease

mutations and post-translational modifications, are likely to be involved [171].

Clinical Manifestations

From a clinical point of view, systemic AL amyloidosis is a truly protean condition [31, 172]. Indeed, depending on the number and types of organs involved, highly heterogeneous clinical manifestations can arise (Fig. 2.3).

A few manifestations, including conspicuous macroglossia, periorbital purpura and the shoulder pad sign (Fig. 2.3), can be regarded as almost pathognomonic (with few exceptions [173]) for systemic AL amyloidosis. They should, therefore, greatly favour a diagnosis of systemic amyloidosis and guide the physician towards a correct typing as AL [31, 172]. Nonetheless, these manifestations are rather uncommon, being present in no more than 15–20 % of cases. Involvement of soft tissues can also manifest as carpal tunnel syndrome due to amyloid deposition within the carpal canal [168]. This condition is often bilateral and can precede the clinical onset of other organ involvement by many years.

In the clinical series of 1339 patients with systemic AL amyloidosis followed at our Center (Table 2.1), the most frequently affected organs are kidneys and heart [174]. Renal involvement [175–178] results almost invariably in proteinuria, which can be prominent and can lead to severe hypoalbuminemia. More than 50 % of AL patients present with nephrotic syndrome at diagnosis. In contrast, renal insufficiency is infrequent at clinical onset, even though approximately 20 % of patients eventually develop terminal kidney failure and require dialysis. Progression of renal damage depends on residual organ function as well as on the severity of proteinuria [178, 179].

Table 2.1 Clinical presentation of AL amyloidosis

Organ or syndrome	Occurrence[a]	Overt clinical presentation	Early red flags
Heart	70 %	• Heart failure • Arrhythmias • Restrictive cardiac wall thickening • Low electrocardiographic voltage • Late gadolinium enhancement at MRI	• NTproBNP>332 ng/L (100 % sensitivity) • BNP>73 ng/L (89 % sensitivity)
Kidney	70 %	• Nephrotic syndrome • Renal failure	• Proteinuria>0.5 g/day (predominantly albumin)
Liver	22 %	• Hepatomegaly without scan defects	• Elevation of ALP or γGT in the absence of other causes
PNS/ANS	14 %	• Symmetric ascending peripheral neuropathy (small fiber, axonal) • Postural hypotension • Bladder and bowel dysfunction	• Neuropathic pain and loss of sensitivity to temperature • Onset of hypotension or resolution of hypertension
Soft tissues	13 %	• Purpura (periorbital) • Macroglossia • Claudication of the jaw • Muscular pseudohypertrophy • Articular deposits	• Carpal tunnel syndrome
General symptoms	74 %	• Malnutrition	• Unexplained fatigue • Weight loss

Adapted from Merlini and Palladini: Differential diagnosis of monoclonal gammopathy of undetermined significance. Hematology Am Soc Hematol Educ Program 2012 with permission from the American Society of Hematology (License Number: 3466630213342)

ALP alkaline phosphatase, *ANS* autonomous nervous system, *γGT* γ-glutamyl transpeptidase and *PNS* peripheral nervous system

[a]Data from 1339 patients diagnosed at the Pavia Amyloidosis Research and Treatment Center

This can, however, be halted by effective therapy [178, 180], which underlines the paramount importance of an early diagnosis and timely treatment initiation. The ability to replace the organ function through dialysis explains why renal involvement in AL has a lesser impact on survival than cardiac involvement. Despite significant morbidities associated with dialysis, most AL patients with renal involvement eventually die because of amyloid-related cardiac dysfunction.

At diagnosis, two-thirds of patients show echocardiographic signs of cardiac amyloidosis, consisting mainly of increased interventricular septum and posterior wall thicknesses, and often reduced internal ventricular chamber dimensions [181, 182]. Amyloid infiltrates within the myocardium may result in a characteristic granular sparkling appearance (Fig. 2.3). Global systolic function, as estimated by ejection fraction, is usually preserved at presentation, but tends to deteriorate with disease progression. Increased ventricular wall thicknesses are paradoxically accompanied by low voltage and a pseudo-infarction pattern with Q waves in precordial leads at ECG examination (Fig. 2.3). Recently, the usefulness of cardiac magnetic resonance [183] and left ventricular strain imaging [184–187], both for the diagnosis of AL cardiomyopathy and for prognostic assessments of AL patients, has been reported. Also, molecular imaging with amyloidotropic radiotracers is emerging as a useful diagnostic tool to investigate amyloid cardiomyopathy [188].

Clinically, amyloid cardiomyopathy manifests as right-sided heart failure. The presence and severity of cardiac involvement strongly influence the prognosis [189]. The severity of heart dysfunction can be quantified through the cardiac biomarkers N-terminal natriuretic peptide type B (NT-proBNP) and cardiac troponins (cTn) [190–193], which form the basis for a prognostic stratification [194–196] and can be used to monitor organ response to therapy [163, 192, 195]. Heart involvement is the leading cause of death in AL: 50 % of patients die due to chronic heart failure and 25 % die from sudden cardiac death due to

fatal arrhythmias. Complex ventricular arrhythmias on 24-h ECG Holter monitoring, including couplets and non-sustained ventricular tachycardia, correlate with sudden death and are an independent prognostic factor [197]. Conduction disturbances are also frequently observed and negatively influence prognosis [198, 199].

Despite the great impact of cardiac involvement on prognosis, an effective treatment can significantly improve the survival of AL patients with cardiac amyloidosis, thus radically modifying the natural history of the disease [200].

Approximately, 22 % of AL patients present with liver involvement, resulting in hepatomegaly and/or elevated serum alkaline phosphatase levels [174, 201]. Jaundice is rare and, when present, often indicates a poor prognosis [202–204]. Rarely, hepatic amyloidosis can lead to spontaneous liver rupture, which is usually fatal [205, 206]. The spleen is generally affected by amyloid deposition, in some cases to a large extent, but splenic involvement is rarely of clinical relevance. When it does occur it leads to hyposplenism [207] and, anecdotally, to splenic rupture [208].

The involvement of the peripheral/autonomous nervous system is seen in about 14 % of patients [174] in the form of a predominantly sensitive, axonal, symmetrical and progressive neuropathy [209]. When peripheral neuropathy is the dominant syndrome, a differential diagnosis between AL and hereditary amyloidosis becomes mandatory. The presence of amyloid autonomic neuropathy manifests as postural hypotension, erectile dysfunction and gastrointestinal symptoms (constipation, diarrhoea or an alternation thereof). The latter symptoms can also be the consequence of amyloid deposition within the gastrointestinal tract, which is clinically evident in less than 10 % of cases. Other sites of amyloid deposition, including cutis, muscle, respiratory tract, genitourinary system and lymph nodes, are less commonly documented.

General symptoms, which are not explained by a specific pattern of organ involvement, are common and include fatigue—which is present in two-thirds of AL patients at presentation and can be rather severe—anorexia and dysgeusia. Unintentional weight loss is observed in more than 50 % of cases and can be masked by or underestimated because of concurrent liquid retention. Malnutrition, as assessed by low body mass index and low serum prealbumin level, is an important prognostic factor in AL [210–212].

Clinical Approach

In 2005, the International Society for Amyloidosis released consensus criteria for the definition of organ involvement and treatment response in AL amyloidosis, an unprecedented tool for physicians involved in the diagnosis and treatment of these patients [213]. These criteria have been subsequently updated and extended [178, 195, 214]. AL amyloidosis should be included in the differential diagnosis of: nondiabetic nephrotic syndrome; nonischemic cardiomyopathy with hypertrophic pattern on echocardiography; increased NT-proBNP in the absence of primary heart disease; hepatomegaly and/or increased alkaline phosphatase levels with no imaging abnormalities of the liver; peripheral and/or autonomic neuropathy; unexplained facial or neck purpura or macroglossia; association of monoclonal component with unexplained fatigue, weight loss, edema or paresthesia.

Diagnosis is based on the histological demonstration of amyloid deposits and determination of the amyloid type. Diagnosis of amyloid as AL in tissue samples necessitates a search for the plasma cell clone responsible for the production of amyloidogenic light chains, which is best achieved by a combination of clinical chemistry and hematologic investigations [215, 216]. However, once the coexistence of a monoclonal gammopathy and systemic amyloidosis has been ascertained, the possibility of a fortuitous combination of non-AL systemic amyloidosis (AA, wild-type ATTR or hereditary) and incidental, unrelated paraproteinemia should formally be taken into account [217–219]. This holds true especially in elderly subjects, due to the remarkable prevalence of monoclonal gammopathies of undetermined significance (MGUS) in this setting [220]. On the other hand, the rare association of systemic AL amyloidosis with the presence of a potentially amyloidogenic mutation has been reported [221, 222]. Since treatment is radically different from one form of systemic amyloidosis to the other, amyloid typing is mandatory in tissue deposits and requires a scrupulous clinical evaluation and appropriate techniques, including immunohistochemistry, immune-electron microscopy, mass-spectroscopy-based methods and genetic testing [105].

Organ dysfunction can be halted, amyloid deposits can be slowly reabsorbed and survival can be significantly extended if the production of amyloidogenic light chains is zeroed or substantially reduced [1]. Possibly, due to the low proliferative profile of the underlying amyloidogenic plasma cell clone, a durable hematologic response to therapy can be achieved and translate into organ response, with a survival of 10 years or more [223, 224]. Based on these observations, the current therapeutic approach to systemic AL amyloidosis aims at eradicating the underlying plasma cell dyscrasia with chemotherapy, using regimens which are mainly adopted from anti-multiple myeloma therapies (Fig. 2.4). However, alternative approaches have also been considered. The anthracycline 4′-iodo-4′-deoxy-doxorubicin was shown to bind to amyloid fibrils both in vitro and in vivo and to promote amyloid clearance [225] (Fig. 2.4), although its clinical efficacy in AL amyloidosis is limited [226, 227]. Other strategies are currently under investigation in preclinical or clinical settings [228], including selective downregulation of the offending immunoglobulin light chain via anti-sense oligonucleotides [229] or small interfering RNA molecules [230–232] or, indirectly, through upregulation of ER quality control mechanisms [233], passive immunotherapy with anti-amyloid antibodies [234, 235] and pharmacological depletion of SAP (Fig. 2.4) [44].

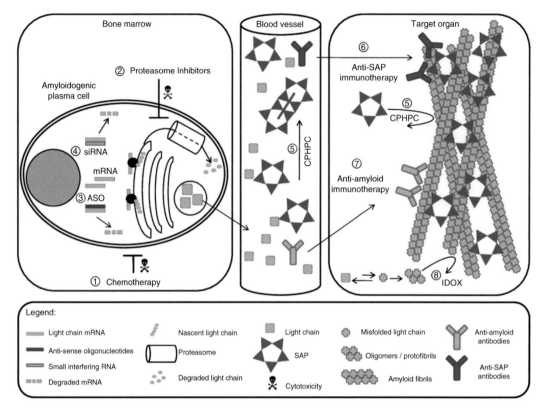

Fig. 2.4 Therapeutic options in AL amyloidosis. Similarly to anti-myeloma therapies, (1) chemotherapy and (2) proteasome inhibitors can be employed to eradicate amyloidogenic plasma cells. (3) Small molecules to increase ER quality control mechanisms can be applied to help attenuating secretion of amyloidogenic light chains. (4) Anti-sense oligonucleotides and (5) small interfering RNAs have been tested, in preclinical settings, to downregulate the production of the amyloidogenic light chains. (6) The palindromic compound (R)-1-[6-[(R)-2-carboxy-pyrrolidin-1-yl]-6-oxo-hexa-noyl]pyrrolidine-2 carboxylic acid (*CPHPC*) can be used to inhibit serum amyloid P component (*SAP*) binding to amyloid fibrils. The compound also crosslinks and dimerizes circulating SAP, favouring its hepatic clearance. This strategy can be combined with the use of (7) anti-SAP antibodies to eliminate visceral amyloid deposits. (8) Passive immunization with amyloid-reactive antibodies could promote the resolution of amyloid deposits. (9) The anthracycline 4'-iodo-4'-deoxy-doxorubicin (*IDOX*) interferes with amyloid fibril growth and promotes amyloid clearance

References

1. Merlini G, Bellotti V. Molecular mechanisms of amyloidosis. N Engl J Med. 2003;349:583–96.
2. Carrell RW, Lomas DA. Conformational disease. Lancet. 1997;350:134–8.
3. Knowles TP, Vendruscolo M, Dobson CM. The amyloid state and its association with protein misfolding diseases. Nat Rev Mol Cell Biol. 2014;15:384–96.
4. Fandrich M, Fletcher MA, Dobson CM. Amyloid fibrils from muscle myoglobin. Nature. 2001;410:165–6.
5. Chiti F, Dobson CM. Protein misfolding, functional amyloid, and human disease. Annu Rev Biochem. 2006;75:333–66.
6. Ryno LM, Wiseman RL, Kelly JW. Targeting unfolded protein response signaling pathways to ameliorate protein misfolding diseases. Curr Opin Chem Biol. 2013;17:346–52.
7. Westermark GT, Westermark P. Serum amyloid A and protein AA: molecular mechanisms of a transmissible amyloidosis. FEBS Lett. 2009;583:2685–90.
8. Corlin DB, Heegaard NH. Beta(2)-microglobulin amyloidosis. Subcell Biochem. 2012;65:517–40.
9. Abrahamson M, Grubb A. Increased body temperature accelerates aggregation of the Leu-68→Gln mutant cystatin C, the amyloid-forming protein in hereditary cystatin C amyloid angiopathy. Proc Natl Acad Sci USA. 1994;91:1416–20.
10. McCutchen SL, Lai Z, Miroy GJ, Kelly JW, Colon W. Comparison of lethal and nonlethal transthyretin variants and their relationship to amyloid disease. Biochemistry. 1995;34:13527–36.

11. Booth DR, et al. Instability, unfolding and aggregation of human lysozyme variants underlying amyloid fibrillogenesis. Nature. 1997;385:787–93.
12. Isaacson RL, Weeds AG, Fersht AR. Equilibria and kinetics of folding of gelsolin domain 2 and mutants involved in familial amyloidosis-Finnish type. Proc Natl Acad Sci USA. 1999;96:11247–52.
13. Raimondi S, et al. Effects of the known pathogenic mutations on the aggregation pathway of the amyloidogenic peptide of apolipoprotein a-I. J Mol Biol. 2011;407:465–76.
14. Valleix S, et al. Hereditary systemic amyloidosis due to Asp76Asn variant beta2-microglobulin. N Engl J Med. 2012;366:2276–83.
15. Rowczenio DM, et al. Online registry for mutations in hereditary amyloidosis including nomenclature recommendations. Hum Mutat. 2014;35:E2403–12.
16. Benson MD. The hereditary amyloidoses. Best Pract Res Clin Rheumatol. 2003;17:909–27.
17. Kim SH, et al. Furin mediates enhanced production of fibrillogenic ABri peptides in familial British dementia. Nat Neurosci. 1999;2:984–8.
18. Chen CD, et al. Furin initiates gelsolin familial amyloidosis in the Golgi through a defect in Ca(2+) stabilization. EMBO J. 2001;20:6277–87.
19. De Strooper B, Vassar R, Golde T. The secretases: enzymes with therapeutic potential in Alzheimer disease. Nat Rev Neurol. 2010;6:99–107.
20. Goate A, Hardy J. Twenty years of Alzheimer's disease-causing mutations. J Neurochem. 2012;120 Suppl 1:3–8.
21. Saraiva MJ. Transthyretin amyloidosis: a tale of weak interactions. FEBS Lett. 2001;498:201–3.
22. Westermark P, Mucchiano G, Marthin T, Johnson KH, Sletten K. Apolipoprotein A1-derived amyloid in human aortic atherosclerotic plaques. Am J Pathol. 1995;147:1186–92.
23. Solomon A, et al. Amyloid contained in the knee joint meniscus is formed from apolipoprotein A-I. Arthritis Rheum. 2006;54:3545–50.
24. Westermark P, Westermark GT, Suhr OB, Berg S. Transthyretin-derived amyloidosis: probably a common cause of lumbar spinal stenosis. Ups J Med Sci. 2014;119:223–8.
25. Connors LH, Lim A, Prokaeva T, Roskens VA, Costello CE. Tabulation of human transthyretin (TTR) variants, 2003. Amyloid. 2003;10:160–84.
26. Obici L, et al. Structure, function and amyloidogenic propensity of apolipoprotein A-I. Amyloid. 2006;13:191–205.
27. Yazaki M, et al. Cardiac amyloid in patients with familial amyloid polyneuropathy consists of abundant wild-type transthyretin. Biochem Biophys Res Commun. 2000;274:702–6.
28. Tsuchiya A, Yazaki M, Kametani F, Takei Y, Ikeda S. Marked regression of abdominal fat amyloid in patients with familial amyloid polyneuropathy during long-term follow-up after liver transplantation. Liver Transpl. 2008;14:563–70.
29. Liepnieks JJ, Zhang LQ, Benson MD. Progression of transthyretin amyloid neuropathy after liver transplantation. Neurology. 2010;75:324–7.
30. Ihse E, Suhr OB, Hellman U, Westermark P. Variation in amount of wild-type transthyretin in different fibril and tissue types in ATTR amyloidosis. J Mol Med. 2011;89:171–80.
31. Obici L, Perfetti V, Palladini G, Moratti R, Merlini G. Clinical aspects of systemic amyloid diseases. Biochim Biophys Acta. 2005;1753:11–22.
32. Obici L, Raimondi S, Lavatelli F, Bellotti V, Merlini G. Susceptibility to AA amyloidosis in rheumatic diseases: a critical overview. Arthritis Rheum. 2009;61:1435–40.
33. Saraiva MJ. Hereditary transthyretin amyloidosis: molecular basis and therapeutical strategies. Expert Rev Mol Med. 2002;4:1–11.
34. Sipe JD, et al. Amyloid fibril protein nomenclature: 2012 recommendations from the Nomenclature Committee of the International Society of Amyloidosis. Amyloid. 2012;19:167–70.
35. Kisilevsky R, Fraser P. Proteoglycans and amyloid fibrillogenesis. Ciba Found Symp. 1996;199:58–67. discussion 68–72, 90–103.
36. Nelson SR, Lyon M, Gallagher JT, Johnson EA, Pepys MB. Isolation and characterization of the integral glycosaminoglycan constituents of human amyloid A and monoclonal light-chain amyloid fibrils. Biochem J. 1991;275(Pt 1):67–73.
37. Pepys MB, et al. Human serum amyloid P component is an invariant constituent of amyloid deposits and has a uniquely homogeneous glycostructure. Proc Natl Acad Sci USA. 1994;91:5602–6.
38. Pepys MB. Amyloidosis. Annu Rev Med. 2006;57:223–41.
39. Hawkins PN, Myers MJ, Lavender JP, Pepys MB. Diagnostic radionuclide imaging of amyloid: biological targeting by circulating human serum amyloid P component. Lancet. 1988;1:1413–8.
40. Hazenberg BP, et al. Diagnostic performance of 123I-labeled serum amyloid P component scintigraphy in patients with amyloidosis. Am J Med. 2006;119(355):e15–24.
41. Tennent GA, Lovat LB, Pepys MB. Serum amyloid P component prevents proteolysis of the amyloid fibrils of Alzheimer disease and systemic amyloidosis. Proc Natl Acad Sci USA. 1995;92:4299–303.
42. Botto M, et al. Amyloid deposition is delayed in mice with targeted deletion of the serum amyloid P component gene. Nat Med. 1997;3:855–9.
43. Pepys MB, et al. Targeted pharmacological depletion of serum amyloid P component for treatment of human amyloidosis. Nature. 2002;417:254–9.
44. Bodin K, et al. Antibodies to human serum amyloid P component eliminate visceral amyloid deposits. Nature. 2010;468:93–7.
45. Cohen AS, Calkins E. Electron microscopic observations on a fibrous component in amyloid of diverse origins. Nature. 1959;183:1202–3.

46. Eanes ED, Glenner GG. X-ray diffraction studies on amyloid filaments. J Histochem Cytochem. 1968; 16:673–7.
47. Termine JD, Eanes ED, Ein D, Glenner GG. Infrared spectroscopy of human amyloid fibrils and immunoglobulin proteins. Biopolymers. 1972;11:1103–13.
48. Petkova AT, et al. A structural model for Alzheimer's beta-amyloid fibrils based on experimental constraints from solid state NMR. Proc Natl Acad Sci USA. 2002;99:16742–7.
49. Jaroniec CP, MacPhee CE, Astrof NS, Dobson CM, Griffin RG. Molecular conformation of a peptide fragment of transthyretin in an amyloid fibril. Proc Natl Acad Sci USA. 2002;99:16748–53.
50. Ritter C, et al. Correlation of structural elements and infectivity of the HET-s prion. Nature. 2005; 435:844–8.
51. Makin OS, Atkins E, Sikorski P, Johansson J, Serpell LC. Molecular basis for amyloid fibril formation and stability. Proc Natl Acad Sci USA. 2005;102:315–20.
52. Nelson R, et al. Structure of the cross-beta spine of amyloid-like fibrils. Nature. 2005;435:773–8.
53. Greenwald J, Riek R. Biology of amyloid: structure, function, and regulation. Structure. 2010;18: 1244–60.
54. Sawaya MR, et al. Atomic structures of amyloid cross-beta spines reveal varied steric zippers. Nature. 2007;447:453–7.
55. Fitzpatrick AW, et al. Atomic structure and hierarchical assembly of a cross-beta amyloid fibril. Proc Natl Acad Sci USA. 2013;110:5468–73.
56. Dobson CM, Karplus M. The fundamentals of protein folding: bringing together theory and experiment. Curr Opin Struct Biol. 1999;9:92–101.
57. Dobson CM. Getting out of shape. Nature. 2002;418:729–30.
58. Chiti F, Dobson CM. Amyloid formation by globular proteins under native conditions. Nat Chem Biol. 2009;5:15–22.
59. Haass C, Selkoe DJ. Soluble protein oligomers in neurodegeneration: lessons from the Alzheimer's amyloid beta-peptide. Nat Rev Mol Cell Biol. 2007;8:101–12.
60. Glabe CG. Structural classification of toxic amyloid oligomers. J Biol Chem. 2008;283:29639–43.
61. Stefani M. Structural polymorphism of amyloid oligomers and fibrils underlies different fibrillization pathways: immunogenicity and cytotoxicity. Curr Protein Pept Sci. 2010;11:343–54.
62. Serio TR, et al. Nucleated conformational conversion and the replication of conformational information by a prion determinant. Science. 2000;289:1317–21.
63. Knowles TP, et al. An analytical solution to the kinetics of breakable filament assembly. Science. 2009;326:1533–7.
64. Hawkins PN, Pepys MB. A primed state exists in vivo following histological regression of amyloidosis. Clin Exp Immunol. 1990;81:325–8.
65. Simons JP, et al. Pathogenetic mechanisms of amyloid A amyloidosis. Proc Natl Acad Sci USA. 2013;110:16115–20.
66. Harris DL, King E, Ramsland PA, Edmundson AB. Binding of nascent collagen by amyloidogenic light chains and amyloid fibrillogenesis in monolayers of human fibrocytes. J Mol Recognit. 2000;13:198–212.
67. Stevens FJ, Kisilevsky R. Immunoglobulin light chains, glycosaminoglycans, and amyloid. Cell Mol Life Sci. 2000;57:441–9.
68. Yan SD, et al. Receptor-dependent cell stress and amyloid accumulation in systemic amyloidosis. Nat Med. 2000;6:643–51.
69. Sousa MM, Cardoso I, Fernandes R, Guimaraes A, Saraiva MJ. Deposition of transthyretin in early stages of familial amyloidotic polyneuropathy: evidence for toxicity of nonfibrillar aggregates. Am J Pathol. 2001;159:1993–2000.
70. Andersson K, Olofsson A, Nielsen EH, Svehag SE, Lundgren E. Only amyloidogenic intermediates of transthyretin induce apoptosis. Biochem Biophys Res Commun. 2002;294:309–14.
71. Lambert MP, et al. Diffusible, nonfibrillar ligands derived from Abeta1-42 are potent central nervous system neurotoxins. Proc Natl Acad Sci USA. 1998;95:6448–53.
72. Hartley DM, et al. Protofibrillar intermediates of amyloid beta-protein induce acute electrophysiological changes and progressive neurotoxicity in cortical neurons. J Neurosci. 1999;19:8876–84.
73. Walsh DM, et al. Naturally secreted oligomers of amyloid beta protein potently inhibit hippocampal long-term potentiation in vivo. Nature. 2002;416:535–9.
74. Liao R, et al. Infusion of light chains from patients with cardiac amyloidosis causes diastolic dysfunction in isolated mouse hearts. Circulation. 2001;104:1594–7.
75. Brenner DA, et al. Human amyloidogenic light chains directly impair cardiomyocyte function through an increase in cellular oxidant stress. Circ Res. 2004;94:1008–10.
76. Shi J, et al. Amyloidogenic light chains induce cardiomyocyte contractile dysfunction and apoptosis via a non-canonical p38alpha MAPK pathway. Proc Natl Acad Sci USA. 2010;107:4188–93.
77. Silveira JR, et al. The most infectious prion protein particles. Nature. 2005;437:257–61.
78. Campioni S, et al. A causative link between the structure of aberrant protein oligomers and their toxicity. Nat Chem Biol. 2010;6:140–7.
79. Kyle RA, et al. Incidence and natural history of primary systemic amyloidosis in Olmsted County, Minnesota, 1950 through 1989. Blood. 1992;79:1817–22.
80. Pinney JH, et al. Systemic amyloidosis in England: an epidemiological study. Br J Haematol. 2013;161:525–32.
81. Merlini G, Stone MJ. Dangerous small B-cell clones. Blood. 2006;108:2520–30.

82. Gertz MA, Kyle RA, Greipp PR. The plasma cell labeling index: a valuable tool in primary systemic amyloidosis. Blood. 1989;74:1108–11.
83. Rajkumar SV, Gertz MA, Kyle RA. Primary systemic amyloidosis with delayed progression to multiple myeloma. Cancer. 1998;82:1501–5.
84. Gertz MA, Kyle RA, Noel P. Primary systemic amyloidosis: a rare complication of immunoglobulin M monoclonal gammopathies and Waldenstrom's macroglobulinemia. J Clin Oncol. 1993;11:914–20.
85. Hofmann-Guilaine C, et al. Association light chain deposition disease (LCDD) and amyloidosis. One case. Pathol Res Pract. 1985;180:214–9.
86. Adami F, et al. Coexistence of primary AL amyloidosis and POEMS syndrome: efficacy of melphalan-dexamethasone and role of biochemical markers in monitoring the diseases course. Am J Hematol. 2010;85:131–2.
87. Adams D, et al. New elements in the diagnosis and the treatment of primary AL amyloid polyneuropathy and neuropathy due to POEMS syndrome. Rev Neurol (Paris). 2011;167:57–63.
88. Cohen AD, et al. Systemic AL amyloidosis due to non-Hodgkin's lymphoma: an unusual clinicopathologic association. Br J Haematol. 2004;124:309–14.
89. Telio D, et al. Two distinct syndromes of lymphoma-associated AL amyloidosis: a case series and review of the literature. Am J Hematol. 2010;85:805–8.
90. Ikee R, Kobayashi S, Hemmi N, Suzuki S, Miura S. Amyloidosis associated with chronic lymphocytic leukemia. Amyloid. 2005;12:131–4.
91. Perfetti V, et al. AL amyloidosis. Characterization of amyloidogenic cells by anti-idiotypic monoclonal antibodies. Lab Invest. 1994;71:853–61.
92. McElroy Jr EA, Witzig TE, Gertz MA, Greipp PR, Kyle RA. Detection of monoclonal plasma cells in the peripheral blood of patients with primary amyloidosis. Br J Haematol. 1998;100:326–7.
93. Perfetti V, et al. Cells with clonal light chains are present in peripheral blood at diagnosis and in apheretic stem cell harvests of primary amyloidosis. Bone Marrow Transplant. 1999;23:323–7.
94. Manske MK, et al. Quantitative analysis of clonal bone marrow CD19+ B cells: use of B cell lineage trees to delineate their role in the pathogenesis of light chain amyloidosis. Clin Immunol. 2006;120:106–20.
95. Solomon A, Macy SD, Wooliver C, Weiss DT, Westermark P. Splenic plasma cells can serve as a source of amyloidogenic light chains. Blood. 2009;113:1501–3.
96. Perfetti V, et al. Membrane CD22 defines circulating myeloma-related cells as mature or later B cells. Lab Invest. 1997;77:333–44.
97. Perfetti V, Vignarelli MC, Casarini S, Ascari E, Merlini G. Biological features of the clone involved in primary amyloidosis (AL). Leukemia. 2001;15:195–202.
98. Perfetti V, et al. The degrees of plasma cell clonality and marrow infiltration adversely influence the prognosis of AL amyloidosis patients. Haematologica. 1999;84:218–21.
99. Paiva B, et al. The clinical utility and prognostic value of multiparameter flow cytometry immunophenotyping in light-chain amyloidosis. Blood. 2011;117:3613–6.
100. Kourelis TV, et al. Coexistent multiple myeloma or increased bone marrow plasma cells define equally high-risk populations in patients with immunoglobulin light chain amyloidosis. J Clin Oncol. 2013;31:4319–24.
101. Pardanani A, et al. Circulating peripheral blood plasma cells as a prognostic indicator in patients with primary systemic amyloidosis. Blood. 2003;101:827–30.
102. Dispenzieri A, et al. Absolute values of immunoglobulin free light chains are prognostic in patients with primary systemic amyloidosis undergoing peripheral blood stem cell transplantation. Blood. 2006;107:3378–83.
103. Wechalekar AD, et al. A new staging system for AL amyloidosis incorporating serum free light chains, cardiac troponin-T and NT-proBNP. Blood. 2009;114. abstr. 2796.
104. Kumar S, et al. A novel prognostic staging system for light chain amyloidosis (AL) incorporating markers of plasma cell burden and organ involvement. Blood. 2009;114. abstr. 2797.
105. Merlini G, Seldin DC, Gertz MA. Amyloidosis: pathogenesis and new therapeutic options. J Clin Oncol. 2011;29:1924–33.
106. Comenzo RL, et al. Mobilized CD34+ cells selected as autografts in patients with primary light-chain amyloidosis: rationale and application. Transfusion. 1998;38:60–9.
107. Fonseca R, et al. Chromosomal abnormalities in systemic amyloidosis. Br J Haematol. 1998;103:704–10.
108. Hayman SR, et al. Translocations involving the immunoglobulin heavy-chain locus are possible early genetic events in patients with primary systemic amyloidosis. Blood. 2001;98:2266–8.
109. Perfetti V, et al. Translocation T(4;14)(p16.3;q32) is a recurrent genetic lesion in primary amyloidosis. Am J Pathol. 2001;158:1599–603.
110. Bochtler T, et al. Hyperdiploidy is less frequent in AL amyloidosis compared with monoclonal gammopathy of undetermined significance and inversely associated with translocation t(11;14). Blood. 2011;117:3809–15.
111. Bochtler T, et al. Gain of chromosome 1q21 is an independent adverse prognostic factor in light chain amyloidosis patients treated with melphalan/dexamethasone. Amyloid. 2014;21:9–17.
112. Weinhold N, et al. Inherited genetic susceptibility to monoclonal gammopathy of unknown significance. Blood. 2014;123:2513–7. quiz 2593.
113. Weinhold N, et al. The CCND1 c.870G>A polymorphism is a risk factor for t(11;14)(q13;q32) multiple myeloma. Nat Genet. 2013;45:522–5.
114. Chubb D, et al. Common variation at 3q26.2, 6p21.33, 17p11.2 and 22q13.1 influences multiple myeloma risk. Nat Genet. 2013;45:1221–5.

115. Weinhold N, et al. Immunoglobulin light-chain amyloidosis shares genetic susceptibility with multiple myeloma. Leukemia. 2014;28:2254–6.

116. Abraham RS, et al. Functional gene expression analysis of clonal plasma cells identifies a unique molecular profile for light chain amyloidosis. Blood. 2005;105:794–803.

117. Zhou P, et al. Clonal plasma cell pathophysiology and clinical features of disease are linked to clonal plasma cell expression of cyclin D1 in systemic light-chain amyloidosis. Clin Lymphoma Myeloma Leuk. 2012;12:49–58.

118. Zhou P, et al. CD32B is highly expressed on clonal plasma cells from patients with systemic light-chain amyloidosis and provides a target for monoclonal antibody-based therapy. Blood. 2008;111:3403–6.

119. Deshmukh M, Elderfield K, Rahemtulla A, Naresh KN. Immunophenotype of neoplastic plasma cells in AL amyloidosis. J Clin Pathol. 2009;62:724–30.

120. Kumar S, Kimlinger TK, Lust JA, Donovan K, Witzig TE. Expression of CD52 on plasma cells in plasma cell proliferative disorders. Blood. 2003; 102:1075–7.

121. Kyle RA, et al. A long-term study of prognosis in monoclonal gammopathy of undetermined significance. N Engl J Med. 2002;346:564–9.

122. Madan S, et al. Clinical features and treatment response of light chain (AL) amyloidosis diagnosed in patients with previous diagnosis of multiple myeloma. Mayo Clin Proc. 2010;85:232–8.

123. Perfetti V, et al. Analysis of V(lambda)-J(lambda) expression in plasma cells from primary (AL) amyloidosis and normal bone marrow identifies 3r (lambdaIII) as a new amyloid-associated germline gene segment. Blood. 2002;100:948–53.

124. Comenzo RL, Zhang Y, Martinez C, Osman K, Herrera GA. The tropism of organ involvement in primary systemic amyloidosis: contributions of Ig V(L) germ line gene use and clonal plasma cell burden. Blood. 2001;98:714–20.

125. Abraham RS, et al. Immunoglobulin light chain variable (V) region genes influence clinical presentation and outcome in light chain-associated amyloidosis (AL). Blood. 2003;101:3801–8.

126. Bellavia D, et al. Utility of Doppler myocardial imaging, cardiac biomarkers, and clonal immunoglobulin genes to assess left ventricular performance and stratify risk following peripheral blood stem cell transplantation in patients with systemic light chain amyloidosis (Al). J Am Soc Echocardiogr. 2011; 24:444–54.

127. Perfetti V, et al. Evidence that amyloidogenic light chains undergo antigen-driven selection. Blood. 1998;91:2948–54.

128. Abraham RS, et al. Analysis of somatic hypermutation and antigenic selection in the clonal B cell in immunoglobulin light chain amyloidosis (AL). J Clin Immunol. 2004;24:340–53.

129. Abraham RS, et al. Novel analysis of clonal diversification in blood B cell and bone marrow plasma cell clones in immunoglobulin light chain amyloidosis. J Clin Immunol. 2007;27:69–87.

130. Hurle MR, Helms LR, Li L, Chan W, Wetzel R. A role for destabilizing amino acid replacements in light-chain amyloidosis. Proc Natl Acad Sci USA. 1994;91:5446–50.

131. Helms LR, Wetzel R. Specificity of abnormal assembly in immunoglobulin light chain deposition disease and amyloidosis. J Mol Biol. 1996;257:77–86.

132. Bellotti V, Merlini G. Toward understanding the molecular pathogenesis of monoclonal immunoglobulin light-chain deposition. Nephrol Dial Transplant. 1996;11:1708–11.

133. Raffen R, et al. Physicochemical consequences of amino acid variations that contribute to fibril formation by immunoglobulin light chains. Protein Sci. 1999;8:509–17.

134. Myatt EA, et al. Pathogenic potential of human monoclonal immunoglobulin light chains: relationship of in vitro aggregation to in vivo organ deposition. Proc Natl Acad Sci USA. 1994; 91:3034–8.

135. Wall J, Murphy CL, Solomon A. In vitro immunoglobulin light chain fibrillogenesis. Methods Enzymol. 1999;309:204–17.

136. Ramirez-Alvarado M, Merkel JS, Regan L. A systematic exploration of the influence of the protein stability on amyloid fibril formation in vitro. Proc Natl Acad Sci USA. 2000;97:8979–84.

137. Wall JS, et al. Structural basis of light chain amyloidogenicity: comparison of the thermodynamic properties, fibrillogenic potential and tertiary structural features of four Vlambda6 proteins. J Mol Recognit. 2004;17:323–31.

138. Baden EM, Randles EG, Aboagye AK, Thompson JR, Ramirez-Alvarado M. Structural insights into the role of mutations in amyloidogenesis. J Biol Chem. 2008;283:30950–6.

139. Schormann N, Murrell JR, Liepnieks JJ, Benson MD. Tertiary structure of an amyloid immunoglobulin light chain protein: a proposed model for amyloid fibril formation. Proc Natl Acad Sci USA. 1995;92:9490–4.

140. Pokkuluri PR, Solomon A, Weiss DT, Stevens FJ, Schiffer M. Tertiary structure of human lambda 6 light chains. Amyloid. 1999;6:165–71.

141. Randles EG, Thompson JR, Martin DJ, Ramirez-Alvarado M. Structural alterations within native amyloidogenic immunoglobulin light chains. J Mol Biol. 2009;389:199–210.

142. Poshusta TL, et al. Mutations in specific structural regions of immunoglobulin light chains are associated with free light chain levels in patients with AL amyloidosis. PLoS One. 2009;4:e5169.

143. Bellotti V, Mangione P, Merlini G. Review: immunoglobulin light chain amyloidosis–the archetype of

structural and pathogenic variability. J Struct Biol. 2000;130:280–9.

144. Sletten K, Natvig JB, Husby G, Juul J. The complete amino acid sequence of a prototype immunoglobulin-lambda light-chain-type amyloid-fibril protein AR. Biochem J. 1981;195:561–72.

145. Omtvedt LA, et al. Glycosylation of immunoglobulin light chains associated with amyloidosis. Amyloid. 2000;7:227–44.

146. Connors LH, et al. Heterogeneity in primary structure, post-translational modifications, and germline gene usage of nine full-length amyloidogenic kappa1 immunoglobulin light chains. Biochemistry. 2007;46:14259–71.

147. Lim A, Wally J, Walsh MT, Skinner M, Costello CE. Identification and location of a cysteinyl post-translational modification in an amyloidogenic kappa1 light chain protein by electrospray ionization and matrix-assisted laser desorption/ionization mass spectrometry. Anal Biochem. 2001;295:45–56.

148. Lavatelli F, et al. A novel approach for the purification and proteomic analysis of pathogenic immunoglobulin free light chains from serum. Biochim Biophys Acta. 2011;1814:409–19.

149. Lavatelli F, et al. Amyloidogenic and associated proteins in systemic amyloidosis proteome of adipose tissue. Mol Cell Proteomics. 2008;7:1570–83.

150. Solomon A, et al. Light chain-associated amyloid deposits comprised of a novel kappa constant domain. Proc Natl Acad Sci USA. 1998;95:9547–51.

151. Klimtchuk ES, et al. The critical role of the constant region in thermal stability and aggregation of amyloidogenic immunoglobulin light chain. Biochemistry. 2010;49:9848–57.

152. Brambilla F, et al. Reliable typing of systemic amyloidoses through proteomic analysis of subcutaneous adipose tissue. Blood. 2012;119:1844–7.

153. Vrana JA, et al. Classification of amyloidosis by laser microdissection and mass spectrometry-based proteomic analysis in clinical biopsy specimens. Blood. 2009;114:4957–9.

154. Vrana JA, et al. Clinical diagnosis and typing of systemic amyloidosis in subcutaneous fat aspirates by mass spectrometry-based proteomics. Haematologica. 2014;99:1239–47.

155. Grogg KL, Aubry MC, Vrana JA, Theis JD, Dogan A. Nodular pulmonary amyloidosis is characterized by localized immunoglobulin deposition and is frequently associated with an indolent B-cell lymphoproliferative disorder. Am J Surg Pathol. 2013;37:406–12.

156. Nasr SH, et al. The diagnosis and characteristics of renal heavy-chain and heavy/light-chain amyloidosis and their comparison with renal light-chain amyloidosis. Kidney Int. 2013;83:463–70.

157. Picken MM. Non-light-chain immunoglobulin amyloidosis: time to expand or refine the spectrum to include light + heavy chain amyloidosis? Kidney Int. 2013;83:353–6.

158. Reixach N, Deechongkit S, Jiang X, Kelly JW, Buxbaum JN. Tissue damage in the amyloidoses: transthyretin monomers and nonnative oligomers are the major cytotoxic species in tissue culture. Proc Natl Acad Sci USA. 2004;101:2817–22.

159. Diomede L, et al. A caenorhabditis elegans-based assay recognizes immunoglobulin light chains causing heart amyloidosis. Blood. 2014;123:3543–52.

160. Mishra S, et al. Human amyloidogenic light chain proteins result in cardiac dysfunction, cell death, and early mortality in zebrafish. Am J Physiol Heart Circ Physiol. 2013;305:H95–103.

161. Comenzo RL, et al. Dose-intensive melphalan with blood stem cell support for the treatment of AL amyloidosis: one-year follow-up in five patients. Blood. 1996;88:2801–6.

162. Dember LM, et al. Effect of dose-intensive intravenous melphalan and autologous blood stem-cell transplantation on al amyloidosis-associated renal disease. Ann Intern Med. 2001;134:746–53.

163. Palladini G, et al. Circulating amyloidogenic free light chains and serum N-terminal natriuretic peptide type B decrease simultaneously in association with improvement of survival in AL. Blood. 2006;107:3854–8.

164. Trinkaus-Randall V, et al. Cellular response of cardiac fibroblasts to amyloidogenic light chains. Am J Pathol. 2005;166:197–208.

165. Monis GF, et al. Role of endocytic inhibitory drugs on internalization of amyloidogenic light chains by cardiac fibroblasts. Am J Pathol. 2006;169:1939–52.

166. Teng J, et al. Different types of glomerulopathic light chains interact with mesangial cells using a common receptor but exhibit different intracellular trafficking patterns. Lab Invest. 2004;84:440–51.

167. Keeling J, Teng J, Herrera GA. AL-amyloidosis and light-chain deposition disease light chains induce divergent phenotypic transformations of human mesangial cells. Lab Invest. 2004;84:1322–38.

168. Prokaeva T, et al. Soft tissue, joint, and bone manifestations of AL amyloidosis: clinical presentation, molecular features, and survival. Arthritis Rheum. 2007;56:3858–68.

169. Perfetti V, et al. The repertoire of lambda light chains causing predominant amyloid heart involvement and identification of a preferentially involved germline gene, IGLV1-44. Blood. 2012;119:144–50.

170. Prokaeva T, Spencer B, et al. Contribution of light chain variable region genes to organ tropism and survival in AL amyloidosis. Amyloid. 2010;17:62. Abstract OP-046.

171. Enqvist S, Sletten K, Stevens FJ, Hellman U, Westermark P. Germ line origin and somatic mutations determine the target tissues in systemic AL-amyloidosis. PLoS One. 2007;2:e981.

172. Falk RH, Comenzo RL, Skinner M. The systemic amyloidoses. N Engl J Med. 1997;337:898–909.

173. Cowan AJ, et al. Macroglossia—not always AL amyloidosis. Amyloid. 2011;18:83–6.

174. Merlini G, Palladini G. Differential diagnosis of monoclonal gammopathy of undetermined significance. Hematol Am Soc Hematol Educ Program. 2012;2012:595–603.
175. Gertz MA, Lacy MQ, Dispenzieri A. Immunoglobulin light chain amyloidosis and the kidney. Kidney Int. 2002;61:1–9.
176. Gertz MA, et al. Clinical outcome of immunoglobulin light chain amyloidosis affecting the kidney. Nephrol Dial Transplant. 2009;24:3132–7.
177. Bergesio F, et al. Renal involvement in systemic amyloidosis: an Italian collaborative study on survival and renal outcome. Nephrol Dial Transplant. 2008;23:941–51.
178. Palladini G, et al. A staging system for renal outcome and early markers of renal response to chemotherapy in AL amyloidosis. Blood. 2014; 124:2325–32.
179. Leung N, et al. Severity of baseline proteinuria predicts renal response in immunoglobulin light chain-associated amyloidosis after autologous stem cell transplantation. Clin J Am Soc Nephrol. 2007;2:440–4.
180. Leung N, et al. Renal response after high-dose melphalan and stem cell transplantation is a favorable marker in patients with primary systemic amyloidosis. Am J Kidney Dis. 2005;46:270–7.
181. Falk RH. Diagnosis and management of the cardiac amyloidoses. Circulation. 2005;112:2047–60.
182. Dubrey SW, Hawkins PN, Falk RH. Amyloid diseases of the heart: assessment, diagnosis, and referral. Heart. 2011;97:75–84.
183. Maceira AM, et al. Cardiovascular magnetic resonance in cardiac amyloidosis. Circulation. 2005;111:186–93.
184. Bellavia D, et al. Independent predictors of survival in primary systemic (Al) amyloidosis, including cardiac biomarkers and left ventricular strain imaging: an observational cohort study. J Am Soc Echocardiogr. 2010;23:643–52.
185. Koyama J, Falk RH. Prognostic significance of strain Doppler imaging in light-chain amyloidosis. JACC Cardiovasc Imaging. 2010;3:333–42.
186. Buss SJ, et al. Longitudinal left ventricular function for prediction of survival in systemic light-chain amyloidosis: incremental value compared with clinical and biochemical markers. J Am Coll Cardiol. 2012;60:1067–76.
187. Quarta CC, et al. Left ventricular structure and function in transthyretin-related versus light-chain cardiac amyloidosis. Circulation. 2014;129:1840–9.
188. Merlini G, Narula J, Arbustini E. Molecular imaging of misfolded protein pathology for early clues to involvement of the heart. Eur J Nucl Med Mol Imaging. 2014;41:1649–51.
189. Merlini G, Palladini G. Amyloidosis: is a cure possible? Ann Oncol. 2008;19 Suppl 4:iv63–6.
190. Palladini G, et al. Serum N-terminal pro-brain natriuretic peptide is a sensitive marker of myocardial dysfunction in AL amyloidosis. Circulation. 2003;107:2440–5.
191. Dispenzieri A, et al. Survival in patients with primary systemic amyloidosis and raised serum cardiac troponins. Lancet. 2003;361:1787–9.
192. Palladini G, et al. The combination of high-sensitivity cardiac troponin T (hs-cTnT) at presentation and changes in N-terminal natriuretic peptide type B (NT-proBNP) after chemotherapy best predicts survival in AL amyloidosis. Blood. 2010;116:3426–30.
193. Dispenzieri A, et al. High sensitivity cardiac troponin T in patients with immunoglobulin light chain amyloidosis. Heart. 2014;100:383–8.
194. Dispenzieri A, et al. Serum cardiac troponins and N-terminal pro-brain natriuretic peptide: a staging system for primary systemic amyloidosis. J Clin Oncol. 2004;22:3751–7.
195. Palladini G, et al. New criteria for response to treatment in immunoglobulin light chain amyloidosis based on free light chain measurement and cardiac biomarkers: impact on survival outcomes. J Clin Oncol. 2012;30:4541–9.
196. Kumar S, et al. Revised prognostic staging system for light chain amyloidosis incorporating cardiac biomarkers and serum free light chain measurements. J Clin Oncol. 2012;30:989–95.
197. Palladini G, et al. Holter monitoring in AL amyloidosis: prognostic implications. Pacing Clin Electrophysiol. 2001;24:1228–33.
198. Perlini S, et al. Prognostic value of fragmented QRS in cardiac AL amyloidosis. Int J Cardiol. 2013; 167:2156–61.
199. Boldrini M, et al. Prevalence and prognostic value of conduction disturbances at the time of diagnosis of cardiac AL amyloidosis. Ann Noninvasive Electrocardiol. 2013;18:327–35.
200. Wechalekar AD, et al. A European collaborative study of treatment outcomes in 346 patients with cardiac stage III AL amyloidosis. Blood. 2013;121: 3420–7.
201. Russo P, et al. Liver involvement as the hallmark of aggressive disease in light chain amyloidosis: distinctive clinical features and role of light chain type in 225 patients. Amyloid. 2011;18 Suppl 1:92–3.
202. Park MA, et al. Primary (AL) hepatic amyloidosis: clinical features and natural history in 98 patients. Medicine (Baltimore). 2003;82:291–8.
203. Peters RA, et al. Primary amyloidosis and severe intrahepatic cholestatic jaundice. Gut. 1994; 35:1322–5.
204. Rubinow A, Koff RS, Cohen AS. Severe intrahepatic cholestasis in primary amyloidosis: a report of four cases and a review of the literature. Am J Med. 1978;64:937–46.
205. Ooi LL, Lynch SV, Graham DA, Strong RW. Spontaneous liver rupture in amyloidosis. Surgery. 1996;120:117–9.
206. Kacem C, Helali K, Puisieux F. Recurrent spontaneous hepatic rupture in primary hepatic amyloidosis. Ann Intern Med. 1998;129:339.

207. Di Sabatino A, Carsetti R, Corazza GR. Post-splenectomy and hyposplenic states. Lancet. 2011;378:86–97.
208. Renzulli P, Schoepfer A, Mueller E, Candinas D. Atraumatic splenic rupture in amyloidosis. Amyloid. 2009;16:47–53.
209. Matsuda M, et al. Peripheral nerve involvement in primary systemic AL amyloidosis: a clinical and electrophysiological study. Eur J Neurol. 2011;18:604–10.
210. Caccialanza R, et al. Nutritional status of outpatients with systemic immunoglobulin light-chain amyloidosis 1. Am J Clin Nutr. 2006;83:350–4.
211. Caccialanza R, et al. Malnutrition at diagnosis predicts mortality in patients with systemic immunoglobulin light-chain amyloidosis independently of cardiac stage and response to treatment. JPEN J Parenter Enteral Nutr. 2014;38:891–4.
212. Sattianayagam PT, et al. A prospective study of nutritional status in immunoglobulin light chain amyloidosis. Haematologica. 2013;98:136–40.
213. Gertz MA, et al. Definition of organ involvement and treatment response in immunoglobulin light chain amyloidosis (AL): a consensus opinion from the 10th International Symposium on Amyloid and Amyloidosis, Tours, France, 18-22 April 2004. Am J Hematol. 2005;79:319–28.
214. Gertz MA, Merlini G. Definition of organ involvement and treatment response in immunoglobulin light chain amyloidosis (AL): a consensus opinion. Amyloid. 2010;17:48–9.
215. Merlini G, et al. The Pavia approach to clinical protein analysis. Clin Chem Lab Med. 2001;39:1025–8.
216. Palladini G, et al. Identification of amyloidogenic light chains requires the combination of serum-free light chain assay with immunofixation of serum and urine. Clin Chem. 2009;55:499–504.
217. Anesi E, et al. Therapeutic advances demand accurate typing of amyloid deposits. Am J Med. 2001;111:243–4.
218. Lachmann HJ, et al. Misdiagnosis of hereditary amyloidosis as AL (primary) amyloidosis. N Engl J Med. 2002;346:1786–91.
219. Palladini G, Obici L, Merlini G. Hereditary amyloidosis. N Engl J Med. 2002;347:1206–7. author reply 1206–7.
220. Kyle RA, Rajkumar SV. Epidemiology of the plasma-cell disorders. Best Pract Res Clin Haematol. 2007;20:637–64.
221. Comenzo RL, Zhou P, Fleisher M, Clark B, Teruya-Feldstein J. Seeking confidence in the diagnosis of systemic AL (Ig light-chain) amyloidosis: patients can have both monoclonal gammopathies and hereditary amyloid proteins. Blood. 2006;107:3489–91.
222. Wechalekar AD, Offer M, Gillmore JD, Hawkins PN, Lachmann HJ. Cardiac amyloidosis, a monoclonal gammopathy and a potentially misleading mutation. Nat Clin Pract Cardiovasc Med. 2009;6:128–33.
223. Kyle RA, et al. Long-term survival (10 years or more) in 30 patients with primary amyloidosis. Blood. 1999;93:1062–6.
224. Palladini G, et al. Treatment with oral melphalan plus dexamethasone produces long-term remissions in AL amyloidosis. Blood. 2007;110:787–8.
225. Merlini G, et al. Interaction of the anthracycline 4′-iodo-4′-deoxydoxorubicin with amyloid fibrils: inhibition of amyloidogenesis. Proc Natl Acad Sci USA. 1995;92:2959–63.
226. Gianni L, Bellotti V, Gianni AM, Merlini G. New drug therapy of amyloidoses: resorption of AL-type deposits with 4′-iodo-4′-deoxydoxorubicin. Blood. 1995;86:855–61.
227. Gertz MA, et al. A multicenter phase II trial of 4′-iodo-4′deoxydoxorubicin (IDOX) in primary amyloidosis (AL). Amyloid. 2002;9:24–30.
228. Merlini G, Wechalekar AD, Palladini G. Systemic light chain amyloidosis: an update for treating physicians. Blood. 2013;121:5124–30.
229. Ohno S, et al. The antisense approach in amyloid light chain amyloidosis: identification of monoclonal Ig and inhibition of its production by antisense oligonucleotides in in vitro and in vivo models. J Immunol. 2002;169:4039–45.
230. Phipps JE, et al. Inhibition of pathologic immunoglobulin-free light chain production by small interfering RNA molecules. Exp Hematol. 2010;38:1006–13.
231. Hovey BM, et al. Preclinical development of siRNA therapeutics for AL amyloidosis. Gene Ther. 2011;18:1150–6.
232. Zhou P, Ma X, Iyer L, Chaulagain C, Comenzo RL. One siRNA pool targeting the lambda constant region stops lambda light-chain production and causes terminal endoplasmic reticulum stress. Blood. 2014;123:3440–51.
233. Cooley CB, et al. Unfolded protein response activation reduces secretion and extracellular aggregation of amyloidogenic immunoglobulin light chain. Proc Natl Acad Sci USA. 2014;111:13046–51.
234. Hrncic R, et al. Antibody-mediated resolution of light chain-associated amyloid deposits. Am J Pathol. 2000;157:1239–46.
235. Solomon A, Weiss DT, Wall JS. Immunotherapy in systemic primary (AL) amyloidosis using amyloid-reactive monoclonal antibodies. Cancer Biother Radiopharm. 2003;18:853–60.

AA Amyloidosis

3

Amanda K. Ombrello and Ivona Aksentijevich

AA amyloidosis, also known as reactive amyloidosis, is a form of amyloidosis that develops in patients with chronic inflammatory states. It is estimated that, worldwide, approximately 45 % of all generalized amyloid cases are AA amyloidosis [1]. Whereas infectious diseases such as tuberculosis, malaria, leprosy, and chronic osteomyelitis were once the leading causes of AA amyloidosis, effective treatments for these infections have brought other causes of AA amyloidosis to the forefront. Within the field of rheumatology, there is a recently characterized group of diseases, known as the hereditary autoinflammatory diseases, which have an increased risk for the development of AA amyloidosis. Historically, AA amyloidosis has also been seen in other rheumatologic diseases such as rheumatoid arthritis (RA), ankylosing spondylitis (AS), and systemic juvenile arthritis (SJIA), although with the therapeutic developments of the past

20 years, the prevalence has decreased significantly. Additionally, AA amyloidosis has been associated with granulomatous diseases such as sarcoidosis and Crohn's disease and malignancies such as mesothelioma and Hodgkin's disease. There have been a number of AA amyloidosis cases described that are associated with intravenous drug use and other infectious conditions such as bronchiectasis and HIV [2–4]. Approximately, 6 % of AA amyloidosis cases have no identified disease association [2].

In the amyloidosis nomenclature, there is often some confusion in distinguishing between amyloidoses that develop due to mutations in the *amyloid fibril protein itself* versus amyloidoses associated with genetic mutations in *non-amyloid proteins*. The former are frequently referred to as hereditary amyloidoses. This is in contrast to familial AA amyloidosis, which develops in patients with diseases that have genetic mutations in *non-amyloid* proteins: these mutations result in upregulation of the inflammatory response of the innate immune system, and this inflammation predisposes patients to the development of AA amyloidosis. The hereditary autoinflammatory diseases are included in this subset [5].

AA amyloid fibrils deposit as a result of an enhanced and prolonged inflammatory state that leads to misfolding of the AA amyloid protein and deposition into tissues. Although the pathogenesis is not completely understood, there

3

A.K. Ombrello, MD (✉)
Inflammatory Disease Section, National Human Genome Research Institute, National Institutes of Health, 10 Center Drive 4 N/208 MSC 1375, Bethesda, MD 20892, USA
e-mail: ombrelloak@mail.nih.gov

I. Aksentijevich, MD
Inflammatory Disease Section, National Human Genome Research Institute, National Institutes of Health, 9000 Rockville Pike, 10-CRC/B2-5235, Bethesda, MD 20892, USA
e-mail: aksentii@mail.nih.gov

© Springer International Publishing Switzerland 2015
M.M. Picken et al. (eds.), *Amyloid and Related Disorders*, Current Clinical Pathology,
DOI 10.1007/978-3-319-19294-9_3

are many factors that influence the risk of developing AA amyloidosis. The precursor protein of the fibrils in AA amyloidosis is an apolipoprotein called serum amyloid A (SAA). In humans, SAA is expressed by three different genes that are localized on chromosome 11p15.1. SAA1 and SAA2 are two SAA isoforms that are acute phase reactants synthesized by the liver that have the ability to form amyloid. Approximately, 80 % of secreted SAA1 and SAA2 are bound to lipoproteins and of that, 90 % are bound to high density lipoprotein [1]. SAA is produced in the liver in response to proinflammatory cytokines such as interleukin (IL)-1, IL-6, and tumor necrosis factor (TNF)-α (alpha) and can rise more than 1,000 fold during inflammation [6].

The exact role of SAA is unknown but, as this protein is highly conserved among species, it has been speculated that SAA plays a role as a chemoattractant and in lipid metabolism [6, 7]. In support of this, is the fact that amyloid deposition occurs initially in organs that are major sites of lipid and cholesterol metabolism such as the kidney, liver, and spleen. Additionally, there are other apolipoproteins such as apolipoprotein AI (apo AI) and apolipoprotein E (apo E) that are present in the SAA bound high density lipoprotein (HDL) fraction. Apo AI and apo E are thought to play significant roles in reverse cholesterol metabolism which involves interaction with peripheral cells, such as macrophages, to facilitate the removal of excess free cholesterol [1]. The liberated cholesterol is transported to the liver for intestinal excretion. Interestingly, other apolipoproteins (Apolipoprotein AI, AII, and AIV) may also be associated with amyloidosis, both hereditary (Apolipoprotein AI and AII) and sporadic (Apolipoprotein AIV).

Under normal circumstances, SAA is secreted by the liver and completely degraded by macrophages. The secreted SAA protein is 104 amino acids in size and is primarily secreted in an α (alpha)-helix structure [8]. Patients with AA amyloidosis have a flaw in the degradation sequence that is not completely understood, which results in incomplete degradation and accumulation of intermediate SAA products. Initially, in these patients, SAA is transferred to the lysosome

where the c-terminal portion of the SAA protein is cleaved allowing the remaining protein to fold into a β (beta) sheet configuration. Deposited amyloid contains only 66–76 amino acids compared to the 104 in secreted SAA [8]. The cleaved fragments polymerize and form fibrils that are deposited in the extracellular space and bind proteoglycans and other proteins such as serum amyloid P. Once bound by the aforementioned components, the fibrils become resistant to proteolysis and deposit in organ tissues [9].

Although organ involvement varies, AA amyloidosis most commonly affects the kidneys with 90 % of patients having some degree of renal involvement [10]. Frequently, renal disease is initially observed when patients present with unexplained proteinuria. If the AA amyloidosis diagnosis is delayed or the patient's underlying inflammatory condition is not suppressed, patients will go on to develop renal failure. Lachmann et al. published an article in 2007 detailing the natural history of AA amyloidosis and found that the median survival after diagnosis was 133 months. Patients with higher SAA levels had a significantly higher risk of death than those with lower SAA concentrations [2]. Gastrointestinal involvement is seen in approximately 20 % of patients; in contrast, testes are frequently involved (87 %). Although associated with AA amyloidosis, amyloid goiter, hepatomegaly, splenomegaly, adrenal involvement, and pulmonary involvement are relatively uncommon findings [9]. Other tissues such as the heart, tongue, and skin are rarely involved.

A diagnosis of AA amyloid is made based on the examination of a tissue biopsy. The tissues most commonly tested include kidney, rectum, abdominal fat pad, and gingiva. Staining with Congo red reveals the characteristic "apple green birefringence" of amyloid deposits under polarized microscopy. For an AA amyloid type diagnosis, immunohistochemistry staining is needed.

There have been a number of risk factors associated with the development of AA amyloidosis. The gene that codes for SAA1 has polymorphisms that when present, carry a three to sevenfold increased risk for the development of AA amyloidosis [11]. Specifically, Caucasian patients with

RA, juvenile arthritis, and patients with autoinflammatory diseases such as familial Mediterranean fever (FMF) who have the SAA1α/α (alpha/alpha) genotype have an increased risk of amyloidosis. In that group of patients, the SAA1γ (gamma) allele is associated with a decreased susceptibility of amyloidosis [11]. Conversely, in Japanese RA patients, the SAA1α/α (alpha/alpha) genotype is associated with a decreased susceptibility of amyloidosis development but the SAA1γ (gamma) genotype carries an increased risk [12]. Additionally, within the autoinflammatory syndromes, there are specific diseases which carry an increased risk for amyloidosis and, within those diseases, specific genetic mutations further increase one's risk for the development of amyloidosis. Further elaboration of the risk of amyloidosis within the autoinflammatory syndromes will be discussed later as each autoinflammatory disease is described.

AA Amyloidosis in Rheumatic Disease

In developed countries, prior to the initiation of therapy with disease modifying antirheumatic drugs (DMARDs) and biologic agents, rheumatoid arthritis was the most common inflammatory disease associated with AA amyloidosis [10]. Studies preceding the biologic era reported the prevalence of AA amyloidosis to be 5–20 %, and increased prevalence was seen in Northern Europeans compared to North Americans [13]. Patients who had a long history of poorly controlled, severe disease with extraarticular manifestations were at the most risk for developing amyloidosis, and the median time from the first symptoms of their rheumatic condition to the diagnosis of amyloidosis was 212 months [10]. The full effect of DMARD and antitumor necrosis factor therapy in rheumatoid arthritis-associated amyloidosis has yet to be fully appreciated, but recent studies are showing a sustained decline in the number of new cases [14].

Juvenile idiopathic arthritis (JIA) is another rheumatic disease that is associated with the development of AA amyloidosis with the highest prevalence in the patients with systemic juvenile arthritis (SJIA) followed by those with polyarticular disease. In the era pre-DMARD and biologic therapy, the prevalence of AA amyloidosis in JIA patients ranged from 1 to 10 % [15]. Higher prevalence was seen in Northern European patients, especially Polish patients who had a prevalence of 10.6 % and lower prevalence was observed in North Americans. The reasons for this discrepancy are not completely clear although it was speculated that selection bias, genetic background, and a tendency toward more early, aggressive therapy in North Americans may have played a role [16, 17]. AA amyloidosis has been observed in JIA patients as early as 1 year after diagnosis; conversely, it has also been seen 25 years after diagnosis [15, 18]. Similar to rheumatoid arthritis, the occurrence of new amyloid cases has significantly decreased in the past 20 years due to the increased efficacy of treatment with DMARDs and biologics [14, 18].

Historically, the incidence of AA amyloidosis in ankylosing spondylitis patients has been estimated at 6 % based on postmortem analysis [19, 20]. However, within the subset of severely affected patients, up to 13 % have developed AA amyloidosis [21]. Patients with a long history of active disease are at the most risk for developing clinical signs of AA amyloidosis. As is the current trend with both rheumatoid arthritis and JIA, the incidence of new cases is on the decline [18].

The Hereditary Autoinflammatory Diseases

The hereditary autoinflammatory diseases define a group of illnesses that are characterized by attacks of seemingly unprovoked recurrent inflammation without significant levels of either autoantibodies or antigen-specific T cells, which are typically found in patients with autoimmune diseases. Whereas autoimmune diseases like systemic lupus erythematosus (SLE) and rheumatoid arthritis (RA) result from a derangement in the adaptive immune system, the autoinflammatory syndromes are a result of malfunctions in the innate immune system [22, 23]. The inflammatory attacks are thus mediated by the cells of innate immunity, namely neutrophils and macrophages. Although seemingly unprovoked, these attacks are often initiated by stress, immunization, or trauma, suggesting that gene–environment interactions play an important role in pathogenesis.

During the past 15 years, major research has been undertaken to understand the pathogenesis of autoinflammatory diseases, which ultimately has led to a new classification of monogenic and polygenic autoinflammatory disorders.

Monogenic Autoinflammatory Diseases

The term autoinflammation was introduced based on the studies of hereditary periodic fever syndromes, a group of Mendelian diseases with similar clinical presentations including recurrent fevers and systemic inflammation. Although there is some variability, common findings include serositis, cutaneous rash, arthritis, and ocular involvement (Table 3.1). The inflammatory attacks are accompanied by intense acute phase response [erythrocyte sedimentation rate (ESR) and c-reactive protein (CRP)] and high levels of SAA. The monogenic autoinflammatory diseases include conditions that are inherited in an autosomal dominant fashion such as the tumor necrosis factor receptor-associated periodic syndrome (TRAPS; MIM191190), the syndrome of pyogenic arthritis with pyoderma gangrenosum and acne (PAPA; MIM604416), and Blau syndrome (also known as early-onset sarcoidosis) (MIM186580). Also inherited in an autosomal dominant fashion is a spectrum of phenotypes caused by mutations in the same gene with the mildest being familial cold autoinflammatory syndrome (FCAS1; MIM120100), followed by Muckle–Wells syndrome (MWS; MIM191900), the most severe neonatal onset multisystem inflammatory disease (NOMID; MIM607115), and familial cold autoinflammatory syndrome 2 (FCAS2; MIM611762). In contrast, familial Mediterranean fever (FMF; MIM249100), Majeed syndrome (MIM609628), hyperimmunoglobulinemia D syndrome (HIDS; MIM260920),

the deficiency of IL-1 receptor antagonist (DIRA; MIM612852), the deficiency of IL-36 receptor antagonist (DITRA/PSORP; MIM 614204), and the proteasome-related autoinflammatory syndromes (PRAAS): Chronic Atypical Neutrophilic Dermatosis with Lipodystrophy and Elevated Temperature Syndrome (CANDLE), Japanese Autoinflammatory Syndrome with Lipodystrophy (JASL; also known as Nakajo–Nishimura Syndrome), and Joint Contractures, Muscle Atrophy, Microcytic Anemia, and Panniculitis Induced Lipodystrophy (JMP) (MIM256040) are inherited as autosomal-recessive traits [22, 24].

More recently, next generation sequencing (NGS) technologies have led to the identification of several causal genes in patients with rare autoinflammatory diseases such as the syndrome of autoinflammation, PLC-γ (gamma)-associated antibody deficiency, and immune dysregulation (APLAID; MIM614878); the recessively inherited HOIL-1 /RBCK1 deficiency and deficiency of ADA2 (DADA2/Polyarteritis nodosa) [25].

As interest and understanding of these diseases have grown, so has the realization that some, but not all, of the hereditary autoinflammatory diseases carry an increased risk for the development of AA amyloidosis.

Familial Mediterranean Fever

Familial Mediterranean fever (FMF) is the most common of the Mendelian autoinflammatory diseases. It is seen most frequently in the Armenian, Arab, Turkish, and Sephardi Jewish populations with carrier frequencies ranging from 1:3 to 1:10 in population-based studies. The disease prevalence is significantly lower due to reduced penetrance of many of the FMF-associated mutations. The high carrier frequency in multiple populations may confer selective advantage and resistance to a yet-unknown endemic pathogen. Typically, carriers for various FMF-associated mutations are asymptomatic but they may actually have subclinical evidence of inflammation or even be periodically symptomatic [26].

Patients with FMF have acute attacks of fever and localized inflammation that commonly

Table 3.1 Clinical manifestations of the hereditary periodic fever syndromes

Disease	Gene	Inheritance	Flare duration	Fever	Cutaneous manifestations	Abdominal manifestations	Pulmonary	Arthritis arthralgias	Neurologic	AA Amyloidosis
FMF	*MEFV*	AR	1–3 days	Yes	Erysipeloid erythema	Pain, constipation, diarrhea	Pleurisy	Yes	No	Yes-10 %
HIDS	*MVK*	AR	3–7 days	Yes	Maculopapular	Pain, vomiting, constipation, diarrhea	Rare	Yes	No	Rare
DIRA	*ILRN*	AR	Continuous	Yes	Pustular neutrophilic	Not known	No	Yes	No	Not described
PRAAS	*PSMB8*	AR	Continuous	Yes	Violaceous annular plaques; Heliotrope rash, periorbital swelling; Lipodystrophy	Truncal obesity; Hyperlipidemia	Rare	Yes	Basal ganglia calcification	Not described
DITRA	*IL36RN*	AR	Days to weeks	Yes	Sterile pustulosis	Cholangitis	Not described	Yes	Not described	Not described
DADA2	*CECR1*	AR	Continuous	Yes	Livedo racemosa; Vasculitis	Portal hypertension; Hepatomegaly; Splenomegaly	Not described	Yes	Lacunar strokes (ischemic and hemorrhagic)	Not described
TRAPS	*TNFRSF1A*	AD	1–4 weeks	Yes	Migratory macular rash, periorbital edema	Pain, constipation, diarrhea	Pleurisy	Yes	No	Yes 14–25 %
FCAS	*NLRP3*	AD	<24 h	Yes	Cold-induced neutrophilic urticarial-like	Nausea	Not seen	Yes	No	Rare
MWS	*NLRP3*	AD	1–3 days	Yes	Neutrophilic urticarial-like	Occasional abdominal pain	Rare	Yes	Sensorineural deafness	Yes 25–33 %

(continued)

Table 3.1 (continued)

Disease	Gene	Inheritance	Flare duration	Fever	Cutaneous manifestations	Abdominal manifestations	Pulmonary	Arthritis arthralgias	Neurologic	AA Amyloidosis
NOMID/CINCA	*NLRP3*	AD	Continuous	Yes	Neutrophilic urticarial-like	Uncommon	Rare	Yes	Aseptic meningitis sensorineural deafness papilledema	Rare
PAPA	*PSTPIP1*	AD	Weeks	Yes	Pyoderma gangrenosum / Cystic acne	Uncommon	Not seen	Yes	No	Not described
APLAID	*PLCG2*	AD	Continuous with periodic worsening	No	Recurrent vesiculobullae / Corneal bullae and ulcerations	Enterocolitis	Recurrent sinopulmonary infection / Interstitial lung disease	Yes	Not described	Not described

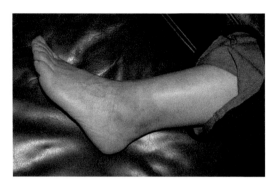

Fig. 3.1 Familial Mediterranean fever. Erysipeloid erythema in a patient with FMF (mutations M694V/M680I)

involve the peritoneum, pleura, skin, or joints. The hallmark cutaneous finding is an erysipeloid erythematous rash on the dorsum of the foot or ankle (Fig. 3.1). Biopsies of the rash show a mixed cellular infiltrate [27]. Attacks begin during childhood with up to 90 % of patients experiencing their initial attack prior to age 20. Attacks typically last 1–3 days and subside spontaneously. Between attacks, patients generally feel well, although there may be some persistent acute phase reactant elevation on laboratory analysis. The quality and severity of attacks can vary from one attack to another and can differ significantly between members of the same family [22, 23].

FMF is an autosomal-recessive disease that results from mutations in the *MEFV* gene. The *MEFV* gene is located on chromosome 16p and contains ten exons that encode the pyrin/marenostrin protein. The FMF-associated mutations are found primarily in exon 10 that encodes the B30.2/PRYSPRY domain at the C terminal end of the protein. The pyrin protein is expressed predominately in neutrophils, but also in synovial fibroblasts and dendritic cells. Pyrin was found to interact with ASC, the apoptosis-associated speck-like protein, with a caspase-recruitment domain (CARD), through cognate pyrin domain (PYD) association and is involved in regulation of the caspase-1 pathway, which results in secretion of IL-1β(beta) [28]. The pyrin protein has also been shown to affect apoptosis and NF-κ(kappa)B activation [28–30]. In the *Infevers* database (fmf.igh.cnrs.fr/infevers), there are currently close to 300 *MEVF* sequence variants

reported; however, only a minority of these are clearly FMF disease-associated mutations [31]. Four mutations (M680I, M694V, M694I, and V726A) account for most disease alleles in various Middle Eastern FMF populations. Mutations affecting the M680 and M694 amino acid residues are associated with early onset of FMF, severe disease, and an increased AA amyloidosis risk in all ethnic groups, whereas the V726A mutation is usually associated with milder FMF. NMR and crystallographic data indicate that severe FMF mutations map close to a putative binding pocket of the PRYSPRY domain, whereas a less severe mutation V726A is located on the opposite side of the domain [24]. Although by definition the diagnosis of FMF would require that two mutations be present (as it is an autosomal-recessive disease), there is a subset of patients who present with typical FMF symptoms but have only one demonstrable mutation in the *MEFV* gene despite sequencing of the entire *MEFV* gene [32, 33]. In addition, there are reports of families with clearly dominantly inherited mutations in *MEFV* who present with FMF-like disease [34, 35]. This could be possibly explained by observation from pyrin knock-in mouse model studies, which suggest that FMF is the result of gain-of-function mutations leading to the activation of IL-1β (beta) pathway [36]. In support of single mutation FMF, analysis of asymptomatic carriers has found evidence for subclinical inflammation as manifested by elevated acute phase reactants [26, 37].

The prevalence of AA amyloidosis in FMF patients in various case series has ranged from 0 % in Armenians living in America to 37 % in the Sephardi Jewish population. A multicenter study published by Touitou et al. found an overall prevalence of 11.4 % [38]. The incidence varied depending on the population frequency of homozygosity for the M694V mutation, male gender, SAA1 α/α (alpha/alpha) genotype, positive family history, and non-compliance with colchicine treatment [38, 39]. The large, multicenter study revealed that country of residence and its infant mortality rate strongly correlated with the development of AA amyloidosis. Patients residing in Armenia, Turkey, and Arabian countries had a three-fold increased risk of developing AA amyloidosis compared to other countries [38]. It is unclear as to why this risk factor is significant, but it has been speculated that environmental factors such as increased poverty levels, standards of health care, and infections may contribute to this finding. Of note, patients born in countries that carry a high risk for developing AA amyloidosis who immigrate to a low-risk country tend to develop AA amyloidosis at the lower rates after emigration. This was initially identified in a group of 100 Armenians with FMF who were living in the United States. None of them developed AA amyloidosis in comparison to the 24 % of FMF patients living in Armenia who had developed amyloidosis at the time of publication [39]. Recent studies from Turkey reported that, as it would have been expected, there has been a significant decrease in the rate of secondary amyloidosis; nevertheless, SAA amyloidosis was still present in 193/2,246 patients (8.6 %) [40] The main reason for this decline is better medical care with increased awareness and treatment of the disease [41]. The multicenter study by Touitou et al. also noted that FMF patients with the M694V/M694V mutations in the *MEFV* gene had a higher risk for AA amyloidosis, especially if they lived in Armenia, Israel, and Arabian countries. FMF patients with the SAA1 α/α (alpha/alpha) genotype have been observed to have a sevenfold increase in the risk for amyloidosis with a notable additional increase in patients who carry two copies of the severe mutation, M694V. One other risk factor identified in the multicenter study was disease duration [42].

The presence of M694V was also reported as the major risk factor for amyloidosis in a comprehensive review of the literature that included 3,505 patients with FMF from Turkey. Among 400 patients with amyloidosis and known genotypes, 47 % had the M694V/ M694V genotype, while an additional 21 % of patients carried at least one M694V mutation. The majority of other high-risk genotypes are also found in the exon 10 of *MEFV*, in particular mutations affecting the M694 and M680 amino acid residues [43]. FMF patients homozygous for the M694V mutation had the highest levels of SAA even during remission (Fig. 3.2). However, it should not go unstated that there are other non-exon ten mutations (S179I) that have been associated with the development of amyloidosis, although these cases are rare [42–44]. The development of amyloidosis in an E148Q patient is especially interesting considering that the carrier frequency of E148Q in certain populations is over 10 %. In general, patients with the E148Q mutation are thought to have milder and atypical FMF-like disease; however, there have been amyloidosis cases described in E148Q/E148Q patients [45]. In most cases, the E148Q variant has been observed in combination with a true FMF-associated mutation, inherited either in *trans* or in *cis* as a "complex allele" [44]. Some studies have suggested a gene dosage effect, with patients who have three or four *MEFV* mutations appearing to have more severe disease and susceptibility to amyloidosis [46].

FMF patients who develop amyloidosis generally have classic FMF with two inherited mutations. It is exceedingly rare, although not unheard of, for patients with single mutation FMF to develop amyloidosis. Such is the case with multiple members of a Spanish family with a H478Y mutation that causes an autosomal dominant form of FMF-like disease. AA amyloidosis has developed in many of the mutation positive members of this family [34].

Although it would seem logical that FMF patients who have frequent, severe attacks would be at the most risk for the development of AA amyloidosis, studies have found that is not always the case. There are patients who have had hundreds of attacks and never develop amyloidosis and there are patients who, at the age of five, passed away from amyloidosis-related complications. Even more intriguing is the subset of FMF patients who are referred to as phenotype II patients [47, 48]. These patients present with AA amyloidosis prior to experiencing their first FMF attack. In phenotype II patients, the distribution of the common *MEFV* mutations is not significantly different from that found in FMF patients with typical symptoms who do or do not develop amyloidosis. Patients homozygous for the M694V mutation have been observed most commonly in the phenotype II [49]. Lane et al.,

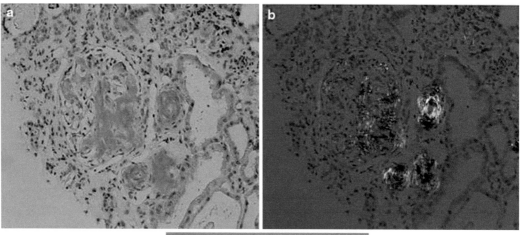

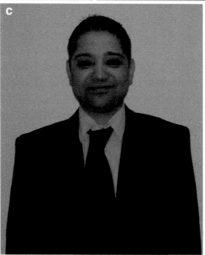

Fig. 3.2 Familial Mediterranean fever-associated AA amyloidosis. *Top left*: Renal biopsy from an FMF patient homozygous for the M694V mutation revealing the presence of amyloid deposits. *Top right*: Renal biopsy revealing the characteristic "apple-green birefringence" pattern on polarized microscopy. *Bottom*: A 24-year-old patient with FMF (M694V/M694V) who underwent renal transplant in 2006 at age 21 secondary to AA amyloidosis. Slides from his renal biopsy are above. He also has biopsy proven AA amyloidosis in his gastrointestinal tract and heart

described 6/24 FMF patients with AA amyloidosis who did not have any symptoms of inflammation prior to diagnostic biopsy. These patients were either heterozygous carriers for one M694V mutation or carried other mild FMF-associated mutations [44]. Although unclear, it seems that secondary genetic or environmental factors play a significant role in the development of AA amyloidosis in patients with FMF [47–49].

The major histocompatibility complex (MHC) has been found to be associated with a number of inflammatory diseases such as Behçet's disease, rheumatoid arthritis, and psoriatic arthritis. In the case of FMF, the MHC class I chain-related gene A (*MICA*) is of specific interest. Analysis of *MICA* in FMF patients has revealed that although certain *MICA* alleles are associated with earlier onset of symptoms (A9 allele) and decreased frequency of attacks (A4 allele), when specifically examining FMF patients with amyloidosis, no significant association has been found [50–52].

A hallmark event for patients with FMF came with the implementation of daily colchicine as primary therapy in the early 1970s [53]. Subsequent studies have shown that compliance with daily colchicine causes a marked decrease in

FMF symptoms in 90 % of patients as well as a decrease in SAA levels [54, 55]. Additionally, Zemer et al. found that colchicine compliance reduced the risk of proteinuria development from 48.9 % in untreated/non-compliant patients to 1.7 % in colchicine compliant patients over the course of 11 and 9 years respectively [56]. A marked decrease in both the frequency of FMF flares as well as new cases of AA amyloidosis has been substantiated in subsequent studies [57, 58]. In recent years, patients who continue to have frequent attacks while on colchicine, patients who have persistently elevated inflammatory markers despite colchicine therapy, and patients who are intolerant to colchicine's side effects, have had the IL-1 receptor antagonist, anakinra added to their regimen. Although large studies have not been conducted using anakinra, preliminary case reports have shown positive results with reduction in clinical symptoms and/or acute phase reactants [59, 60]. Anakinra had a strong effect in suppressing inflammation in FMF patients with amyloidosis and may change the prognosis of these patients [61].

Regarding FMF patients with amyloidosis who have undergone renal transplantation, a study was completed that compared long-term outcomes between FMF patients and patients transplanted for other conditions. Overall graft and patient survival was comparable to that of the non-FMF group and, with continuation of colchicine, amyloid infiltration of the transplanted kidney was held to 5 % [62]. At 5 years after transplantation, patient survival was at 89 %, while recurrence was noted only in 1/18 patients [62].

Since albuminuria is an early finding in FMF amyloidosis, patients should undergo periodic urinalyses, especially those who are at high risk. In one large series, the sensitivity of renal biopsy for detecting amyloidosis in FMF was 88 %, followed by rectal biopsy at 75 %, liver biopsy at 48 %, and gingival biopsy at 19 % [63]. Many physicians prefer rectal biopsy because it is relatively noninvasive. The sensitivity of bone marrow biopsy in a more recent small series was found to be 80 %, and the sensitivity of testicular biopsy is about 87 % [64, 65].

Tumor Necrosis Factor Receptor-Associated Periodic Syndrome

TRAPS was initially described clinically in a family of Irish/Scottish descent. At that time, it was given the appropriate name of familial Hibernian fever [66]. Additional cases of patients not of Irish or Scottish descent coupled with the discovery of the mutated gene being the *TNFRSF1A* gene, brought about its change in name to TRAPS [67]. Patients with TRAPS typically present within the first decade of life. They frequently have a history of prolonged fever episodes lasting for at least 3 days but commonly lasting many weeks. Additional clinical findings include abdominal pain frequently associated with constipation, diarrhea and bowel obstruction. Analysis of the abdominal cavity during flares has revealed sterile peritonitis. Other symptoms include periorbital edema, conjunctivitis and localized myalgias (Fig. 3.3). On imaging, affected muscle groups show focal areas of edema [22, 23]. Cutaneous findings include an erythematous macular rash that on biopsy contains superficial and deep perivascular infiltrates of mononuclear cells [68]. Patients often report the rash migrates distally during its course and clinically, can resemble cellulitis. Patients can also report erythematous annular patches. Arthralgias are fairly common but frank arthritis is relatively rare. Attacks are commonly associated with stress or physical exertion. During attacks, there is marked elevation in the acute phase reactants (ESR, CRP, SAA) as well as leukocytosis and thrombocytosis. In the interim period between attacks, acute phase reactants may return to normal or, in some cases, remain mildly elevated [22, 23].

TRAPS is an autosomal dominant disorder caused by missense mutations in the *TNFRSF1A* gene that is located on chromosome 12p13. The *TNFRSF1A* gene encodes the 55-kDa TNF receptor protein (also known as TNFR1, p55, CD120a) [22]. To date, there are more than 60 disease-associated mutations listed in the *Infevers* database and almost all of them are found in exons 2–4 that encode the first two cysteine rich domains (CRD1-CRD2) of the extracellular

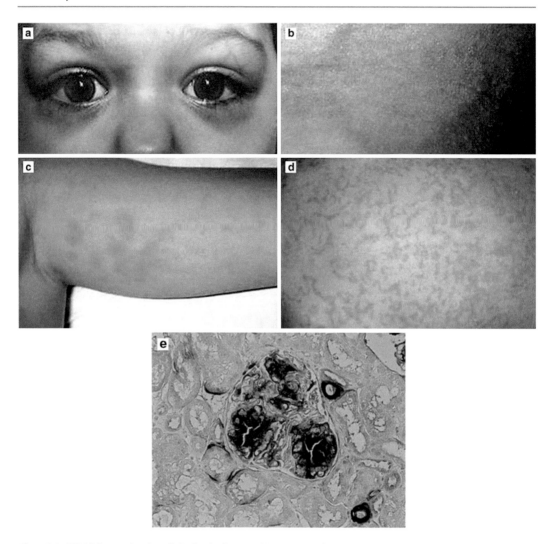

Fig. 3.3 TRAPS-associated clinical findings. (**a**) Periorbital edema in a young girl with a C52F mutation in *TNFRSF1A*. (**b**) An erythematous annular patch. (**c**) Erythematous patches. (**d**) Generalized erythematous patches and plaques. Renal biopsy of the patient in (**a**) showing amyloid deposits in the glomeruli. This patient underwent renal transplant secondary to TRAPS-related AA amyloidosis at the age of 13. (**a–d** reprinted with permission from Toro JR, Aksentijevich I, Hull K, Dean J, Kastner DL. Tumor necrosis factor receptor-associated periodic syndrome: a novel syndrome with cutaneous manifestations. Arch Dermatol. 2000;136:1487–1494. Copyright © (2000) American Medical Association. All rights reserved)

domain of TNFR1. Mutations associated with the most severe and penetrant disease phenotype and confer the highest risk to develop SAA amyloidosis affect cysteine residues that participate in the assembly of disulfide bonds important for TNFR1 folding [67]. Likewise, another common TRAPS-associated mutation, T50M, involves a highly conserved intra chain hydrogen bond critical for the folding of the extracellular domain of TNFR1. As a result of these structural changes induced by TRAPS mutations, the mutant receptor accumulates within the cell triggering innate immune responses and the production of various pro-inflammatory cytokines [69]. The wild type protein, made by the normal allele since TRAPS is caused by heterozygous mutations, is expressed on the cell surface and further amplifies the inflammatory loop. The real challenges in the diagnosis of TRAPS are patients who carry low-penetrance variants such as R92Q and

P46L. Although these variants were initially reported as associated with TRAPS, further studies have questioned their clinical significance. The allele frequency of R92Q is in the range from 1 to 10 % in Caucasians, while the P46L variant is found at a frequency of close to 20 % in African and African-American patients. Testing patients for TNFR1 mutations identify many of them to have these variants; however, the phenotype of these patients is not similar to TRAPS patients with structural mutations, and thus the clinical significance of these variants is still controversial [70, 71].

It is estimated that between 14 and 25 % of patients with TRAPS develop AA amyloidosis [66]. Patients who have cysteine mutations appear to have an increased risk (the probability of developing life-threatening amyloidosis is 24 % versus 2 % for noncysteine residue substitutions) above that of TRAPS in general although there are non-cysteine mutation TRAPS patients who have developed amyloidosis [71, 72]. The highest risk factor for SAA amyloidosis in TRAPS patients is a positive family history, thus patients who have members with AA amyloidosis should be followed closely for the development of proteinuria and aggressively treated to normalize acute phase reactants [44]. This study by Lane et al., reported that, in 9/12 patients with TRAPS, a family history for amyloidosis is a more significant risk factor for amyloidosis than actual genotype. Only 5/12 patients carried a cysteine mutation or T50M. This series also demonstrated that in patients with established AA amyloidosis without severe renal impairment at the time of diagnosis, effective treatment of the underlying disease can lead to a regression of amyloid deposits. The outcome of renal transplantation in these patients was good.

The treatment of TRAPS has proven challenging. Originally, as many of the symptoms were similar to FMF, patients were prescribed colchicine but had little or no response to the medication. Colchicine has also not been found to affect the development of amyloidosis in TRAPS [72]. Tapering courses of corticosteroids have been found to be effective at ameliorating symptoms and inflammation; however, as corticosteroids have many potential adverse effects, they should be reserved for patients who have infrequent disease flares [72].

Biologic therapies have been met with some success in TRAPS patients. The soluble p75 TNFR:Fc fusion protein, etanercept, has been introduced for treatment of TRAPS based on the observation of reduced levels of the soluble p55 protein in the serum of TRAPS patients and has been successful in reducing the severity and frequency of attacks in some patients [72, 73]. There have also been patients with AA amyloidosis who have had a favorable renal response to etanercept. Conversely, there have been multiple reports of patients responding negatively to infliximab and adalimumab with resultant paradoxical reactions [74, 75]. Therefore, of the anti-TNF alpha agents, only the use of etanercept is supported.

The use of the IL-1 receptor antagonist, anakinra, has been met with substantial success in patients with TRAPS and AA amyloidosis. Patients report a marked decrease in the severity of attacks as well as decreased frequency. Acute phase reactants also show a marked decrease and sometimes, complete normalization [76]. Regression of proteinuria has been seen in some amyloidosis patients with daily administration of anakinra [77].

Cryopyrin-Associated Periodic Fever Syndromes

Within the spectrum of autoinflammatory disorders exist three clinically distinct diseases that have mutations in the NLRP3 gene. NLRP3 is also known as CIAS1 (cold-induced autoinflammatory syndrome 1) or NALP3. The three diseases are: familial cold autoinflammatory syndrome (FCAS), Muckle–Wells syndrome (MWS) and neonatal onset multisystem inflammatory disease (NOMID) that is also known as chronic infantile neurologic cutaneous and articular (CINCA) syndrome.

Cryopyrin-associated periodic fever syndromes (CAPS)-disease associated mutations are inherited in an autosomal dominant fashion or as de novo mutations in patients with the most severe disease, NOMID. Initially, up to 40 % of patients with CAPS were reported as mutation-negative by standard sequencing. The majority of these patients have subsequently been found to carry somatic mosaic mutations in *NLRP3*. The estimates of the level of somatic mosaicism vary widely, ranging from as low as 4.2 % up to 35.8 %, and mutant myeloid cells are predominantly responsible for driving inflammation in mosaic patients [78].

NLRP3 encodes the cryopyrin/NLRP3 protein located on chromosome 1q44 [79]. Cryopyrin is a component of a multi-protein complex known as the NLRP3 inflammasome. The NLRP3 inflammasome acts as an intracellular sensor for various pathogen-associated molecular patterns (PAMPS) and danger-associated molecular patterns (DAMPS). The disease causing mutations lead to a constitutively activated inflammasome, causing an increase in caspase-1 activation and secretion of IL-1 and IL-18 (Fig. 3.4). CAPS-associated mutations are subtle missense nucleotide changes found almost exclusively in exon 3 that encodes the NACHT/NBS domain. Interestingly, mutations affecting the same or adjacent residues can cause very different phenotypes. To date there are 172 *NLRP3* gene variants published in *Infevers*; however, only about half of them are true disease-associated mutations. Although the majority of mutations are specific for one of the cryopyrinopathies, there are a number of mutations that have an associated overlap clinical phenotype particularly in the range of FCAS/MWS or MWS/NOMID. The clinical significance of variants such as V198M, Q703K, and R488K is still under discussion, because they are found at low allele frequencies in the general population or sometimes in unaffected patients.

Familial cold autoinflammatory syndrome is generally the least severe of the cryopyrinopathies. First described in 1940, clinical characteristics include recurrent episodes of urticarial rash, fever, conjunctivitis, and arthralgias that are triggered by exposure to cold temperatures and develop in infancy [80] (Fig. 3.5a). The episodes are brief and self-limited and typically begin 1–3 h after exposure with resolution occurring within 24 h [23]. There is a marked inflammatory response during episodes that may or may not persist after the episode resolves. AA amyloidosis rarely occurs in FCAS and, if it develops, it is typically in older patients [81].

First described in 1962, patients with Muckle–Wells syndrome have a clinical constellation of fevers, myalgias, arthralgias, urticarial-like rash, and progressive sensorineural hearing loss [82]. Ophthalmologic involvement manifests with conjunctivitis, episcleritis, or iridocyclitis [83]. Biopsies of the skin rash show a perivascular and interstitial infiltrate of neutrophils and lymphocytes in the papillary dermis [84] (Fig. 3.5b). Unlike FCAS, MWS attacks are not precipitated by cold exposure, and other precipitating factors are not well understood. Attacks are typically 24–48 h in duration but laboratory abnormalities may persist in quiescent times. This disease presents in childhood and may present during the first few days of life. AA amyloidosis is quite common in MWS, affecting up to one-third of the patients [22].

NOMID/CINCA is the most severe cryopyrinopathy. Patients commonly present immediately after birth and the disease almost universally presents in infancy. A non-pruritic, urticaria-like rash is typically present at birth. Other disease manifestations include short stature and a disabling arthritis that can result in a characteristic bony overgrowth pattern. Neurologic symptoms found in patients include: chronic aseptic meningitis, optic disc edema, cerebral atrophy, seizures, mental retardation, and headaches [85, 86]. Generally, patients have ongoing, continuous symptoms with exacerbated attacks and, historically, approximately 20 % of patients died prior to reaching adulthood [85]. There have been NOMID patients who develop AA amyloidosis as they get older although cases are not as frequent as those with MWS, possibly due to a shortened life span in these patients [85].

The discovery of IL-1 mediated inflammation in these patients was the foundation for a breakthrough in therapy targeting the IL-1 pathway. Prior to the development of the various IL-1 antagonist medications, the cryopyrinopathies were difficult to treat. Limited success was with

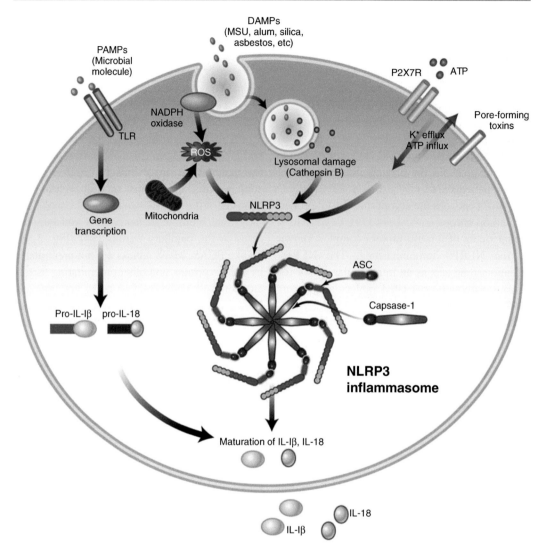

Fig. 3.4 NLRP3 inflammasome. The NLRP3 protein is an intracellular sensor for many pathogen-associated molecular patterns (PAMPs) and danger-associated molecular patterns (DAMPs). The NLRP3 inflammasome assembly is formed and activated by various signals including: reactive oxygen species (ROS), cathepsin B which is released from damaged lysosomes, or by pore formation in the plasma membrane that facilitates the influx of ATP and/or efflux of K+. As a result, activated caspase-1 units cleave the pro-IL1β (beta) and pro IL-18 cytokines into the mature cytokines IL-1β (beta) and IL-18. Subsequent release of IL-1β (beta) and IL-18 results in inflammation. Patients with cryopyrinopathies have gain-of-function mutations which cause constitutive activation of the NLRP3 inflammasome

administration of nonsteroidal anti-inflammatory drugs, colchicine, corticosteroids, and various DMARDs. However, that all changed with the targeting of the IL-1 pathway. Both the IL-1 receptor antagonist, anakinra, and the soluble IL-1 receptor decoy, rilonacept, have had remarkable success in treating the cryopyrinopathies. Often within hours of starting treatment, patients experience a dramatic improvement [87–90]. Laboratory response is also significant with normalization of the ESR, CRP, and SAA levels. The CAPS patients afflicted with AA amyloidosis have also had a positive response to IL-1 blockade with reported normalization of proteinuria and attenuation of renal disease [44, 91–93]. The long-acting, fully human IgG1 anti-Il-1β (beta)

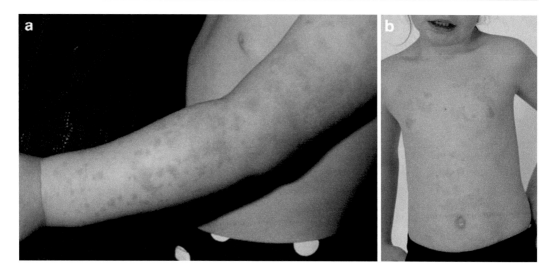

Fig. 3.5 *Left* (**a**) Characteristic cold-induced urticarial-like rash in a 1-year-old patient with FCAS. *Right* (**b**) Urticarial rash present in an 11-year-old girl with Muckle–Wells Syndrome

monoclonal antibody, canakinumab, has also provided sustained clinical remissions in patients [94, 95].

Hyper IgD Syndrome

Hyper IgD Syndrome (HIDS) is another autoinflammatory disease that presents in early childhood. Hyper IgD Syndrome is a mild disease in the spectrum of Mevalonate Kinase deficiencies (MKD). Patients present with chills, high fevers, abdominal pain, and lymphadenopathy. Other manifestations of disease include skin rash, arthralgias, diarrhea, and vomiting. Attacks are often provoked by stress and, during the first year of life, parents may report their child having prolonged fevers after immunizations (Fig. 3.6). HIDS attacks typically last approximately 4–6 days and can recur every 4–6 weeks. The attacks tend to decrease in severity and frequency as a patient ages [23]. Laboratory features include an acute phase response (elevated CRP and ESR) and markedly elevated IgD (and often IgA), although cases with normal IgD have been described. Inflammatory markers including SAA are high during attacks and may remain elevated in the intercurrent period. However, AA amyloidosis is rarely seen in this disease with very few

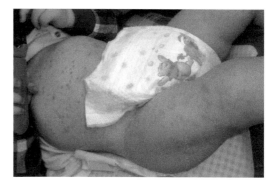

Fig. 3.6 Characteristic maculopapular rash in a 16-month-old boy with HIDS following immunizations

cases reported in the literature [22, 23, 96]. Of the four patients with amyloidosis and MKD, none of them were previously diagnosed as having HIDS and none of them had been previously treated. These patients received the molecular diagnosis of MKD after being diagnosed with amyloidosis [44].

HIDS is an autosomal-recessive disease that involves loss of function mutations in the *MVK* gene that encodes the mevalonate kinase enzyme (MK). Mevalonate kinase catalyzes an early step in the biosynthesis of cholesterol and non-sterol isoprenoids leading to a reduction in enzymatic activity. The result is an increase in mevalonic acid levels in urine and blood samples during active disease. Severe *MVK* mutations that completely abolish enzyme activity are identified in patients with mevalonic aciduria who present with recurrent fever, mental retardation, dysmorphic features, and developmental abnormalities [97]. HIDS-associated mutations are milder loss-of-function mutations that likely affect stability and/or folding of the MK protein rather than the catalytic properties of the enzyme. *Infevers* lists over 75 mutations resulting in the clinical phenotype.

The most frequently occurring *MVK* mutations are V377I and I268T with V377I accounting for up to 75 % of HIDS carrier chromosomes, and thus an initial diagnostic screen for HIDS should target these two mutations. It is unclear how exactly mevalonate kinase deficiency results in an autoinflammatory disease. Initial hypotheses suggested that accumulation of mevalonic acid was responsible for inflammation in HIDS patients, but more recent studies showed that the lack of isoprenoid products, small GTPase Rac1, could give rise to activated caspase-1 and hence excessive IL-1β (beta) secretion [98].

There have been a wide variety of medications used in HIDS patients to attempt to prevent and abort attacks. High dose corticosteroids used at the time of an attack reduces the severity and duration of attacks with over 50 % of patients responding at least partially to this medication. Colchicine has been ineffective in the treatment of HIDS attacks. Interestingly, a small study showed improvement with the use of simvastatin [99]. The use of biologic medications such as etanercept and anakinra at the onset of an attack has shown promising results. Although there are no randomized trials to support their use, small studies have shown partial to good responses to both medications [100–102].

Other Monogenic Autoinflammatory Diseases

There are other autoinflammatory diseases which have been well recognized based on characteristic clinical findings associated with genetic mutations but that have not been associated with AA amyloidosis. They include both dominantly and recessively inherited diseases (Table 3.1). These conditions are very rare so one cannot exclude the possibility of developing AA amyloidosis but, as of yet, no association has been made.

Polygenic and Complex Autoinflammatory Disease

What has become increasingly evident in the past decade is that diseases which were once thought to be purely "autoimmune" in nature have components of autoinflammatory disease as well. For instance, Behçet's disease has a strong association with HLA-B51, which would indicate a role of the adaptive immune system. Behçet's disease has been increasingly recognized as autoinflammatory as some of the clinical characteristics are similar to those seen in the monogenic autoinflammatory diseases. Likewise, uric acid has been shown to activate the NLRP3 inflammasome, which supports an autoinflammatory basis for gout. Monosodium urate (MSU) and calcium pyrophosphate dihydrate (CPPD) crystals cause an increase in caspase-1 activation and IL-1β (beta); IL-18 secretion in LPS stimulated mouse macrophages and conversely mice deficient for inflammasome components were defective in crystal-induced IL-1β (beta) secretion [103]. MSU crystal-recruited monocytes differentiate into proinflammatory M1-like macrophages in a peritoneal murine model of gout producing more IL-1 along with other cytokines and chemokines [104].

These findings provide a new concept that the innate immune system may play a critical role in the triggering of crystal-induced acute inflammation. Not surprisingly IL-1inhibitors appear to be beneficial in treatment of gout. Other conditions that have been considered polygenic autoinflammatory diseases include: SJIA, adult-onset Still's disease, periodic fever with aphthous stomatitis, pharyngitis, and adenitis (PFAPA) and recurrent idiopathic pericarditis.

Behçet's disease has been associated with AA amyloidosis with frequencies ranging from 0.01 to 4.8 % of patients [105]. A cumulative review done by Akpolat et al. in 2002 showed a male predominance in patients developing AA amyloidosis. AA amyloidosis patients commonly had vascular involvement. Interestingly, the study revealed that patients who developed AA amyloidosis tended to come from the Middle East and Mediterranean regions, which implicated genetic/environmental factors. AA amyloidosis has yet to be described in patients with PFAPA or idiopathic pericarditis.

Inflammatory Bowel Disease

Although seen less frequently than in the hereditary periodic fever syndromes, the risk of AA amyloidosis has been well established in patients with Crohn's disease. It is estimated that AA amyloidosis occurs in approximately 1 % of patients in the United States and up to 3 % in Northern European patients but that AA amyloidosis-induced complications are a major cause of mortality in Crohn's patients [106, 107]. Conversely, AA amyloidosis presenting in ulcerative colitis patients is extremely rare with estimated prevalence of 0.07 % [106, 107]. In general, the Crohn's disease patients have a long-standing history of aggressive, poorly controlled disease; however, there are reports of early onset amyloidosis as well as development of AA amyloidosis in patients with well-controlled inflammatory markers [106–108]. Other noted associations include patients with histories of suppurative complications like fistulas and abscesses as well as being of the male gender. There has not been an association of AA amyloidosis and extraintestinal manifestations of Crohn's [106, 107].

In the past decade, treatment of Crohn's related amyloidosis has primarily been with the chimeric anti-tumor necrosis factor alpha monoclonal antibody, infliximab. Infliximab has had positive results in the overall treatment of Crohn's disease with patients achieving clinical remission on the medication. Regarding the effectiveness of infliximab in the treatment of amyloidosis, there are a number of case reports documenting

attenuation of the amyloidotic effect with administration [109, 110]. In a study by Sattianayagam et al., 15/24 patients reached end-stage renal disease after a median time of 6.3 years from development of renal dysfunction. Six patients proceeded to renal transplantation and five grafts were functional at 0.8, 3.2, 4.2, 20.1, and 24.6 years after transplantation. One graft failed 14.5 years post-transplantation in a patient with sustained inflammation [111]. Although there are some case reports documenting improvement of renal function after surgical resection of diseased bowel, there has not been significant evidence to support this [112, 113].

The pathogenesis of inflammatory bowel disease (IBD) is poorly understood. Many studies have suggested an abnormal mucosal immune system, both innate and adaptive, as a contributing factor. Defective antigen presentation and altered immune response to antigens are just two of the many proposed mechanisms [114–116]. Failure of the immune system to function properly when exposed to pathogens can result in a prolonged inflammatory response with granuloma formation as the bacteria are unable to be cleared. The innate immune system also plays a potentially significant role in the development of IBD through the interaction of the toll-like receptors (TLRs). Gram-negative bacteria are a major component of the intestinal flora, and lipopolysaccharide (LPS) is the main antigen of gram-negative bacteria. LPS is the primary ligand for TLR4 which, when bound, acts along with the NOD2 (nucleotide-binding oligomerization domain) protein to induce a proinflammatory cytokine response through the nuclear factor kappa B (NF-κ(kappa)B) system [117]. Regarding genetics and the innate immune system, there has been a susceptibility gene to Crohn's disease known as *NOD2* or *CARD15* that encodes for the nucleotide-binding oligomerization domain protein 2 (NOD2). In particular, three variants (R702W, G908R, and 1007 fs) have been associated with susceptibility to Crohn's disease in multiple populations [118]. As previously mentioned, wild-type NOD2 activates

NF-κ(kappa)B and macrophages in response to bacterial LPS. Mutant forms of NOD2 show reduced response to stimulation with LPS, but this reduced response allows for reduced microbial clearance and attenuation of other inflammatory pathways [119].

Sarcoidosis and Sinus Histiocytosis with Massive Lymphadenopathy

Sarcoidosis is a multisystem disease of unknown etiology that results in non-caseating granulomatous deposition in affected organs. Considering that, prior to effective treatment, granulomatous infections such as tuberculosis and leprosy carried a high risk for developing AA amyloidosis, and biopsies from Crohn's disease patients often reveal granulomas, one might be led to infer that sarcoidosis patients would also be at increased risk for developing AA amyloidosis. This finding has not been substantiated as, in the literature, there are very few documented reports of AA amyloidosis in sarcoid [120, 121]. Interestingly, though, patients with active sarcoidosis have significantly elevated SAA levels when compared to controls [122]. When examining sarcoid patients further, it was observed that the levels of SAA were the highest in patients with active disease. Additionally, SAA1 isoforms were found in sarcoidosis patients but were absent in the control samples [123]. Sarcoid granulomas have been found to have increased expression of IL-1β (beta) which may partly attribute to this elevation in SAA [124].

Along a similar vein, sinus histiocytosis with massive lymphadenopathy (SHML) or Rosai–Dorfman disease, is a rare histiocytic proliferative disorder of unknown etiology. Patients typically have painless swelling of lymph nodes (most commonly cervical) and varying forms of extranodal involvement. Histiocytic cells have been found to synthesize IL-1, IL-6, and TNF-α (alpha) which can induce proliferation of SAA by the liver [125]. Interestingly, only one case of AA amyloidosis associated with SHML can be found in the literature [126].

AA Amyloidosis and Obesity

There is emerging evidence that obese people carry an increased risk for the development of AA amyloidosis. Studies have shown that in obese people, SAA is produced by adipocytes, resulting in chronically elevated levels of SAA [127, 128]. Adipocytes treated with SAA release inflammatory cytokines as well as having decreased secretion of adiponectin [129]. There is a report of a morbidly obese patient developing AA amyloidosis in the absence of any other known inflammatory condition. This report supports the theory that chronic production of SAA by adipocytes can contribute to the development of AA amyloidosis [130]. Further investigation is needed to provide additional evidence of this observation.

Summary

AA amyloidosis is a form of systemic amyloidosis that develops in patients with chronic inflammatory states. With effective treatments, infections that were once the leading cause of AA amyloidosis have become an infrequent cause in developed countries. Although rheumatic diseases such as rheumatoid arthritis, systemic juvenile arthritis, and ankylosing spondylitis are still the primary underlying conditions predisposing patients to the development of AA amyloidosis, marked advancements in treatments for these conditions over the past 20 years have resulted in a declining number of new cases. The monogenic autoinflammatory diseases, or hereditary periodic fever syndromes, have become well-recognized contributors to the conditions predisposing patients to developing AA amyloidosis. Unique to familial Mediterranean fever, the use of colchicine has been shown to be an effective treatment for the inflammatory disease and, additionally, helps to reduce a patient's risk of developing amyloidosis. As is the case with rheumatic diseases, new biologic medications that suppress the inflammatory immune response are being used to treat autoinflammatory conditions. As AA amyloidosis generally develops in patients after years of unopposed inflammation, it should not go unmentioned that very young patients with SJIA, FMF, and TRAPS can develop this complication early in life. There should be a low threshold for AA amyloid evaluation in these patients if new-onset proteinuria is observed on a routine urinalysis.

In patients diagnosed with AA amyloidosis, biologic medications such as antitumor necrosis factor medications, IL-1 inhibitors, and IL-6 inhibitors are being used to try and reduce the inflammatory state. There is also an international trial currently being conducted using the molecule eprodisate disodium in patients with AA amyloidosis. By binding the amyloidogenic precursor proteins, eprodisate disodium attempts to prevent the deposition of amyloid in organs, hence preserving renal function.

The understanding of the pathogenesis of AA amyloidosis and the conditions that predispose patients to its development continues to expand. However, there are still 6 % of cases that occur "sporadically," which enforces the need for us to continue pursuing new genetic diagnoses of conditions which have been previously unrecognized/uncharacterized.

References

1. Rocken C, Shakespeare A. Pathology, diagnosis and pathogenesis of AA amyloidosis. Virchows Arch. 2002;440(2):111–22.
2. Lachmann HJ, Goodman HJB, Gilbertson AJ, et al. Natural history and outcome in systemic AA amyloidosis. N Engl J Med. 2007;356:2361–71.
3. Connolly JO, Gillmore JD, Lachmann HJ, Davenport A, Hawkins PN, Woolfson RG. Renal amyloidosis in intravenous drug users. Q J Med. 2006;99:737–42.
4. Akcay S, Akman B, Ozdemir H, Eyuboglu FO, Karacan O, Ozdemir N. Bronchiectasis-related amyloidosis as a cause of chronic renal failure. Ren Fail. 2002;24(6):815–23.
5. Picken M. New insights into systemic amyloidosis: the importance of diagnosis of specific type. Curr Opin Nephrol Hypertens. 2007;16:196–203.
6. Uhlar CM, Whitehead AS. Serum amyloid A, the major vertebrate acute-phase reactant. Eur J Biochem. 1999;265:501–23.
7. Xu L, Badolato R, Murphy WJ, et al. A novel biologic function of serum amyloid A. Induction of T lymphocyte migration and adhesion. J Immunol. 1995;155:1184–90.
8. Stevens FJ. Hypothetical structure of human serum amyloid A protein. Amyloid. 2004;11:71–80.
9. Van der Hilst JCH. Recent insights into the pathogenesis of type AA amyloidosis. ScientificWorldJournal. 2011;11:641–50.
10. Gertz MA, Kyle RA. Secondary systemic amyloidosis: response and survival in 64 patients. Medicine (Baltimore). 1991;70:246–56.
11. Booth DR, Booth SE, Gillmore JD, Hawkins PN, Pepys MB. SAA₁ alleles as risk factors in reactive systemic AA amyloidosis. Amyloid. 1998;5:262–5.
12. Baba S, Masago SA, Takahashi T, et al. A novel allelic variant of serum amyloid A, SAA1 gamma: genomic evidence, evolution, frequency, and implication as a risk factor for reactive systemic AA amyloidosis. Hum Mol Genet. 1995;4:1083–7.
13. Dhillon V, Woo P, Isenberg D. Amyloidosis in the rheumatic disease. Ann Rheum Dis. 1989;48:696–701.
14. Immonen K, Finne P, Gronhagen-Riska C, et al. A marked decline in the incidence of renal replacement therapy for amyloidosis associated with inflammatory rheumatic diseases—data from nationwide registries in Finland. Amyloid. 2011;18:25–8.
15. David J, Vouyiouka O, Ansell BM, Hall A, Woo P. Amyloidosis in chronic juvenile arthritis: a morbidity and mortality study. Clin Exp Rheum. 1993;11:85–90.
16. Filipowicz-Sosnowska AM, Roztropowicz-Denisiewicz K, Rosenthal CJ, Baum J. The amyloidosis of juvenile rheumatoid arthritis—comparative studies in Polish and American children. Arthritis Rheum. 1978;21(6):699–703.
17. David J, Woo P. Reactive amyloidosis. Arch Dis Child. 1992;67(3):258–61.
18. Immonen K, Savolainen A, Kautiainen H, Hakala M. Longterm outcome of amyloidosis associated with juvenile idiopathic arthritis. J Rheumatol. 2008;35:907–12.
19. Singh G, Kumari N, Aggarwal A, Krishnani N, Misra R. Prevalence of subclinical amyloidosis in ankylosing spondylitis. J Rheumatol. 2007;34:371–3.
20. Gratacos J, Orellana C, Sanmarti R, et al. Secondary amyloidosis in ankylosing spondylitis. A systematic survey of 137 patients using abdominal fat aspiration. J Rheumatol. 1997;24:912–5.
21. Lehtinen K. Mortality and causes of death in 398 patients admitted to hospital with ankylosing spondylitis. Ann Rheum Dis. 1993;52:174–6.
22. Kastner DL, Aksentijevich I. Intermittent and periodic arthritis syndromes. In: Koopman WJ, Moreland LW, editors. Arthritis and allied conditions: a textbook of rheumatology. 15th ed. Philadelphia, PA: Lippincott Williams & Wilkins; 2005. p. 1411–61.
23. Barron K, Athreya B, Kastner D. Periodic fever syndrome and other inherited autoinflammatory diseases. In: Cassidy JT, Petty RE, Laxer RM, Lindsley CB, editors. Textbook of pediatric rheumatology.

6th ed. Philadelphia, PA: Saunders Elsevier; 2011. p. 642–60.

24. Masters SL, Simon A, Aksentijevich I, Kastner DL. Horror autoinflammaticus: the molecular pathophysiology of autoinflammatory disease. Annu Rev Immunol. 2009;27:621–68.

25. Boisson B, Laplantine E, Prando C, et al. Immunodeficiency, autoinflammation and amylopectinosis in humans with inherited HOIL-1 and LUBAC deficiency. Nat Immunol. 2012;13:1178–86.

26. Ozen S, Bakkaloglu A, Yilmaz E, et al. Mutations in the gene for familial Mediterranean fever: do they predispose to inflammation? J Rheumatol. 2003;30(9):2014–8.

27. Barzilai A, Langevitz P, Goldberg I, et al. Erysipelas-like erythema of familial Mediterranean fever: clinicopathologic correlation. J Am Acad Dermatol. 2000;42:791–5.

28. Chae JJ, Komarow HD, Cheng J, et al. Targeted disruption of pyrin, the FMF protein, causes heightened sensitivity to endotoxin and a defect in macrophage apoptosis. Mol Cell. 2003;11:591–604.

29. Masumoto J, Dowds TA, Schaner P, et al. ASC is an activating adaptor for NF-κ(kappa)B and caspase-8 dependent apoptosis. Biochem Biophys Res Commun. 2003;303:69–73.

30. Stehlik C, Fiorentino L, Dorfleutner A, et al. The PAAD/PYRIN family protein ASC is a dual regulator of a conserved step in nuclear factor κ(kappa)B activation pathways. J Exp Med. 2002;196:1605–15.

31. Touitou I, Lesage S, McDermott M, et al. Infevers: an evolving mutation database for auto-inflammatory syndromes. Hum Mutat. 2004;24:194–8.

32. Marek-Yagel D, Berkun Y, Padeh S, et al. Clinical disease among patients heterozygous for familial Mediterranean fever. Arthritis Rheum. 2009;60: 1862–6.

33. Booty MG, Chae JJ, Masters SL, et al. Familial Mediterranean fever with a single MEFV mutation. Where is the second hit? Arthritis Rheum. 2009;60:1851–61.

34. Aldea A, Campistol JM, Arostegui JI, et al. A severe autosomal-dominant periodic inflammatory disorder with renal AA amyloidosis and colchicine resistance associated to the MEFV H478Y variant in a Spanish kindred: an unusual familial Mediterranean fever phenotype or another MEFV-associated periodic inflammatory disorder? Am J Med Genet A. 2004;124A(1):67–73.

35. Stoffels M, Szperl A, Simon A, et al. MEFV mutations affecting pyrin amino acid 577 cause autosomal dominant autoinflammatory disease. Ann Rheum Dis. 2014;73(2):455–61.

36. Chae JJ, Cho YH, Lee GS, et al. Gain of function pyrin mutations induce NLRP3 protein-independent interleukin-1β (beta) activation and severe autoinflammation in mice. Immunity. 2011;34(5):755–68.

37. Lachmann HJ, Sengul B, Yavuzsen TU, et al. Clinical and subclinical inflammation in patients with familial Mediterranean fever and in heterozygous carriers of MEFV mutations. Rheumatology. 2006;45:745–50.

38. Touitou I, Sarkisian T, Medlej-Hashim M, et al. Country as the primary risk factor for renal amyloidosis in familial Mediterranean fever. Arthritis Rheum. 2007;56:1706–12.

39. Schwabe AD, Peters RS. Familial Mediterranean fever in Armenians. Analysis of 100 cases. Medicine. 1974;53:453–62.

40. Kasifoglu T, Bilge SY, Sari I, et al. Amyloidosis and its related factors in Turkish patients with familial Mediterranean fever: a multicenter study. Rheumatology. 2014;53(4):741–5.

41. Akse-Onal V, Sag E, Ozen S, et al. Decrease in the rate of secondary amyloidosis in Turkish children with FMF: are we doing better? Eur J Pediatr. 2010;169:971–4.

42. Livneh A, Langevitz P, Shinar Y, et al. MEFV mutation analysis in patients suffering from amyloidosis of familial Mediterranean fever. Amyloid. 1999;6:1–6.

43. Akpolat T, Ozkaya O, Ozen S. Homozygous M694V as a risk factor for amyloidosis in Turkish FMF patients. Gene. 2012;492(1):285–89.

44. Lane T, Loeffler JM, Rowczenio DM, et al. AA amyloidosis complicating the hereditary periodic fever syndromes. Arthritis Rheum. 2013;65(4):1116–21.

45. Topaloglu R, Ozaltin F, Yilmaz E, et al. E148Q is a disease-causing MEFV mutation: a phenotypic evaluation in patients with familial Mediterranean fever. Ann Rheum Dis. 2005;64:750–2.

46. Gershoni-Baruch R, Brik R, Shinawi M, Livneh A. The differential contribution of MEFV mutant alleles to the clinical profile of familial Mediterranean fever. Eur J Hum Genet. 2002;10(2):145–9.

47. Sohar E, Gafni J, Pras M, Heller H. Familial Mediterranean fever a survey of 470 cases and review of the literature. Am J Med. 1967;43(2):227–53.

48. Kutlay S, Yilmaz E, Koytak ES, et al. A case of familial Mediterranean fever with amyloidosis as the first manifestation. Am J Kidney Dis. 2001;38(6), E34.

49. Balci B, Tinaztepe K, Yilmaz E, et al. MEFV gene mutations in familial Mediterranean fever phenotype II patients with renal amyloidosis in childhood: a retrospective clinicopathological and molecular study. Nephrol Dial Transplant. 2002;17:1921–3.

50. Turkcapar N, Tuncah T, Kutlay S, et al. The contribution of genotypes at the MICA gene triplet repeat polymorphisms and MEFV mutations to amyloidosis and course of the disease in the patients with familial Mediterranean fever. Rheumatol Int. 2007;27: 545–51.

51. Touitou I, Picot MC, Domingo C, et al. The MICA region determines the first modifier locus in familial Mediterranean fever. Arthritis Rheum. 2001;44(1):163–9.

52. Medlej-Hashim M, Delague V, Chouery E, et al. Amyloidosis in familial Mediterranean fever

patients: correlation with *MEFV* genotype and *SAA1* and *MICA* polymorphisms effects. BMC Med Genet. 2004;5:4.

53. Goldfinger SE. Colchicine for familial Mediterranean fever. N Engl J Med. 1972;287(25):1302.

54. Zemer D, Revach M, Pras M, et al. A controlled trial of colchicine in preventing attacks of familial Mediterranean fever. N Engl J Med. 1974;291(18):932–4.

55. Duzova A, Bakkaloglu A, Besbas N, et al. Role of A-SAA in monitoring subclinical inflammation and in colchicine dosage in familial Mediterranean fever. Clin Exp Rheumatol. 2003;21(4):509–14.

56. Zemer D, Pras M, Sohar E, Modan M, Cabili S, Gafni J. Colchicine in the prevention and treatment of the amyloidosis of familial Mediterranean fever. N Engl J Med. 1986;314(16):1001–5.

57. Livneh A, Zemer D, Langevitz P, Laor A, Sohar E, Pras M. Colchicine treatment of AA amyloidosis of familial Mediterranean fever. Arthritis Rheum. 1994;37(12):1804–11.

58. Sevoyan MK, Sarkisian TF, Beglaryan AA, Shahsuvaryan G, Armenian H. Prevention of amyloidosis in familial Mediterranean fever with colchicine: a case-control study in Armenia. Med Princ Pract. 2009;18:441–6.

59. Meinzer U, Quartier P, Alexandra JF, Hentgen V, Retornaz F, Kone-Paut I. Interleukin-1 targeting drugs in familial Mediterranean fever: a case series and a review of the literature. Semin Arthritis Rheum. 2011;41(2):265–71.

60. Chae JJ, Wood G, Masters SL, et al. The B30.2 domain of pyrin, the familial Mediterranean fever protein, interacts directly with caspase-1 to modulate IL-1β (beta) production. Proc Natl Acad Sci USA. 2006;103(26):9982–7.

61. Stankovic Stojanovic K, Delmas Y, Torres PU, et al. Dramatic beneficial effect of interleukin-1 inhibitor treatment in patients with familial Mediterranean fever complicated with amyloidosis and renal failure. Nephrol Dial Transplant. 2012;27(5):1898–901.

62. Abedi AS, Nakhjavani JM, Etemadi J. Long-term outcome of renal transplantation in patients with familial Mediterranean fever amyloidosis: a single-center experience. Tranplant Proc. 2013;45(10):3502–4.

63. Blum A, Sohar E. The diagnosis of amyloidosis. Ancillary procedures. Lancet. 1962;1:721–4.

64. Sungur C, Sungur R, Ruacan S, et al. Diagnostic value of bone marrow biopsy in patients with renal disease secondary to familial Mediterranean fever. Kidney Int. 1993;44:834–6.

65. Ozdemir BH, Ozdemir OG, Ozdemir FN, Ozdemir AI. Value of testis biopsy in the diagnosis of systemic amyloidosis. Urology. 2002;59(2):201–5.

66. Williamson LM, Hull D, Mehta R, Reeves WG, Robinson BH, Toghill PJ. Familial Hibernian fever. Q J Med. 1982;51(204):469–80.

67. McDermott MF, Aksentijevich I, Galon J, et al. Germline mutations in the extracellular domains of the 55 kDa TNF receptor, TNFR1, define a family of dominantly inherited autoinflammatory syndromes. Cell. 1999;97(1):133–44.

68. Toro JR, Aksentijevich I, Hull K, Dean J, Kastner DL. Tumor necrosis factor receptor associated periodic syndrome: a novel syndrome with cutaneous manifestations. Arch Dermatol. 2000;136:1487–94.

69. Simon A, Park H, Maddipati R, et al. Concerted action of wild-type and mutant TNF receptors enhances inflammation in TNF receptor 1-associated periodic fever syndrome. Proc Natl Acad Sci USA. 2010;107(21):9801–6.

70. Pelagatti MA, Meini A, Caorsi R, et al. Long-term clinical profile of children with the low-penetrance R92Q mutation of the *TNFRSF1A* gene. Arthritis Rheum. 2011;63(4):1141–50.

71. Aksentijevich I, Galon J, Soares M, et al. The tumor-necrosis-factor receptor-associated periodic syndrome: new mutations in *TNFRSF1A*, ancestral origins, genotype-phenotype studies, and evidence for further genetic heterogeneity of periodic fevers. Am J Hum Genet. 2001;69:301–14.

72. Hull KM, Drewe E, Aksentijevich I, et al. The TNF receptor-associated periodic syndrome (TRAPS): emerging concepts of an autoinflammatory disorder. Medicine (Baltimore). 2002;81(5):349–68.

73. Drewe E, McDermott EM, Powell PT, Isaacs JD, Powell RJ. Prospective study of anti-tumour necrosis factor receptor superfamily 1B fusion protein, and case study of anti-tumour necrosis factor receptor superfamily 1A fusion protein, in tumour necrosis factor associated periodic syndrome (TRAPS): clinical and laboratory findings in a series of seven patients. Rheumatology. 2003;42:235–9.

74. Drewe E, Powell RJ, McDermott EM. Comment on: failure of anti-TNF therapy in TNF receptor 1-associated periodic syndrome (TRAPS). Rheumatology (Oxford). 2007;46:1865–6.

75. Jacobelli S, Andre M, Alexandra JF, Dode C, Papo T. Failure of anti-TNF therapy in TNF receptor 1-associated periodic syndrome (TRAPS). Rheumatology (Oxford). 2007;46:1211–2.

76. Gattorno M, Pelagatti MA, Meini A, et al. Persistent efficacy of anakinra in patients with tumor necrosis factor receptor-associated periodic syndrome. Arthritis Rheum. 2008;58(5):1516–20.

77. Obici L, Meini A, Cattlini M, et al. Favourable and sustained response to anakinra in tumour necrosis factor receptor-associate periodic syndrome (TRAPS) with or without AA amyloidosis. Ann Rheum Dis. 2011;70(8):1511–2.

78. Tanaka N, Izawa K, Saito MK, et al. High incidence of NLRP3 somatic mosaicism in patients with chronic infantile neurologic, cutaneous, articular syndrome: results of an international multicenter collaborative study. Arthritis Rheum. 2011;63(11):3625–32.

79. Hoffmann HM, Mueller JL, Broide DH, Wanderer AA, Kolodner RD. Mutation of a new gene encoding a putative pyrin-like protein causes familial cold autoinflammatory syndrome and Muckle-Wells syndrome. Nat Genet. 2001;29:301–5.

80. Kile RM, Rusk HA. A case of cold urticarial with an unusual family history. JAMA. 1940;114:1067–8.

81. Hoffman HM, Wanderer AA, Broide DH. Familial cold autoinflammatory syndrome: phenotype and genotype of an autosomal dominant periodic fever. J Allergy Clin Immunol. 2001;108:615–20.

82. Muckle TJ, Wells M. Urticaria, deafness, and amyloidosis: a new heredo-fammilial syndrome. Q J Med. 1962;31:235–48.

83. Neven B, Peieur AM, Quartier dit Maire P. Cryopyrinopathies: update on pathogenesis and treatment. Nature. 2008;4(9):481–9.

84. Lieberman A, Grossman ME, Silvers DN. Muckle-Wells syndrome: case report and review of cutaneous pathology. J Am Acad Dermatol. 1998;39:290–1.

85. Prieur AM, Griscelli C, Lampert F, et al. A chronic, infantile, neurological, cutaneous and articular (CINCA) syndrome. A specific entity analysed in 30 patients. Scand J Rheumatol. 1987;66:57–68.

86. Hashkes PJ, Lovell DJ. Recognition of infantile-onset multisystem inflammatory disease as a unique entity. J Pediatr. 1997;130(4):513–5.

87. Hoffman HM, Throne ML, Amar NJ, et al. Efficacy and safety of rilonacept (interleukin-1 trap) in patients with cryopyrin-associated periodic syndromes results from two sequential placebo-controlled studies. Arthritis Rheum. 2008;58(8):2443–52.

88. Kuemmerle-Deschner JB, Tyrrell PN, Koetter I, et al. Efficacy and safety of anakinra therapy in pediatric and adult patients with the autoinflammatory Muckle-Wells syndrome. Arthritis Rheum. 2011;63(3):840–9.

89. Goldbach-Mansky R, Daily NJ, Canna SW, et al. Neonatal-onset multisystem inflammatory disease responsive to interleukin-1 beta inhibition. N Engl J Med. 2006;355:581–92.

90. Goldbach-Mansky R, Shroff SD, Wilson M, et al. A pilot study to evaluate the safety and efficacy of the long-acting interleukin-1 inhibitor rilonacept (interleukin-1 trap) in patients with familial cold autoinflammatory syndrome. Arthritis Rheum. 2008;58:2432–342.

91. Thornton BD, Hoffman HM, Bhat A, Don BR. Successful treatment of renal amyloidosis due to familial cold autoinflammatory syndrome using and interleukin 1 receptor antagonist. Am J Kidney Dis. 2007;49(3):477–81.

92. Neven B, Marvillet I, Terrada C, et al. Long-term efficacy of the interleukin-1 receptor antagonist anakinra in ten patients with neonatal-onset multisystem inflammatory disease/chronic infantile neurologic, cutaneous, articular syndrome. Arthritis Rheum. 2010;62(1):258–67.

93. Leslie KS, Lachmann HJ, Bruning E, et al. Phenotype, genotype, and sustained response to anakinra in 22 patients with autoinflammatory disease associated with *CIAS-1/NALP3* mutations. Arch Dermatol. 2006;142:1591–7.

94. Kuemmerle-Deschner JB, Ramos E, Blank N, et al. Canakinumab (ACZ885, a fully human IgG1 anti-IL-1β (beta) mAb) induces sustained remission in pediatric patients with cryopyrin-associated periodic syndrome (CAPS). Arthritis Res Ther. 2011; 13(1):R34.

95. Lachmann HJ, Kone-Paut I, Kuemmerle-Deschner JB, et al. Use of canakinumab in the cryopyrin-associated periodic syndrome. N Engl J Med. 2009;360:2416–25.

96. Van der Hilst JCH, Drenth JPH, Bodar EJ, et al. Serum amyloid A serum concentrations and genotype do not explain low incidence of amyloidosis in hyper-IgD syndrome. Amyloid. 2005;12(2):115–9.

97. Haas D, Hoffman GF. Mevalonate kinase deficiencies: from mevalonic aciduria to hyperimmunoglobulinemia D syndrome. Orphanet J Rare Dis. 2006;1:13.

98. Normand S, Massonnet B, Delwail A, et al. Specific increase in caspase-1 activity and secretion of IL-1 family cytokines: a putative link between mevalonate kinase deficiency and inflammation. Eur Cytokine Netw. 2009;20:101–7.

99. Simon A, Drewe E, van der Meer JWM, et al. Simvastatin treatment for inflammatory attacks of the hyperimmunoglobulinemia D and periodic fever syndrome. Clin Pharmacol Ther. 2004;75:476–83.

100. van der Hilst JCH, Bodar EJ, Barron KS, et al. Long-term follow-up, clinical features, and quality of life in a series of 103 patients with hyperimmunoglobulinemia D syndrome. Medicine. 2008;87(6): 301–10.

101. Takada K, Aksentijevich I, Mahadevan V, Dean JA, Kelley RI, Kastner DL. Favorable preliminary experience with etanercept in two patients with the hyperimmunoglobulinemia D and periodic fever syndrome. Arthritis Rheum. 2003;48(9):2645–51.

102. Bodar EJ, van der Hilst JCH, Drenth JPH, van der Meer JWM, Simon A. Effect of etanercept and anakinra on inflammatory attacks in the hyper-IgD syndrome: introducing a vaccination provocation model. Neth J Med. 2005;63(7):260–4.

103. Martinon F, Petrilli V, Mayor A, Tardivel A, Tschopp J. Gout-associated uric acid crystals activate the NALP3 inflammasome. Nature. 2006;440:237–41.

104. Martin WJ, Shaw O, Liu X, Steiger S, Harper JL. Monosodium urate monohydrate crystal-recruited noninflammatory monocytes differentiate in M1-like proinflammatory macrophages in a peritoneal murine model of gout. Arthritis Rheum. 2011;63(5):1322–32.

105. Akpolat T, Akkoyunlu M, Akpolat I, Dilek M, Odabas AR, Ozen S. Renal Behçet's disease: a cumulative analysis. Semin Arthritis Rheum. 2002;31(5):317–37.

106. Greenstein AJ, Sachar DB, Nannan Pandy AK, et al. Amyloidosis and inflammatory bowel disease. A 50 year experience with 25 patients. Medicine. 1992;71(5):261–70.

107. Wester AL, Vatn MH, Fausa O. Secondary amyloidosis in inflammatory bowel disease: a study of 18 patients admitted to Rikshospitalet University Hospital, Oslo, from 1962-1998. Inflamm Bowel Dis. 2001;7(4):295–300.

108. Basturk T, Ozagari A, Ozturk T, Kusaslan R, Unsal A. Crohn's disease and secondary amyloidosis: early complication? A case report and review of the literature. J Ren Care. 2009;35(3):147–50.

109. Fidalgo C, Calado J, Cravo M. Secondary amyloidosis in a patient with long duration Crohn's disease treated with infliximab. BioDrugs. 2010;24(Supp 1):15–7.

110. Iizuka M, Sagara S, Etou T. Efficacy of scheduled infliximab maintenance therapy on systemic amyloidosis associated with Crohn's disease. Inflamm Bowel Dis. 2011;17(7):E67–8.

111. Sattianayagam PT, Gillmore JD, Pinney JH, et al. Inflammatory bowel disease and systemic AA amyloidosis. Dig Dis Sci. 2013;58(6):1689–97.

112. Fitchen JH. Amyloidosis and granulomatous ileocolitis. Regression after surgical removal of the involved bowel. N Engl J Med. 1975;292(7):352–3.

113. Manelstam P, Simmons DE, Mitchell B. Regression of amyloid in Crohn's disease after bowel resection. A 19-year follow-up. J Clin Gastroenterol. 1989;11(3):324–6.

114. Bene L, Falus A, Baffy N, Fulop AK. Cellular and molecular mechanisms in the two major forms of inflammatory bowel disease. Pathol Oncol Res. 2011;17(3):463–72.

115. Niess JH. Role of mucosal dendritic cells in inflammatory bowel disease. World J Gastroenterol. 2008;14:5138–48.

116. Kraus TA, Toy L, Chan L, et al. Failure to induce oral tolerance in Crohn's disease and ulcerative colitis patients: possible genetic risk. Ann NY Acad Sci. 2004;1029:225–38.

117. Cario E, Rosenberg IM, Brandwein SL, Beck PL, Reinecker HC, Podolsky DK. Lipopolysaccharide activates distinct signaling pathways in intestinal epithelial cell lines expressing toll-like receptors. J Immunol. 2000;164:966–72.

118. Adler J, Rangwalla SC, Dwamena BA, Higgins PDR. The prognostic power of the NOD2 genotype for complicated Crohn's disease: a meta-analysis. Am J Gastroenterol. 2011;106:699–712.

119. Maeda S, Hsu LC, Liu H, et al. Nod2 mutation in Crohn's disease potentiates NF-κ (kappa) B activity and IL-1β (beta) processing. Science. 2005;300: 1584–7.

120. Rainfray M, Meyrier A, Valeyre D, Tazi A, Battesti JP. Renal amyloidosis complicating sarcoidosis. Thorax. 1998;43:422–3.

121. Komatsuda A, Wakui H, Ohtani H, et al. Amyloid A-type renal amyloidosis in a patient with sarcoidosis: report of a case and review of the literature. Clin Nephrol. 2003;60(4):284–8.

122. Rothkrantz-kos S, van Dieijen-Visser MP, Mulder PGH, Drent M. Potential usefulness of inflammatory markers to monitor respiratory functional impairment in sarcoidosis. Clin Chem. 2003;49(9): 1510–7.

123. Bargagli E, Magi B, Olivieri C, Bianchi N, Landi C, Rottoli P. Analysis of serum amyloid A in sarcoidosis patients. Respir Med. 2011;105:775–80.

124. Devergne O, Emilie D, Peuchmaur M, Crevon MC, D'Agay MF, Galanaud P. Production of cytokines in sarcoid lymph nodes: preferential expression of interleukin-1 beta and interferon-gamma genes. Hum Pathol. 1992;23(3):317–23.

125. Foss HD, Herbst H, Araujo I, et al. Monokine expression in Langerhans' cell histiocytosis and sinus histiocytosis with massive lymphadenopathy (Rosai-Dorfman disease). J Pathol. 1996; 179:60–5.

126. Rocken C, Wieker K, Grote HJ, Muller G, Franke A, Roessner A. Rosai-Dorfman disease and generalized AA amyloidosis: a case report. Hum Pathol. 2000;31:621–4.

127. Poitou C, Viguerie N, Cancello R, et al. Serum amyloid A: production by human white adipocyten and regulation by obesity and nutrition. Diabetologia. 2005;48:519–28.

128. Upragarin N, Landman WJ, Gaastra W, Gruys E. Extrahepatic production of acute phase serum amyloid A. Histol Histopathol. 2005;20:1295–307.

129. Faty A, Ferre P, Commans S. The acute phase protein serum amyloid A induces lipolysis and inflammation in human adipocytes through distinct pathways. PLoS One. 2012;7(4):e34031.

130. Alsina E, Martin M, Panadés M, Fernández E. Renal AA amyloidosis secondary to morbid obesity? Clin Nephrol. 2009;72(4):312–4.

Leukocyte Cell-Derived Chemotaxin 2 Amyloidosis (ALECT2)

4

Oana Madalina Mereuta, Chris P. Larsen, and Ahmet Dogan

Introduction

Amyloidosis caused by deposition of leukocyte cell-derived chemotaxin 2 (ALECT2) has been recently described [1] and has emerged as a frequent form of systemic amyloidosis in the USA, with predominant involvement of kidney and liver [1–5]. The disease has a strong ethnic bias with up to 92 % of ALECT2 patients reported in the literature being Hispanic subjects (particularly Mexican) [2–7]. Aside from Hispanics, Punjabis, First Nations people in British Columbia, and Native Americans appear to be more frequently affected by ALECT2 amyloidosis than Caucasians [8]. There are a

O.M. Mereuta, MD, PhD
Department of Pathology, Memorial Sloan Kettering Cancer Center, 1275 York Avenue, New York, NY 10065, USA
e-mail: mereutao@mskcc.org

C.P. Larsen, MD
Nephropath, 10810 Executive Center Drive, Little Rock, AR 72211, USA
e-mail: chris.larsen@nephropath.com

A. Dogan, MD, PhD (✉)
Departments of Pathology and Laboratory Medicine, Memorial Sloan Kettering Cancer Center, 1275 York Avenue, New York, NY 10065, USA
e-mail: dogana@mskcc.org

number of reasons such a common type systemic amyloidosis has only recently been described. These include relatively restricted geographical and ethnic distribution, relatively indolent clinical course with only late stage end-organ damage and lack of analytical tools that could determine the amyloid type accurately. Introduction of laser microdissection (LMD) and nano-flow liquid chromatography/tandem mass spectrometry (MS)-based proteomic analysis (LMD/MS) for classification of amyloidosis has been important in determining true incidence of ALECT2 amyloidosis as LMD/MS can identify the amyloid-type in an unbiased version and does not require type-specific reagents used by immunoassays [2, 9].

Based on two retrospective analysis of kidney biopsy specimens containing amyloid proteins, ALECT2 was the most common type after immunoglobulin light chain, AL-type (so-called primary amyloidosis) and AA amyloidosis (so-called secondary amyloidosis), with a frequency of up to 0.2 % in the total kidney biopsies and up to 10 % in the renal amyloid samples [3, 4]. The restricted geographic distribution is clearly evident in that ALECT2 is the most common type of amyloidosis diagnosed in the Southwest portion of the United States, being even more common than AL amyloidosis [4]. Outside the kidney, LECT2 amyloid deposits have been noted in liver, spleen, adrenal, and colon specimens (Figs. 4.1 and 4.2) but frequently do not appear to cause functional organ damage at these sites [2, 5]. ALECT2 has been officially recognized as a unique type of amyloidosis by International Society of Amyloidosis [10].

Overview of LECT2 Biology and ALECT2 Pathogenesis

First described in studies searching for proteins with leukocyte chemotactic activity [11], LECT2 protein was well characterized before its discovery as an amyloid fibril precursor. It was also shown to

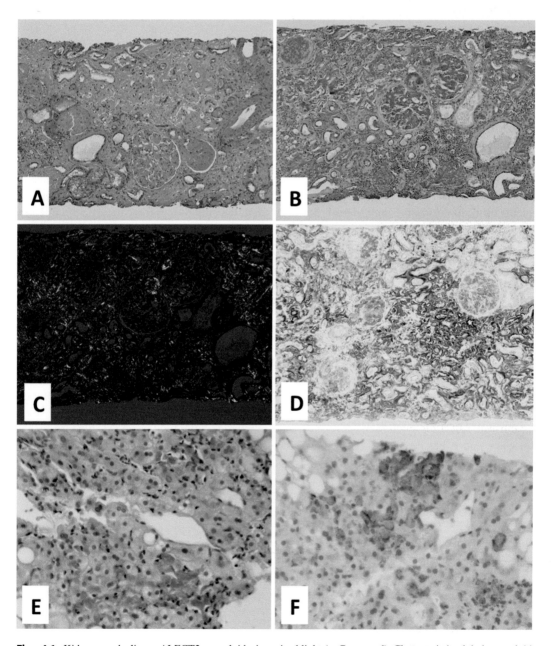

Fig. 4.1 Kidney and liver ALECT2 amyloidosis. Eosinophilic amyloid deposits in the kidney with glomerular, interstitial, and vascular involvement (**a**, H&E) stain with Congo red (**b**). Congo red stain viewed under polar-ized light (**c**, Congo red). Characteristic globular amyloid deposition in the liver (**e**, Congo red). Amyloid deposits are strongly immunoreactive for LECT2 antibody (**d** and **f**, Immunoperoxidase)

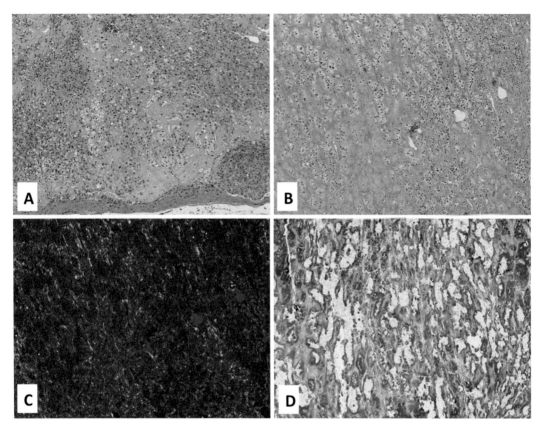

Fig. 4.2 Adrenal gland ALECT2 amyloidosis. Eosinophilic extracellular deposits (**a**, H&E) stain with Congo red (**b**) and show appropriate color change under polarized light (**c**, Congo red). Immunohistochemistry shows that the deposits are positive for LECT2 antibody (**d**, Immunoperoxidase)

be involved in the restructuring of cartilage and, therefore, was named chondromodulin [12].

The in vivo function of LECT2 has yet to be established. LECT2 is synthesized principally by the liver, and it has been shown that increased expression of LECT2 may occur with hepatocellular tumors [13]. LECT2 is also a cytokine involved in the regulation of hepatocyte activity and functions as an immunomodulator [14]. LECT2 mRNA was specifically detected in adult and fetal liver but not in other tissues [15]. Initial immunohistochemical (IHC) studies using polyclonal antisera demonstrated that LECT2 is physiologically synthesized by a variety of cells other than hepatocytes and endothelial cells and becomes positively stainable under pathological conditions in cells originally negative [16]. But more recent IHC and mRNA in-situ hybridiza-

tion assays have failed to identify expression outside liver tissue. LECT2 expression may be related to the cell cycle and damage/repair process [17, 18].

The pathogenesis of ALECT2 amyloidosis still needs to be elucidated. It has been suggested that an increased expression of LECT2 or other factors involved in the metabolism of LECT2 or a genetic defect in LECT2 catabolic pathway/LECT2 transport may result in an increased local tissue concentration of LECT2 leading to the initiation of fibril formation [1, 2]. LECT2 has extensive β-structure, and the entire secreted LECT2 protein is incorporated into the amyloid fibrils suggesting that the proteolytic degradation is not necessary for fibril formation [19]. LECT2 serum levels are elevated in hepatic disorders [20, 21] but no increased levels have been detected so far in ALECT2 amyloidosis [2, 22].

The human LECT2 gene (*LECT2*) is found on chromosome 5q31.1 by fluorescence in situ hybridization, in close proximity to cytokine genes, including interleukin (IL)-4, IL-5, and IL-9. *LECT2* consists of four exons and three introns [23]. The gene codes for 151 amino acids (MW 16,376 Da) including an 18 amino acid signal peptide [1]. Genetic analysis performed in 35 patients with kidney involvement and one case of hepatic amyloidosis did not detect *LECT2* mutations [1, 2, 4, 5, 24]. Although ALECT2 amyloidosis does not appear to be caused by genetic mutations, homozygosity for a non-synonymous single nucleotide variant in exon 3 seems to be required for disease. All 35 patients sequenced thus far show homozygosity for the G nucleotide at position 172 (SNP rs31517) resulting in replacement of isoleucine by valine at position 40 of mature protein. This is a common polymorphism which has previously been demonstrated to be a risk factor for the progression of rheumatoid arthritis [25]. It has been hypothesized that the polymorphism might increase the amyloidogenic propensity of LECT2. It is also possible that the polymorphism might segregate with another causative mutation though this is considered less likely since this variant is homozygous in patients of varying ethnicities [2]. The preponderance of disease in certain ethnicities as well as the description in siblings [4] suggests a genetic etiology. If this is the case then ALECT2 might be considered a digenic disease in which homozygosity for the common SNP rs31517 is required in addition to some other yet-unknown variant.

The possibility of an ethnic background as a predisposing factor in the development of amyloidosis had been raised for the first time in an autopsy study performed at Los Angeles County-University of Southern California Medical Center [26]. The study included 467 patients with amyloidosis found among 52,370 autopsies. Classification of amyloidosis (AA vs. other types) was accomplished by using the potassium permanganate CR staining method and a specific anti-AA antiserum, supplemented by the anatomical distribution of the amyloid in some instances.

The study found a statistically significant increase in amyloidosis among Hispanic patients as compared with Caucasians. Interestingly, the increase was mostly among the non-AA amyloid cases (negative for anti-AA antibody) and not anatomically compatible with senile cardiac (systemic) amyloidosis defined by the heart as the principal organ involved and the confinement of amyloid in other organs to small blood vessels. Hispanics accounted for 76 % of these cases as compared with 18.5 % for Caucasians. The cases did not fit the inheritance or clinical patterns of familial amyloidosis so these cases were considered principally AL-type. Because of the technical limitations of the study, we can only assume that most of these Hispanic patients could have been affected by ALECT2 amyloidosis, but this hypothesis cannot be supported without an accurate amyloid typing of the specimens. However, the findings suggest that the frequency of amyloidosis may vary significantly in different ethnic groups.

The main clinical and pathological features of ALECT2 amyloidosis involving the kidney and the liver are summarized in Table 4.1.

Renal ALECT2 Amyloidosis

ALECT2 amyloidosis represents the third most common form of amyloidosis involving the kidney. ALECT2 is commonly recognized to be an important cause of end-stage renal disease affecting mainly Hispanic patients who typically present with slowly progressive renal insufficiency with or without proteinuria [3, 4, 6, 7]. It is not known whether LECT2 deposition in the kidney is a slow process that begins early in life and remains undetected until significant accumulation has occurred, or whether the deposition of the aberrant protein is a more rapid process that begins later in life. However, most of the patients maintain renal function until late in life [4]. It has been also suggested that amyloid deposition in other organs like liver, spleen, and even heart may occur in later stages of the renal disease, especially if the patient's life is extended by dialysis [19]. There is a better survival in renal ALECT2 amyloidosis compared to AL and AA

Table 4.1 Main clinicopathological features of ALECT2 amyloidosis involving the kidney and the liver: summary of the largest case series of ALECT2 published to date

	Larsen et al. [3]	Murphy et al. [2, 22][a]	Dogan et al. [24]	Said et al. [6]	Said et al. [7]	Larsen et al. [4]	Mereuta et al. [5]	Hutton et al. [8]
Study period (years)	8.5	N/A	N/A	5	6	5	4	4
Biopsy specimens (N)	21,598	10	30	474	72	23,650	130	4
Amyloidosis cases, N (%)	285(1.3)	10(100)	30(100)	474(100)	72(100)	414(1.8)	130(100)	4(100)
ALECT2 cases, N (%)	7(2.5)	10(100)	30(100)	13(2.7)	72(N/A)	40(9.7)	32(25)	4(100)
Organ involved (N)	Kidney (7)	Kidney (10)	Kidney (24) Spleen (7/7) Liver (4/7) Adrenals (6/7)[b]	Kidney	Kidney	Kidney	Liver	Kidney
Median age, years (range)	67.8(58–84)	68(58–84)	65(40–78)	N/A	65.5(43–88)	70.4(52–86)	60.5(33–79)	65(56–78)
Hispanic ethnicity, N(%)	5(71)	7(70)	20(67)	N/A	66(91.7)	35(88)	28(88)	–
Other ethnicity (N)	Caucasian (1) Native American (1)	Caucasian (1) Middle Eastern (1) Native American (1)	Punjabi (6) Arab (2) Caucasian (2)	N/A	Middle Eastern (3) Native American (1) African (1) Caucasian (1)	Native American (3)[c] Middle Eastern (1) Caucasian (1)	Caucasian (4)	First Nations from Northern British Columbia, Canada (4)

(continued)

Table 4.1 (continued)

	Larsen et al. [3]	Murphy et al. [2, 22]ᵃ	Dogan et al. [24]	Said et al. [6]	Said et al. [7]	Larsen et al. [4]	Mereuta et al. [5]	Hutton et al. [8]
Main presentation, N(%)	N/A	Renal insufficiency 10(100) Proteinuria 3(30)	Renal insufficiency 24(100) Proteinuria 24(100) Incidental (other organs)	N/A	Renal insufficiency 64(91.4) Proteinuria 52(78.8)	Renal insufficiency 27(68) Proteinuria 13(33)	Liver dysfunctionᵈ 12(38) Incidental 7(22)	Renal insufficiency 4(100) Proteinuria 3(75)
Morphology (N)	Interstitial (7) Mesangium (6) GBM (4) Arterioles (7) Arteries (5)	Interstitial (10) Mesangium (9) GBM (5) Arterioles (9) Arteries (6)	Interstitial/vascular (kidney) Globular (liver) Vascular/stromal (other organs)	Interstitial (13)	Interstitial (72) GBM (66) Vascular (60)	Interstitial (40) Glomerular (35) Arterioles (33) Arteries (23) Medullary (13)	Portal/globular (32)	Interstitial (4) Mesangium (4) Arterioles (4) Arterial (4)
LECT2 gene analysis (N)ᵉ	No LECT2 mutation (2)	No LECT2 mutation (2)	No LECT2 mutation (10)	N/A	N/A	No LECT2 mutation (10)	No LECT2 mutation (10)ᶠ	N/A

N/A data not available, GBM glomerular basement membrane
ᵃSeven cases previously reported [3]
ᵇAmyloid deposits revealed by ¹²³I Serum Amyloid P component (SAP) scintigraphy in seven cases
ᶜThere was a high density of ALECT2 amyloidosis from the Southwest USA including New Mexico, Arizona and far West Texas (2 % of total biopsies and 54 % of amyloidosis cases from this area were ALECT2 patients). Two of the patients in this series are siblings
ᵈIn ALECT2 amyloidosis, elevated liver functions tests, in particular elevation of alkaline phosphatase, was the most frequent abnormality
ᵉAll cases tested show homozygosity for the G nucleotide at position 172 (SNP rs31517) resulting in replacement of isoleucine by valine at position 40 of mature protein
ᶠOne case of hepatic and nine cases of renal ALECT2 amyloidosis previously reported [24]

forms due to the absence of cardiac involvement in ALECT2 patients [7]. No specific treatment for ALECT2 is available but a reliable diagnosis on renal biopsies is required in order to avoid any mistreatment. Renal transplantation is considered for patients with end-stage kidney disease. Early data in five patients transplanted for ALECT2 shows that after a mean of 20 months post-transplant, there was no graft loss, though one did show recurrence of disease [7].

There are consistent morphological features of renal amyloid deposition in ALECT2. There is a preferential interstitial deposition within the cortex. A minimal glomerular and vascular involvement is often present (Figs. 4.1a–c and 4.2a–c). The medulla is not involved by amyloid deposition in most cases. This aspect differentiates ALECT2 from other forms of amyloidosis with distinctive morphologic patterns such as AApoAIV (apolipoprotein AIV), with predominantly medullary involvement and AFib (fibrinogen A α chain), which typically shows florid deposition restricted to the glomeruli. Strikingly, congophilic amyloid was also described in ALECT2 [4]. IHC studies show strong staining for antibodies directed against LECT2 within the amorphous material (Figs. 4.1d and 4.2d), whereas stains for AA, lambda, kappa, fibrinogen, and immunoglobulins are negative). Ultrastructural examination shows evidence of small, non-branching, overlapping fibrils within the cortical interstitium of all patients and within the mesangium of patients with glomerular involvement [4].

Hepatic ALECT2 Amyloidosis

The liver is a frequent site of involvement by systemic amyloidosis where 60–90 % of cases have been reported to show liver involvement at autopsy [27]. Although AL is the most common type of hepatic amyloid, ALECT2 may account for 25 % of hepatic amyloidosis cases [5]. Therefore, a correct diagnosis of hepatic ALECT2 amyloidosis is fundamental and bears clinical significance.

Hepatic ALECT2 amyloidosis exhibits a number of unique clinical and pathological features. Similar to renal ALECT2 amyloidosis, most of the patients are of Hispanic ethnicity. The diagnosis of hepatic ALECT2 is often incidentally discovered during evaluations for conditions unrelated to the liver or was associated with other liver diseases such as chronic viral hepatitis and steatohepatitis. Interestingly, the patients usually have no evidence of kidney disease at the time of presentation [5]. These findings suggest that hepatic ALECT2 amyloidosis may not cause a clinically significant liver disease which makes the diagnosis more difficult to establish. Nevertheless, a case of hepatic ALECT2 amyloidosis causing portal hypertension with recurrent esophageal variceal bleeding has been recently reported [28].

Hepatic ALECT2 amyloidosis presents with a characteristic pathological pattern. The ALECT2-involved liver specimens contain unusual globular amyloid deposits located in the periportal parenchyma or at the periphery of the portal triad and sometimes around central venules (Fig. 4.1e) [5, 29]. This histological pattern was described previously in the liver and gastrointestinal tract, but its significance was unclear [30–35]. Kanel et al. [30] suggested that globular amyloid deposits represent a distinct presentation of hepatic amyloidosis, meanwhile the findings of Makhlouf and Goodman [32] support the idea that globular hepatic amyloid is an early form of liver involvement in systemic amyloidosis. Furthermore, in some cases amyloid was documented also in other organs such as spleen, kidney, adrenal gland, heart, gallbladder, pancreas, thyroid, or abdominal fat pad. Thus, the globular liver deposition was indicative for a systemic involvement. Recognition of the characteristic globular pattern of ALECT2 amyloid deposition helps one to consider ALECT2 amyloidosis in the differential diagnosis of hepatic amyloidosis because it contrasts distinctly with the perisinusoidal amyloid deposition pattern that typifies hepatic AL amyloidosis [5].

The etiology of hepatic ALECT2 amyloidosis is currently unknown. ALECT2 amyloid deposits stain positively by IHC (Fig. 4.1f), but normal liver, hepatocytes in ALECT2 and other types of hepatic amyloidosis, and other normal and neoplastic tissues including hepatocellular carcinoma are negative. LECT2 mRNA is strongly and uniformly expressed in hepatocytes in ALECT2 amyloidosis. Hepatocytes in normal liver and AL amyloidosis are negative or exhibit weak/focal LECT2 mRNA expression, and there is variable expression in hepatocellular carcinoma. Therefore, upregulation of LECT2 expression, either constitutively (controlled by yet undefined genetic factors) or secondary to hepatocellular damage, is hypothesized to be the most likely cause of ALECT2 amyloidosis [5].

Conclusions

ALECT2 amyloidosis is a frequent cause of renal and hepatic amyloidosis and especially should be considered in Hispanic patients with renal or hepatic amyloidosis. These cases may not be easily recognized or may be misdiagnosed as AL or AA amyloidosis based on the clinical context [36, 37]. Therefore, accurate typing of amyloid deposits either by LMD/MS analysis or immunohistochemistry in specialist centers is essential before any management decision is made for renal and hepatic amyloidosis patients in order to avoid incorrect and unnecessarily toxic therapies.

References

1. Benson MD, James S, Scott K, Liepnieks JJ, Kluve-Beckerman B. Leukocyte chemotactic factor 2: a novel renal amyloid protein. Kidney Int. 2008;74(2):218–22.
2. Murphy CL, Wang S, Kestler D, et al. Leukocyte chemotactic factor 2 (LECT2)-associated renal amyloidosis: a case series. Am J Kidney Dis. 2010;56(6):1100–7.
3. Larsen CP, Walker PD, Weiss DT, Solomon A. Prevalence and morphology of leukocyte chemotactic factor 2-associated amyloid in renal biopsies. Kidney Int. 2010;77(9):816–9.
4. Larsen CP, Kossmann RJ, Beggs ML, Solomon A, Walker PD. Clinical, morphologic and genetic features of renal leukocyte chemotactic factor 2 amyloidosis. Kidney Int. 2014;86(2):378–82.
5. Mereuta OM, Theis JD, Vrana JA, et al. Leukocyte cell-derived chemotaxin 2 (LECT2)-associated amyloidosis is a frequent cause of hepatic amyloidosis in the United States. Blood. 2014;123(10):1479–82.
6. Said SM, Sethi S, Valeri AM, et al. Renal amyloidosis: origin and clinicopathologic correlations of 474 recent cases. Clin J Am Soc Nephrol. 2013;8(9):1515–23.
7. Said SM, Sethi S, Valeri AM, et al. Characterization and outcomes of renal leukocyte chemotactic factor 2-associated amyloidosis. Kidney Int. 2014;86(2):370–7.
8. Hutton HL, DeMarco ML, Magil AB, Taylor P. Renal leukocyte chemotactic factor 2 (LECT2) amyloidosis in First Nations people in Northern British Columbia, Canada: a report of 4 cases. Am J Kidney Dis. 2014;64(5):790–2.
9. Vrana JA, Gamez JD, Madden BJ, Theis JD, Bergen 3rd HR, Dogan A. Classification of amyloidosis by laser microdissection and mass spectrometry-based proteomic analysis in clinical biopsy specimens. Blood. 2009;114(24):4957–9.
10. Sipe JD, Benson MD, Buxbaum JN, et al. Amyloid fibril protein nomenclature: 2010 recommendations from the nomenclature committee of the International Society of Amyloidosis. Amyloid. 2010;17:101–4.
11. Yamagoe S, Yamakawa Y, Matsuo Y, et al. Purification and primary amino acid sequence of a novel neutrophil chemotactic factor LECT2. Immunol Lett. 1996;52:9–13.
12. Hiraki Y, Inoue H, Kondo J, et al. A novel growthpromoting factor derived from fetal bovine cartilage, chondromodulin II. Purification and aminoacid sequence. J Biol Chem. 1996;271:22657–62.
13. Ovejero C, Cavard C, Périanin A, et al. Identification of the leukocyte cell-derived chemotaxin 2 as a direct target gene of β-catenin in the liver. Hepatology. 2004;40:167–76.
14. Segawa Y, Itokazu Y, Inoue N, Saito T, Suzuki K. Possible changes in expression of chemotaxin LECT2 mRNA in mouse liver after concanavalin A-induced hepatic injury. Biol Pharm Bull. 2001;24(4):425–8.
15. Yamagoe S, Mizuno S, Suzuki K. Molecular cloning of human and bovine LECT2 having a neutrophil chemotactic activity and its specific expression in the liver. Biochim Biophys Acta. 1998;1396(1):105–13.
16. Yamagoe S, Akasaka T, Uchida T, et al. Expression of a neutrophil chemotactic protein LECT2 in human hepatocytes revealed by immunochemical studies using polyclonal and monoclonal antibodies to a recombinant LECT2. Biochem Biophys Res Commun. 1997;237(1):116–20.
17. Nagai H, Hamada T, Uchida T, Yamagoe S, Suzuki K. Systemic expression of a newly recognized protein, LECT2, in the human body. Pathol Int. 1998;48(11):882–6.
18. Uchida T, Nagai H, Gotoh K, et al. Expression pattern of a newly recognized protein, LECT2, in

hepatocellular carcinoma and its premalignant lesion. Pathol Int. 1999;49(2):147–51.

19. Benson MD. LECT2 amyloidosis. Kidney Int. 2010;77:757–9.

20. Sato Y, Watanabe H, Kameyama H, et al. Serum LECT2 level as a prognostic indicator in acute liver failure. Transplant Proc. 2004;36(8):2359–61.

21. Sato Y, Watanabe H, Kameyama H, et al. Changes in serum LECT 2 levels during the early period of liver regeneration after adult living related donor liver transplantation. Transplant Proc. 2004;36(8):2357–8.

22. Murphy C, Wang S, Kestler D, Larsen C, Benson D, Weiss D, Solomon A. Leukocyte chemotactic factor 2 (LECT2)-associated renal amyloidosis. Amyloid. 2011;18 Suppl 1:223–5.

23. Yamagoe S, Kameoka Y, Hashimoto K, Mizuno S, Suzuki K. Molecular cloning, structural characterization, and chromosomal mapping of the human LECT2 gene. Genomics. 1998;48(3):324–9.

24. Dogan A, Theis JD, Vrana JA, et al. Clinical and pathological phenotype of leukocyte cell-derived chemotaxin-2 (LECT2) amyloidosis (ALECT2) (abstract OP-058). Amyloid. 2010;17 Suppl 1:69–70.

25. Kameoka Y, Yamagoe S, Hatano Y, Kasama T, Suzuki K. Val58Ile polymorphism of the neutrophil chemoattractant LECT2 and rheumatoid arthritis in the Japanese population. Arthritis Rheum. 2000; 43(6):1419–20.

26. Buck FS, Koss MN, Sherrod AE, Wu A, Takahashi M. Ethnic distribution of amyloidosis: an autopsy study. Mod Pathol. 1989;2(4):372–7.

27. Buck FS, Koss MN. Hepatic amyloidosis: morphologic differences between systemic AL and AA types. Hum Pathol. 1991;22:904–7.

28. Damlaj M, Amre R, Wong P, How J. Hepatic ALECT2-amyloidosis causing portal hypertension and recurrent variceal bleeding: a case report and review of the literature. Am J Clin Pathol. 2014;141(2):288–91.

29. Chandan VS, Shah SS, Lam-Himlin DM, et al. Globular hepatic amyloid is highly sensitive and specific for LECT2 amyloidosis. Am J Surg Pathol. 2015;39:558–64.

30. Kanel GC, Uchida T, Peters RL. Globular hepatic amyloid-an unusual morphologic presentation. Hepatology. 1981;1:647–52.

31. Agaram N, Shia J, Klimstra DS, et al. Globular hepatic amyloid: a diagnostic peculiarity that bears clinical significance. Hum Pathol. 2005;36:845–49.

32. Makhlouf HR, Goodman ZD. Globular hepatic amyloid: an early stage in the pathway of amyloid formation. A study of 20 new cases. Am J Surg Pathol. 2007;31(10):1615–21.

33. Pilgaard J, Fenger C, Schaffalitzky de Muckadell OB. Globular amyloid deposits in the liver. Histopathology. 1993;23(5):479–80.

34. Demirhan B, Bilezikci B, Kiyici H, Boyacioglu S. Globular amyloid deposits in the wall of the gastrointestinal tract: report of six cases. Amyloid. 2002;9(1):42–6.

35. Hemmer PR, Topazian MD, Gertz MA, Abraham SC. Globular amyloid deposits isolated to the small bowel: a rare association with AL Amyloidosis. Am J Surg Pathol. 2007;31:141–5.

36. Comenzo RL. LECT2 makes the amyloid list. Blood. 2014;123(10):1436–7.

37. Picken MM. Alect2 amyloidosis: primum non nocere (first, do not harm). Kidney Int. 2014;86:229–32.

The Hereditary Amyloidoses

5

Merrill D. Benson

Introduction

The hereditary amyloidoses are a group of fibril
deposition diseases which are usually systemic
with multiple organ system pathology. Each disease is designated by the fibril precursor protein
that is the principle constituent of the amyloid
deposits. While considered rare, in the aggregate,
hereditary amyloidosis is relatively common.
Diagnostically, there are two challenges which
face both the clinician and the pathologist: The
first is to be aware that amyloidosis may be at the
root of the patient's signs and symptoms. The
second is to determine the type of amyloidosis
that is involved. The diagnosis of amyloidosis
can only be confirmed by tissue biopsy, and while
a biopsy may be to confirm the clinician's suspicion that amyloidosis is the cause of the illness,
in many cases, biopsies are done to determine the
cause of an organ's dysfunction which may be
seen in a number of different diseases. In these
cases, the histologic demonstration of amyloidosis is often a surprise. The job of the pathologist
is to recognize amyloid when it is present. This is
not always that easy. Variations in fibril deposition patterns and inconsistencies in amyloid
staining by histochemical dyes can make the
diagnosis of amyloidosis difficult. It is important
to remember that amyloid is a generic term and at
least 26 different proteins can give tissue deposits
that meet the pathology criteria for amyloidosis
[1]. Some of these proteins give fibrils which
stain readily with Congo red, the principal dye
for recognizing amyloid deposits, but others do
not. Sometimes, variations in histologic staining
can give a hint as to which type of amyloidosis is
involved. Distribution of fibril deposition may
also give a clue as to the type of hereditary amyloidosis that is involved.

Hereditary amyloidosis may be either systemic or localized. Localized types of hereditary
amyloidoses include procalcitonin in medullary
carcinoma of the thyroid, kerato-epithelin in corneal dystrophy, some cardiac atria amyloid in
which there are mutations in atrial natriuretic
peptide, Alzheimer disease with mutations in the
$A\beta$-protein or presenilin, spongiform encephalopathies due to mutations in prion protein, and
hereditary British or Danish dementia caused by
mutations in the ABriPP or ADanPP protein.

Seven different proteins are currently recognized as causing hereditary systemic amyloidosis
(Table 5.1) [2]. While most of these proteins are
characterized by specific organ system involvement (kidney, heart, peripheral nerve), the fact

M.D. Benson, MD (✉)
Department of Pathology and Laboratory Medicine,
Indiana University School of Medicine,
Van Nuys Medical Science Building, 635 Barnhill
Drive, MS-128, Indianapolis, IN 46202-5126, USA
e-mail: mdbenson@iupui.edu

© Springer International Publishing Switzerland 2015
M.M. Picken et al. (eds.), *Amyloid and Related Disorders*, Current Clinical Pathology,
DOI 10.1007/978-3-319-19294-9_5

Table 5.1 Mutant proteins other than transthyretin associated with autosomal dominant systemic amyloidosis

Protein	cDNA change[a]	Amino acid change[b]	Codon change	Clinical features
Transthyretin				
Apolipoprotein AI	*Greater than 120 mutations[c]*			
	148G→C	Gly26Arg	GGC26CGC	PN, Nephropathy
	172G→A	Glu34Lys	GAA34AAA	Nephropathy
	178T→G	Ser36Ala	TCC36GCC	Nephropathy
	251T→G	Leu60Arg	CTG60CGG	Nephropathy
	220T→C/A	Trp50Arg	TGG50CGG/AGG	Nephropathy
	del250-284insGTCAC	del60-71insVal/Thr	del60-71ins GTCAC	Hepatic
	251T→G	Leu60Arg	CTG60CGG	Nephropathy
	263T→C	Leu64Pro	CTC64CCC	Nephropathy
	del280-288	del70-72	del70-72GAGTTCTGG	Nephropathy
	284T→A	Phe71Tyr	TTC71TAC	Palatal mass
	294insA(fs)	Asn74Lys(fs)	AAC74AAAC(fs)	Nephropathy
	296T→C	Leu75Pro	CTG75CCG	Hepatic
	341T→C	Leu90Pro	CTG90CCG	Cardiomyopathy, cutaneous, laryngeal
	532insGC(fs)	Ala154(fs)	GCC154GGC(fs)	Nephropathy
	535delC	His155Met(fs)	535delC	Nephropathy
	562G→T	Ala164Ser	GCC164TCC	Nephropathy
	581T→C	Leu170Pro	CTG170CCG	Laryngeal
	590G→C	Arg173Pro	CGC173CCC	Cardiomyopathy, cutaneous, laryngeal
	593T→C	Leu174Ser	TTG174TCG	Cardiomyopathy
	595G→C	Ala175Pro	GCX175CCX[d]	Laryngeal
	604T→A	Leu178His	TTG178CAT	Cardiomyopathy, laryngeal
	391-393delLys107del		delAAG	Aortic intima
Gelsolin	594G→A	Gly167Arg	GGG167AGC	Nephropathy
	633C→A	Asn184Lys	AAC184AAA	Nephropathy
	640G→A	Asp187Asn	GAC187AAC	PN, lattice corneal dystrophy
	640G→T	Asp187Tyr	GAC187TAC	PN
Cystatin C	280T→A	Leu68Gln	CTG68CAG	Cerebral hemorrhage

Protein			
Fibrinogen A	1718G→T	Arg554Leu	CGT554CTT	Nephropathy
	1633G→A	Glu526Lys	GAG526AAG	Nephropathy
	1634A→T	Glu526Val	GAG526GTG	Nephropathy
	1629delG	Glu524Glu(fs)	GAG524GA_	Nephropathy
	1627G→A	Glu524Lys	GAG524AAG	Nephropathy
	1622delT	Val522Ala(fs)	GTC522G_C	Nephropathy
	1676A→T	Glu540Val	GAA540GTA	Nephropathy
	del1606-1620 ATGTTAGGA	GAGTTTinsCA		Nephropathy
	1618-1622delTTGT	Phe521Ser(fs)		Nephropathy
	del1636-1650insCA1649-1650			Nephropathy
	1712C→A	Pro552His	CCT552CAT	Nephropathy
	1720-1721del/insTT	Gly555Phe	GGT555TTT	Nephropathy
	1670C→A	Thr538Lys	ACA538AAA	Nephropathy, neuropathy
	1632delT	Thr525fs	ACT525AC_	Nephropathy
Lysozyme	214T→A	Tyr54Asn	TAT54AAT	Cardiomyopathy
	221T→C	Ile56Thr	ATA56ACA	Nephropathy, petechiae
	253G→C	Asp67His	GAT67CAT	Nephropathy
	244T→C/A	Trp64Arg	TGG64CGG/AGG	Nephropathy/hepatic
	223T→A	Phe57Ile	TTT57ATT	Nephropathy
	254A→G	Asp67Gly	GAT67GGT	Nephropathy
	413T→A	Trp112Arg	TGG112AGG	Nephropathy, GI
Apolipoprotein AII	301T→G	Stop78Gly	TGA78GGA	Nephropathy
	302G→C	Stop78Ser	TGA78TCA	Nephropathy
	301T→C	Stop78Arg	TGA78CGA	Nephropathy
	301T→A	Stop78Arg	TGA78AGA	Nephropathy
	302G→T	Stop78Leu	TGA78TTA	Nephropathy

PN Peripheral Neuropathy, fs Frame Shift
[a]cDNA numbering is from initiation codon (ATG)
[b]Amino acids numbered for N-terminus of mature protein
[c]List of most TTR mutations (3)
[d]Deduced

that they usually are associated with deposits in blood vessel walls throughout the body attests to the fact that these diseases are truly systemic. The amyloid fibril precursor protein is synthesized in one organ (in most cases the liver), but amyloid deposits are found in other organ systems. In hereditary localized amyloidosis, the amyloid precursor protein is synthesized in the organ in which the amyloid deposits are found. This is true for atrial natriuretic factor, procalcitonin, and islet amyloid polypeptide (IAPP, amylin). The type of amyloidosis in localized forms is easier to determine because of the specific organ involved; however, it is important to remember that the systemic forms of amyloidosis may be associated with deposits in many of the organs that can be involved with localized amyloidosis. The localized forms (except for the Alzheimer and prion diseases) are often incidental findings and not a primary factor in the person's health. The systemic forms of hereditary amyloidosis are much more life threatening and deserve in-depth review.

Types of Hereditary Amyloidosis

First, a few words on nomenclature: As with many scientific fields, the nomenclature for the amyloidoses can present difficulties in communication even for those steeped in the history of amyloid. In science, the first descriptions of proteins are usually given names which may relate to the functionality, site of synthesis, or structural characteristics. Later, with developing knowledge, there is usually a tendency to try to improve communication by introducing more appropriate terms and organizing them in a more consistent fashion. This often leads to problems. There are several points in amyloid history which exemplified these problems: (1) The disease we now call reactive amyloidosis was for many years, and even today, called "secondary" to indicate that it occurred in patients who had a primary, usually inflammatory, disease. For the pathologist, it was often referred to as "typical" amyloidosis since the staining with Congo red was usually consistent from one case to another. (2) Immunoglobulin

light chain-associated amyloidosis in the past, and to this day, was often called "primary" amyloidosis. "Primary," of course, has the same meaning as idiopathic or essential, indicating that there is no predisposing condition that explains the development of amyloidosis. This form of amyloidosis was often referred to by the pathologist as "atypical" since the histologic staining pattern with Congo red often varies from case to case, perhaps the result of the varying structures of immunoglobulin light chain fibril components. The use of "primary" has been problematic, however, because you will find some articles describing "primary" familial amyloidosis: an attempt to explain a disease with hereditary characteristics but for which a cause was not known. Now that we have identified many gene mutations that cause hereditary amyloidosis, the use of the word "primary" in this context should be discouraged. It is not only the clinician that has problems with nomenclature, but the basic scientist is also presented with the conundrum of nomenclature problems. Serum amyloid A 2 (SAA 2) which is the amyloid producing SAA in mice is now SAA 1.1 to adhere to the convention of the human gene designation. Islet amyloid-associated peptide and amylin are continuing to have their differences for students of Islets of Langerhans amyloidosis. Even transthyretin (TTR) is still referred to by its old name, prealbumin, which was a name derived from the fact that it traveled faster toward the anode than albumin in protein electrophoresis. Many pathology clinical laboratories still measure "prealbumin" levels and do not have a clue as to what TTR is.

The International Amyloid Society has a Nomenclature Committee which has established suggested designations for the different types of amyloid, and this is updated on a periodic basis for both human and animal systems [1]. In the list of nomenclature scheme, different types of amyloidosis are referred to by first the letter "A" followed by the precursor protein for that type of amyloidosis. As an example, immunoglobulin light chain amyloidosis becomes AL, transthyretin amyloidosis becomes ATTR, reactive or serum amyloid A amyloidosis becomes AA, and apolipoprotein AI amyloidosis becomes AApoAI. More specific

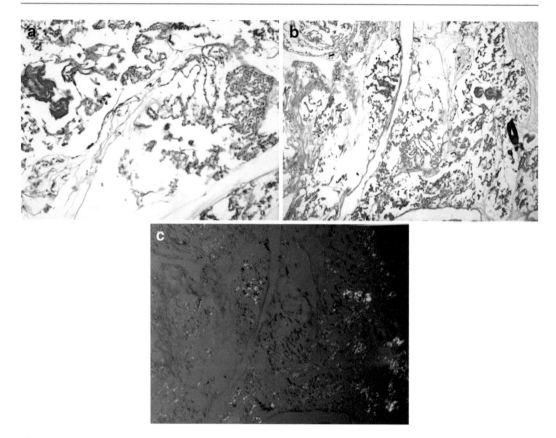

Fig. 5.1 **a** Vitrectomy specimen from a patient with TTR Ile84Ser amyloidosis showing fibrillar strands and globules of amyloid. H&E original magnification ×200. **b** Vitrectomy specimen as in (**a**) stained with *Congo red.* **c** Section in (**b**) viewed between two crossed polars showing typical *green birefringence* of amyloid. Original magnification ×100

designations may be used if felt necessary for better communication. An example would be ALλ or ALκ or ATTR Val30Met to indicate a specific protein mutation.

Transthyretin amyloidosis is the most common form of systemic hereditary amyloidosis. Greater than 120 mutations in transthyretin (also known as prealbumin) are associated with amyloidosis with peripheral neuropathy and cardiomyopathy being the most common clinical manifestations [3]. It is truly a systemic disease with amyloid deposits in vascular walls throughout the body, and a number of transthyretin mutations are associated with deposits in the vitreous of the eye (Fig. 5.1) and the leptomeninges (Fig. 5.2).

Transthyretin is a prominent plasma protein present normally at approximately 25 mg/dl in the blood [4]. It is synthesized principally by hepatocytes although some synthesis is a feature of the choroid plexus and the retinal pigment epithelium of the eye. Transthyretin is a single chain protein of 127 amino acid residues [5]. The protein typically folds into seven or eight β-structured sheets in two planes, and then four monomers form a tetramer which is present in the blood as a 56-kDa transport protein for thyroid hormone and retinal-binding protein/vitamin A [6]. Transthyretin has extensive β-structure and, like immunoglobulin light chains, would be expected to be a prime candidate for amyloid β-fibril formation. While there are greater than 120 transthyretin mutations associated with amyloidosis, only a few of the mutations exist in extended kindreds, and due to incomplete penetrance of the genetic defect, many cases appear "sporadic" when in fact more detailed family history will disclose the genetic basis of the disease.

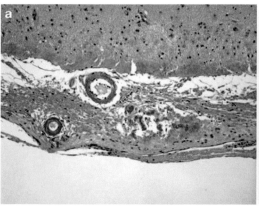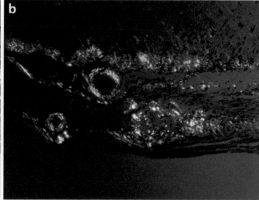

Fig. 5.2 **a** Leptomeningeal and brain biopsy from patient with TTR Gly53Arg amyloidosis showing amyloid deposits, in leptomeninges, and blood vessel walls. (**b**) Same section as (**a**) viewed between crossed polars demonstrating typical *green birefringence* of amyloid. Original magnification ×100

Transthyretin amyloidosis is an autosomal dominant trait as would be expected from a defect in a structural protein. The most frequently identified transthyretin mutations include Val30Met which is common in Portugal, Sweden, Japan, and the USA [7–9], Leu58His which is common in the USA but originated in Germany [10], Thr60Ala which is common in the USA but originated in Ireland [11], Ser77Tyr which was first discovered in the USA but probably originated in Germany [12], Ile84Ser which was discovered in a kindred in the USA but probably originated in Switzerland [13], and Val122Ile which is present in approximately 3 % of African-Americans in the USA and probably originated in the west coast of Africa [14]. Each of these mutations is now worldwide and not limited to just one country. Many of the other mutations have been described in single individuals or single families and, once identified and reported in the scientific literature, tend not to be subject of further research. Now that new forms of treatment for transthyretin amyloidosis may be on the horizon, identification and classification of the transthyretin amyloidoses have become more important. It should be pointed out that wild-type TTR can undergo fibrillogenesis in older patients, who develop senile systemic amyloidosis (SSA). Although it affects primarily myocardium (sometimes termed "senile cardiac amyloidosis"), there is also systemic involvement of the vessels and,

not uncommonly, clinical (and pathologic) evidence of pulmonary and carpal tunnel involvement; the involvement of other sites, frequently seen at autopsy, is usually not clinically apparent. It is estimated that 25 % of octogenarians may be affected by senile cardiac amyloidosis, predominantly males. Overall, the progression of ATTR derived from the wild-type transthyretin is slower. Although, ultimately, heart failure ensues, it does so at a slower rate than in hereditary ATTR (in particular, certain "cardiotrophic" mutations) or AL with cardiac involvement [14, 15].

Transthyretin

Transthyretin amyloidosis was originally called familial amyloidotic polyneuropathy (FAP) because the first mutation to be discovered, Val30Met, is associated principally with neuropathy, although cardiac pathology and renal pathology are commonly seen [7] (Fig. 5.3). The neuropathy is axonal with usual presentation of neuropathic symptoms in the lower extremities and slowly progressive involvement of more proximal nerves. Carpal tunnel syndrome, a compression neuropathy at the wrist, is common but unfortunately early diagnosis by histologic evaluation of tissue from carpal tunnel release is not routinely done. When peripheral nerve is biopsied (usually the sural nerve), the neuropathy is often fairly advanced (Fig. 5.4) [16]. Even so, amyloid deposits may not be demonstrated due to the sporadic nature of amyloid deposition in peripheral nerve. If deposits are identified by staining with Congo red or metachromatic dyes, immunohistochemistry with antitransthyretin antibody will usually indicate the type of amyloidosis. When cardiac amyloidosis is present, sampling error is much less of a problem, and

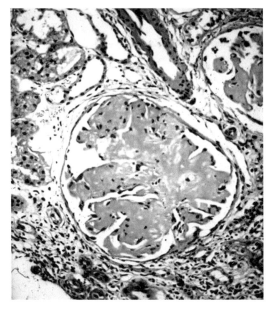

Fig. 5.3 Renal biopsy from a patient with TTR Val30Met amyloidosis who presented with renal failure showing glomerular deposition of amyloid. Original magnification 160×

endomyocardial biopsy is usually diagnostic (Fig. 5.5). More definitive characterization of amyloid deposits can be obtained by analysis with amino acid sequencing or mass spectrometric analysis of biopsy tissue [17, 18]. Confirmation of the hereditary nature of transthyretin amyloidosis relies on DNA analysis [19]. While multiple RFLPs have been used in the past, present DNA analysis involves direct nucleotide sequencing of DNA usually obtained for peripheral blood white cells. The transthyretin gene has four exons: The first exon codes for only the first three amino terminal amino acid residues. No mutation in this exon has been found. The other three exons share fairly equally the amyloid-associated mutations with multiple mutations occurring at a number of sites. The clinician can obtain transthyretin sequence analysis from a number of commercial laboratories and, because transthyretin amyloidosis continues to be a prominent area of research, a number of the research centers continue to offer specialized service in this area.

Apolipoprotein AI

ApoAI is probably the second most common systemic hereditary amyloidosis [20, 21]. At least 20 different mutations have been associated with ApoAI amyloidosis, and kindreds have been identified in the USA, Spain, South Africa,

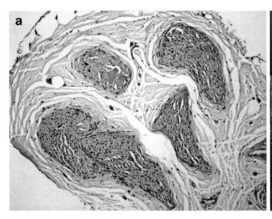
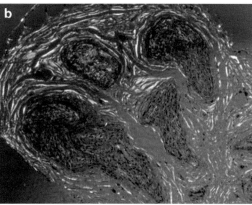

Fig. 5.4 a Sural nerve biopsy from a patient with TTR Thr49Ala amyloidosis showing amorphous amyloid deposits within nerve trunks and blood vessel walls. *Congo red,* original magnification ×100. **b** Same section as (**a**) viewed between crossed polars showing typical *green birefringence* of amyloid. Note deposits in walls of endoneurial vessels

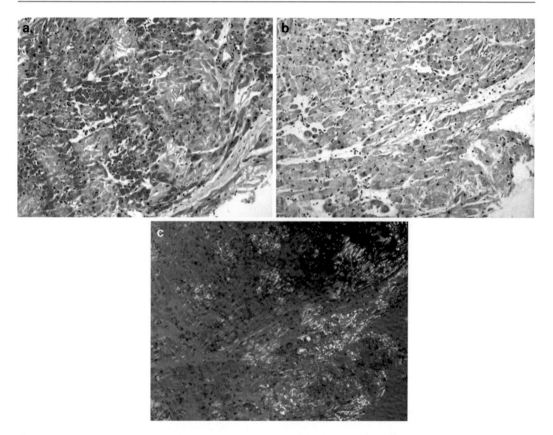

Fig. 5.5 **a** Endomyocardial biopsy from a patient with TTR Ser50Arg amyloidosis demonstrating amorphous amyloid deposits between myocardial fibrils. H&E ×100. **b** Section of same biopsy as in (**a**) stained with *Congo red* viewed in bright light. **c** Section of biopsy in (**a, b**) viewed between crossed polars showing typical *green birefringence* of amyloid

Germany, Italy, and the UK (Table 5.1). ApoAI is the major protein constituent of HDL. It is synthesized in the liver and small intestine. The pathogenesis of amyloid formation from apolipoprotein is very intriguing. Unlike transthyretin, only a portion of the ApoAI molecule is incorporated into amyloid fibrils. ApoAI is a single chain 243 amino acid residue protein. Only the amino terminal (approximately 93) residues have been identified in amyloid fibrils. ApoAI has mainly α-helical structure, so formation of β-pleated sheet amyloid fibrils must entail considerable tertiary structural rearrangement of the ApoAI fibril precursor [22]. An even more fascinating aspect of ApoAI amyloidosis is that the disease phenotype varies with the location of the gene mutation. Mutations in the amino terminal portion of ApoAI from residue 1 to 75, whether due to single amino acid substitutions or nucleotide deletions and insertions, are associated with renal pathology and/or hepatic amyloid deposition [23]. The renal pathology is fairly characteristic. Unlike immunoglobulin light chain, amyloid A, and some of the other hereditary amyloid diseases, the glomerulus is usually spared from ApoAI amyloid deposition (Fig. 5.6). The amyloid deposits in interstitial and medullary areas of the kidney. The clinical presentation is notable

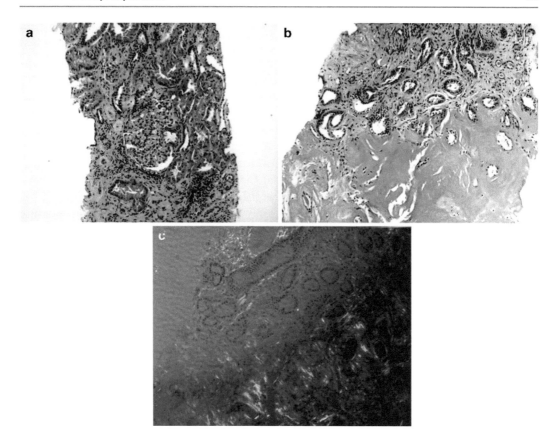

Fig. 5.6 a Renal biopsy from a patient with ApoAI Gly26Arg amyloidosis presenting with elevated serum creatinine but minimal proteinuria. Note lack of glomerular involvement. H&E magnification ×100. **b** Same renal biopsy as in (**a**) showing dense amyloid deposition at corticomedullary junction. **c** Section shown in (**b**) stained with *Congo red* and viewed through crossed polars

for the lack of proteinuria in the face of increasing renal insufficiency as measured by serum creatinine. For renal pathologists whose typical studies are focused on glomerular disease, ApoAI renal amyloid can be a diagnostic challenge. A similar picture may be seen in approximately 5 % of patients with AA (secondary) amyloidosis in which medullary amyloid deposition is a prominent feature. Hepatic deposition of amyloid is observed in patients with some of the amino terminal ApoAI mutations. The most notable is the Leu75Pro mutation which is usually an incidental finding at the time of cholecystectomy or liver

biopsy for other reasons than amyloid suspicion (Fig. 5.7). This particular syndrome is very slowly progressive and, while sometimes associated with renal impairment, does not appear to shorten longevity [24]. Only the Gly26Arg ApoAI amyloidosis is associated with peripheral neuropathy, and this manifestation has not been observed in all affected families (Fig. 5.8) [20]. Mutations in ApoAI from residue 90 on toward the carboxyl terminus of the molecule present the most fascinating feature of this disease [23, 25]. The typical presentation is with subepithelial laryngeal, cutaneous, and cardiac amyloid depo-

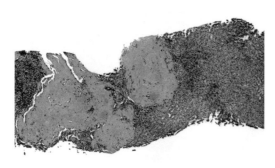

Fig. 5.7 Liver biopsy from a patient with ApoAI Arg75Pro amyloidosis with nodular deposition of amyloid. Congo red magnification ×40

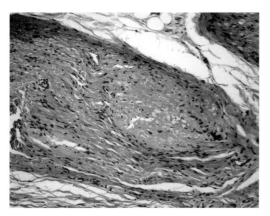

Fig. 5.8 Peripheral nerve of a patient with ApoAI Gly26Arg amyloidosis showing amorphous amyloid deposition within the nerve trunk. H&E ×100

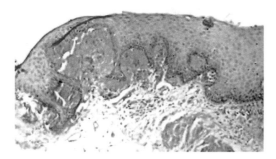

Fig. 5.9 *Congo red* stained section of laryngeal biopsy from a patient with ApoAI Arg173Pro amyloidosis showing dense subepithelial deposits. Congo red ×100

sition. Patients develop vocal hoarseness in early adult years (Fig. 5.9). A characteristic dusky coarse skin texture is often observed in the axillae and the nape of the neck (Fig. 5.10). Subsequently, restrictive cardiomyopathy leads to heart failure and death (Fig. 5.11), although one mutation (Leu170Pro) has been reported in an individual with only laryngeal amyloid and no evidence of more systemic deposition. This syndrome is associated with a number of mutations in the carboxyl terminal portion of ApoAI, but analysis of the amyloid fibril deposits reveals that only the amino terminal portion of the molecule is incorporated into the fibrils. It is obvious that catabolic processing of the mutated protein goes astray with the formation of inert amyloid fibril deposits.

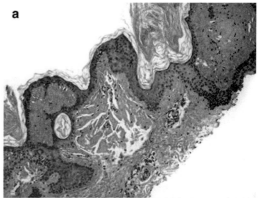

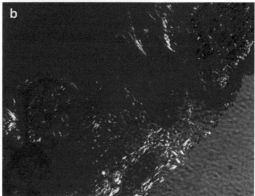

Fig. 5.10 a Skin biopsy from a patient with ApoAI Arg173Pro amyloidosis stained with *Congo red* showing subepithelial amyloid deposits. **b** Same skin biopsy specimen as Fig. 5.10a viewed between crossed polars

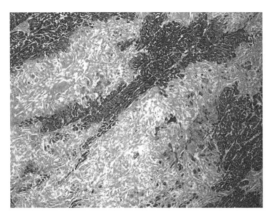

Fig. 5.11 Section of postmortem heart demonstrating marked loss of myocardial fibers and replacement with amyloid. Heart failure from restrictive cardiomyopathy is the usual cause of death in this disease. H&E ×40

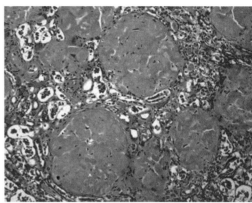

Fig. 5.12 Renal biopsy from a patient with fibrinogen Aα-chain Glu526Val amyloidosis showing typical histology with obliteration of glomerular architecture, loss of tubules, and appearance of glomeruli collapsing on one another. H&E ×100

Fibrinogen Aα-Chain

Fibrinogen Aα-chain amyloidosis is one of the easier forms of amyloidosis to recognize histologically. It typically gives glomerular deposition of amyloid with atrophy of the tubules and collapse of glomeruli on each other (Fig. 5.12). The clinical disease is rapidly progressive with proteinuria and hypertension, followed by azotemia. Fourteen mutations in fibrinogen Aα-chain have been described (Table 5.1). The most common, Glu526Val, which is relatively common in the USA but probably originated in Germany, is also found in many European countries [26, 27]. Penetrance of this condition is variable and the lack of informative family history can make the clinical diagnosis difficult. In many patients, the amyloid is detected by kidney biopsy, and in these cases the differentiation from AL and AA amyloidosis is imperative. Fibrinogen Aα- chain is synthesized by the liver and is a major component of the blood coagulation system. Only a carboxyl terminal fragment of the Aα-chain is incorporated into amyloid fibrils and, in all cases described thus far, this region has contained the altered amino acid residues. The fact that only a portion of fibrinogen Aα-chain is present in the

amyloid fibril probably explains why immunohistochemistry may not be very informative in this form of amyloidosis. In addition, at least three fibrinogen Aα-chain mutations involve single nucleotide deletions which result in out of frame transcriptions coding for an entirely new peptide which, of course, would not be recognized by antisera raised to the native protein. While DNA analysis by RFLP is available for some of the mutations, direct nucleotide sequencing is required to ascertain the genetic defect in many patients. This analysis usually requires the help of laboratories in amyloid research centers.

Gelsolin

Gelsolin amyloidosis may be associated with two mutations that occur at the same amino acid site in the protein. The most common Asp187Asn is found in families in Finland and occasionally in the USA and Japan [28]. The disease is characterized by peripheral neuropathy which causes facial palsy and lattice corneal dystrophy (Fig. 5.13). Amyloid deposition can be confirmed by histology of cornea tissue obtained at the time of cornea transplant. The deposits are indistinguishable from some of the localized forms of lattice dystrophy.

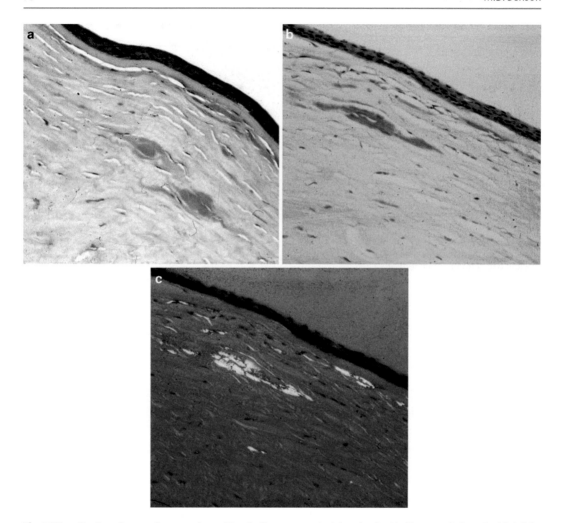

Fig. 5.13 **a** Section of cornea from a patient with gelsolin amyloidosis Asp187Asn showing amyloid deposits within the stroma of the cornea. H&E ×200. **b** Same cornea tissue as in (**a**) stained with *Congo red* viewed with bright light. **c** Section in Fig. 5.13b viewed between crossed polars showing typical *green birefringence* of amyloid

Gelsolin amyloidosis is truly a systemic disease and deposits are found in heart, kidney, and other tissues. Although usually not life threatening, patients homozygous for the Asp187Asn mutation have been reported to have accelerated systemic disease [29]. A second gelsolin mutation is Asp187Tyr which has been reported in kindreds in Denmark and Czechoslovakia with similar phenotype to the Finnish disease [30]. Recently, two more mutations in gelsolin have been discovered, one at amino acid position 167 (Gly→Arg) and the other at position 184 (Asn→Lys) (Table 5.1). Both are associated with nephropathy.

Lysozyme

Seven different mutations in the bacteriolytic enzyme, lysozyme, have been found associated with amyloidosis (Table 5.1). While amyloid deposits may be found in many organ systems, lysozyme amyloidosis is particularly nephropathic [31]. The histology is relatively typical of this disease with vascular, interstitial, and glomerular deposition (Fig. 5.14). The glomerular amyloid deposits are much less extensive than those seen in fibrinogen Aα-chain amyloidosis. Lysozyme amyloidosis tends to be a relatively

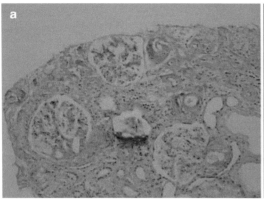

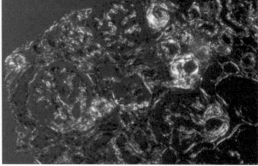

Fig. 5.14 a Renal biopsy from a patient with lysozyme amyloidosis (Phe57Ile) stained with *Congo red* showing amyloid deposition in glomeruli, interstitium, and vascu-lar structures. **b** Same section of renal biopsy as (**a**) viewed between crossed polars showing typical *green birefringence* of amyloid. H&E ×100

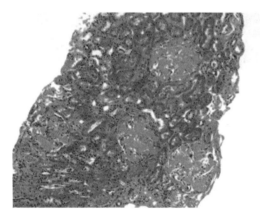

Fig. 5.15 Renal biopsy from a patient with ApoAII amy-loidosis with stop to Gly mutation showing dense deposi-tion of amyloid within glomeruli. H&E ×100

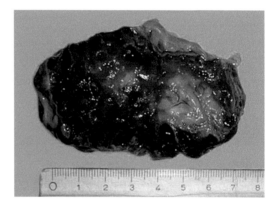

Fig. 5.16 Gross specimen of kidney removed after sev-eral years of dialysis for ApoAII amyloidosis

slowly progressive disease, and kidney transplan-tation may prolong life for 20 or more years [32]. Rarely, ALys can cause massive hepatic amyloi-dosis and has been associated with liver rupture.

minal 21 amino acid residue extension of the pro-tein is found in the amyloid fibril protein. Five different stop-codon mutations have been identified in families: four from the USA and one in Spain.

Apolipoprotein AII

ApoAII amyloidosis is also primarily nephropathic with extensive glomerular deposition of amyloid (Figs. 5.15, 5.16, 5.17) [33]. In far advanced cases, amyloid deposits are found in many organ systems. It is a relatively slowly progressive disease, and renal transplantation may prolong life for 10 or more years [34]. The inherited defect is in the stop codon for the ApoAII gene such that a carboxyl ter-

Cystatin C

Cystatin C amyloidosis is seen in families in Iceland that have a mutation in the cystatin gene that gives a Leu68Gln amino acid change [35, 36]. These patients develop cerebral amyloid angiopa-thy which is very similar to the more prevalent Aβ (Alzheimer protein) cerebral angiopathy. Patients die in their early adult to mid-age of recurrent cerebral hemorrhages.

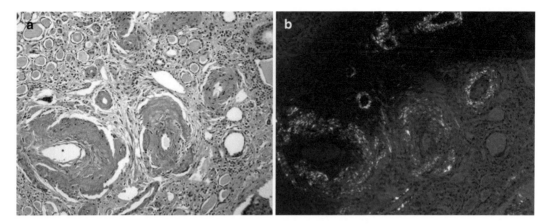

Fig. 5.17 (**a**) Section of nephrectomy specimen from a patient with ApoAII amyloidosis similar to the specimen in Fig. 5.16. Notice complete lack of glomerular structures and only remaining amyloid is within vascular walls. Congo red ×100. (**b**) Same section as Fig. 5.17a viewed between crossed polars showing typical *green birefringence* of amyloid

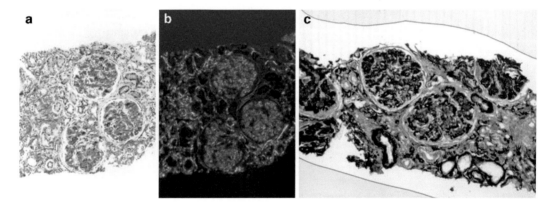

Fig. 5.18 (**a**) Renal biopsy of a patient with Lect2 amyloidosis showing glomerular, interstitial, and vascular deposition of amyloidosis. (**b**) Same biopsy section as Fig. 5.18a viewed between crossed polars with dense deposition of amyloid. (**c**) Same biopsy section as Fig. 5.18a, b treated with anti-Lect2 antibody using an antigen-retrieval technique showing specific staining of glomerular vessel and interstitial amyloid deposits. Slide developed with diaminobenzidine ×100

Lect2

Lect2 is a newly identified form of systemic amyloidosis which is noted for renal pathology [37]. Since its initial discovery, a large number of cases have been identified mainly from those renal biopsies for which no satisfactory diagnosis could be made. Unfortunately, several of these patients had been treated with chemotherapy on the misguided assumption that their renal amyloidosis was of AL (immunoglobulin light chain) origin. There is no evidence at the present time that Lect 2 amyloidosis is a hereditary form of amyloidosis, although a disproportionate number of patients have been identified of Hispanic ori-

gin and a few from the Punjab. Leukocyte chemotactic factor 2 (Lect2) is a normal serum protein that is synthesized principally by the liver. No specific function for the protein has been verified, although basic studies have suggested it may be a cartilage modulating factor (alternatively named chondromodulin). It may be overexpressed in certain liver diseases such as hepatocellular carcinoma, but whether increased synthesis is relative to generation of amyloidosis is not known. The renal pathology is highlighted by glomerular, vascular, and interstitial deposition of amyloid and can be fairly typical of the disease (Fig. 5.18). Most of the cases that have been reviewed have been fairly advanced with this tricompartmental distribution of amyloid deposition. Where the initial amyloid occurs and its phases of progression toward end-stage renal diseases are yet to be clarified. It is truly a systemic form of amyloidosis, and we have seen significant hepatic as well as renal deposition.

Conclusion

While the various types of genetically determined amyloidosis are relatively uncommon, it is extremely important that both the treating physician and the pathologist who interpret tissue biopsies are aware of these diseases. Determination of the correct type of amyloidosis can aid with prediction of organ system involvement and prognosis. Most important is to avoid a misdiagnosis as the standard treatment for the more common AL (immunoglobulin light chain, "primary") amyloidosis is chemotherapy. It is imperative to confirm the type of amyloidosis before going down the therapeutic pathway.

References

1. Sipe JD, Benson MD, Buxbaum JN, et al. Amyloid fibril protein nomenclature: 2010 recommendations from the nomenclature committee of the International Society of Amyloidosis. Amyloid. 2010;17(3–4):101–4.
2. Benson MD. Other systemic forms of amyloidosis. In: Gertz MA, Rajkumar SV, editors. Amyloidosis: diagnosis and treatment, Chapter 15. New York, Dordrecht, Heidelberg, London: Humana Press—Springer Science + Business Media, LLC; 2010. p. 205–25.
3. Zeldenrust SR, Benson MD. Familial and senile amyloidosis caused by transthyretin. In: Ramirez-Alvarado M, Kelly J, Dobson C, editors. Protein misfolding diseases: current and emerging principles and therapies, Part IV, Chap. 36. Hoboken, NJ: Wiley; 2010. p. 795–815.
4. Robbins J. Thyroxine-binding proteins. Prog Clin Biol Res. 1976;5:331–55.
5. Kanda Y, Goodman DS, Canfield RE, Morgan FJ. The amino acid sequence of human plasma prealbumin. J Biol Chem. 1974;249(21):6796–805.
6. Blake CCF, Geisow MJ, Oatley SJ. Structure of prealbumin: secondary, tertiary and quaternary interactions determined by Fourier refinement at 1.8 Å (angstrom). J Mol Biol. 1978;121(3):339–56.
7. Andrade C. A peculiar form of peripheral neuropathy. Familial atypical generalized amyloidosis with special involvement of the peripheral nerves. Brain. 1952;75(3):408–27.
8. Andrade C, Araki S, Block WD, et al. Hereditary amyloidosis. Arthritis Rheum. 1970;13(6):902–15.
9. Holmgren G, Bergstrom S, Drugge U, et al. Homozygosity for the transthyretin-Met30-gene in seven individuals with familial amyloidosis with polyneuropathy detected by restriction enzyme analysis of amplified genomic DNA sequences. Clin Genet. 1992;41(1):39–41.
10. Mahloudji M, Teasdall RD, Adamkiewicz JJ, Hartmann WH, Lambird PA, McKusick VA. The genetic amyloidoses. With particular reference to hereditary neuropathic amyloidosis, type II (Indiana or Rukavina type). Medicine. 1969;48(1):1–37.
11. Benson MD, Wallace MR, Tejada E, Baumann H, Page B. Hereditary amyloidosis. Description of a new American kindred with late onset cardiomyopathy. Arthritis Rheum. 1987;30(2):195–200.
12. Wallace MR, Dwulet FE, Williams EC, Conneally PM, Benson MD. Identification of a new hereditary amyloidosis prealbumin variant, Tyr-77, and detection of the gene by DNA analysis. J Clin Invest. 1988;81(1):189–93.
13. Falls HF, Jackson JH, Carey JG, Rukavina JG, Block WD. Ocular manifestations of hereditary primary systemic amyloidosis. Arch Ophthalmol. 1955;54(5):660–4.
14. Gorevic PD, Prelli FC, Wright J, Pras M, Frangione B. Systemic senile amyloidosis. Identification of a new prealbumin (transthyretin) variant in cardiac tissue: immunologic and biochemical similarity to one form of familial amyloidotic polyneuropathy. J Clin Invest. 1989;83(3):836–43.
15. Ng B, Connors LH, Davidoff R, Skinner M, Falk RH. Senile systemic amyloidosis presenting with heart failure: a comparison with light chain-associated amyloidosis. Arch Intern Med. 2005;165(12):1425–9.
16. Benson MD, Kincaid JC. Invited review: the molecular biology and clinical features of amyloid neuropathy. Muscle Nerve. 2007;36(4):411–23.
17. Benson MD, Breall J, Cummings OW, Liepnieks JJ. Biochemical characterization of amyloid by endomyocardial biopsy. Amyloid. 2009;16(1):9–14.
18. Vrana JA, Gamez JD, Madden BJ, Theis JD, Bergen 3rd HR, Dogan A. Classification of amyloidosis by laser microdissection and mass spectrometry-based proteomic analysis in clinical biopsy specimens. Blood. 2009;114(24):4957–9.
19. Benson MD. Amyloidosis. In: Scriver CR, Beaudet AL, Sly WS, Valle D, Childs B, Kinzler KW, Vogelstein B, editors. The metabolic and molecular bases of inherited disease, Part 22, Chap. 209, Connective tissue, vol. 4. 8th ed. New York: McGraw Hill Book Co; 2001. p. 5345–78.
20. Van Allen MW, Frohlich JA, Davis JR. Inherited predisposition to generalized amyloidosis. Neurology. 1969;19(1):10–25.
21. Nichols WC, Dwulet FE, Liepnieks J, Benson MD. Variant apolipoprotein AI as a major constituent of a human hereditary amyloid. Biochem Biophys Res Commun. 1988;156(2):762–8.

22. Nichols WC, Gregg RE, Brewer HB, Benson MD. A mutation in apolipoprotein A-I in the Iowa type of familial amyloidotic polyneuropathy. Genomics. 1990;8(2):318–23.

23. Hamidi Asl K, Liepnieks JJ, Nakamura M, Parker F, Benson MD. A novel apolipoprotein A-1 variant, Arg173Pro, associated with cardiac and cutaneous amyloidosis. Biochem Biophys Res Commun. 1999; 257(2):584–8.

24. Obici L, Palladini G, Giorgetti S, et al. Liver biopsy discloses a new apolipoprotein A-I hereditary amyloidosis in several unrelated Italian families. Gastroenterology. 2004;126(5):1416–22.

25. Hamidi Asl L, Liepnieks JJ, Hamidi Asl K, et al. Hereditary amyloid cardiomyopathy caused by a variant apolipoprotein AI. Am J Pathol. 1999;154(1): 221–7.

26. Uemichi T, Liepnieks JJ, Benson MD. Hereditary renal amyloidosis with a novel variant fibrinogen. J Clin Invest. 1994;93(2):731–6.

27. Uemichi T, Liepnieks JJ, Yamada T, Gertz MA, Bang N, Benson MD. A frame shift mutation in the fibrinogen Aα-chain gene in a kindred with renal amyloidosis. Blood. 1996;87(10):4197–203.

28. Meretoja J. Familial systemic paramyloidosis with lattice dystrophy of the cornea, progressive cranial neuropathy, skin changes and various internal symptoms. Ann Clin Res. 1969;1(4):314–24.

29. Maury CPJ, Kere J, Tolvanen R, de la Chapelle A. Homozygosity for the Asn187 gelsolin mutation in Finnish-type familial amyloidosis is associated with severe renal disease. Genomics. 1992;13(3):902–3.

30. de la Chapelle A, Tolvanen R, Boysen G, et al. Gelsolin-derived familial amyloidosis caused by asparagine or tyrosine substitution for aspartic acid at residue 187. Nat Genet. 1992;2(2):157–60.

31. Pepys MB, Hawkins PN, Booth DR, et al. Human lysozyme gene mutations cause hereditary systemic amyloidosis. Nature. 1993;362(6420):553–7.

32. Yazaki M, Farrell SA, Benson MD. A novel lysozyme mutation Phe57Ile associated with hereditary renal amyloidosis. Kidney Int. 2003;63(5):1652–7.

33. Benson MD, Liepnieks JJ, Yazaki M, et al. A new human hereditary amyloidosis: the result of a stop-codon mutation in the apolipoprotein AII gene. Genomics. 2001;72(3):272–7.

34. Magy N, Liepnieks JJ, Yazaki M, Kluve-Beckerman B, Benson MD. Renal transplantation for apolipoprotein AII amyloidosis. Amyloid. 2003;10(4):224–8.

35. Gudmundsson G, Hallgrimsson J, Jonasson TA, Bjarnason O. Hereditary cerebral hemorrhage with amyloidosis. Brain. 1972;95(2):387–404.

36. Ghiso J, Pons-Estel B, Frangione B. Hereditary cerebral amyloid angiopathy: the amyloid fibrils contain a protein which is a variant of cystatin C, an inhibitor of lysosomal cysteine proteases. Biochem Biophys Res Commun. 1986;136(2):548–54.

37. Benson MD, James S, Scott K, Liepnieks JJ, Kluve-Beckerman B. Leukocyte chemotactic factor 2: a novel renal protein. Kidney Int. 2008;74(2):218–22.

Dialysis-Associated Amyloidosis

6

Paweena Susantitaphong, Laura M. Dember, and Bertrand L. Jaber

Introduction

Dialysis-associated amyloidosis is a unique type of amyloidosis, affecting patients with chronic kidney disease treated with dialysis. It does not affect persons with normal or mildly impaired kidney function. Even though it is rarely a cause of death, dialysis-associated amyloidosis can lead to debilitating complications [1, 2]. Periarticular tissue and bone are the most common sites of amyloid deposition [1, 2]. Beta-2 microglobulin (β2m) is the amyloidogenic protein in dialysis-associated amyloidosis. The β2m amyloid deposits in tissue eventually cause symptoms and signs related to amyloidosis. The typical clinical manifestations are carpal tunnel syndrome, chronic arthropathy, spondyloarthropathies, subchondral bone cysts, and fractures.

β2m is the light chain component of the major histocompatibility complex (MHC) class-1 molecule. All cells that express MHC class-1 molecules synthesize β2m, which covalently binds to the heavy chain at the cell surface where it provides a stabilizing function [3]. When the MHC complex is shed from the cell surface, β2m dissociates from the heavy chain and enters the blood circulation or other body fluids, such as synovial fluid, as a glycosylated polypeptide with a molecular weight of 11,815 Da. β2m is cleared from the blood by the kidney where it is freely filtered through the glomerulus and almost fully reabsorbed and catabolized by the proximal tubule [4].

The average production rate of β2m is estimated at 2.4 mg/kg/day, but its generation rate may increase in chronic inflammatory states, infections, and lymphoproliferative disorders [5]. The normal serum β2m concentration is 1.5–3.0 mg/L. However, in patients with chronic kidney failure, the serum level may increase 10–60-fold reaching 20–50 mg/L, as a result of both increased production from chronic inflammation and decreased renal elimination, and dialyzer clearance [6].

P. Susantitaphong, MD
Division of Nephrology, Department of Medicine,
St. Elizabeth's Medical Center, Tufts University
School of Medicine, 736 Cambridge Street,
Boston, MA 02135, USA

Extracorporeal Multiorgan Support Dialysis Center,
Division of Nephrology, Department of Medicine,
King Chulalongkorn Memorial Hospital,
Chulalongkorn University, Bangkok, Thailand
e-mail: pesancerinus@hotmail.com

L.M. Dember, MD
Renal-Electrolyte and Hypertension Division,
Perelman School of Medicine, University of
Pennsylvania, Philadelphia, PA, USA
e-mail: ldember@upenn.edu

B.L. Jaber, MD, MS (✉)
Division of Nephrology, Department of Medicine,
St. Elizabeth's Medical Center, Tufts University
School of Medicine, 736 Cambridge Street,
Boston, MA 02135, USA
e-mail: bertrand.jaber@steward.org

© Springer International Publishing Switzerland 2015
M.M. Picken et al. (eds.), *Amyloid and Related Disorders*, Current Clinical Pathology,
DOI 10.1007/978-3-319-19294-9_6

While β2m is the major component of the amyloid deposits, in vitro and in vivo studies indicate that other molecules also play an important role in the pathogenesis of dialysis-associated amyloidosis. Some of these molecules include glycosaminoglycans, proteoglycans, apolipoprotein E, serum amyloid P component, phospholipids, and free fatty acids [7]. Knowledge about dialysis-associated amyloidosis might help pathologists identify this disorder and help clinicians provide better care for their patients.

A recent report of an autosomal dominant form of β2m amyloidosis in individuals with normal kidney function and normal circulating levels of β2m but with an inherited mutation producing a single amino acid alteration (Asp76Asn) suggests that a minor alteration in the amino acid sequence of β2m can render the protein amyloidogenic in a concentration-independent manner. The amino acid alteration also affects the tissue distribution of amyloid deposits with involvement in Asp76Asn β2m disease of nerves, gastrointestinal tract, heart, and liver rather than osteoarticular tissues [8].

Epidemiology

The incidence of dialysis-associated amyloidosis in the United States is not known as there are no large epidemiological or histological studies investigating this complication of long-term dialysis. However, a small study from Germany suggests that the incidence of carpal tunnel syndrome in the dialysis population, a known manifestation of dialysis-associated amyloidosis, is declining [9]. Although a definitive diagnosis can only be made histologically, tissue acquisition for this purpose is rarely attempted. In clinical practice, β2m amyloid osteoarticular deposits are usually diagnosed based on clinical and radiological findings. There has been little attempt to identify dialysis-associated amyloidosis that is not clinically apparent. Therefore, subclinical β2m amyloidosis may be more frequent than we realize [2].

The clinical syndrome of β2m amyloid osteoarthropathy is unusual in individuals who have been dialysis-dependent for fewer than 5 years and is

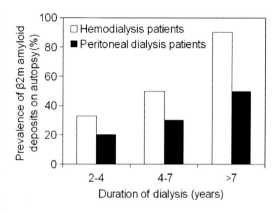

Fig. 6.1 Prevalence of β2 mamyloid deposits at autopsy according to duration of dialysis. The autopsy was performed on osteoarticular specimens obtained from 54 deceased patients who had received long-term hemodialysis and 26 deceased patients who had received peritoneal dialysis [10, 11]

most commonly seen after 10 years of dialysis (Fig. 6.1). However, an autopsy registry report from Belgium suggests that β2m amyloid deposits are present more often and earlier than is clinical disease. Examination of multiple joints obtained at autopsy from 54 patients with kidney failure treated with maintenance hemodialysis and age-matched control subjects revealed β2m amyloid deposits, as evidenced by Congo red positivity and anti-β2m immunostaining, in 48 % of the hemodialysis patients. The prevalence of amyloid deposits was 21 % among patients who had been dialyzed for less than 2 years, a population in whom clinically evident dialysis-associated amyloidosis is extremely rare. However, the prevalence of amyloid deposits increased progressively with duration of dialysis reaching 33 %, 50 %, 90 %, and 100 % at 2–4 years, 4–7 years, 7–13 years, and greater than 13 years, respectively [10]. In a similar study performed in 26 patients treated with peritoneal dialysis, the prevalence of β2m amyloid deposits was 20 %, 30 %, and 50 % for those on dialysis for less than 2 years, 2–4 years, and 4–7 years, respectively [11]. Thus, the prevalence was similar for peritoneal dialysis and hemodialysis patients matched for duration of kidney failure. Taken together, these studies suggest that β2m amyloid deposits occur early in chronic kidney failure, and well in advance of the development of clinically evident disease.

Pathophysiology

Although the mechanisms underlying β2m amyloid fibril formation and deposition have not been fully elucidated, significant advances have been achieved. Native β2m is the major structural component of β2m amyloid fibrils. In addition, just as with other types of amyloidosis, there are several other associated molecules including glycosaminoglycans (GAGs), particularly heparan sulfate and chondroitin sulfate, proteoglycans (PGs) such as chondroitin sulfate proteoglycan, apolipoprotein E (ApoE), serum amyloid P component, alpha2-macroglobulin, and plasma proteinase inhibitors [12].

In the clinical setting, the earliest deposition of β2m amyloid is observed in the cartilage tissue that contains numerous PGs such as aggrecan, biglycan, decorin, and lumican [12]. Decorin is also the component of the tendinous tissue present in the carpal tunnel. Several in vitro and in vivo studies that have helped elucidate the potential roles of these molecules in the formation of β2m amyloid fibrils will be reviewed.

In vitro studies suggest that there are three phases of β2m amyloid fibril formation: nucleation, extension, and stabilization. β2m amyloid fibril formation occurs at a low pH in vitro. Partial unfolding of β2m is thought to be a prerequisite to its assembly into amyloid fibrils. A pH of 2.0–3.0 appears to be optimal for promoting the extension of β2m amyloid fibrils. Indeed, some

PGs, especially biglycan, can induce the polymerization of acid-denatured β2m amyloid fibrils. Moreover, low concentration of trifluoroethanol and very small concentration of sodium dodecyl sulfate can induce partial unfolding of β2m amyloid fibrils, resulting in the extension of β2m amyloid fibrils at a neutral pH as well as fibril stabilization. Some GAGs, especially heparin, can also enhance fibril extension in the presence of trifluoroethanol at neutral pH [13]. Finally, ApoE, GAGs, and PGs can form stable complexes with fibrils playing a role in the stabilization of β2m amyloid fibrils.

A hypothesized model for the deposition of β2m amyloid fibrils in vivo has been proposed [12] (Fig. 6.2), whereby fibril formation takes place through a nucleation-dependent polymerization model, followed by several molecular interactions that lead to stabilization of the fibrils, rendering them resistant to proteolysis.

The earliest stage of β2m amyloid deposition occurs in the cartilage, followed by extension to the capsule and synovium. To explain this specific tissue involvement, it is important to gain understanding of the biochemical composition and physiology of these tissues. In the joint space, the synovial fluid is composed primarily of hyaluronan and sulfated GAGs and is produced by synovial fibroblasts, recirculating into the blood stream via the lymphatic system. The synovial membrane consists of an interstitium or subintima filled with GAGs, matrix proteins, and

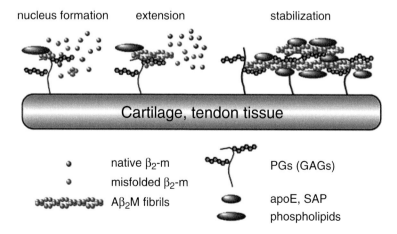

Fig. 6.2 A hypothetical in vivo model for the molecular mechanisms incriminated in the deposition of β2m amyloid fibrils. Modified with permission from [12]

fibroblasts. Synoviocytes are classified as macrophage-like and fibroblast-like resident cells based on morphology and function. Macrophage-like synoviocytes tend to produce cytokines (e.g., interleukin-1β [IL-1β] and tumor necrosis factor-α [TNF-α]), whereas fibroblast-like synoviocytes produce matrix proteins (e.g., fibronectin, laminin, and collagen), GAGs (both nonsulfated [hyaluronan] and sulfated [e.g., chondroitin-6 sulfate, dermatan sulfate, and heparin sulfate]), and matrix metalloproteinases (MMPs) (e.g., collagenase and stromelysin). In the normal joint, the majority of the cells residing in the synovial intimal lining are fibroblast-like, but this ratio may vary in inflammatory joint disorders. Macrophage-like synoviocytes in the intimal lining appear to originate from the bone marrow, whereas intimal fibroblasts-like cells originate from the subintima [14]. The cartilage is composed of chondrocytes, type-2 collagen, and GAGs, the most abundant of which is aggregan.

β2m has specific affinity for collagen, which is dose-dependent. This may explain its predilection to deposit in articular structures where collagen is abundant and also explain why in situ, heparan sulfate is the most common GAG component of β2m amyloid. Interestingly, native β2m in solution is a highly soluble monomeric protein, which is incapable of amyloid generation under physiological conditions at neutral pH. However, β2m amyloid proteins obtained from patients undergoing treatment with chronic dialysis are not uniformly water soluble suggesting heterogeneity in terms of superstructure [15]. Other factors may be involved after β2m deposition, including modification by advanced glycation endproducts (AGEs) [16] such as imidazolone, carboxymethyl lysine, and pentosidine, molecules known to accumulate in uremia.

Advanced glycation endproducts have proinflammatory properties and induce macrophage chemotaxis with the release of pro-inflammatory cytokines, thereby contributing to joint inflammation. Furthermore, AGE-modified β2m appears to interact with the AGE receptor present on monocytes and macrophages, thus stimulating the release of platelet-derived growth factors,

IL-6, TNF-α, and IL-1β. AGE-modified β2m can also induce bone resorption by stimulating collagenase synthesis, leading to collagen degradation and connective tissue breakdown, resulting in the creation of a potential nidus for β2m deposition. Moreover, AGE-modified β2m can decrease the synthesis of type-1 collagen by fibroblasts. After deposition, β2m activates synovial fibroblasts to produce MMPs such as stromelysin, which cause articular destruction [17]. Serum stromelysin is elevated in patients with dialysis-associated amyloidosis, thereby linking β2m-deposition with destructive arthropathy [18]. Moreover, β2m stimulates mRNA and protein synthesis of IL-6 by osteoblasts, a potent bone-resorbing cytokine. Therefore, theoretically both hormonal and local regulatory factors can aggravate the deleterious effects of β2m on bone resorption [17]. β2m also appears to have osteoclastogenic effects that may be relevant for the bone cystic formations observed in β2m amyloidosis [19]. Interestingly, one study detected non-fibrillar β2m aggregates in the spleen and heart, which suggests that accumulation of the protein may precede amyloidogenesis, at least in the nonskeletal tissues [20].

In summary, the clinical manifestations of dialysis-associated amyloidosis are likely the result of complex in situ inflammatory reactions, induced by monocytes and macrophages, synovial cells, osteoblasts, and osteoclasts in response to β2m, AGE, and AGE-modified β2m. Inflammatory local bone destruction can also precipitate the migration of inflammatory cells, resulting in the release of more cytokines and further tissue destruction [16]. The pathogenesis of β2m amyloidosis is summarized in Fig. 6.3.

Risk Factors

Although the retention of β2m is a prerequisite for the development of β2m amyloidosis [21], there are other patient- and dialysis-related risk factors. Advanced age and duration of dialysis are important predictors of this complication. Indeed, β2m amyloidosis is seen earlier in older patients despite shorter duration of dialysis.

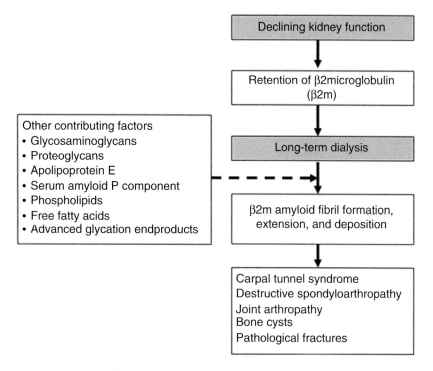

Fig. 6.3 Proposed pathogenesis of β2m amyloidosis (Reprinted with permission from [12])

In one study from Japan, among patients receiving dialysis for 20–24, 25–29, and ≥ 30 years, the incidence of orthopedic surgical interventions related to dialysis-associated amyloidosis was 25 %, 66 %, and 78 %, respectively [22]. Carboxymethyl lysine, which is an AGE found on proteins and lipids as a result of oxidative stress and chemical glycation, accumulates with aging and in uremia, and serum levels have been shown to predict development of the carpal tunnel syndrome, a clinical manifestation of dialysis-associated amyloidosis [23]. Measures of oxidative stress, including levels of superoxide dismutase and malonyldialdehyde, have also been associated with dialysis-associated amyloidosis [24].

In terms of dialysis-related factors, cellulose-based dialyzer membranes, previously used in conventional hemodialysis, have small pores that are impermeable to β2m and are considered less compatible with blood components resulting in activation of several inflammatory pathways including the complement system [25]. These dialyzers were believed to increase the intradialytic generation of β2m, thereby contributing to further accumulation of this molecule. Synthetic polymers, which were subsequently developed, are more permeable to β2m and are known as high-flux dialyzers. These filters also possess more biocompatible properties and have a lower complement-activating potential. Although the removal of circulating β2m can be enhanced by the use of high-flux dialyzers, and other novel therapies such as hemodiafiltration, frequent hemodialysis, and hemoperfusion, β2m continues to accumulate over time. The predicted annual net retention of β2m according to varying duration and frequency of high-flux hemodialysis is shown in Fig. 6.4. The use of high-flux dialyzer would be expected to delay but not prevent the development of β2m amyloidosis. An additional potential dialysis-related contributor to β2m accumulation is the contamination of dialysate water with bacterial products. This can induce host inflammatory responses during dialysis including cytokine production, which may accelerate the course of

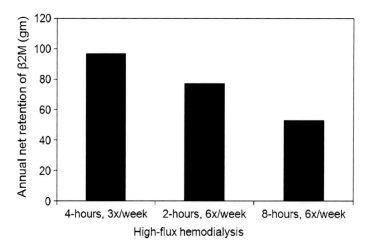

Fig. 6.4 Predicted annual retention of β2 microglobulin according to session length and frequency of high-flux hemodialysis

dialysis-associated amyloidosis. Several studies have demonstrated that the use of ultrapure dialysate, which has undergone a terminal filtration process aimed at removal of bacterial products, results in a reduction of cytokine production and circulating levels of IL-6 and C-reactive protein [26]. However, the potential long-term salutary effect of this strategy on the development of β2m amyloidosis is at present unknown, although in a recent cross-sectional study of 147 patients, the prevalence of suspected or confirmed dialysis-associated amyloidosis was 68 % among patients dialyzed with low-flux dialyzers compared to 28 % among those dialyzed with high-flux dialyzers and against ultrapure dialysate [23].

In summary, advanced age, the uremic milieu, and dialysis-related variables including dialyzer characteristics and the dialysate water purity may impact the molecular composition of the cartilage and other connective tissues, providing optimal conditions for β2m amyloid fibril formation and the resulting associated morbidity [27].

Clinical Manifestations

Carpal Tunnel Syndrome

The carpal tunnel syndrome is the most common presentation of β2m amyloidosis [28] and is usually bilateral and progressive. The clinical manifestations are the result of entrapment of the median nerve. Typical presentations include paresthesias of the palmar surface of the thumb, forefinger, and third and medial half of the fourth fingers. The pain is usually exacerbated by dialysis and is worse at night or during activities that impinge on the nerve such as wrist flexion or extension. Atrophy of the hand muscles may eventually occur. However, it is also important to consider other causes of the carpal tunnel syndrome, including other types of amyloid (e.g., light chain amyloid [AL] and transthyretin amyloid [ATTR]) as well as ischemic or traumatic median nerve injury as a result of the ipsilateral creation of an arteriovenous fistula or graft.

Scapulohumeral and Other Arthropathies

β2m amyloid fibrils commonly deposit in and around the rotator cuff. This results in shoulder pain that is worse while in the supine position and impairment with daily activities including getting dressed. Chronic arthralgias of the shoulders, knees, and hips have also been reported, spanning from minor discomfort to loss of range of motion with severe debilitating pain. Chronic joint effusion can also develop, which tend to be pauci-cellular.

Bone Cysts and Pathological Fractures

Subchondral bone cysts and articular erosions are pathognomonic findings of β2m amyloidosis. These lesions can multiply and enlarge in size on serial imaging studies, mimicking cancer-related bone lytic lesions, and can result in pathological fractures, including hip fractures [29].

Destructive Spondyloarthropathy

Destructive spondyloarthropathy is associated with symptoms related to myelopathy or radioculopathy with pain and stiffness of the spine. The cervical spine is most frequently affected (85 %), followed by the lumbar (10 %) and thoracic (5 %) spine. Involvement of the second cervical vertebrae can result in life threatening vertical subluxation of the odontoid process. This potential complication should be suspected and ruled out in patients on long-term dialysis with chronic neck pain being scheduled for surgery that would require endotracheal intubation for general anesthesia.

Visceral Involvement

Autopsy data demonstrate that β2m amyloidosis can also involve visceral tissues. Visceral amyloid deposition occurs late (after more than 15 years of hemodialysis). The heart is the most commonly involved organ, followed by the gastrointestinal system (with bowel infarction and perforation), lung, and spleen [30, 31]. Nonfibrillar deposits of β2m have also been detected in the heart and spleen extracts [20].

Interestingly, whereas vascular and interstitial amyloid deposits are demonstrable in visceral organs, they are rarely observed in the vessels of osteoarticular tissues. Subendothelial amyloid nodules protruding into the vessel lumen have also been described, leading to tissue ischemia and occasionally wall perforation [32]. Involvement of the genitourinary tract includes the development of kidney and bladder calculi containing β2m deposits, which can cause obstruction [33].

Clinical Diagnosis

The clinical diagnosis of β2m amyloidosis is primarily suspected on the basis of the history. Patients rarely display symptoms until they have received dialysis for at least 5 years [34], presenting with symptoms of the carpal tunnel syndrome, shoulder pain, and typically, cervical radioculopathy or myelopathy.

On physical examination, findings of the carpal tunnel syndrome include diminished pin-prick sensation in the median nerve distribution or thenar muscle atrophy. The Hoffman-Tinel test and Phalen test may increase the sensitivity and specificity of early detection of the carpal tunnel syndrome. Joint swelling can be found in chronic arthropathy, and limited shoulder range of motion may reflect amyloid-related rotator cuff tears. Cervical tenderness and radioculopathy usually reflect more destructive spondyloarthropathy, and some patients may develop pathological fracture of long bones [29]. β2m amyloid deposition in the myocardium may result in congestive heart failure, and its accumulation in bowel tissue has been associated with reports of intestinal obstruction and bleeding.

Differential Diagnosis

If β2m amyloidosis is suspected based on Congo red positivity of tissue; other types of amyloidoses such as AA, AL or ATTR cannot be excluded until the presence of β2m in the deposits is confirmed by immunostaining using anti-β2m antibodies or by proteomic methods. Furthermore, other causes of bone disease in dialysis patients need to be ruled out including that associated with secondary hyperparathyroidism.

Clinical Investigations

Radiological Imaging

Plain X-Rays

Radiolucencies of various sizes within the cortical and medullary bone are the characteristic findings (Fig. 6.5a) [35]. Fine sclerotic margins are usually present without matrix calcification.

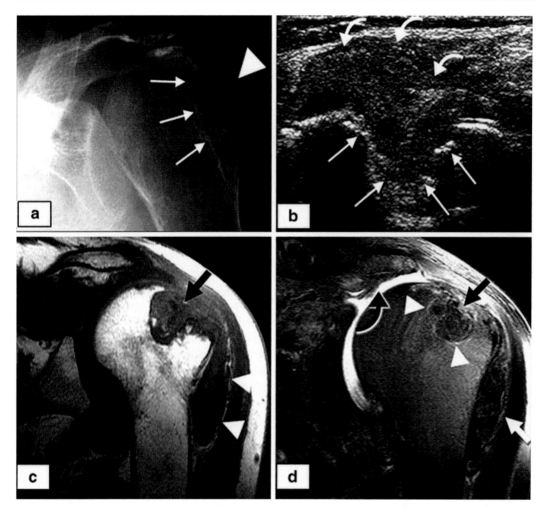

Fig. 6.5 (**a**) Conventional radiograph showing a well-defined cystic lesion (*arrowhead*) with sclerotic rim (*arrows*) in the superior–posterior humeral head. (**b**) Ultrasound of the shoulder showing erosion of the humeral head (*straight arrows*) and communicating with the joint space. Erosions are filled with echogenic amyloid tissue (*curved arrows*). (**c**) Coronal T1-weighted magnetic resonance image showing osteolysis in the superior–posterior humeral head and communicating with the joint (*arrow*). Low-signal-intensity tissue representing amyloid deposition appears within the lesion. Amyloid deposits are also visible within the subdeltoid bursa between the deltoid muscle and humerus (*arrowheads*). (**d**) Corresponding T2-weighted magnetic resonance image of the same lesions that are characteristic for amyloidosis. Signal of amyloid tissue (*straight arrows*) remains low with the exception of a small rim of high intensity around intraosseous lesion (*arrowheads*). Complete rupture of the supraspinatus tendon (*curved arrow*) is apparent. Reprinted with permission from [35]

The cysts are typically bilateral, locating in the periarticular bones and ligamentous areas. A large amount of deposits may result in pathological fracture. In addition, periarticular soft tissue masses, erosive changes, joint destruction, subluxation, and dislocation can also be observed.

Secondary hyperparathyroidism-associated brown tumors are other causes of lytic bone lesions observed in long-term dialysis patients. However, brown tumors tend to co-localize with subperiosteal and subchondral bone resorption. Moreover, brown tumors are not associated with para-articular lesions.

Scintigraphy

Scintigraphy with I^{123} radiolabeled serum amyloid P, iodohippurate sodium I^{131} β2m, or In^{111} β2m is an imaging technique that assesses the total body burden of amyloid deposits in long-term dialysis patients. Of note however, scintigraphy with In^{111} radiolabeled β2m tracer, which uses recombinant human β2m, has been shown to provide higher quality images while reducing total radiation exposure [36]. Unfortunately, these imaging techniques are not widely available in clinical practice and remain experimental.

Ultrasonography

Ultrasound has been used for the diagnosis of scapulohumeral joint disease by demonstrating tendon thickness, accumulation of joint fluid, and presence of amyloid deposits, in the form of echogenic pads of material between muscle layers and in intra- and peri-articular areas (Fig. 6.5b) [35]. In one study, the presence of a rotator cuff thickness of greater than 8 mm coupled to echogenic pads found between the rotator cuff muscle layers was shown to correlate with clinical or histological evidence of β2m amyloidosis, with a sensitivity of 72–79 % and specificity of 79–100 % [37].

X-Ray Computed Tomography

X-ray computed tomography can identify pseudotumors, representing intermediate attenuation and pseudocystic lesions in the juxta-articular bone. It is the best imaging study to detect small osteolytic lesions and may be useful to assess the distribution and extension of destructive changes.

Magnetic Resonance Imaging

Typical magnetic resonance imaging characteristics of β2m amyloid lesions are detected on long T1 and short T2 relaxation times, showing low-to-intermediate signal intensity. This imaging study can be helpful to differentiate destructive amyloid-related spondyloarthropathies from infectious processes, which typically feature a low signal on T1 and a high signal on T2 (Fig. 6.5c and d) [35].

Tissue Biopsy

Histopathological examination is the gold standard technique for diagnosing β2m amyloidosis. The diagnosis is made on the basis of positive Congo red staining with typical green-yellow birefringence under polarized light, coupled to positive immunostaining of Congo red-positive deposits with an anti-β2m antibody [38, 39] (Fig. 6.6) or by proteomic methods.

Since β2m amyloidosis involves the cartilaginous components of the joints in the early stages of the disease, it is not readily accessible by biopsy. Synovial fragments obtained from arthroscopy have been used to identify Congo red-positive deposits with limited success. Unfortunately, the yield of other investigations such as subcutaneous fat and rectal biopsies is even lower.

Three pathological stages of β2m amyloid have been described [38]. In stage 1, the β2m amyloid deposits are found only on the cartilage surface as a thin rim of amyloid along the joint space or as small globular-like deposits deeper in the cartilage. In stage 2, the β2m amyloid deposits involve capsules and synovia with evidence of proliferation and hyperplasia of the synovial lining, which is not associated with infiltration of macrophages. In stage 3, large β2m amyloid deposits are detected along with recruitment of macrophages. This stage is associated with marginal bone erosions on plain X-rays.

Treatment

Supportive Treatment

Nonsteroidal anti-inflammatory drugs, intra-articular injection of steroids, and low-dose oral corticosteroids can be used to ameliorate symptoms of joint pain and inflammation. In addition to physical therapy, wrist splints, cervical collars, lumbar corsets, knee braces, and immobilization for spondyloarthropathies are also helpful.

When the disease is resistant to medical therapy or patients experience significant disability, surgical therapy should be considered. Surgical

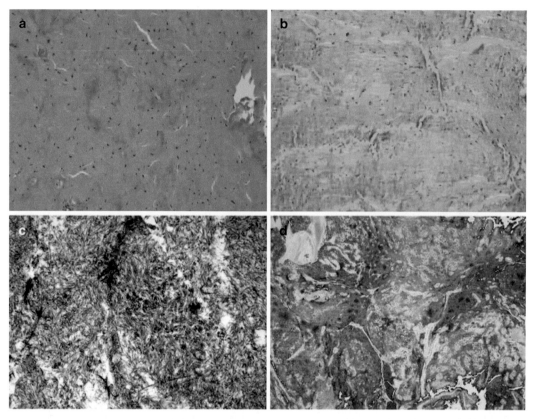

Fig. 6.6 Tissue biopsy specimen obtained from a shoulder nodule. (**a**) Histopathology showing areas of acellular glassy pink amorphous material typically seen in amyloidosis. (**b**) Congo red stain showing apple-green birefrin-gence consistent with amyloid. (**c**) Electron microscopy showing typical nonbranching amyloid fibrils. (**d**) Positive immunohistochemistry stain confirming β2-microglobulin amyloidosis. Reprinted with permission from [39]

interventions including carpal tunnel decompression, total joint replacement, and laminectomy with spinal stabilization may be the best available treatment choice to alleviate pain and restore function. Unfortunately, relapses after surgery due to ongoing accumulation of β2m amyloid deposits are common.

Specific Treatment

Although novel extracorporeal treatment modalities such as online hemodiafiltration [40, 41], hemofiltration [42], frequent hemodialysis [43, 44], and direct hemoperfusion using the selective β2m adsorption Lixelle column [45, 46] have all

be shown to enhance removal of β2m [47, 48], alleviate pain in some instances, reduce the radiolucency of bone cysts, and improve objective quality of life measures [29], they do not provide a cure for the disease. In a large survey of 345 Japanese patients with dialysis-associated amyloidosis on dialysis for an average of 26 years, and receiving treatment with the β2m adsorption Lixelle column for an average of 3.5 years, 91 % felt that their amyloidosis-related symptoms did not worsen, and the treating physicians felt that the treatment was effective or partially effective in 73 % of the patients [49]. These findings suggest that the Lixelle column might arrest the progression of dialysis-associated amyloidosis.

Doxycycline, a member of the tetracycline family of antibiotics, has been shown to inhibit formation of several types of amyloid fibrils in vitro or in animal models. Because tetracyclines achieve high tissue concentrations in the skeletal system, the use of doxycline for β2m amyloidosis is particularly appealing. In a recent case series, three patients with dialysis-associated amyloidosis had reductions in articular pain and improvements in range of motion with daily administration of doxycycline despite the persistence of amyloid deposits by magnetic resonance imaging [50]. The efficacy and safety of this promising therapy require further study.

Successful kidney transplantation remains the only effective treatment of dialysis-associated amyloidosis as it provides rapid resolution of symptoms including joint pain. Following kidney transplantation, new amyloid formation should cease with restoration of kidney function. However, consistent with the known tissue stability of all types of amyloid deposits, histological demonstration of β2m amyloid and radiological findings such as bone cysts persist during long-term follow-up despite improvement in symptoms [51].

Prevention

Dialysis Modality

The main determinants of β2m removal during dialytic therapies include the treatment modality (i.e., hemodialysis, peritoneal dialysis, hemofiltration, or hemodiafiltration), the dialyzer solute clearance characteristics, the treatment duration, and the ultrafiltration volume [52]. In clinical practice, most patients receive hemodialysis thrice weekly using high-flux dialyzers, which have been shown in post-hoc analyses, to reduce all-cause and cardiovascular mortality compared with low-flux dialyzers particularly among patients who had survived more than 3.7 years of dialysis [53, 54]. These observations argue for a potential link between the vascular β2m amyloid deposits and the epidemic of cardiovascular disease in the dialysis population [2]. High-

molecular-weight cut-off (50–60 kDa) dialyzers have been shown to be more effective at decreasing circulating levels of β2m than standard high-flux dialyzers [55, 56]. Furthermore, compared to low-flux hemodialysis, convective dialytic therapies, as defined by the use of high-flux hemodialysis, hemofiltration, or hemodiafiltration, have been shown to enhance the removal of β2m and decrease circulating levels of β2m, pentosidine, and superoxide dismutase [57]. The potential prevention of dialysis-associated amyloidosis using these dialytic therapies requires further study.

Ultrapure Dialysate

Studies have demonstrated that the production of cytokines by blood leukocytes correlates with the bacterial count and endotoxin level in the dialysate, and with the use of high-dialyzers that are more permeable to soluble bacterial products, thereby increasing the synthesis of β2m. The Association for the Advancement of Medical Instrumentation defines ultrapure dialysate according to a bacterial count limit of less than 0.1 colony forming units/ml and an endotoxin level of less than 0.03 endotoxin unit/ml. The use of ultrapure dialysate has been shown to decrease circulating levels of β2m and pentosidine [58], and the prevalence of dialysis-related amyloidosis may be lower among patients dialyzed with high-flux dialyzers and against ultrapure dialysate compared to those dialyzed with low-flux dialyzers [23], which is in support of this hypothesis. Although to date, there is no clinical trial demonstrating a clear benefit of ultrapure dialysate in terms of reduction in the rate of dialysis-associated amyloidosis, ultrapure dialysate should be considered in the setting of dialysis modalities that are designed to enhance the removal of β2m such as high-flux hemodialysis or hemodiafiltration, and which utilize dialyzers that are highly permeable to high-molecular weight solutes, including dialysate bacterial contaminants, thereby increasing generation of β2m through activation of the immune system.

Conclusion

In conclusion, the incidence of dialysis-associated amyloidosis and the precise mechanisms of β2m amyloidogenesis remain poorly understood. Histological evidence of β2m amyloid deposition is demonstrable early in the course of the disease in a substantial proportion of patients with kidney failure and is not restricted to osteoarticular tissue. Therefore, early detection especially in high-risk patients may be important to prevent or delay disease progression and development of debilitating complications. Supportive treatment modalities include the use of high-flux hemodialysis, hemofiltration, hemodiafiltration, ultrapure dialysate, and selective β2m adsorption with the Lixelle hemoperfusion column. The future development of β2m fibrillogenesis inhibitors is another promising treatment strategy [59]. For now, however, the most effective treatment is kidney transplantation, although not available to the majority of the patients.

References

1. Sergio R, Acchiardo M. Chapter 79—dialysis amyloidosis, section 25- dialysis amyloidosis. Handbook of Dialysis Therapy 4th ed. In: Allen R, Nissenson M, Richard N, Fine MD, editors. Saunders: Elsevier; 2007. p 1041–7.
2. Dember LM, Jaber BL. Dialysis-related amyloidosis: late finding or hidden epidemic? Semin Dial. 2006;19(2):105–9. Epub 2006/03/23.
3. Harris HW, Gill 3rd TJ. Expression of class I transplantation antigens. Transplantation. 1986;42(2):109–17.
4. Bernier GM, Conrad ME. Catabolsm of human beta-2-microglobulin by the rat kidney. Am J Physiol. 1969;217(5):1359–62. Epub 1969/11/01.
5. Miyata T, Jadoul M, Kurokawa K, Van Ypersele de Strihou C. Beta-2 microglobulin in renal disease. J Am Soc Nephrol. 1998;9(9):1723–35. Epub 1998/09/04.
6. Drueke TB, Massy ZA. Beta2-microglobulin. Semin Dial. 2009;22(4):378–80. Epub 2009/08/28.
7. Yamamoto S, Kazama JJ, Narita I, Naiki H, Gejyo F. Recent progress in understanding dialysis-related amyloidosis. Bone. 2009;45 Suppl 1:S39–42. Epub 2009/03/24.
8. Valleix S, Gillmore JD, Bridoux F, Mangione PP, Dogan A, Nedelec B, et al. Hereditary systemic amyloidosis due to Asp76Asn variant beta2-microglobulin. N Engl J Med. 2012;366(24):2276–83. Epub 2012/06/15.
9. Schwalbe S, Holzhauer M, Schaeffer J, Galanski M, Koch KM, Floege J. Beta 2-microglobulin associated amyloidosis: a vanishing complication of long-term hemodialysis? Kidney Int. 1997;52(4):1077–83. Epub 1997/11/05.
10. Jadoul M, Garbar C, Noel H, Sennesael J, Vanholder R, Bernaert P, et al. Histological prevalence of beta 2-microglobulin amyloidosis in hemodialysis: a prospective post-mortem study. Kidney Int. 1997;51(6):1928–32. Epub 1997/06/01.
11. Jadoul M, Garbar C, Vanholder R, Sennesael J, Michel C, Robert A, et al. Prevalence of histological beta2-microglobulin amyloidosis in CAPD patients compared with hemodialysis patients. Kidney Int. 1998;54(3):956–9. Epub 1998/09/12.
12. Naiki H, Yamamoto S, Hasegawa K, Yamaguchi I, Goto Y, Gejyo F. Molecular interactions in the formation and deposition of beta2-microglobulin-related amyloid fibrils. Amyloid. 2005;12(1):15–25. Epub 2005/08/04.
13. Yamamoto S, Hasegawa K, Yamaguchi I, Tsutsumi S, Kardos J, Goto Y, et al. Low concentrations of sodium dodecyl sulfate induce the extension of beta 2-microglobulin-related amyloid fibrils at a neutral pH. Biochemistry. 2004;43(34):11075–82. Epub 2004/08/25.
14. Moe SM, Chen NX. The role of the synovium and cartilage in the pathogenesis of beta(2)-microglobulin amyloidosis. Semin Dial. 2001;14(2):127–30. Epub 2001/03/27.
15. Heegaard NH. beta(2)-microglobulin: from physiology to amyloidosis. Amyloid. 2009;16(3):151–73. Epub 2009/08/07.
16. Niwa T. Dialysis-related amyloidosis: pathogenesis focusing on AGE modification. Semin Dial. 2001;14(2):123–6. Epub 2001/03/27.
17. Tran M, Rutecki GW, Sprague SM. The pathogenesis of beta(2)-microglobulin-induced bone lesions in dialysis-related amyloidosis. Semin Dial. 2001;14(2):131–3. Epub 2001/03/27.
18. Naganuma T, Sugimura K, Uchida J, Tashiro K, Yoshimura R, Takemoto Y, et al. Increased levels of serum matrix metalloproteinase-3 in haemodialysis patients with dialysis-related amyloidosis. Nephrology (Carlton). 2008;13(2):104–8. Epub 2008/02/16.
19. Kazama JJ, Maruyama H, Gejyo F. Osteoclastogenesis and osteoclast activation in dialysis-related amyloid osteopathy. Am J Kidney Dis. 2001;38(4 Suppl 1):S156–60. Epub 2001/09/29.
20. Stoppini M, Mangione P, Monti M, Giorgetti S, Marchese L, Arcidiaco P, et al. Proteomics of beta2-microglobulin amyloid fibrils. Biochim Biophys Acta. 2005;1753(1):23–33. Epub 2005/09/13.
21. Gejyo F, Homma N, Suzuki Y, Arakawa M. Serum levels of beta 2-microglobulin as a new form of amyloid protein in patients undergoing long-term hemodialysis. N Engl J Med. 1986;314(9):585–6. Epub 1986/02/27.

22. Yamamoto S, Kazama JJ, Maruyama H, Nishi S, Narita I, Gejyo F. Patients undergoing dialysis therapy for 30 years or more survive with serious osteoarticular disorders. Clin Nephrol. 2008;70(6):496–502. Epub 2008/12/04.

23. Schiffl H. Impact of advanced dialysis technology on the prevalence of dialysis-related amyloidosis in long-term maintenance dialysis patients. Hemodial Int. 2014;18(1):136–41. Epub 2013/05/31.

24. Celik G, Capraz I, Yontem M, Bilge M, Unaldi M, Mehmetoglu I. The relationship between the antioxidant system, oxidative stress and dialysis-related amyloidosis in hemodialysis patients. Saudi J Kidney Dis Transpl. 2013;24(6):1157–64. Epub 2013/11/16.

25. Jaradat MI, Moe SM. Effect of hemodialysis membranes on beta 2-microglobulin amyloidosis. Semin Dial. 2001;14(2):107–12. Epub 2001/03/27.

26. Schiffl H, Lang SM, Stratakis D, Fischer R. Effects of ultrapure dialysis fluid on nutritional status and inflammatory parameters. Nephrol Dial Transplant. 2001;16(9):1863–9. Epub 2001/08/28.

27. Gejyo F, Narita I. Current clinical and pathogenetic understanding of beta2-m amyloidosis in long-term haemodialysis patients. Nephrology (Carlton). 2003;8(Suppl):S45–9. Epub 2004/03/12.

28. Danesh F, Ho LT. Dialysis-related amyloidosis: history and clinical manifestations. Semin Dial. 2001;14(2):80–5. Epub 2001/03/27.

29. Bataille S, Fernandez C, Zink JV, Brunet P, Berland Y, Burtey S. The Case | A hip fracture in a hemodialysis patient. Pathologic right-hip fracture from beta2-microglobulin amyloidosis. Kidney Int. 2013;83(6):1211–2. Epub 2013/06/04.

30. Gal R, Korzets A, Schwartz A, Rath-Wolfson L, Gafter U. Systemic distribution of beta 2-microglobulin-derived amyloidosis in patients who undergo long-term hemodialysis. Report of seven cases and review of the literature. Arch Pathol Lab Med. 1994;118(7):718–21. Epub 1994/07/01.

31. Choi HS, Heller D, Picken MM, Sidhu GS, Kahn T. Infarction of intestine with massive amyloid deposition in two patients on long-term hemodialysis. Gastroenterology. 1989;96(1):230–4. Epub 1989/01/01.

32. Zhou H, Pfeifer U, Linke R. Generalized amyloidosis from beta 2-microglobulin, with caecal perforation after long-term haemodialysis. Virchows Arch A Pathol Anat Histopathol. 1991;419(4):349–53. Epub 1991/01/01.

33. Esslimani M, Serre I, Granier M, Robert M, Baldet P, Costes V. Urogenital amyloidosis: clinico-pathological study of 8 cases. Ann Pathol. 1999;19(6):487–91. Epub 2000/01/05. Amylose urogenitale: etude anatomo-clinique a propos de 8 cas.

34. Saito A, Gejyo F. Current clinical aspects of dialysis-related amyloidosis in chronic dialysis patients. Ther Apher Dial. 2006;10(4):316–20. Epub 2006/08/17.

35. Kiss E, Keusch G, Zanetti M, Jung T, Schwarz A, Schocke M, et al. Dialysis-related amyloidosis revisited. AJR Am J Roentgenol. 2005;185(6):1460–7. Epub 2005/11/24.

36. Ketteler M, Koch KM, Floege J. Imaging techniques in the diagnosis of dialysis-related amyloidosis. Semin Dial. 2001;14(2):90–3. Epub 2001/03/27.

37. Kay J, Benson CB, Lester S, Corson JM, Pinkus GS, Lazarus JM, et al. Utility of high-resolution ultrasound for the diagnosis of dialysis-related amyloidosis. Arthritis Rheum. 1992;35(8):926–32. Epub 1992/08/11.

38. Jadoul M, Garbar C, van Ypersele de Strihou C. Pathological aspects of beta(2)-microglobulin amyloidosis. Semin Dial. 2001;14(2):86–9. Epub 2001/03/27.

39. Mendoza PD, Fenves AZ, Punar M, Stone MJ. Subcutaneous beta2-microglobulin amyloid shoulder nodulesin a long-term hemodialysis patient. Proc (Bayl Univ Med Cent). 2010;23(2):139–41. Epub 2010/04/17.

40. Lornoy W, Becaus I, Billiouw JM, Sierens L, Van Malderen P, D'Haenens P. On-line haemodiafiltration. Remarkable removal of beta2-microglobulin. Long-term clinical observations. Nephrol Dial Transplant. 2000;15 Suppl 1:49–54. Epub 2000/03/29.

41. Rabindranath KS, Strippoli GF, Daly C, Roderick PJ, Wallace S, MacLeod AM. Haemodiafiltration, haemofiltration and haemodialysis for end-stage kidney disease. Cochrane Database Syst Rev. 2006;4: CD006258. Epub 2006/10/21.

42. Jaber BL, Zimmerman DL, Teehan GS, Swedko P, Burns K, Meyer KB, et al. Daily hemofiltration for end-stage renal disease: a feasibility and efficacy trial. Blood Purif. 2004;22(6):481–9. Epub 2004/11/04.

43. Raj DS, Ouwendyk M, Francoeur R, Pierratos A. beta(2)-microglobulin kinetics in nocturnal haemodialysis. Nephrol Dial Transplant. 2000;15(1):58–64. Epub 1999/12/23.

44. Leypoldt JK, Cheung AK, Deeter RB, Goldfarb-Rumyantzev A, Greene T, Depner TA, et al. Kinetics of urea and beta-microglobulin during and after short hemodialysis treatments. Kidney Int. 2004;66(4):1669–76. Epub 2004/10/02.

45. Kutsuki H. beta(2)-Microglobulin-selective direct hemoperfusion column for the treatment of dialysis-related amyloidosis. Biochim Biophys Acta. 2005;1753(1):141–5. Epub 2005/09/20.

46. Yamamoto Y, Hirawa N, Yamaguchi S, Ogawa N, Takeda H, Shibuya K, et al. Long-term efficacy and safety of the small-sized beta2-microglobulin adsorption column for dialysis-related amyloidosis. Ther Apher Dial. 2011;15(5):466–74. Epub 2011/10/07.

47. Lin CL, Yang CW, Chiang CC, Chang CT, Huang CC. Long-term on-line hemodiafiltration reduces predialysis beta-2-microglobulin levels in chronic hemodialysis patients. Blood Purif. 2001;19(3):301–7. Epub 2001/03/13.

48. Thomas G, Jaber BL. Convective therapies for removal of middle molecular weight uremic toxins in end-stage renal disease: a review of the evidence. Semin Dial. 2009;22(6):610–4. Epub 2009/12/19.

49. Gejyo F, Amano I, Ando T, Ishida M, Obayashi S, Ogawa H, et al. Survey of the effects of a column for adsorption of beta2-microglobulin in patients with

dialysis-related amyloidosis in Japan. Ther Apher Dial. 2013;17(1):40–7. Epub 2013/02/06.

50. Montagna G, Cazzulani B, Obici L, Uggetti C, Giorgetti S, Porcari R, et al. Benefit of doxycycline treatment on articular disability caused by dialysis related amyloidosis. Amyloid. 2013;20(3):173–8. Epub 2013/06/06.

51. Campistol JM. Dialysis-related amyloidosis after renal transplantation. Semin Dial. 2001;14(2):99–102. Epub 2001/03/27.

52. Leypoldt JK. Kinetics of beta-microglobulin and phosphate during hemodialysis: effects of treatment frequency and duration. Semin Dial. 2005;18(5):401–8.

53. Cheung AK, Rocco MV, Yan G, Leypoldt JK, Levin NW, Greene T, et al. Serum beta-2 microglobulin levels predict mortality in dialysis patients: results of the HEMO study. J Am Soc Nephrol. 2006;17(2):546–55. Epub 2005/12/31.

54. Locatelli F, Martin-Malo A, Hannedouche T, Loureiro A, Papadimitriou M, Wizemann V, et al. Effect of membrane permeability on survival of hemodialysis patients. J Am Soc Nephrol. 2009;20(3):645–54. Epub 2008/12/19.

55. Haase M, Bellomo R, Baldwin I, Haase-Fielitz A, Fealy N, Morgera S, et al. Beta2-microglobulin removal and plasma albumin levels with high cut-off hemodialysis. Int J Artif Organs. 2007;30(5):385–92. Epub 2007/06/07.

56. Lee D, Haase M, Haase-Fielitz A, Paizis K, Goehl H, Bellomo R. A pilot, randomized, double-blind, crossover study of high cut-off versus high-flux dialysis membranes. Blood Purif. 2009;28(4):365–72. Epub 2009/09/05.

57. Susantitaphong P, Siribamrungwong M, Jaber BL. Convective therapies versus low-flux hemodialysis for chronic kidney failure: a meta-analysis of randomized controlled trials. Nephrol Dial Transplant. 2013;28(11):2859–74. Epub 2013/10/02.

58. Susantitaphong P, Riella C, Jaber BL. Effect of ultrapure dialysate on markers of inflammation, oxidative stress, nutrition and anemia parameters: a meta-analysis. Nephrol Dial Transplant. 2013;28(2):438–46. Epub 2013/01/08.

59. Regazzoni L, Colombo R, Bertoletti L, Vistoli G, Aldini G, Serra M, et al. Screening of fibrillogenesis inhibitors of beta2-microglobulin: integrated strategies by mass spectrometry capillary electrophoresis and in silico simulations. Anal Chim Acta. 2011;685(2):153–61. Epub 2010/12/21.

Localized Amyloidoses and Amyloidoses Associated with Aging Outside the Central Nervous System

7

Per Westermark

Introduction

Local deposition of amyloid, without any systemic distribution, is a biochemically, histologically, and clinically very heterogeneous group of alterations (Table 7.1). The importance of some of these forms is still very unclear although there is increasing evidence that many of these deposits are signaling a pathological process that may be involved in local tissue injury. Only in a few types is the amyloid itself of evident pathogenic impact. Localized amyloid deposits are much more common than the systemic amyloidoses. They are particularly frequent in association with aging and already at the age of about 60 years; virtually everyone has amyloid deposits in one or more tissues. Some of the localized amyloid forms occur in conjunction with specific diseases and may also be involved in their pathogenesis. Usually, it is clear from the appearance of the amyloid and its localization what type it is. However, the localized amyloids may sometimes create real problems in surgical pathology and may be difficult to discriminate from systemic

amyloidosis. This is a very important distinction to make since, although the systemic forms are almost always a threat to the patient, many of the localized amyloids are innocent, as far as we know.

Generally, there is a distinction in pathogenesis between localized and systemic amyloidosis in that the fibril protein in the former is synthesized close to the deposition site, while in the latter, the fibril precursor is produced in one or several organs, and then transported in soluble form by the blood plasma to the site where amyloid fibrils form, by mechanisms that are not yet understood. An exception may be the amyloid in atherosclerotic plaques and in cardiac valves, which, although localized, originates from the plasma.

There are many reports in the scientific literature on single organ manifestations of systemic amyloidosis, and sometimes these forms are claimed to be examples of localized amyloidosis. Thus, the cardiac manifestation of wild-type transthyretin (senile systemic) amyloidosis has been called senile cardiac amyloidosis in some publications. Careful analysis of such cases, however, shows a more widely spread amyloidosis, at least affecting arteries in many organs (see below).

The morphology of the localized amyloids does not differ from that of the systemic. Both have the same hyaline appearance in routine

P. Westermark (✉)
Department of Immunology, Genetics and Pathology,
Rudbeck Laboratory, Uppsala University,
Uppsala SE 751 85, Sweden
e-mail: Per.Westermark@igp.uu.se

Table 7.1 The extracerebral localized amyloid forms

Main location	Amyloid protein	Mother protein	Prevalence	Associated state or disease
Different organs	AL	Monoclonal immunoglobulin light chain	Rare	Local monoclonal plasma cell clone
Different organs	AH	Monoclonal immunoglobulin heavy chain	Very rare	Local monoclonal plasma cell clone
Islets of Langerhans	AIAPP	IAPP	Common	Aging, type 2 diabetes
Anterior pituitary	APro	Prolactin	Common	Aging
Parathyroid glands	?	?	Common	Aging
Cardiac atria	AANF	Atrial natriuretic factor (peptide)	Common	Aging, atrial fibrillation?
Endocrine tumors	Varying	Polypeptide hormones	Common in many tumors	Tumors
Seminal vesicles	ASem1	Semenogelin 1	Common	Aging
Skin[a]	AGal7	Galectin-7	Rare	Lichen amyloidosus, macular amyloidosis
Skin	AIns	Insulin	Rare?	Iatrogenic at site of injection
Skin	AEnf	Enfuvirtide	Rare	Iatrogenic at site of injection
Skin tumors	?	?	Common	Tumors and dysplasia
Calcifying epithelial odontogenic tumor; unerupted tooth follicles	AOAAP	Odontogenic ameloblast-associated protein	Common in tumors	Tumors
Thoracic aorta, other arteries	AMed	Lactadherin	Common	Aging, aortic aneurysm, and dissection?
Arterial intima Cardiac valves	AApoAI, +?	Apolipoprotein AI	Common	Atherosclerosis
Joints, cartilage[b]	AApoAI, ATTR	Apolipoprotein AI, transthyretin	Common	Aging
Cornea	AKer ALac	Kerato-epithelin Lactoferrin?	Rare Rare	Corneal dystrophies
Corpora amylacea of lung, prostate	?	?	Common	Aging

[a]Not yet included in the official list of amyloid proteins
[b]May sometimes be a part of systemic rather than localized amyloidosis

sections and vary in their affinity for Congo red and the appearance of yellow to green birefringence. Their principal ultrastructural morphology is also similar. The pathogenesis of localized amyloid deposits may vary between the biochemical types, but certain possible mechanisms may be mentioned. Overexpression of the fibril protein is probably often of importance and is particularly evident in some polypeptide hormone-producing tumors and in localized AL amyloidosis. In the latter, there is a local produc-tion of a monoclonal, amyloidogenic immunoglobulin light chain. Aberrant processing or abnormal cleavage of a precursor may release an amyloidogenic segment, normally buried in a larger molecule. The loss of chaperone molecules may cause a fibrillogenic molecule to misfold and aggregate into amyloid fibrils. Since amyloidogenesis in general is a nucleation-dependent process [1], seeding may be a mechanism but this has so far not been definitely shown. Changes in the microenvironment, e.g., salt concentration or pH, may also theoretically play a role. However, in general, very little is known about the pathogenesis of the localized amyloidoses.

Localized AL Amyloidosis

There are probably few conditions that have resulted in so many case reports as localized AL amyloidosis. It is uncommon but not extremely rare and can cause some diagnostic problems, particularly in the sense that it has to be distinguished from the systemic form. The amyloid deposits often cause a tumor-like process, where the type is sometimes known as "amyloidoma," and the microscopic diagnosis is usually a surprise. In most cases, the alteration is initially suspected to be a tumor and the diagnosis becomes clear only after microscopic analysis of a biopsy, where more or less cell-free hyaline areas are seen. A Congo red stained section, examined in polarized light, reveals the amyloid diagnosis. A more diffuse localized pulmonary amyloidosis has also been described, but the AL nature was not proven [2]. Diffuse pulmonary amyloidosis should always be suspected of being part of a systemic disease [3]. Among the localized forms, localized AL amyloidosis is probably the one that is most easily mistaken for systemic amyloidosis. The distinction is very important since, although systemic amyloidosis is often life-threatening, in most cases, localized AL amyloidosis is not. Localized AL amyloid can develop at any site, including the central nervous system, or even multiple sites of the same organ, e.g., bronchi. Deposits are most commonly seen in the respiratory tract (paranasal sinuses-larynx—bronchi-lungs), the urinary tract (renal pelvis-urethra), skin, and conjunctiva. In the urinary tract, the bladder is most commonly involved, followed by the ureter, the urethra, and the renal pelvis [4]. There is most often one mass, but bilateral amyloid deposits may occur, e.g., in the bronchi or in the conjunctiva. These lesions are still designated as localized. As in systemic AL amyloidosis, the amyloid is composed of a monoclonal immunoglobulin light chain, which is usually C-terminally truncated [5]. This specific light chain, varying from case to case, is synthesized at the site of deposition by a local clone of plasma cells that are usually benign. Why this happens is not clear but, initially, it may be a result of antigenic stimulation causing a chronic inflammation [6]. Sometimes, clonality is quite obvious from an immunohistochemical staining for light chains (Fig. 7.1), but very often there is a mixture of kappa- and lambda-producing plasma cells, making the clonality less evident. However, clonality may be demonstrated by analysis of immunoglobulin heavy chain gene rearrangements [7–9]. There is not the same strong predominance of lambda chains as in systemic AL amyloidosis, and localized AL kappa amyloidosis is comparably common. The reason for this is unknown but may point to important differences in pathogenesis. Marginal zone lymphoma of mucosa-associated lymphoid tissue (MALT) often contains deposits of amyloid, and the distinction between this neoplasm and "amyloidoma" is not always sharp [10, 11].

The microscopic findings vary with the localization. Deposits may be quite small, as is often seen in the larynx and in the conjunctiva. On the other hand, deposits at some other locations, such as the lungs or urinary bladder, may be quite large. Typically, there are almost acellular amyloid areas intermingled with spots with

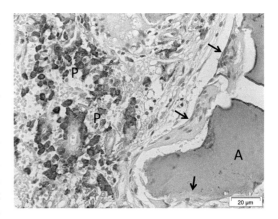

Fig. 7.1 Localized amyloid in the lung, immunolabeled with pwlam, a monoclonal antibody against amyloid proteins of AL lambda type [183]. Amyloid (*A*) and plasma cells (*P*) are strongly labeled. Close to the amyloid are several multinucleated giant cells (*arrows*), a characteristic finding in localized AL amyloid

inflammatory cells, notably plasma cells (Fig. 7.1). An almost constant feature of localized AL amyloidosis is the presence of multinucleated giant cells of foreign body type, mentioned in many of the great number of case reports of this kind of lesion. These cells are usually interpreted as a sign of tissue reaction of the deposited material. However, as an alternative, it is possible that the giant cells directly participate in the generation of fibrils by processing the monoclonal immunoglobulin light chain, produced by plasma cells in the vicinity [12, 13]. Amyloid, close to giant cells, is often more brightly stained with Congo red and shows a particularly bright green birefringence, probably indicating extensive organization of the fibrils (Fig. 7.2). Calcifications and metaplastic bone formation are commonly found, particularly in bronchial deposits.

Appearance of abnormal nodules, bleedings, and results of obstruction are the most common symptoms of localized AL amyloidosis. Localized AL amyloidosis of the urinary tract most commonly presents with macroscopic hematuria, but other symptoms such as anuria or acute renal failure may occur [4]. Very often, the lesions are initially strongly suspected for cancer. This is particularly true for lesions in the tracheabronchial region and in the urinary tract. The rare localized AL amyloidosis of the breast is also very easily mistaken for malignancy and may

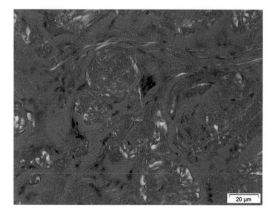

Fig. 7.2 Localized AL amyloid, stained with Congo red and examined under polarized light for birefringence. A strongly birefringent amyloid deposit is apparent

even show micro-calcifications visible at X-ray examination [14]. In most cases, localized amyloidosis is not life threatening, but there are exceptions. In the respiratory tract, where the deposits often are multiple and bilateral [15], the amyloid can cause severe hemorrhages and even death [16, 17]. In most instances, the condition is long-lasting and not curable but may be kept under control by repeated endoscopical intervention [4, 15, 18]. However, a more radical surgical treatment is sometimes necessary and may even include cystectomy for urinary bladder amyloid or nephrectomy for localized amyloidosis in the renal pelvis. The risk of progression to systemic amyloidosis is very small [4], but AL amyloid tumors may appear in patients with systemic amyloidosis [19]. A careful clinical investigation is therefore important.

Amyloid in Endocrine Organs and Tumors

Small deposits are common in certain endocrine organs and their tumors. In general, these amyloid deposits are composed of specific polypeptide hormones or fragments thereof. The importance of the deposits themselves may vary, but it is likely that most of them are fairly innocent, at least when small. However, there is strong evidence that some of them are pathogenically important, both when appearing as large deposits and during their formation, then as toxic oligomers. The best studied example is the amyloid in the islets of Langerhans, but there are other deposits which may play a pathogenic role.

Islet of Langerhans

Localized amyloid deposits, restricted to the islets of Langerhans, are very commonly seen. Such amyloid may appear as an age-dependent phenomenon and is found in >10 % of subjects over the age of 70 years. Usually, the deposits are quite small, not detectable in routine stained sections and not affecting more than a few percentages of the islets in the pancreatic body and tail.

When more pronounced, a "hyalinization" of the islets may be obvious (Fig. 7.3a) and may then also be noticed in H&E stained sections. Extensive and widespread islet amyloid deposits often occur in conjunction with type 2 diabetes (not type 1; exception, see below).

Islet amyloid is the most typical pancreatic lesion found in type 2 diabetes and seen in >90 % of individuals. The deposits are restricted to the islets, and no amyloid occurs in the exocrine parenchyma (Fig. 7.3b). The amyloid deposits occur in close association with the insulin-producing beta cells, which may show some degenerative signs. Although islets may become more or less converted into amyloid, there are always some endocrine cells left in the masses, which may be shown by the application of antibodies against the major islet polypeptide hormones (Fig. 7.3c). A common finding is an irregular involvement of different parts of the pancreas. Generally, most amyloid is seen in the body and tail. Sometimes, small lobules of the pancreas contain a lot of islet amyloid while other parts may be spared.

Although islet amyloid does not occur in the type 1 diabetic pancreas, it has recently become a topic of interest in this form of diabetes. Islet amyloid develops frequently and rapidly in normal human islets, transplanted into the portal system of type 1 diabetic individuals [20] and may constitute an important cause of the gradually decreasing function of these islets.

The fibril protein in islet amyloid is islet amyloid polypeptide (IAPP, or amylin), which is a product of the beta cells. IAPP was discovered by analysis of amyloid deposits taken from an insulinoma [21, 22] and, subsequently, from islet material [23, 24]. IAPP is stored together with insulin in the secretory vesicles, and the two polypeptides are released together at exocytosis.

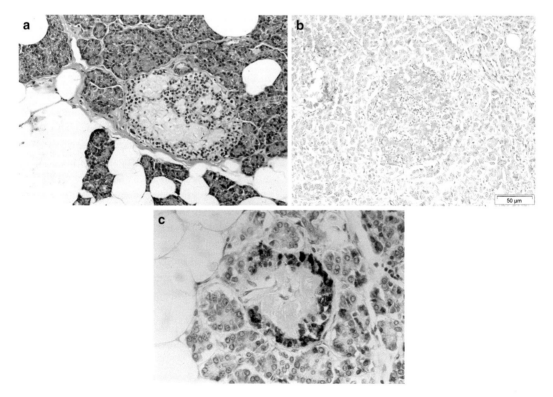

Fig. 7.3 (**a**) An H&E stained section of pancreas from a type 2 diabetic individual. In this routine section, large amounts of amyloid already are apparent in the islets. (**b**) An example of a similar islet, stained with Congo red. Note the residual endocrine cells. (**c**) An amyloid-rich islet immunolabeled with antibodies against insulin. In spite of the large masses of amyloid, there are many heavily granulated, albeit defective beta cells

As in the case of insulin, IAPP is expressed as a prohormone, which is then processed by the two converting enzymes PC 1/3 and PC2 at double basic amino acid residues (for review, see [25]). The processing takes place in the golgi and in the secretory vesicles. The concentration of IAPP is much lower than insulin and the plasma levels are less than 10 % of that of insulin. IAPP is a 37 amino acid residue peptide belonging to the calcitonin gene-related peptide family (which also contains calcitonin, adrenomedullin, and intermedin). IAPP is a very fibrillogenic peptide that is difficult to keep non-aggregated in solution. Insulin is an inhibitor of the fibrillogenesis and may be an important physiological chaperone within the beta cell. IAPP's physiological role is not fully understood, but it has both para- and autocrine effects on islet cells and peripheral effects [25].

It is not understood why IAPP forms amyloid in type 2 diabetes. Overexpression of IAPP is probably important but other factors, including loss of balance with insulin production and aberrant processing of proIAPP, may be involved in the pathogenesis. The effect of the amyloid has been a matter of discussion for many years, but there is an increasing understanding that the deposition of islet amyloid is followed by a loss of insulin-producing beta cells [26]. Therefore, the IAPP amyloid is suspected of playing an important role in the gradual loss of beta cell function during the course of type 2 diabetes. Whether islet amyloid is involved in the initial stages of type 2 diabetes is less well understood. As with the situation in Alzheimer's disease, it is not known whether it is the mature amyloid fibrils that are pathogenically important. There is increasing evidence that prefibrillar IAPP aggregates (oligomers) exert toxic effects on the beta cell, leading to beta cell death [25]. However, recent studies have indicated that beta cell death is due to intracellular aggregation of IAPP, affecting autophagic pathways rather than extracellular aggregates exerting toxic effects [27, 28]. It is possible that the mature amyloid fibrils are more inert since there are always endocrine cells remaining in direct contact with the amyloid (Fig. 7.3c).

Parathyroid Glands

Amyloid in the parathyroid glands probably belongs to the least studied forms and almost all papers on the subject are fairly old. Microdeposits are, however, commonly found both in normal and hyperplastic glands as well as in adenomas [29, 30]. Amyloid is found in follicles and may have a laminated structure. Also, intracellular amyloid may occur [31]. Parathyroid glands are often involved in systemic amyloidosis but the distribution is different, with a major involvement of vessels. In apparently normal parathyroid glands, the prevalence of localized amyloid increases with age and there is no sex difference [29].

The nature of the parathyroid amyloid is not known but the small parathyroid hormone (84 amino acid residues) may be a good candidate, and labeling with antibodies against parathormone has been reported [30].

Amyloid in the Cardiac Atria

In the older literature, cardiac amyloid deposits associated with aging were regarded as one entity, starting in the atria and sometimes subsequently spreading to the ventricles [32]. However, in 1979, it was shown that there is one distinctive localized form of amyloid specific for the cardiac atria and that deposits in the ventricles are different [33] and part of a systemic amyloidosis, most often wt ATTR (senile systemic) amyloidosis in which wild-type transthyretin constitutes the fibrils [34]. This latter form may also involve the atria, as may all kinds of systemic amyloidosis.

Localized atrial amyloidosis, also termed isolated atrial amyloidosis (IAA), is always limited to the atria. The fibril protein is atrial natriuretic factor (or peptide) (ANF) [35, 36], a 28 amino acid residue polypeptide hormone, expressed by atrial myocytes. ANF is stored as a 126 amino acid residue prohormone in cytoplasmic vesicles in the myocytes. When released, the prohormone is cleaved to yield the mature peptide by the cardiomyocyte membrane protease corin [37]. There is immunohistochemical evidence that the

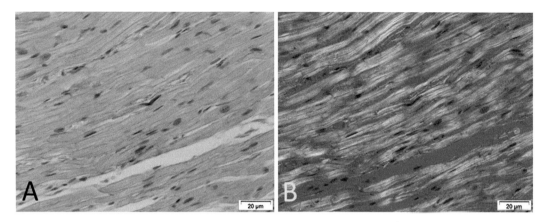

Fig. 7.4 Typical appearance of AANF amyloid in cardiac atria. (**a**) in ordinary light and (**b**) under polarized light

propeptide, or a part thereof, is also associated with the amyloid fibrils [38].

AANF amyloid only affects the atria, including the auricles and the myocardial sleeves of pulmonary veins [33, 39, 40]. The amyloid is not evenly spread but often patchy. Most commonly, both atria are affected [39, 41]. The distribution is quite typical, with fine streaks covering individual cardiomyocytes (Fig. 7.4) and often the subendocardial layer. There are often amyloid deposits within the walls of small vessels [33], and this should not be taken as evidence for systemic disease. Most of the amyloid is extracellular, but intracellular deposits have been found within cardiomyocytes [42, 43]. The amyloid never forms the large, homogeneous deposits seen in many other biochemical forms of amyloidosis and will be missed if special stains are not applied to sections.

AANF amyloid is one of the most prevalent senile types of amyloidosis and both prevalence and severity increase with age [39]. The published prevalence numbers vary, and it has been found in up to 90 % in octogenarians [44]. One has to be careful when examining atria for AANF amyloid since the atria are easily overstained with Congo red or other amyloid dyes. This fact probably explains some very high prevalence numbers in the literature.

Atrial AANF amyloidosis is more common in women than men and affects the left atrium more commonly than the right [44, 45]. The pathogenesis is unknown but increased expression of proANF is most probably of importance, and the presence of AANF amyloid deposits is particularly common in subjects with atrial fibrillation and in patients undergoing mitral valve replacement [44, 46, 47]. AANF amyloid was found in 90 % of patients with severe congestive heart failure undergoing heart transplantation [48]. Whether or not the amyloid itself is of pathogenic importance for the diseases is unclear, but it is reasonable to believe that the intra- and extracellular aggregates may influence electric impulse conduction.

From a practical point of view, AANF amyloid must be distinguished from deposits of systemic amyloidosis. Usually, the pure morphological criteria are enough to make this distinction. If there is any problem, immunohistochemical labeling with antibodies against ANF (which are commercially available) may be applied and will solve the issue.

Pituitary Gland

Occurrence of small amyloid deposits in the pituitary is a well-known phenomenon in association with aging, and this amyloid belongs to the "classical" senile forms. The deposits are limited to the adenohypophysis where they appear as small, elongated, and thin streaks between capillaries and epithelial cells [49] (Fig. 7.5). Intracellular aggregates may also exist [31]. Age-related pituitary amyloid is a very common autopsy finding

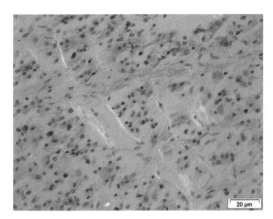

Fig. 7.5 Adenohypophysis of an elderly individual. Amyloid is a very common finding but may be difficult to recognize due to its loose arrangement and weak affinity for Congo red. Partially crossed polars

and, in Japanese material, it was found in more than 90 % of cases over 70 years of age [50]. Similar figures have been found by others.

By purification, amino acid sequence analysis, and further immunohistochemistry, the main fibrillar protein was identified as being derived from prolactin [51]. Prolactin, one of the major pituitary hormones, is comprised of 198 amino acid residues; there were no indications of cleaved protein products in the amyloid.

Nothing is known regarding abnormalities associated with the formation of pituitary amyloid nor is there any evidence of a functional consequence.

Amyloid in Endocrine Tumors

"Amyloid stroma" is a typical finding in some kinds of polypeptide hormone-producing tumors. An analysis of well-characterized endocrine tumors showed that certain hormone-producing cells are associated with amyloid, particularly those giving rise to C-cell tumor medullary carcinoma of the thyroid and insulinoma of the pancreas [52]. Other endocrine tumors may also contain amyloid, and it is possible that there are other hormones that are amyloid-forming in addition to those presently known. In addition, there are occasional

reports on tumors without known endocrine activity that have an amyloid stroma [53]. It is possible that such tumors produce an aberrant peptide.

Medullary Carcinoma of the Thyroid

Medullary thyroid carcinoma is a tumor derived from the calcitonin-producing C-cells. It constitutes about 5 % of the thyroid carcinomas. Deposition of amyloid in the stroma is a fairly typical finding and was seen in 82 % of tumors in a large series of medullary carcinomas [54] and is one of the useful markers for this carcinoma. There may be conspicuous amounts of amyloid in some tumors (Fig. 7.6). Fine needle aspiration biopsies stained with Congo red may assist in the diagnosis of medullary thyroid carcinoma.

Analysis of the fibrils in one medullary carcinoma showed procalcitonin as the main protein [55]. Studies by others have revealed only mature calcitonin [56]. Antibodies against the hormone can be used to label this amyloid form. Calcitonin-derived amyloid has only been described in tumors.

Interestingly, two different studies, analyzing large series, have shown that medullary thyroid carcinomas with amyloid have a better prognosis than tumors without [57, 58]. A possible reason is that aggregated calcitonin, either as oligomeric aggregates or as mature fibrils, exert a toxic effect on tumor cells and, thereby, kill them [59]. If this is the case, the same thing should be true of other tumors with amyloid as well, e.g., insulinomas, but no such studies seem to have been performed.

Insulinoma of the Pancreas

Insulinomas are derived from islet beta cells and typically produce insulin as well as other beta cell peptides, including the amyloidogenic IAPP. In a study of 12 insulinomas, 7 had amyloid deposits, some large amounts [52]. IAPP was originally purified from the amyloid of an amyloid-rich insulin-producing tumor [21, 22]. A very large insulinoma, in 70 % consisting of amyloid, has been described [60] as well as other giant insulinomas with amyloid [61].

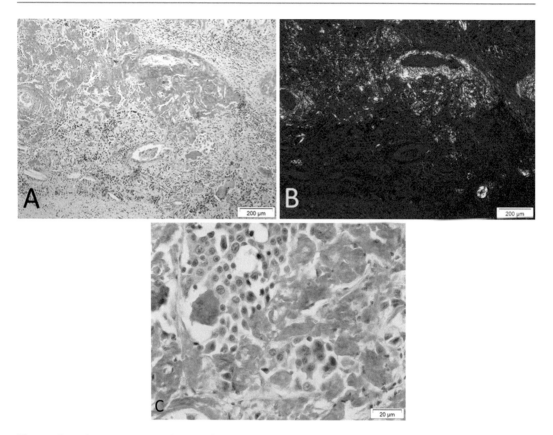

Fig. 7.6 Lymph node metastasis of a medullary carcinoma, rich in amyloid. (**a**) Congo red in ordinary light and (**b**) the same field between crossed polars. (**c**) is a close-up showing tumor cells in close contact with amyloid

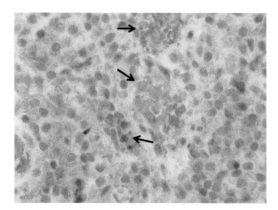

Fig. 7.7 Amyloid-rich insulinoma, immunolabeled with antibodies against IAPP. The amyloid (*arrows*) is strongly IAPP-positive while tumor cells vary in their reaction with the antibody

Similar to the amyloid in the islets of Langerhans, the amyloid found in insulinomas consists of IAPP (Fig. 7.7). It is not clear whether proIAPP is an important ingredient in some cases. Aggregated IAPP in a pre-amyloid form is toxic against cells in vitro. It is therefore possible that the formation of amyloid is of benefit to the patient. However, an elevated production of IAPP from a malignant insulinoma was associated with the development of diabetes, putatively dependent upon the effects of IAPP on islet release of insulin [62].

Pituitary Adenoma

There is an unusually large number of case reports on amyloid in pituitary adenomas. One reason may be that the amyloid sometimes forms fairly large globules (or sphaeroids), which are easily seen already in routine sections [63, 64]. Most commonly, amyloid (with globules) is reported in prolactinomas [64–67], but it has also been described in adenomas producing growth hormone [68] and melanocorticotropin [69].

Amyloid at Sites of Peptide Injection

Insulin

As was demonstrated in the 1940s, by repeated heating and freezing, insulin can easily be converted into amyloid-like fibrils in vitro [70]. In later years, there have been an increasing number of reports showing that amyloid may develop at the sites of repeated subcutaneous insulin injection [71–74]. Initially this was believed to be due to the use of foreign insulin (porcine or bovine), but nowadays only human insulin is used. As seen by a recent publication, insulin amyloid formation is not rare [75]. The amyloid appears as subcutaneous nodules, which may become quite large. Histological examination reveals amyloid masses with a typical Congo red staining reaction. Sometimes, foreign body giant cells may be present. A correct diagnosis can be obtained by immunohistochemistry.

It is important to think about the possibility of iatrogenic insulin amyloid when there are localized deposits subcutaneously in the abdomen. Putatively, this kind of amyloidosis may be a pitfall since it may easily be mistaken for a manifestation of systemic amyloidosis, particularly since the abdominal subcutaneous adipose tissue is a commonly used site for the diagnosis of systemic disease. Alternatively, due to its nodular appearance, the insulin amyloid may be mistaken for a localized AL amyloidosis.

Enfuvirtide

Enfuvirtide is a 36 amino acid residue synthetic anti-HIV peptide, acting through inhibition of binding between the virus particle and CD4+ cells. It is particularly rich in leucine, glutamic acid, and glutamine. Two cases of enfuvirtide-derived localized amyloid deposition have been described [75].

Localized Amyloid Deposits in the Skin

The skin is one of the principal sites for localized AL amyloidosis, described above, but other forms of amyloid deposits are even more common. Small, or sometimes very small, amyloid deposits occur subepidermally in the two related and, most probably, biochemically identical amyloid forms, lichen amyloidosus (LA) and macular amyloidosis (MA). LA, MA, and some related variants are in the dermatological literature collectively often referred to as "primary localized cutaneous amyloidosis" (PLCA). LA appears as slightly elevated, irregular papules, or plaques, often affecting the shins, but it may also appear elsewhere. Amyloid is seen as irregular, small masses in the papillary dermis. Very often the amyloid is seen to contain a number of macrophages with engulfed melanin (melanophages) (Fig. 7.8). There is no amyloid in the reticular dermis or in the walls of blood vessels. Transepidermal elimination of amyloid may occur [76]. The deposits are moderately Congophilic. MA appears as irregular areas with a rippled hyperpigmentation, and is most commonly encountered on the upper back, between the shoulder blades or over one of them. In this

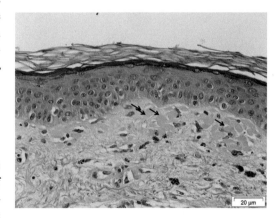

Fig. 7.8 Macular amyloidosis stained with H&E. Amyloid (*arrows*) appears as small, often sharply demarcated corpuscles. Note the many melanophages, a typical feature of lichen amyloidosus and macular amyloidosis

form, the amyloid is sometimes so scanty that the deposits are difficult to see, particularly since their affinity for Congo red is weak and green birefringence is difficult to demonstrate. Staining methods other than Congo red are therefore often used, e.g., the fluorescent dye thioflavin S (or T). In Japan, the dye Pagoda red (Dylon, Japan) is often used, although its properties when complexed with amyloid are less well known than Congo red. Also, in MA, melanophages are quite typical and are of help for diagnosis. There are usually no other inflammatory cells, unless there are secondary changes due to scratching. LA and MA are closely related and are sometimes seen in the same patient where they are then referred to as "biphasic amyloidosis." Both types tend to run a chronic course and generate an intractable pruritus.

In addition to LA and MA, there are other very rare clinical forms of localized subepidermal amyloidosis, sometimes with the appearance of poikiloderma [77].

Morphological studies on the origin of the amyloid have indicated a close relationship between the basal cell layer and the amyloid fibrils, strongly indicating a keratinocyte origin of the fibril protein [78]. A direct, secretory mechanism has been suggested from electron microscopic findings [79, 80] as an alternative to the possibility that the amyloid derives from degenerative keratinocytes [81]. Most studies on the biochemical nature of the fibrils in LA and MA have been performed by the application of antibodies against known proteins. These studies have repeatedly reported reactions with antibodies against basic keratin variants, and CK5 antibodies have been suggested for diagnostic work [82, 83]. A pathogenesis involving processing of keratin from apoptotic keratinocytes has also been suggested [84]. However, recent research including mass spectrometric analysis of extracted amyloid has indicated that the fibril protein is not derived from keratin but from galectin-7 [85, 86]. Galectin-7 is a carbohydrate binding protein specifically expressed by keratinocytes. It is a small protein of 136 residues arranged as a β-sandwich [87], which makes it a good amyloid fibril protein candidate.

LA and MA are relatively rare in the Western world but are more prevalent in Southeast Asia and in South America. It has been repeatedly suggested that LA and MA may be induced by long-term scratching, particularly with a nylon towel or brush. This may be doubtful since these conditions sometimes do not produce itching. There is often a family history, and also a connection between LA and multiple endocrine neoplasia syndrome 2A has been established [88, 89]. The mutated gene is RET located on chromosome 10. A linkage study in Chinese families with LA and/or MA has indicated a locus on chromosome 1 [90] and another in a Brazilian family identified a mutated oncostatin M (OSM) receptor β which is a receptor for OSM and interleukin-31 [91]. A number of families with LA and mutations in the interleukin-31 receptor protein genes have been described [92]. Interleukin-31 is involved in the genesis of itching, but the precise connection between mutations in this gene and the pathogenesis of amyloid is still unknown. The recent discoveries of amyloid protein and mutations in LA and MA indicate that the pathogenesis may be complicated.

MA belongs to a group of related conditions which, in addition, include notalgia paresthetica and macular posterior pigmentary incontinence (also called "posterior pigmented pruritic patch") [93]. These latter conditions have similarities in symptoms and clinical appearance but lack amyloid. Interestingly, macular posterior pigmentary incontinence (without amyloid) was present in several members of a kindred with multiple endocrine neoplasia syndrome 2A [94].

Amyloid in Skin Tumors

Small amyloid deposits are exceedingly common in certain skin tumors, particularly basal cell carcinomas, and in precancerous lesions such as actinic keratosis and Bowen's disease. In a Swedish study of 260 basal cell carcinomas, Olsen and Westermark found amyloid in 75 % of tumors [95] while Looi found amyloid in 66 % of sections of tumors with different ethnic origins [96]. Those of the nodular type, particularly,

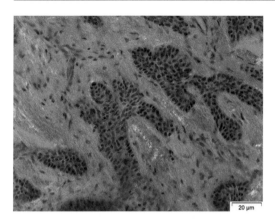

20 µm

Fig. 7.9 Amyloid in a basal cell carcinoma. Congo red with partially crossed polars

develop amyloid [95, 97] (Fig. 7.9). Basal cell papillomas (seborrhoic keratosis) also often contain amyloid, but somewhat less frequently [95]. Amyloid may also occur in other skin tumors. The amyloid is situated in the tumor stroma and is, in most cases, scant, but tumors with more pronounced amyloid infiltration do occur. The affinity for Congo red is relatively weak in most cases.

In actinic keratosis and Bowen's disease, amyloid is commonly found in the papillary dermis [98] where the deposits resemble those found in macular amyloidosis. Also, some other skin lesions, such as porokeratosis, may demonstrate similar amyloid deposits [99].

The nature of the amyloid fibril protein is not known, but it is probably the same in all of these tumors. It has hitherto been believed that it is a keratinocyte protein, and keratin has been suspected from immunohistochemical results [100]; however, direct biochemical characterization is still lacking.

Calcifying Epithelial Odontogenic Tumor

Calcifying epithelial odontogenic (Pindborg) tumor is a rare mandibular or maxillar benign neoplasm that typically contains amyloid deposits in association with the tumor cells [101]. Analysis of the purified main protein revealed a

previously unknown sequence, showing that the amyloid is unique [102]. The 264 amino acid residue protein has been given the name "odontogenic ameloblast-associated protein" and the amyloid protein, therefore, AOAAP. OAAP is believed to be important in odontogenesis and, remarkably, small amyloid deposits of AOAAP can be found in unerupted tooth follicles [103]. OAAP is expressed in other tissues as well but is not known to form amyloid deposits and has been suggested as a breast cancer biomarker [104].

Wild-type Transthyretin (Senile Systemic) Amyloidosis and Peripheral Vascular Amyloid

Wild-type Transthyretin Amyloidosis

Wild-type transthyretin (wt ATTR) amyloidosis (senile systemic amyloidosis[1]) is a systemic amyloid variant that is included in this chapter since it was, in the past, often called senile cardiac amyloidosis, indicating a localized form [106]. This misinterpretation depended on the fact that, when pronounced, the cardiac deposits are strongly predominating (Fig. 7.10a) although there is a more general arterial occurrence of amyloid deposits, in many other organs [107]. Particularly in the lungs, there may be quite widely dispersed amyloidosis, which often has a typical appearance of small nodules in alveolar vessels [107, 108] (Fig. 7.10b). There are very often fairly large amounts of amyloid in the renal medulla, particularly the papillae, while the glomeruli are spared [109]. When the disease gives rise to clinical symptoms, these are usually cardiac although carpal tunnel syndrome may be the first manifestation, depending on deposition of amyloid in the tissue around the median nerve [110, 111]. Whether wt ATTR amyloid deposits can occur in the carpal tunnel

[1]A decision was taken at the latest meeting of the Nomenclature Committee of the International Society of Amyloidosis to replace the name "senile systemic amyloidosis (SSA)" with "wild-type transthyretin amyloidosis" which is a more exact description of the condition [105].

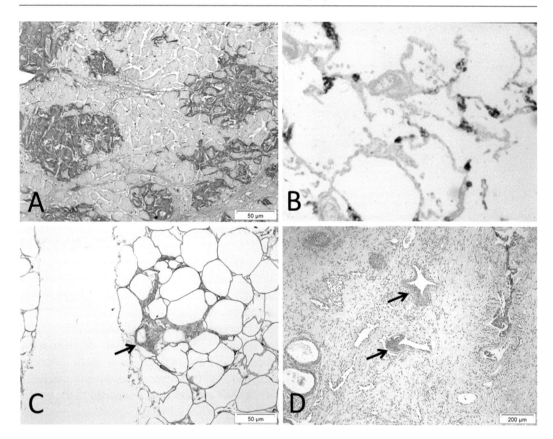

Fig. 7.10 Senile systemic amyloidosis. (**a**) shows a cardiac section with moderate amounts of amyloid, immunolabeled with antibodies against a transthyretin-derived polypeptide. (**b**) shows a lung section, labeled with the same antibodies. In (**c**), immunoreactive amyloid (*arrow*) is demonstrated in subcutaneous adipose tissue. Vascular amyloid deposits (*arrows*), as a sign of senile systemic amyloidosis is a not uncommon finding in prostate samples (**d**)

as a strict local phenomenon is not known. There is also novel research that indicates that deposits in the spinal canal in wt ATTR amyloidosis may cause spinal stenosis [112, 113]. When pronounced, the cardiac amyloid causes a restrictive cardiomyopathy and, typically, the diagnosis is established after endomyocardial biopsies on a patient with unexplained cardiomyopathy and enlarged heart [106]. The biochemical nature of the amyloidosis may be obtained by immunohistochemistry or by western blot on an extract of amyloid-containing tissue, e.g., subcutaneous adipose tissue [114] (Fig. 7.10c) or prostate (Fig. 7.10d).

The amyloid fibril protein in wt ATTR amyloidosis is only wild-type transthyretin [34]. Although full length protein is present in the amyloid, fragments predominate [34, 115]. These

N-terminally truncated transthyretin fragments start at positions 46, 49, and 52 [34, 116].

The appearance of the deposits in the myocardium is often quite typical. When the amyloid is sparse and probably non-symptomatic, small but distinctive amyloid spots appear between muscle cells (Fig. 7.10a). These spots tend to increase in size and number and may finally coalesce into more diffuse amyloid infiltration. The conduction system is relatively spared [117] which may be an important difference from Swedish ATTRM30V amyloidosis [118, 119]. The amyloid seems to be strictly extracellular, in contrast to some other forms, including familial ATTRV30M amyloidosis where some amyloid may be seen intracellularly [116].

Wt ATTR amyloidosis is by far the most common form of systemic amyloidosis, found in

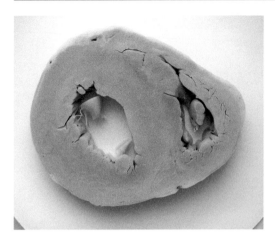

Fig. 7.11 Cross section of a heart from a patient with severe senile systemic amyloidosis. The heart is evenly infiltrated with amyloid

25 % of individuals above the age of 80 [41] and 37 % above the age of 85 [120]. In most cases, there are only small, but sometimes widely spread, vascular deposits; however, in some individuals, mostly men, a severe disease may develop (Fig. 7.11). Earlier, wt ATTR amyloidosis was almost only diagnosed at autopsy [117], but its diagnosis during life is now increasingly common. It is also evident that the disease is not restricted to the very old; in quite a few cases, the cardiomyopathy has been found in patients in their 60s and even earlier. Distinction of this entity from systemic AL amyloidosis is important since wt ATTR amyloidosis usually runs a much more slowly progressive course [121–123] and is treated differently.

Aorta and Other Arteries

Congophilic angiopathy is a well-known, usually Aβ-derived, cerebral, amyloid form, but amyloid deposits restricted to vessels are also common outside the brain and are of a different biochemical nature. Typically, segments of vessels, mainly small arteries, have pronounced amyloid deposits, replacing most of, or the whole of, the media layer. Such deposits are most commonly parts of a systemic amyloidosis rather than tissue-limited.

There are amyloid forms that may be found in different sites in the body but are limited to the vascular walls. In a way, these forms fall between the systemic and localized amyloids but, for practical reasons, they are generally classified as localized. At least the most common of them, AMed amyloid, has a fibril protein, which is synthesized at the place of deposition, similar to other localized amyloid types. Amyloid appearing in atherosclerotic plaques may be an exception in that the fibril protein might be derived from the blood plasma.

Faint deposits of amyloid in arteries, particularly the aorta and associated with aging, have been known for a long time. With the introduction of immunohistochemistry, it was found that the aging aorta is the target of three common and biochemically distinct forms of amyloid, which form deposits principally in the adventitia, media, or intima [124]. The adventitial deposits were found to be a manifestation of senile systemic amyloidosis (wild-type transthyretin derived) while the two others were confined to the vessel walls.

Medin (AMed) Amyloid

Localized amyloid of the medial layer of the aorta and, to some degree, of some other large arteries, is probably the most common of all human amyloid forms [41, 125, 126]. It is most prevalent in the thoracic aorta and, to a lesser extent, in the abdominal part [127]. Small deposits are commonly seen in other large arteries [127], particularly the temporal artery where amyloid deposits form along the internal elastic lamina [128, 129]. It may be found as small deposits in major cerebral arteries [127]. In aortic sections, the amyloid occurs as many small, discrete patches, commonly associated with elastic membranes but also, evidently, within smooth muscle cells (Fig. 7.12). The amyloid is somewhat faintly stained with Congo red and may be seen most easily with partially crossed polarizers, which results in an increased red color. The green birefringence is evident but weak. Above the age of 50–60 years, amyloid deposits in the thoracic aortic media are seen to a varying degree in virtually everyone [124].

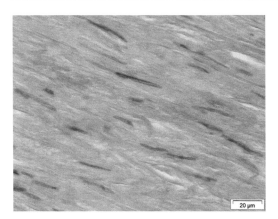

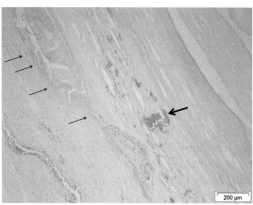

Fig. 7.12 Medin-derived amyloid in the aortic media of an elderly subject. This is an extremely common finding. Note that some amyloid seems to be intracellular. Congo red stain, viewed in ordinary light

Fig. 7.13 Complicated atherosclerotic plaque in the aorta. Amyloid appears both as strongly stainable particles (*thick arrow*) and as more diffuse and weakly stained material (*thin arrows*)

The amyloid protein in localized amyloid of the arterial media is a 50 amino acid residue peptide, called medin [130], and the amyloid is, therefore, termed AMed amyloidosis [105]. It is an internal fragment of the 364 amino acid residue glycoprotein lactadherin, also called BA46 or milk fat globule-EGF factor 8. Lactadherin has amino acid sequence similarity with coagulation factors 5 and 8 and has an integrin binding site at the N-terminal sequence. Lactadherin is a multifunctional protein with roles that include protection against rotavirus infection [131, 132] and the ability to promote phagocytosis of apoptotic cells [133]. Lactadherin may compete with the coagulation factors mentioned above and, thereby, inhibit coagulation [134]. There is evidence that it also acts as a linker protein between elastic laminae and smooth muscle cells [135]. The medin domain is important in this latter function. It is not known whether the cleavage of lactadherin to yield medin is physiological and no normal function for medin has so far been described. Lactadherin is expressed by a number of cells in addition to smooth muscle cells. These include macrophages, endothelial cells, and breast epithelium. In fact, the protein was discovered as a milk component.

The importance of AMed amyloid is not clear. Given its very high prevalence in aging, it has been regarded as innocent. However, it has not been ruled out that aggregated AMed is pathogenically important in certain conditions. AMed amyloid is very commonly seen associated with the internal elastic membrane of the temporal artery, a site where inflammation seems to start at giant cell arteritis. It has therefore been suggested that medin, or lactadherin, act as autoantigens in this disorder [129]. It can be noted that the rare giant cell aortitis affects the thoracic aorta, the segment with most AMed amyloid [136]. Aggregated medin is toxic to smooth muscle cells and may be involved in the pathogenesis of thoracic aortic aneurysm and dissection, either as mature fibrils or as prefibrillar aggregates [137]. In these disorders, there is a loss of smooth muscle cells [138].

Amyloid in Atherosclerotic Plaques and Cardiac Valves

Localized amyloid deposits are common in advanced atherosclerotic lesions [124]. In particular, strongly Congophilic amyloid material is seen close to calcifications but more diffuse and faintly stainable amyloid may occur in necrotic parts of the plaques (Fig. 7.13). In a study of 63 patients over the age of 50, this kind of amyloid was found in 35 % of cases [124].

In one patient with a large amount of material, from which it was possible to purify the main protein, the amyloid fibril protein was found to be derived from apolipoprotein A–I [139]. It is possible that there are other components as well since antibodies against apolipoprotein A–I only partially label the amyloid. This form of amyloidosis may be an exception from the rule that the amyloid protein in localized amyloid is synthesized at the site of deposition. It should be stressed that systemic amyloid, at least when derived from the fibrinogen α-chain, may be deposited in atheromatous plaques [140].

Amyloid deposits of the same appearance and with a close association to calcifications are also very commonly found in surgically removed heart valves, particularly the aortic valve [141, 142]. A biochemical identity is supported by antigenic studies [143].

The importance of the amyloid in the atherosclerotic intima and in the cardiac valves is unknown. However, it cannot be ruled out that aggregated amyloid proteins are important in the pathogenesis of atherosclerosis.

Amyloid in the Seminal Vesicles

Amyloid deposits, often quite pronounced, are common in the seminal vesicles in association with aging. It is a typical "senile" form, rare before the age of 50 but then occurring in increased prevalence to about 20 % after the age of 75 [144]. It is a fairly common finding in association with radical prostatectomy specimens [145]. The abnormality is almost always bilateral [144] and involves also the vasa deferentia and ejaculatory ducts [145] but not the epididymis or the prostate. The deposits are typically subepithelial and can grow to considerable masses, thereby narrowing the lumina [144] (Fig. 7.14). When pronounced, deposits are also found intraluminally [146, 147]. There is no involvement of the muscle layer, and no amyloid is seen in the vessel walls, which may help to distinguish it from systemic amyloidosis.

The amyloid fibril protein was found to be a 14 kDa product of seminal vesicle epithelial cells, [147] and amino acid sequence analysis identified it as being derived from the larger (52 kDa) semenogelin I [148], which is one of the

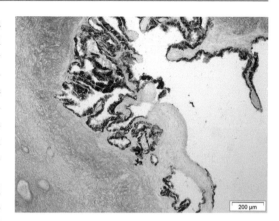

Fig. 7.14 Typical appearance of amyloid in a seminal vesicle. The amyloid is subepithelial while the epithelium was desquamated (autopsy specimen). Section immunolabeled with antibodies against the fibril protein ASemI

main epithelial secretory proteins produced by the vesicles. The expression of this protein is restricted to the vesicles, explaining the localized character of this form of amyloid. The subepithelial position of the amyloid may seem surprising given the origin of an exocrine protein, but reabsorption of secreted protein with retrograde transepithelial transport has been described in the seminal vesicles [149].

The importance of the amyloid is unknown, but hemospermia has been described in several cases [150, 151]. Given the ability of amyloid, or pre-amyloid aggregates, to induce apoptosis, a protection against spreading of prostatic carcinoma was hypothesized. No such effect was found, however [152]. For the general pathologist, it is most important to know that the deposits are not any part of a systemic amyloidosis.

Corneal Amyloid

Familial systemic AGel amyloidosis (Finnish type) is associated with lattice dystrophy of the cornea [153]. Lattice dystrophy has also been described in a patient with AH amyloidosis [154]. In addition, there are a number of different corneal dystrophy conditions in which abnormal material is deposited at different sites in the cornea, and this abnormal material may contain small amyloid aggregates without any systemic involvement [155]. Lattice dystrophies are characterized by irregular, branching lines, detectable at slit lamp examination while gelatinous drop-like corneal dystrophy appears as mulberry-like, protruding, subepithelial depositions [156]. There are also granular forms of corneal dystrophy and all forms may lead to gradual visual impairment. Most types of corneal dystrophy with amyloid are familial and dominantly inherited. Sporadic, local corneal amyloid deposits may also develop as a result of a variety of lesions, including repeated trauma, e.g., trichiasis [157].

Several of the familial corneal dystrophies have been shown to be associated with mutations in the gene for kerato-epithelin (also called transforming growth factor-beta-induced protein ig-h3 or RGD-containing collagen-associated protein) [158]. This is a 660 amino acid residue adhesion protein, that is highly expressed by the corneal epithelium [159]. C-terminal fragments of kerato-epithelin have been extracted from corneal amyloid [160], and amyloid may label immunohistochemically with antibodies against this region [160]. The amyloid in gelatinous drop-like corneal dystrophy is of a different nature, and a number of mutations have been identified in the gene for tumor-associated calcium signal transducer 2 (TACSTD2) [161, 162], which is a 323 amino acid residue cell surface receptor [163]. Also lactoferrin has been identified in corneal amyloid [164].

Amyloid may appear at different levels of the cornea. Deposits may involve the subepitelial layer and the stroma but can also be seen close to the Descemet's membrane. At least in the gelatinous drop-like conditions, amyloid may affect the Bowman's membrane and the overlying epithelium. The described forms of amyloid have not been found elsewhere in the eye.

Amyloid in Joints, Ligaments, and Tendons

The involvement of joints in systemic amyloidoses, particularly of the Aβ2M-type, is well known, but localized amyloid in joints, tendons, ligaments, and cartilage is much more common and underappreciated. These deposits are hardly visible without special stains. In particular, the hip joints, knee joints, invertebral discs, and ligamentum flavum have been studied. Analysis of autopsy materials from the hip [165] and knee [166] joints as well as the intervertebral (Fig. 7.15) and sternoclavicular discs [167, 168] revealed a surprisingly high prevalence of amyloid; in the case of knee joints, it was found in 93 % of cases. Small amyloid deposits occurred in the fibrous tissue, in the synovia, and also in the cartilage. In the synovia, a thin amyloid layer can occur just beneath the synovial cell layer. Given the high prevalence at autopsy, it is not

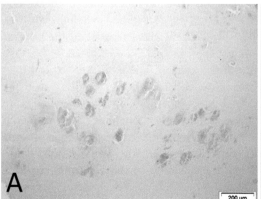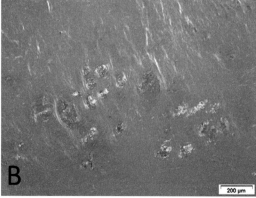

Fig. 7.15 Amyloid deposits in a degeneratively altered vertebral disc. At least some of the amyloid is of transthyretin origin. (**a**), Congo red in ordinary light and (**b**) between crossed polars

Fig. 7.16 ATTR amyloid deposits in ligamentum flavum in a patient undergoing surgery for lumbar spinal stenosis. Congo red and immunolabeling with antibodies against TTR

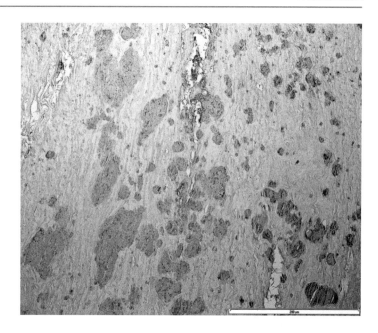

surprising that amyloid deposits may be found in surgical materials from the same locations [169–172] as well as other sites [173].

Analysis of amyloid from meniscus revealed apolipoprotein A–I as a major fibril protein [174]. In another study, amyloid in surgical material associated with rotator cuff tears and lumbar canal stenosis showed immunoreaction with antibodies against transthyretin [175, 176]. Gene analysis showed no mutation. Likewise, several communications have described the analysis of amyloid-containing material removed during surgery for carpal tunnel syndrome in the elderly; these studies also demonstrated the wild-type origin of the amyloid [110, 175]. Wild-type transthyretin is the fibril protein found in senile systemic amyloidosis, which may be associated with carpal tunnel syndrome as the presenting symptom [177]. Wt ATTR (senile systemic) amyloidosis is very common in the elderly and systemic deposits may be quite sparse. Therefore, at present, it is not possible to determine whether the transthyretin deposits commonly found in joints and ligaments constitute a localized form of amyloidosis or are part of a systemic disease. ATTR amyloid deposits in ligamentum flavum can be quite extensive (Fig. 7.16).

As with many of the "senile" forms of localized amyloid, the possible pathogenic importance of the deposits in joints, ligaments, and tendons is unknown. As with the other forms, it is not impossible that the protein aggregates exert some form of toxic effect on cells and thereby participate in degenerative processes.

Additional Localized Aggregates with Amyloid Properties

Fibrillar intracellular aggregates with amyloid staining properties occur in some cells outside the central nervous system. In addition to the epithelial cells in the choroid plexus [178–181], such fibrils have been described in the adrenal cortex [181] (Fig. 7.17a) and in Sertoli cells [31]. The biochemical characteristics of the proteins are not known.

Lastly, corpora amylacea are extracellular spheroids with amyloid properties that are found in certain tissues in association with aging. Particularly common are corpora amylacea in the lungs (Fig. 7.17b) and in the prostate (Fig. 7.17c and d). The prostate protein has been determined to be the S100A8/A9 protein [182].

There is nothing known regarding the pathogenesis or importance of these different aggregates.

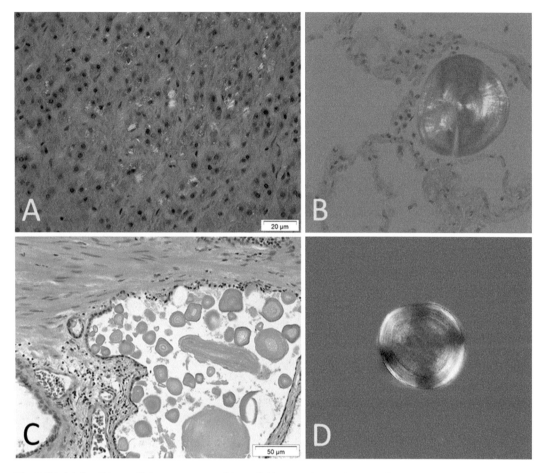

Fig. 7.17 (**a**) Small intracellular aggregates, with amyloid properties, in the adrenal cortex. (**b**) Examples of corpora amylacea in the lung (**b**) and prostate (**c** and **d**). Congo red with crossed polars in (**b**) and (**d**), and H&E in (**c**)

References

1. Rochet J-C, Lansbury PTJ. Amyloid fibrillogenesis: themes and variations. Curr Opin Struct Biol. 2000;10:60–8.
2. Rubinow A, Celli BR, Cohen AS, Rigden BG, Brody JS. Localized amyloidosis of the lower respiratory tract. Am Rew Resp Dis. 1978;118:603–11.
3. Utz JP, Swensen SJ, Gertz MA. Pulmonary amyloidosis. The Mayo clinic experience from 1980 to 1993. Ann Intern Med. 1996;124:407–13.
4. Monge M, Chauveau D, Cordonnier C, Noël LH, Presne C, Makdassi R, Jauréguy M, Lecaque C, Renou M, Grünfeld JP, et al. Localized amyloidosis of the genitourinary tract: report of 5 new cases and review of the literature. Medicine (Baltimore). 2011;90:212–22.
5. Linke RP, Gerhard L, Lottspeich F. Brain-restricted amyloidoma of immunoglobulin λ-light chain origin clinically resembling multiple sclerosis. Biol Chem Hoppe Seyler. 1992;373:1201–9.
6. Merrimen JL, Alkhudair WK, Gupta R. Localized amyloidosis of the urinary tract: case series of nine patients. Urology. 2006;67:904–9.
7. Hagari Y, Mihara M, Hagari S. Nodular localized cutaneous amyloidosis: detection of monoclonality of infiltrating plasma cells by polymerase chain reaction. Br J Dermatol. 1996;135:630–3.
8. Hagari Y, Mihara M, Konohana I, Ueki H, Yamamoto O, Koizumi H. Nodular localized cutaneous amyloidosis: further demonstration of monoclonality of infiltrating plasma cells in four additional Japanese patients. Br J Dermatol. 1998;138:652–4.
9. Setoguchi M, Hoshii Y, Kawano H, Ishihara T. Analysis of plasma cell clonality in localized AL amyloidosis. Amyloid. 2000;7:41–5.
10. Ryan RJ, Sloan JM, Collins AB, Mansouri J, Raje NS, Zukerberg LR, Ferry JA. Extranodal marginal zone lymphoma of mucosa-associated lymphoid

tissue with amyloid deposition: a clinicopathologic case series. Am J Clin Pathol. 2012;137:51–64.

11. Grogg KL, Aubry MC, Vrana JA, Theis JD, Dogan A. Nodular pulmonary amyloidosis is characterized by localized immunoglobulin deposition and is frequently associated with an indolent B-cell lymphoproliferative disorder. Am J Surg Pathol. 2013; 37:406–12.

12. Olsen KE, Sletten K, Sandgren O, Olsson H, Myrvold K, Westermark P. What is the role of giant cells in localized AL amyloidosis? Amyloid. 1999; 6:89–97.

13. Westermark P. Localized AL amyloidosis: a suicidal neoplasm? Ups J Med Sci. 2012;117:244–50.

14. Charlot M, Seldin DC, O'hara C, Skinner M, Sanchorawala V. Localized amyloidosis of the breast: a case series. Amyloid. 2011;18:72–5.

15. Piazza C, Cavaliere S, Foccoli P, Toninelli C, Bolzoni A, Peretti G. Endoscopic management of laryngo-tracheobronchial amyloidosis: a series of 32 patients. Eur Arch Otorhinolaryngol. 2003; 260:349–54.

16. Paccalin M, Hachulla E, Cazalet C, Tricot L, Carreiro M, Rubi M, Grateau G, Roblot P. Localized amyloidosis: a survey of 35 French cases. Amyloid. 2005;12:239–45.

17. Mäkitie AA, Vala U, Kronlund H, Kääriäinen M, Pettersson T. Laryngeal amyloidosis as a cause of death. Amyloid. 2013;20:58.

18. Wierzbicka M, Budzyński D, Piwowarczyk K, Bartochowska A, Marszałek A, Szyfter W. How to deal with laryngeal amyloidosis? Experience based on 16 cases. Amyloid. 2012;19(4):177–81.

19. Abdallah A-O, Westfall C, Brown H, Muzaffar J, Atrash S, Nair B. Unilateral conjunctival AL kappa amyloidosis with trace evidence of systemic amyloidosis. Am J Case Rep. 2012;13:102–5.

20. Westermark GT, Westermark P, Berne C, Korsgren O. Widespread amyloid deposition in transplanted human pancreatic islets. N Engl J Med. 2008;359:977–9.

21. Westermark P, Wernstedt C, Wilander E, Sletten K. A novel peptide in the calcitonin gene related peptide family as an amyloid fibril protein in the endocrine pancreas. Biochem Biophys Res Commun. 1986;140:827–31.

22. Westermark P, Wernstedt C, Wilander E, Hayden DW, O'Brien TD, Johnson KH. Amyloid fibrils in human insulinoma and islets of Langerhans of the diabetic cat are derived from a neuropeptide-like protein also present in normal islet cells. Proc Natl Acad Sci USA. 1987;84:3881–5.

23. Westermark P, Wernstedt C, O'Brien TD, Hayden DW, Johnson KH. Islet amyloid in type 2 human diabetes mellitus and adult diabetic cats contains a novel putative polypeptide hormone. Am J Pathol. 1987;127:414–7.

24. Cooper GJ, Willis AC, Clark A, Turner RC, Sim RB, Reid KBM. Purification and characterization of a peptide from amyloid-rich pancreases of type 2 diabetic patients. Proc Natl Acad Sci USA. 1987;84:8628–32.

25. Westermark P, Andersson A, Westermark GT. Islet amyloid polypeptide, islet amyloid and diabetes mellitus. Physiol Rev. 2011;91:795–826.

26. Jurgens CA, Toukatly MN, Fligner CL, Udayasankar J, Subramanian SL, Zraika S, Aston-Mourney K, Carr DB, Westermark P, Westermark GT, et al. β-cell loss and β-cell apoptosis in human type 2 diabetes are related to islet amyloid deposition. Am J Pathol. 2011;178:2632–40.

27. Shigihara N, Fukunaka A, Hara A, Komiya K, Honda A, Uchida T, Abe H, Toyofuku Y, Tamaki M, Ogihara T, et al. Human IAPP-induced pancreatic β cell toxicity and its regulation by autophagy. J Clin Invest. 2014;124:3634–44.

28. Kim J, Cheon H, Jeong YT, Quan W, Kim KH, Cho JM, Lim YM, Oh SH, Jin SM, Kim JH, et al. Amyloidogenic peptide oligomer accumulation in autophagy-deficient β cells induces diabetes. J Clin Invest. 2014;124:3311–24.

29. Anderson TJ, Ewen SWB. Amyloid in normal and pathological parathyroid glands. J Clin Pathol. 1974;27:656–63.

30. Harach HR, Jasani B. Parathyroid hyperplasia in multiple endocrine neoplasia type 1: a pathological and immunohistochemical reappraisal. Histopathology. 1992;20:305–13.

31. Bohl J, Steinmetz H, Störkel S. Age-related accumulation of congophilic fibrillar inclusions in endocrine cells. Virchows Arch A. 1991;419:51–8.

32. Hodkinson HM, Pomerance A. The clinical significance of senile cardiac amyloidosis: a prospective clinico-pathological study. Q J Med. 1977; 46:381–7.

33. Westermark P, Johansson B, Natvig JB. Senile cardiac amyloidosis: evidence of two different amyloid substances in the ageing heart. Scand J Immunol. 1979;10:303–8.

34. Westermark P, Sletten K, Johansson B, Cornwell GG III. Fibril in senile systemic amyloidosis is derived from normal transthyretin. Proc Natl Acad Sci USA. 1990;87:2843–5.

35. Johansson B, Wernstedt C, Westermark P. Atrial natriuretic peptide deposited as atrial amyloid fibrils. Biochem Biophys Res Commun. 1987; 148:1087–92.

36. Linke RP, Voigt C, Störkel FS, Eulitz M. N-terminal amino acid sequence analysis indicates that isolated atrial amyloid is derived from atrial natriuretic peptide. Virchows Arch B. 1988;55:125–7.

37. Yan W, Wu F, Morser J, Wu Q. Corin, a transmembrane cardiac serine protease, acts as a pro-atrial natriuretic peptide-converting enzyme. Proc Natl Acad Sci USA. 2000;97:8525–9.

38. Pucci A, Wharton J, Arbustini E, Grasso M, Diegoli M, Needleman P, Vigano M, Polak JM. Atrial amyloid deposits in the failing human heart display both

atrial and brain natriuretic peptide-like immunoreactivity. J Pathol. 1991;165:235–41.

39. Steiner I, Hájková P. Patterns of isolated atrial amyloid: a study of 100 hearts on autopsy. Cardiovasc Pathol. 2006;15:287–90.

40. Steiner I, Hájková P, Kvasnicka J, Kholová I. Myocardial sleeves of pulmonary veins and atrial fibrillation: a postmortem histopathological study of 100 subjects. Virchows Arch. 2006;449:88–95.

41. Cornwell GG III, Murdoch WL, Kyle RA, Westermark P, Pitkänen P. Frequency and distribution of senile cardiovascular amyloid. Am J Med. 1983;75:618–23.

42. Johansson B, Westermark P. The relation of atrial natriuretic factor to isolated atrial amyloid. Exp Mol Pathol. 1990;52:266–78.

43. Takahashi M, Hoshii Y, Kawano H, Gondo T, Yokota T, Okabayashi H, Shimada I, Ishihara T. Ultrastructural evidence for the formation of amyloid fibrils within cardiomyocytes in isolated atrial amyloid. Amyloid. 1998;5:35–42.

44. Röcken C, Peters B, Juenemann G, Saeger W, Klein HU, Huth C, Roessner A, Goette A. Atrial amyloidosis: an arrhythmogenic substrate for persistent atrial fibrillation. Circulation. 2002;106:2091–7.

45. Steiner I. The prevalence of isolated atrial amyloid. J Pathol. 1987;153:395–8.

46. Looi L-M. Isolated atrial amyloidosis. A clinicopathologic study indicating increased prevalence in chronic heart disease. Hum Pathol. 1993;24:602–7.

47. Leone O, Boriani G, Chiappini B, Pacini D, Cenacchi G, Martin Suarez S, Rapezzi C, Bacchi Reggiani ML, Marinelli G. Amyloid deposition as a cause of atrial remodelling in persistent valvular atrial fibrillation. Eur Heart J. 2004;25:1237–41.

48. Millucci L, Ghezzi L, Bernardini G, Braconi D, Tanganelli P, Santucci A. Prevalence of isolated atrial amyloidosis in young patients affected by congestive heart failure. ScientificWorldJournal. 2012;2012:293863.

49. Störkel S, Bohl J, Schneider H-M. Senile amyloidosis: principles of localization in a heterogeneous form of amyloidosis. Virchows Arch. 1983; 44:145–61.

50. Tashima T, Kitamoto T, Tateishi J, Ogomori K, Nakagaki H. Incidence and characterization of age related amyloid deposits in the human anterior pituitary gland. Virchows Arch A. 1988;412:323–7.

51. Westermark P, Eriksson L, Engström U, Eneström S, Sletten K. Prolactin-derived amyloid in the aging pituitary gland. Am J Pathol. 1997;150:67–73.

52. Westermark P, Grimelius L, Polak JM, Larsson L-I, van Noorden S, Wilander E, Pearse AGE. Amyloid in polypeptide hormone-producing tumors. Lab Invest. 1977;37:212–5.

53. David R, Buchner A. Amyloid stroma in a tubular carcinoma of palatal salivary gland. Cancer. 1978;41:1836–44.

54. Harach HR, Wilander E, Grimelius L, Bergholm U, Westermark P, Falkmer S. Chromogranin A immunoreactivity compared with argyrophilia, calcitonin immunoreactivity, and amyloid as tumour markers in the histopathological diagnosis of medullary (C-cell) thyroid carcinoma. Pathol Res Pract. 1992;188:123–30.

55. Sletten K, Westermark P, Natvig JB. Characterization of amyloid fibril proteins from medullary carcinoma of the thyroid. J Exp Med. 1976;143:993–8.

56. Khurana R, Agarwal A, Bajpai VK, Verma N, Sharma AK, Gupta RP, Madhusudan KP. Unraveling the amyloid associated with human medullary thyroid carcinoma. Endocrinology. 2004;145:5465–70.

57. Bergholm U, Adami HO, Auer G, Bergström R, Bäckdahl M, Grimelius L, Hansson G, Ljungberg O, Wilander E. Histopathologic characteristics and nuclear DNA content as prognostic factors in medullary thyroid carcinoma. A nationwide study in Sweden. The Swedish MTC Study Group. Cancer. 1989;64:135–42.

58. Scopsi L, Sampietro G, Boracchi P, Del Bo R, Gullo M, Placucci M, Pilotti S. Multivariate analysis of prognostic factors in sporadic medullary carcinoma of the thyroid. A retrospective study of 109 consecutive patients. Cancer. 1996;78:2173–83.

59. Westermark GT. Endocrine amyloid. In: Sipe JD, editor. Amyloid proteins. The beta sheet conformation and disease. Wiley-VCH: Weinheim; 2005. p. 723–54.

60. Mittendorf EA, Liu YC, McHenry CR. Giant insulinoma: case report and review of the literature. J Clin Endocrinol Metab. 2005;90:575–80.

61. Callacondo D, Arenas JL, Ganoza AJ, Rojas-Camayo J, Quesada-Olarte J, Robledo H. Giant insulinoma: a report of 3 cases and review of the literature. Pancreas. 2013;42:1323–32.

62. Stridsberg M, Berne C, Sandler S, Wilander E, Öberg K. Inhibition of insulin secretion, but normal peripheral insulin sensitivity, in a patient with a malignant endocrine pancreatic tumour producing high amounts of an islet amyloid polypeptide-like molecule. Diabetologia. 1993;36:843–9.

63. Landolt AM, Kleihues P, Heitz PU. Amyloid deposits in pituitary adenomas. Differentiation in two types. Arch Pathol Lab Med. 1987;111:453–8.

64. Hinton DR, Polk RK, Linse KD, Weiss MH, Kovacs K, Garner JA. Characterization of spherical amyloid protein from a prolactin-producing pituitary adenoma. Acta Neuropathol. 1997;93:43–9.

65. Paetau A, Partanen S, Mustajoki P, Valtonen S, Pelkonen R, Wahlström T. Prolactinoma of the pituitary containing amyloid. Acta Endocrinol. 1985;109:176–80.

66. Kubota T, Kuroda E, Yamashima T, Tachibana O, Kabuto M, Yamamoto S. Amyloid formation in prolactinoma. Arch Pathol Lab Med. 1986; 110(1):72–5.

67. Levine SN, Ishaq S, Nanda A, Wilson JD, Gonzalez-Toledo E. Occurrence of extensive spherical amyloid deposits in a prolactin-secreting pituitary macroadenoma: a radiologic-pathologic correlation. Ann Diagn Pathol. 2013;17:361–6.
68. Iwase T, Nishizawa S, Baba S, Hinokuma K, Sugimura H, Nakamura S, Uemura K, Shirasawa H, Kino I. Intrasellar neuronal choristoma associated with growth hormone-producing pituitary adenoma containing amyloid deposits. Hum Pathol. 1995; 26:925–8.
69. Bilbao JM, Kovacs K, Horvath E, Higgins HP, Horsey WJ. Pituitary melanocorticotrophinoma with amyloid deposition. J Can Sci Neurol. 1975;2(3):199–202.
70. Waugh DF. A fibrous modification of insulin. I. The heat precipitate of insulin. J Am Chem Soc. 1946; 68:247–50.
71. Störkel S, Schneider H-M, Müntefering H, Kashiwagi S. Iatrogenic, insulin-dependent, local amyloidosis. Lab Invest. 1983;48:108–11.
72. Dische FE, Wernstedt C, Westermark GT, Westermark P, Pepys MB, Rennie JA, Gilbey SG, Watkins PJ. Insulin as an amyloid-fibril protein at sites of repeated insulin injections in a diabetic patient. Diabetologia. 1988;31:158–61.
73. Shikama Y, Kitazawa J, Yagihashi N, Uehara O, Murata Y, Yajima N, Wada R, Yagihashi S. Localized amyloidosis at the site of repeated insulin injection in a diabetic patient. Intern Med. 2010;49:397–401.
74. Yumlu S, Barany R, Eriksson M, Röcken C. Localized insulin-derived amyloidosis in patients with diabetes mellitus: a case report. Hum Pathol. 2009;40:1655–60.
75. D'Souza A, Theis JD, Vrana JA, Dogan A. Pharmaceutical amyloidosis associated with subcutaneous insulin and enfuvirtide administration. Amyloid. 2014;21:71–5.
76. Westermark P. Amyloidosis of the skin: a comparison between localized and systemic amyloidosis. Acta Derm Venereol. 1979;59:341–5.
77. Chandran NS, Goh BK, Lee SS, Goh CL. Case of primary localized cutaneous amyloidosis with protean clinical manifestations: lichen, poikiloderma-like, dyschromic and bullous variants. J Dermatol. 2011;38:1066–71.
78. Black MM, Heather CJ. The ultrastructure of lichen amyloidosus with special reference to the epidermal changes. Br J Dermatol. 1972;87:117–22.
79. Norén P, Westermark P. Two different pathogenetic pathways in lichen amyloidus and macular amyloidosis. Arch Dermatol Res. 1986;278:206–13.
80. Lee Y-S, Fong P-H. Macular and lichenoid amyloidosis: a possible secretory product of stimulated basal keratinocytes. An ultrastructural study. Pathology. 1991;23:322–6.
81. Kumakiri M, Hashimoto K. Histogenesis of primary localized cutaneous amyloidosis: sequential change of epidermal keratinocytes to amyloid via filamentous degeneration. J Invest Dermatol. 1979; 73:150–62.
82. Huilgol SC, Ramnarain N, Carrington P, Leigh IM, Black MM. Cytokeratins in primary cutaneous amyloidosis. Australas J Dermatol. 1998;39:81–5.
83. Apaydin R, Gürbüz Y, Bayramgürler D, Müezzinoglu B, Bilen N. Cytokeratin expression in lichen amyloidosus and macular amyloidosis. J Eur Acad Dermatol Venereol. 2004;18:305–9.
84. Kobayashi H, Hashimoto K. Amyloidogenesis in organ-limited cutaneous amyloidosis: an antigenic identity between epidermal keratin and skin amyloid. J Invest Dermatol. 1983;80:66–72.
85. Westermark P, Murphy CL, Eulitz M, Wallgren-Pettersson C, Udd B, Hellman U, Ihse E, Weiss DT, Solomon A. Galectin 7-associated cutaneous amyloidosis. Amyloid. 2010;17 Suppl 1:71.
86. Miura Y, Harumiya S, Ono K, Fujimoto E, Akiyama M, Fujii N, Kawano H, Wachi H, Tajima S. Galectin-7 and actin are components of amyloid deposit of localized cutaneous amyloidosis. Exp Dermatol. 2013;22:36–40.
87. Leonidas DD, Vatzaki EH, Vorum H, Celis JE, Madsen P, Acharya KR. Structural basis for the recognition of carbohydrates by human galectin-7. Biochemistry. 1998;67:13930–40.
88. Kousseff BG, Espinoza C, Zamore GA. Sipple syndrome with lichen amyloidosis as a paracrinopathy: pleiotropy, heterogeneity, or a contiguous gene? J Am Acad Dermatol. 1991;25:651–7.
89. Verga U, Fugazzola L, Cambiaghi S, Pritelli C, Alessi E, Cortelazzi D, Gangi E, Beck-Peccoz P. Frequent association between MEN 2A and cutaneous lichen amyloidosis. Clin Endocrinol (Oxf). 2003;59:156–61.
90. Lin MW, Lee DD, Lin CH, Huang CY, Wong CK, Chang YT, Liu HN, Hsiao KJ, Tsai SF. Suggestive linkage of familial primary cutaneous amyloidosis to a locus on chromosome 1q23. Br J Dermatol. 2005;152:29–36.
91. Arita K, South AP, Hans-Filho G, Sakuma TH, Lai-Cheong J, Clements S, Odashiro M, Odashiro DN, Hans-Neto G, Hans NR, et al. Oncostatin M receptor-beta mutations underlie familial primary localized cutaneous amyloidosis. Am J Hum Genet. 2008;82:73–80.
92. Tanaka A, Lai-Cheong JE, van den Akker PC, Nagy N, Millington G, Diercks GF, van Voorst Vader PC, Clements SE, Almaani N, Techanukul T, et al. The molecular skin pathology of familial primary localized cutaneous amyloidosis. Exp Dermatol. 2010;19:416–23.
93. Westermark P, Ridderström E, Vahlquist A. Macular posterior pigmentary incontinence: its relation to macular amyloidosis and notalgia paresthetica. Acta Derm Venereol. 1996;76:302–4.
94. Bugalho MJGM, Limbert E, Sobrinho LG, Clode AL, Soares J, Nunes JFM, Pereira MC, Santos MA. A kindred with multiple endocrine neoplasia

type 2A associated with pruritic skin lesions. Cancer. 1992;70:2664–7.

95. Olsen K, Westermark P. Amyloid in basal cell carcinoma and seborrheic keratosis. Acta Derm Venereol. 1994;74:273–5.

96. Looi LM. Localized amyloidosis in basal cell carcinoma. A pathologic study. Cancer. 1983;52:1833–6.

97. Satti MB, Azzopardi JG. Amyloid deposits in basal cell carcinoma of the skin. A pathologic study of 199 cases. J Am Acad Dermatol. 1990;22:1082–7.

98. Hashimoto K, King LE. Secondary localized cutaneous amyloidosis associated with actinic keratosis. J Invest Dermatol. 1973;61:293–9.

99. Ginarte M, León A, Toribio J. Disseminated superficial porokeratosis with amyloid deposits. Eur J Dermatol. 2005;15:298–300.

100. Apaydin R, Gürbüz Y, Bayramgürler D, Bilen N. Cytokeratin contents of basal cell carcinoma, epidermis overlying tumour, and associated stromal amyloidosis: an immunohistochemical study. Amyloid. 2005;12:41–7.

101. Pindborg JJ. A calcifying epithelial odontogenic tumor. Cancer. 1958;11:838–43.

102. Solomon A, Murphy CL, Weaver K, Weiss DT, Hrncic R, Eulitz M, Donnell RL, Sletten K, Westermark GT, Westermark P. Calcifying epithelial odontogenic (Pindborg) tumor-associated amyloid consists of a novel human protein. J Lab Clin Med. 2003;142:348–55.

103. Murphy CL, Kestler DP, Foster JS, Wang S, Macy SD, Kennel SJ, Carlson ER, Hudson J, Weiss DT, Solomon A. Odontogenic ameloblast-associated protein nature of the amyloid found in calcifying epithelial odontogenic tumors and unerupted tooth follicles. Amyloid. 2008;15:89–95.

104. Siddiqui S, Bruker CT, Kestler DP, Foster JS, Gray KD, Solomon A, Bell JL. Odontogenic ameloblast associated protein as a novel biomarker for human breast cancer. Am Surg. 2009;75:769–75.

105. Sipe JD, Benson MD, Ikeda S, Merlini G, Saraiva MJ, Westermark P. Updated nomenclature 2014: amyloid fibril proteins and clinical classification of the amyloidoses. Amyloid. 2014;21:221–4.

106. Benson MD, Breall J, Cummings OW, Liepnieks JJ. Biochemical characterization of amyloid by endomyocardial biopsy. Amyloid. 2009;16:9–14.

107. Pitkänen P, Westermark P, Cornwell GG III. Senile systemic amyloidosis. Am J Pathol. 1984;117: 391–9.

108. Ueda M, Ando Y, Haraoka K, Katsuragi S, Terasaki Y, Sugimoto M, Sun X, Uchino M. Aging and transthyretin-related amyloidosis: pathologic examinations in pulmonary amyloidosis. Amyloid. 2006;13(1):24–30.

109. Westermark P, Bergström J, Solomon A, Murphy C, Sletten K. Transthyretin-derived senile systemic amyloidosis: clinicopathologic and structural consideration. Amyloid. 2003;10 Suppl 1:48–54.

110. Sekijima Y, Uchiyama S, Tojo K, Sano K, Shimizu Y, Imaeda T, Hoshii Y, Kato H, S-i I. High prevalence of wild-type transthyretin deposition in patients with idiopathic carpal tunnel syndrome: a common cause of carpal tunnel syndrome in the elderly. Hum Pathol. 2011;42:1785–91.

111. Gioeva Z, Urban P, Meliss RR, Haag J, Axmann HD, Siebert F, Becker K, Radtke HG, Röcken C. ATTR amyloid in the carpal tunnel ligament is frequently of wildtype transthyretin origin. Amyloid. 2013; 20:1–6.

112. Westermark P, Westermark GT, Suhr OB, Berg S. Transthyretin-derived amyloidosis: probably a common cause of lumbar spinal stenosis. Ups J Med Sci. 2014;119:223–8.

113. Yanagisawa A, Ueda M, Sueyoshi T, Okada T, Fujimoto T, Ogi Y, Kitagawa K, Tasaki M, Misumi Y, Oshima T, et al. Amyloid deposits derived from transthyretin in the ligamentum flavum as related to lumbar spinal canal stenosis. Mod Pathol. 2015; 28:201–7.

114. Westermark P, Davey E, Lindbom K, Enqvist S. Subcutaneous fat tissue for diagnosis and studies of systemic amyloidosis. Acta Histochem. 2006;108:209–13.

115. Felding P, Fex G, Westermark P, Olofsson B-O, Pitkänen P, Benson L. Prealbumin in Swedish patients with senile systemic amyloidosis and familial amyloidotic polyneuropathy. Scand J Immunol. 1985;21:133–40.

116. Bergström J, Gustavsson Å, Hellman U, Sletten K, Murphy CL, Weiss DT, Solomon A, Olofsson B-O, Westermark P. Amyloid deposits in transthyretin-derived amyloidosis: cleaved transthyretin is associated with distinct amyloid morphology. J Pathol. 2005;206:224–32.

117. Johansson B, Westermark P. Senile systemic amyloidosis: a clinico-pathological study of twelve patients with massive amyloid infiltration. Int J Cardiol. 1991;32:83–92.

118. Eriksson A, Eriksson P, Olofsson B-O, Thornell L-E. The cardiac atrioventricular conduction system in familial amyloidosis with polyneuropathy. A clinico-pathologic study of six cases from Northern Sweden. Acta Pathol Microbiol Immunol Scand A. 1983;91:343–9.

119. Eriksson A, Eriksson P, Olofsson B-O, Thornell L-E. The sinoatrial node in familial amyloidosis with polyneuropathy. A clinico-pathological study of nine cases from northern Sweden. Virchows Arch A. 1984;402:239–46.

120. Tanskanen M, Kiuru-Enari S, Tienari P, Polvikoski T, Verkkoniemi A, Rastas S, Sulkava R, Paetau A. Senile systemic amyloidosis, cerebral amyloid angiopathy, and dementia in a very old Finnish population. Amyloid. 2006;13:164–9.

121. Kyle RA, Spittell PC, Gertz MA, Li CY, Edwards WD, Olson LJ, Thibodeau SN. The premortem

recognition of systemic senile amyloidosis with cardiac involvement. Am J Med. 1996;101:395–400.

122. Ng B, Connors LH, Davidoff R, Skinner M, Falk RH. Senile systemic amyloidosis presenting with heart failure: a comparison with light chain-associated amyloidosis. Arch Intern Med. 2005; 165:1425–9.

123. Rapezzi C, Merlini G, Quarta CC, Riva L, Longhi S, Leone O, Salvi F, Ciliberti P, Pastorelli F, Biagini E, et al. Systemic cardiac amyloidoses: disease profiles and clinical courses of the 3 main types. Circulation. 2009;120:1203–12.

124. Mucchiano G, Cornwell GG III, Westermark P. Senile aortic amyloid. Evidence of two distinct forms of localized deposits. Am J Pathol. 1992;140: 871–7.

125. Schwartz P. Amyloidosis, cause and manifestation of senile deterioration. Springfield, IL: C.C. Thomas; 1970.

126. Battaglia S, Trentini GP. Aortenamyloidose im Erwachsenenalter. Virchows Arch A. 1978;378: 153–9.

127. Peng S, Glennert J, Westermark P. Medin-amyloid: a recently characterized age-associated arterial amyloid form affects mainly arteries in the upper part of the body. Amyloid. 2005;12:96–102.

128. Muckle TJ. Giant cell inflammation compared with amyloidosis of the internal elastic lamina in temporal arteries. Arthritis Rheum. 1988;31:1186–9.

129. Peng S, Westermark P, Näslund J, Häggqvist B, Glennert J, Westermark P. Medin and medin-amyloid in ageing inflamed and non-inflamed temporal arteries. J Pathol. 2002;196:91–6.

130. Häggqvist B, Näslund J, Sletten K, Westermark GT, Mucchiano G, Tjernberg LO, Nordstedt C, Engström U, Westermark P. Medin: an integral fragment of aortic smooth muscle cell-produced lactadherin forms the most common human amyloid. Proc Natl Acad Sci USA. 1999;96:8669–74.

131. Yolken RH, Peterson JA, Vonderfecht SL, Fouts ET, Midthun K, Newburg DS. Human milk mucin inhibits rotavirus replication and prevents experimental gastroenteritis. J Clin Invest. 1992;90:1984–91.

132. Newburg DS, Peterson JA, Ruiz-Palacios M, Matson DO, Morrow AL, Shults J, de Lourdes GM, Chaturvedi P, Newburg SO, Scallan CD, et al. Role of human-milk lactadherin in protection against symptomatic rotavirus infection. Lancet. 1998; 351:1160–4.

133. Hanayama RM, Miwa K, Shinohara A, Iwamatsu A, Nagata S. Identification of a factor that links apoptotic cells to phagocytes. Nature. 2002;417:182–7.

134. Shi J, Gilbert GE. Lactadherin inhibits enzyme complexes of blood coagulation by competing for phospholipid-binding sites. Blood. 2003;101: 2628–36.

135. Larsson A, Peng S, Persson H, Rosenbloom J, Abrams WR, Wassberg E, Thelin S, Sletten K, Gerwins P, Westermark P. Lactadherin binds to

elastin—a starting point for medin amyloid formation? Amyloid. 2006;13:78–85.

136. Zehr KJ, Mathur A, Orszulak TA, Mullany CJ, Schaff HV. Surgical treatment of ascending aortic aneurysms in patients with giant cell aortitis. Ann Thorac Surg. 2005;79:1512–7.

137. Peng S, Larsson A, Wassberg E, Gerwins P, Thelin S, Fu X, Westermark P. Role of aggregated medin in the pathogenesis of thoracic aortic aneurysm and dissection. Lab Invest. 2007;87:1195–205.

138. López-Candales A, Holmes DR, Liao S, Scott MJ, Wickline SA, Thompson RW. Decreased vascular smooth muscle cell density in medial degeneration of human abdominal aortic aneurysms. Am J Pathol. 1997;150:993–1007.

139. Westermark P, Mucchiano G, Marthin T, Johnson KH, Sletten K. Apolipoprotein A1-derived amyloid in human aortic atherosclerotic plaques. Am J Pathol. 1995;147:1186–92.

140. Stangou AJ, Banner NR, Hendry BM, Rela M, Portmann B, Wendon J, Monaghan M, Maccarthy P, Buxton-Thomas M, Mathias CJ, et al. Hereditary fibrinogen A alpha-chain amyloidosis: phenotypic characterization of a systemic disease and the role of liver transplantation. Blood. 2010;115:2998–3007.

141. Goffin YA, Murdoch W, Cornwell GG III, Sorenson GD. Microdeposits of amyloid in sclerocalcific heart valves: a histochemical and immunofluorescence study. J Clin Pathol. 1983;36:1342–9.

142. Kristen AV, Schnabel PA, Winter B, Helmke BM, Longerich T, Hardt S, Koch A, Sack FU, Katus HA, Linke RP, et al. High prevalence of amyloid in 150 surgically removed heart valves—a comparison of histological and clinical data reveals a correlation to atheroinflammatory conditions. Cardiovasc Pathol. 2010;19:228–35.

143. Yokota T, Okabayashi H, Ishihara T, Takahashi M, Iwata T, Yamashita Y, Miyamoto AT, Ushino F. Dystrophic amyloid of the cardiac valves and atherosclerotic aorta has the same antigenicity. Pathol Int. 1995;45:85–6.

144. Pitkänen P, Westermark P, Cornwell GG III, Murdoch W. Amyloid of the seminal vesicles. A distinctive and common localized form of senile amyloidosis. Am J Pathol. 1983;110:64–9.

145. Kee KH, Lee MJ, Shen SS, Suh JH, Lee OJ, Cho HY, Ayala AG, Ro JY. Amyloidosis of seminal vesicles and ejaculatory ducts: a histologic analysis of 21 cases among 447 prostatectomy specimens. Ann Diagn Pathol. 2008;12:235–8.

146. Goldman H. Amyloidosis of seminal vesicles and vas deferens: primary localized cases. Arch Pathol. 1963;75:94–8.

147. Cornwell GG III, Westermark GT, Pitkänen P, Westermark P. Epithelial origin of the amyloid of seminal vesicles in elderly men. J Pathol. 1992;167:297–303.

148. Linke RP, Joswig R, Murphy CL, Wang S, Zhou H, Gross U, Röcken C, Westermark P, Weiss DT,

Solomon A. Senile seminal vesicle amyloid is derived from semenogelin I. J Lab Clin Med. 2005;145:187–93.

149. Mata LR, Maunsbach AB. Absorption of secretory protein by the eithelium of hamster seminal vesicle as studied by electron microscope autoradiography. Biol Cell. 1982;46:65–73.

150. Botash RJ, Poster RB, Abraham JL, Makhuli ZM. Senile seminal vesicle amyloidosis associated with hematospermia: demonstration by endorectal MRI. J Comput Assist Tomogr. 1997;21:748–9.

151. Furuya S, Masumori N, Furuya R, Tsukamoto T, Isomura H, Tamakawa M. Characterization of localized seminal vesicle amyloidosis causing hemospermia: an analysis using immunohistochemistry and magnetic resonance imaging. J Urol. 2005;173:1273–7.

152. Erbersdobler A, Kollermann J, Graefen M, Röcken C, Schlomm T. Seminal vesicle amyloidosis does not provide any protection from invasion by prostate cancer. BJU Int. 2009;103:324–6.

153. Meretoja J. Familial systemic paramyloidosis with lattice dystrophy of the cornea, progressive cranial neuropathy, skin changes and various internal symptoms. A previously unrecognized heritable syndrome. Ann Clin Res. 1969;1:314–24.

154. Pradhan MA, Henderson RA, Patel D, McGhee CN, Vincent AL. Heavy-chain amyloidosis in TGFBI-negative and gelsolin-negative atypical lattice corneal dystrophy. Cornea. 2011;30:1163–6.

155. Klintworth GK. Corneal dystrophies. Orphanet J Rare Dis. 2009;4:7.

156. Kawasaki S, Kinoshita S. Clinical and basic aspects of gelatinous drop-like corneal dystrophy. Dev Ophthalmol. 2011;48:97–115.

157. Lin P-Y, Kao S-C, Hsueh K-F, Chen WY-K, Lee S-M, Lee F-L, Shiuh W-M. Localized amyloidosis of the cornea secondary to trichiasis: clinical course and pathogenesis. Cornea. 2003;22:491–4.

158. Munier FL, Korvatska E, Djemaï A, Le Paslier D, Zografos L, Pescia G, Schorderet DF. Kerato-epithelin mutations in four 5q31-linked corneal dystrophies. Nat Genet. 1997;15:247–51.

159. Escribano J, Hernando N, Ghosh S, Crabb J, Coca-Prados M. cDNA from human ocular ciliary epithelium homologous to beta ig-h3 is preferentially expressed as an extracellular protein in the corneal epithelium. J Cell Physiol. 1994;160:511–21.

160. Stix B, Leber M, Bingemer P, Gross C, Rüschoff J, Fändrich M, Schorderet DF, Vorwerk CK, Zacharias M, Roessner A, et al. Hereditary lattice corneal dystrophy is associated with corneal amyloid deposits enclosing C-terminal fragments of keratoepithelin. Invest Ophthalmol Vis Sci. 2005;46:1133–9.

161. Tsujikawa M, Kurahashi H, Tanaka T, Nishida K, Shimomura Y, Tano Y, Nakamura Y. Identification of the gene responsible for gelatinous drop-like corneal dystrophy. Nat Genet. 1999;21:420–3.

162. Tsujikawa M. Gelatinous drop-like corneal dystrophy. Cornea. 2012;31:S37–40.

163. Ripani E, Sacchetti A, Corda D, Alberti S. Human Trop-2 is a tumor-associated calcium signal transducer. Int J Cancer. 1998;76:671–6.

164. Ando Y, Nakamura M, Katsuragi S, Terazaki H, Nozawa T, Okuda T, Misumi S, Matsunaga N, Hata K, Tajiri T, et al. A novel localized amyloidosis associated with lactoferrin in the cornea. Lab Invest. 2002;82:757–66.

165. Ladefoged C, Christensen HE. Congophilic substance with green dichroism in hip joints in autopsy material. Acta Pathol Microbiol Scand A. 1980;88:55–8.

166. Ladefoged C. Amyloid deposits in the knee joint at autopsy. Ann Rheum Dis. 1986;45:668–72.

167. Goffin YA, Thoua Y, Potvliege PR. Microdeposition of amyloid in the joints. Ann Rheum Dis. 1981;40:27–33.

168. Ladefoged C. Amyloid in intervertebral discs. A histopathological investigation of intervertebral discs from 30 randomly selected autopsies. Appl Pathol. 1985;3:96–104.

169. Ryan LM, Liang G, Kozin F. Amyloid arthropathy: possible association with chondrocalcinosis. J Rheumatol. 1982;9:273–8.

170. Ladefoged C. Amyloid in osteoarthritic hip joints: deposits in relation to chondromatosis, pyrophosphate, and inflammatory cell infiltrate in the synovial membrane and fibrous capsule. Ann Rheum Dis. 1983;42:659–64.

171. Ladefoged C, Fedders O, Petersen OF. Amyloid in intervertebral discs: a histopathological investigation of surgical material from 100 consecutive operations on herniated discs. Ann Rheum Dis. 1986;45:239–43.

172. Mihara S, Kawai S, Gondo T, Ishihara T. Intervertebral disc amyloidosis: histochemical, immunohistochemical and ultrastructural observations. Histopathology. 1994;25:415–20.

173. Mohr W, Kuhn C, Linke RP, Wessinghage D. Deposition of amyloid of unknown origin in articular cartilage. Virchows Arch B. 1991;60:259–62.

174. Solomon A, Murphy CL, Kestler DP, Coriu D, Weiss DT, Makovitzky J, Westermark P. Amyloid contained in the knee joint meniscus is formed from apolipoprotein A-I. Arthritis Rheum. 2006;54:3545–50.

175. Sueyoshi T, Ueda M, Jono H, Irie H, Sei A, Ide J, Ando Y, Mizuta H. Wild-type transthyretin-derived amyloidosis in various ligaments and tendons. Hum Pathol. 2011;42:1259–64.

176. Sueyoshi T, Ueda M, Sei A, Misumi Y, Oshima T, Yamashita T, Obayashi K, Shinriki S, Jono H, Shono M, et al. Spinal multifocal amyloidosis derived from wild-type transthyretin. Amyloid. 2011;18:165–8.

177. Takei Y, Hattori T, Gono T, Tokuda T, Saitoh S, Hoshii Y, S-i I. Senile systemic amyloidosis

presenting as bilateral carpal tunnel syndrome. Amyloid. 2002;9:252–5.

178. Gellerstedt N. Uber das Vorkommen von Sekretkapillaren im Epithel des Plexus chorioideus. Zbl Allg Path Path Anat. 1932;56:164–7.

179. Biondi G. Ein neuer histologischer Befund am Epithel des Plexus corioideus. Z Ges Neurol Psychatry. 1933;144:161–5.

180. Eriksson L, Westermark P. Intracellular neurofibrillary tangle-like aggregations. A constantly present amyloid alteration in the aging choroid plexus. Am J Pathol. 1986;25:124–9.

181. Eriksson L, Westermark P. Age-related accumulation of amyloid inclusions in adrenal cortical cells. Am J Pathol. 1990;136:461–6.

182. Yanamandra K, Alexeyev O, Zamotin V, Srivastava V, Shchukarev A, Brorsson AC, Tartaglia GG, Vogl T, Kayed R, Wingsle G, et al. Amyloid formation by the pro-inflammatory S100A8/A9 proteins in the ageing prostate. PLoS One. 2009;4, e5562.

183. Westermark GT, Sletten K, Westermark P. Alkalidegradation of amyloid: an ancient method useful for making monoclonal antibodies against amyloid fibril proteins. Scand J Immunol. 2009;70:535–40.

Amyloid Deposition in the Central Nervous System

8

Fausto J. Rodriguez, Maria M. Picken, and John M. Lee

Introduction

Amyloidoses are protein conformational disorders that lead to aggregation and formation of insoluble fibrils with a β-pleated sheet structure. The latter is responsible for their physicochemical properties and staining characteristics, most notably their fibrillary ultrastructure and affinity to Congo red stain. Among the many proteins that can undergo fibrillogenesis, only a subset is known to cause amyloid deposition within the central nervous system (CNS) (Table 8.1). Deposition of amyloid in the CNS leads to cognitive decline, dementia, stroke, or a combination of these. CNS amyloid deposition is, in most instances, localized to the brain and its coverings but conversely, systemic amyloidoses, with some exceptions, are largely extracerebral because of the blood–brain barrier. This chapter contains a brief overview of CNS amyloidoses.

In Alzheimer's disease (AD), the most prevalent of the cerebral amyloidoses, there is formation of plaques in the neuropil and deposition of amyloid in small- and medium-sized blood vessels. The deposits are derived from the amyloid β precursor protein (AβPP), an intrinsic transmembrane protein. In Alzheimer's disease plaques are deposited throughout the brain, but are primarily encountered in neocortex and hippocampus. Two major types of plaques are distinguished on routine analysis: neuritic and diffuse. Neuritic plaques consist of an amyloid β protein core (which is Congo red positive) and dystrophic neurites (phosphorylated tau protein positive abnormal neuronal processes). Diffuse plaques consist of amorphous deposits of Aβ protein, which are generally negative for Congo red and no tau protein is detected. Although AD is the most prevalent among the cerebral amyloidoses, several other amyloidoses are also found in the CNS including deposits derived from prion protein, cystatin C, and ABriPP. In rare patients with familial transthyretin (TTR) or familial Finnish amyloidosis, a meningovascular and oculoleptomeningeal

F.J. Rodriguez, MD (✉)
Department of Pathology, Division of
Neuropathology, Johns Hopkins Hospital,
Sheikh Zayed Tower, Room M2101, 1800 Orleans
Street, Baltimore, MD 21231, USA
e-mail: frodrig4@jhmi.edu

M.M. Picken, MD, PhD
Department of Pathology, Loyola University Medical
Center, Loyola University Chicago, Building 110,
Room 2242, 2160 South First Avenue,
Maywood, IL 60153, USA
e-mail: mpicken@luc.edu; MMPicken@aol.com

J.M. Lee, MD, PhD
Department of Pathology and Laboratory Medicine,
NorthShore University Health System,
Room 1914, 2650 Ridge Avenue, Evanston,
IL 60201, USA
e-mail: JLee9@northshore.org

© Springer International Publishing Switzerland 2015
M.M. Picken et al. (eds.), *Amyloid and Related Disorders*, Current Clinical Pathology,
DOI 10.1007/978-3-319-19294-9_8

Table 8.1 Summary of CNS amyloidoses

Type	Pathology	Genetics	Clinical
Aβ	Diffuse plaques Neuritic plaques/NFTs CAA (mild)	Down's AβPP Swe690/691 AβPP V717	Dementia
Aβ	CAA (severe)	AβPP Dutch mutations	Lobar hemorrhages, ± dementia
BR12	Plaques, NFTs, CAA	*BR12* gene chromosome 13	Dementia
Prions (PrP)	Plaques/spongiform changes	sCJD fCJD vCJD GSS	Rapid dementia, ± ataxia, cortical blindness
TTR	Leptomeningeal CAA	Transthyretin gene mutations chromosome 18	Seizures, hemorrhages, ± dementia
Gelsolin	CAA, colocalizes with Lewy bodies	Gelsolin gene mutations Chromosome 9	Finnish hereditary amyloidosis, lattice corneal dystrophy, cranial and peripheral neuropathy
Cystatin C	CAA can be colocalized in Aβ plaques of AD (wild type)	Icelandic mutation	Lobar hemorrhages
AL	Amyloidoma, lepomeningeal CAA	Sporadic type	Tumor-like lesions, focal hemorrhages

AD Alzheimer's disease, *Aβ* amyloid β, *TTR* transthyretin, *AL* light chain amyloid, *BR12* British amyloid protein, *CAA* cerebral amyloid angiopathy, *AβPP* amyloid β precursor protein, *sCJD* sporadic Creutzfeldt–Jakob disease, *fCJD* familial Creutzfeldt–Jakob disease, *vCJD* variant Creutzfeldt–Jakob disease, *GSS* Gerstmann–Straussler–Sheinker

amyloidosis may develop, derived from mutants of the TTR and gelsolin genes, respectively.

Amyloid-Associated Neurodegenerative Diseases

There are a number of neurodegenerative diseases that can lead to amyloid deposition in the brain. The most common of these is AD, where both diffuse and neuritic plaques are deposited in the brain parenchyma (Fig. 8.1a–d). The plaques consist of extracellular deposits of Aβ- protein. The latter results from a cleavage product of AβPP, encoded for a gene in chromosome 21, containing 40 or 42 amino acids through the action of β and γ secretases in a pathologic amyloidogenic pathway. In the "amyloid cascade hypothesis" of AD, Aβ-protein deposition plays a central role in AD pathogenesis [1]. In support of this hypothesis, there is an increase in Aβ deposition in individuals that have one or more copies of the APOe4 allele, in Down's syndrome, and in familial variants of AD leading to early dementia.

However, this hypothesis is not uniformly accepted, and some investigators propose that phosphorylated tau accumulation maybe the primary event in AD pathogenesis [2].

The age-related neuritic core amyloid plaque counts found in the brain are an important component for a pathologic diagnosis of AD. The presence of a few neuritic plaques in an individual 80 or 90 years of age, without dementia, may be considered to be an age-related change but, in a 40-year-old individual, they may represent early onset and/or familial AD. In AD, in addition to amyloid plaques in the neuropil, amyloid deposition occurs in small- and medium-sized blood vessels, resulting in cerebral amyloid angiopathy (CAA) [3]. However, CAA may occur in the absence of AD pathology (see section below; [3]). Mutations in the AβPP protein lead to the Swedish familial variants of AD that are associated with a double mutation adjacent to the β-amyloid secretase (BACE) cleavage site in the N terminus of Aβ. Another group of familial variants of AD involves the V717 mutations, adjacent to presenilin (or γ-secretase) sites near

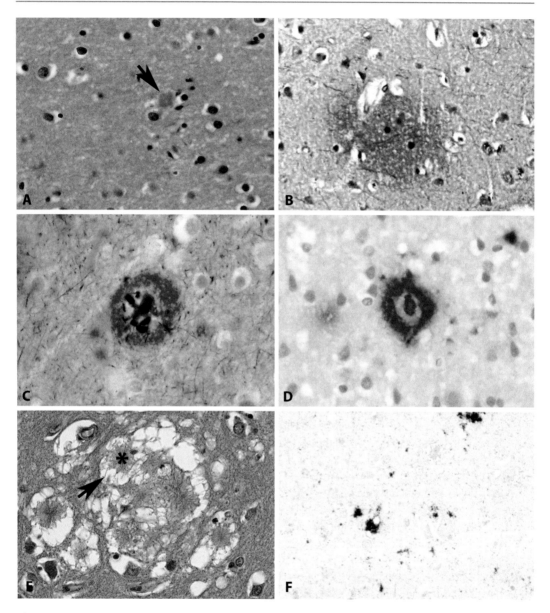

Fig. 8.1 Amyloid deposition in neurodegenerative disorders. One of the hallmarks of Alzheimer disease is the formation of amyloid plaques, extracellular deposits of Aβ protein that may be identified in H&E sections (*arrow*) (**a**). Neocortical diffuse amyloid plaque. These plaques contain pre-amyloidotic deposits of β-amyloid (Aβ protein) that are detectable by immunohistochemistry (not shown). The deposits are silver positive (Bielschowsky stain) but Congo red negative (not shown) (**b**). Neuritic plaques are characterized by a dark amyloid core surrounded by a halo, with associated thickened neuronal processes (neurites) (Hirano method) (**c**). Aβ protein is highlighted in these plaques by immunohistochemistry (**d**). A variety of amyloid containing plaques may develop in prion disease; florid plaques are typical of variant-CJD and are composed of a delicate fibrillary core (*asterisk*) rimmed by spongiotic change (*arrow*) (**e**). In prion disease, plaques and other deposits contain prion-related protein (PrP) which may be recognized by immunohistochemistry (**f**)

the C terminus of the Aβ moiety. Interestingly, in Down's syndrome individuals, who have an extra copy of the gene encoding AβPP protein secondary to trisomy 21, it was found that the initial Aβ fibril formation begins intracellularly before the formation of extracellular plaques.

In addition to amyloid plaque deposition, several intracellular inclusions in CNS neurodegenerative disorders also possess at least some of the properties of amyloid. Among them, the phosphorylated tau-rich neurofibrillary tangles (NFT) have a fibrillar structure and Congo red affinity with birefringence under polarized light. Lewy bodies, composed of α-synuclein, are also the defining pathology in Lewy body disease, which may coexist with AD. Both of these proteins are considered amyloidogenic proteins. In fact, gelsolin, another CNS amyloidogenic protein, has been found to colocalize with both brainstem and cortical Lewy bodies [4]. More recently, TDP43 inclusions and skeins in frontotemporal lobar degeneration and amyotrophic lateral sclerosis have also been found to have similar properties as amyloid [5, 6].

Postmortem brain sections, taken to make a diagnosis of AD, typically include the following: frontal cortex, temporal cortex, hippocampus, entorhinal cortex, and the midbrain [7, 8]. The latter is necessary to identify additional coexisting or alternative pathologies to AD, particularly Lewy body/Parkinson's disease and rare tauopathies. The routine stains used are H & E and a silver stain such as the modified Bielschowsky or Hirano. Although Congo red stains of cortical sections can be performed for the assessment of CAA and plaques, immunohistochemistry against Aβ protein is used more frequently and is more sensitive. Other immunostains routinely used in the evaluation of neurodegenerative disorders include α-synuclein (for Lewy bodies), tau paired helical filament (PHF1) staining for NFT and neuritic changes, and more recently TDP43 used in the evaluation of frontotemporal lobar degenerations. Historically, only silver stains were used to determine a semiquantitative age-related plaque score to indicate definite AD, possible AD, probable AD, and/or no AD [7, 8, 9, 10, 11–13]. More recent consensus guidelines from the National Institute on Aging-Alzheimer's Association incorporate a more systematic ("ABC") approach that includes evaluation of the geographic extent Aβ-amyloid protein deposits (A), in addition to staging of neurofibrillary tangles (B) and number of neuritic plaques (C) [14]. In this approach, a larger number of anatomic brain regions are examined, and the contribution of non-AD pathology is also taken into consideration.

A variety of inherited disorders may also be associated with neurodegeneration and amyloid deposition. A recently discovered form of CNS amyloidosis, called familial British dementia (FBD) or familial Danish dementia (FDD), is caused by mutations in the *BR12* gene located on chromosome 13 [15]. In FBD, the findings are somewhat similar to classic AD, where CAA and neurofibrillary pathology are found, in addition to parenchymal amyloid deposition. This is less so in FDD. An interesting finding is that there may be a role for wild-type BR12 protein in the pathogenesis of AD itself since, in FDD the amyloid deposition is associated with Aβ [15].

In addition to Aβ protein in AD, prion protein (PrP) in prion disease is frequently amyloidogenic in the CNS. Prion disorders include Creutzfeldt–Jakob disease (CJD), of both the sporadic and familial forms, as well as variant CJD, which is related to bovine spongiform encephalopathy. A variety of plaques may be encountered in these disorders [16], specifically in all cases of kuru, Gerstmann–Straussler–Sheinker (GSS) disease, and variant CJD, but only in 10–15% of sporadic CJD. Plaques in these disorders are composed of prion protein (PrP), variably deposited in the form of amyloid. These include unicentric (kuru plaques), multicentric plaques (characteristic of GSS disease), florid plaques (typical of variant CJD) (Fig. 8.1e, f) [17], and diffuse plaques. Autopsy precautions are necessary in the examination of these specimens [18], and cases in the USA should be reported and sent to the National Prion Disease Surveillance Center at Case Western Reserve University (Sponsored by the American Association of Neuropathologists, AANP).

Cerebral Amyloid Angiopathy

The most common form of CAA is found in conjunction with AD [3, 19, 20, 21]. Although most cases of AD have CAA, it is usually focal (in the temporal and occipital lobes) and mild. CAA in AD, or aging, is predominantly caused by deposition of the Aβ40 isoform in the vessels

(Fig. 8.2). Therefore, the ratio of Aβ40 to Aβ42 levels is a major determinant of the extent and severity of CAA [3]. The V717I β-APP and presenilin mutations, which primarily produce more

Aβ42 isoforms, lead to less severe CAA. There are, however, specific mutations in the Aβ protein that can cause CAA almost exclusively and lead to minimal parenchymal Aβ deposition [3].

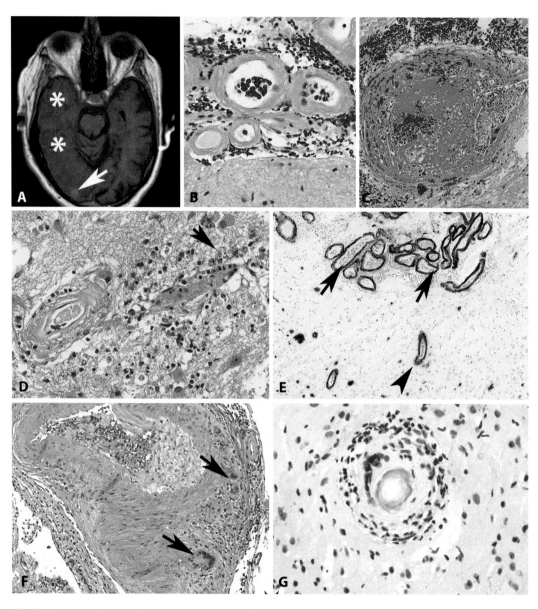

Fig. 8.2 Pathologic features of cerebral amyloid angiopathy. A frequent clinical presentation of amyloid angiopathy is intracerebral hemorrhage (*arrow*), although brain edema often confused with mass-like lesions (*asterisk*) may also develop (T1 weighted axial magnetic resonance image) (**a**). Amyloid angiopathy frequently involves leptomeningeal arteries, which may identified by eosinophilic mural thickening on H&E sections (**b**). Thrombosis and associated ischemia may occur in some cases (**c**). The presence of perivascular hemosiderin-laden macrophages (*arrow*) may be a clue to amyloid angiopathy (**d**). The best method to confirm the presence of amyloid angiopathy is through Aβ protein immunohistochemistry, which identifies leptomeningeal vessels (*arrows*) and superficial parenchymal vessels (*arrowhead*) (**e**). In Aβ-related angitis (ABRA), a giant cell inflammatory response (*arrows*) is associated with amyloid angiopathy (**f**). Small amyloid-containing intraparenchymal vessel is surrounded by multinucleated giant cells (Congo red) (**g**)

These include the Dutch-type mutation of the Aβ sequence (E22Q Aβ; HCHWA-D) and the Arctic mutation in the APP sequence (E693G; APP) [3]. Although there may be little parenchymal deposition of amyloid, these individuals can still present with dementia and other cognitive deficits, secondary to vascular and neurofibrillary pathology. CAA of various types demonstrate similar pathology, with thickening of basal lamina by amyloid and smooth muscle cell loss leading to vessel rupture [22].

A particularly severe form of CAA results from cystatin C (Icelandic) mutations [23], as well as mutations that give rise to the FBD and familial Danish dementia (FDD) [15]. Mutations in the gelsolin protein gene can also lead to a severe CNS CAA (Finnish hereditary amyloidosis) [3, 24]. Numerous mutations in the TTR protein (which usually causes a systemic amyloidosis including involvement of peripheral nerves and heart) can also lead to CNS CAA [25, 26]. The primary vessels involved are usually the superficial leptomeningeal (please see also Fig. 5.2). In addition to the leptomeninges, the eye can also have pathological deposition of mutated TTR protein, where the amyloid leads to vitreous opacity, keratoconjunctivitis, and/or glaucoma (see Fig. 5.1). Patients with amyloidosis derived from gelsolin (AGel) can develop lattice corneal dystrophy, with amyloid deposits within the stroma of the cornea (see Fig. 5.13 and Chaps. 5 and 7).

Clinical attention to CAA is more often in the form of intracerebral lobar hemorrhage, frequently multiple. However, in some instances CAA presents with infarcts or diffuse edema mimicking neoplasms. Therefore, brain specimens obtained during clot removal or brain biopsies that appear normal at first glance should be evaluated for the presence of CAA. Histologic clues include thickening of small to medium sized vessels in leptomeninges and superficial brain parenchyma (Fig. 8.2a–d). Veins and/or capillaries may also be rarely involved. "Double barreling" and an "onion-skin" appearance may be present. Perivascular hemosiderin-laden macrophages may be a subtle clue. Immunohistochemistry for Aβ protein is confirmatory in virtually all cases and used more commonly than Congo red special stains (Fig. 8.2e).

A perivascular inflammatory response with increased microglia and complement activation may be a feature of any CAA subtype [3]. In recent years, a form of CNS vasculitis associated with CAA has been increasingly recognized under the term Aβ-related angitis, in which amyloid angiopathy is identified in association with overt granulomatous inflammation [27] (Fig. 8.2f–g). Angiodestruction and leptomeningeal chronic inflammation may be present. Compared to conventional CAA, patients with Aβ-related angitis are younger, have fewer hemorrhages, and a better outcome [28].

Although prions can cause significant parenchymal amyloid deposition, CAA is less likely to occur in most sporadic or familial prion diseases, except for the subtypes that have mutations leading to stop codons in the prion protein gene [29].

Tumefactive and Neoplasia-Associated CNS Amyloidosis

Tumefactive amyloid deposits in the CNS (amyloidomas) are composed of light chain amyloid (AL) and typically form in the absence of systemic plasma cell dyscrasia [30–32] (Fig. 8.3). These aggregates of AL amyloid are predominantly lambda light chain derived, which may be tested in formalin-fixed tissues by immunohistochemistry and more accurately by mass spectrometry-based proteomics [33]. The deposits may be extra-axial or intraparenchymal and usually exhibit an indolent clinical course. On imaging studies, the deposits take the form of contrast enhancing masses, single or multiple, involving the white matter, periventricular regions, and/or choroid plexus [31]. A subset of cases affect the trigeminal ganglion (Fig. 8.3a, b). Large, amorphous parenchymal aggregates and variable mural vessel involvement are typical (Fig. 8.3c). An associated hypocellular infiltrate of monotypic plasma cells may be identified. Dural-based or orbital marginal zone lymphomas, plasma-cell rich low grade neoplasms that may mimic meningiomas at the clinical level, are also associated with intracranial kappa or lambda light chain amyloid deposition (Fig. 8.3a, d, e) [34]. The differential diagnosis of tumefactive amyloid deposits in the brain mainly involves immunoglobulin

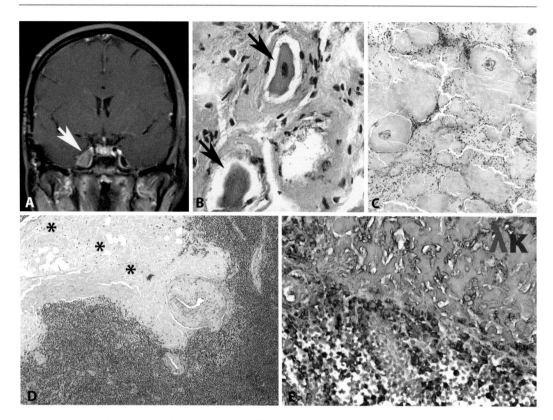

Fig. 8.3 Tumefactive and Neoplasia-Associated CNS Amyloidosis. Tumor-like accumulations of light-chain derived (AL) amyloid are known as amyloidomas and may form indolent intraparenchymal or extra-axial (*arrow*) masses (coronal post-contrast T1-weighted magnetic resonance image) (**a**). Involvement of the tri-geminal ganglion by an amyloidoma in A, histologically confirmed by the identification of residual ganglion cells (*arrows*) (**b**). Intraparenchymal brain involvement by amyloidomas take the form of multiple nodules (Congo red) (**c**). In some instances, overt amyloid deposition may occur in association with marginal zone lymphomas, including those involving the dura and orbit (**d**). Lambda light chain restriction in marginal zone lymphoma demonstrated in plasma cells (*lower* figure) and adjacent amyloid deposit (*upper* figure) (lambda light chain: red chromogen; kappa light chain: brown chromogen) (**e**)

deposition, particularly light chain deposition disease (LCDD), which in contrast to amyloidoma, is Congo red negative, PAS positive, and often associated with a lymphoid neoplasm [33, 35] (Fig. 8.4a–d). Extracerebral deposits in LCDD disease usually contain kappa light chains. Although pathologic light chain deposits in brain may also be composed of kappa light chain [33, 36], several instances of lambda-containing light chain disease have been described in the brain [37–40]. Regardless of the specific aggregate subtype, the identification of light-chain derived deposits in the CNS on biopsy material should trigger a thorough, systematic clinical evaluation for lymphoid neoplasia and plasma cell dyscrasias.

Systemic Amyloidosis and CNS Involvement

In case of systemic amyloidosis caused by AL deposition, AA, and dialysis-associated amyloidosis (derived from β_2-microglobulin), the affected areas of the brain are usually those regions that lack the blood–brain barrier. These include the area postrema in the floor of the fourth ventricle, the infundibulum of the hypothalamus, the pineal gland, the dura and particularly the choroid plexus [41, 42] (Fig. 8.4e–f). Rare instances of CNS AL vascular deposition associated with or without monoclonal gammopathies have been described [43, 44].

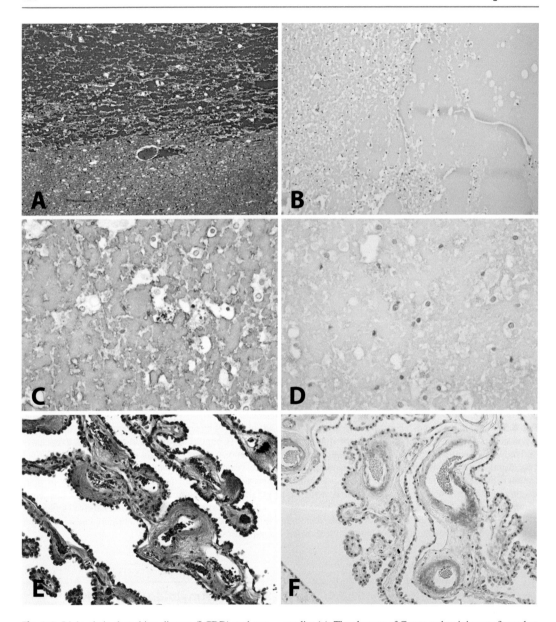

Fig. 8.4 Light chain deposition disease (LCDD) and secondary AL amyloid involvement. The main differential diagnosis of amyloid deposition in the central nervous system is immunoglobulin deposition, particularly light-chain deposition disease, which may form large proteinaceous deposits which have increased eosinophilia and often a crystalline quality (**a**). The absence of Congo red staining confirms that the deposit is not amyloid (Congo red) (**b**). In contrast to amyloidoma, this example contains kappa light chain (**c**), but not lambda (**d**). Involvement by systemic AL amyloid in the CNS usually occurs in areas lacking a blood brain barrier, particularly the choroid plexus (H&E, **e**; Congo red, **f**)

Pituitary Amyloid

Amyloid deposition in the pituitary is associated with aging or adenomas. In the former, the deposits are limited to the adenohypophysis in between glands and, in the latter, amyloid may form fairly large globules (or spheroids). These are usually associated with prolactin-secreting adenomas (prolactinomas), but may also be seen with other adenomas subtypes (Fig. 8.5a–d). Rarely, amyloid deposition may be associated with non-hematopoeitic, non-endocrine neoplasms. For

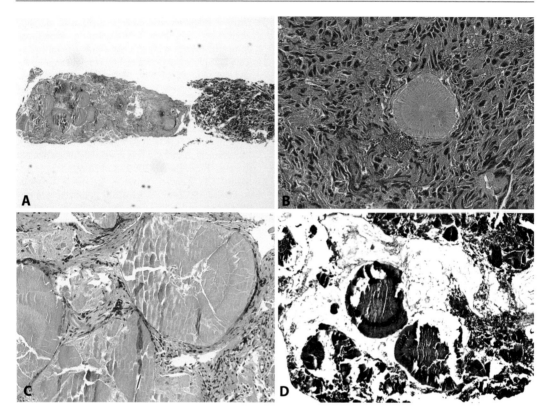

Fig. 8.5 Prolactinoma associated with amyloid stones. Amyloid deposition may also occur in non-hematolymphoid neoplasms, particularly prolactinomas. This may take the form of aggregates of amyloid "stones" (**a** *left*) or in association with pituitary tissue (**a** *right*). Amyloid deposits may be focal (**b**) or the dominant feature (**c**). Amyloid stones in prolactinoma contain prolactin, which may be highlighted by immunohistochemistry (**d**)

example, a curious case of gelsolin amyloid deposition associated with pituicytoma has been reported [45].

References

1. Hardy JA, Higgins GA. Alzheimer's disease: the amyloid cascade hypothesis. Science. 1992;256(5054):184–5.
2. Mann DM, Hardy J. Amyloid or tau: the chicken or the egg? Acta Neuropathol. 2013;126(4):609–13. doi:10.1007/s00401-013-1162-1.
3. Revesz T, Holton JL, Lashley T, Plant G, Frangione B, Rostagno A, Ghiso J. Genetics and molecular pathogenesis of sporadic and hereditary cerebral amyloid angiopathies. Acta Neuropathol. 2009;118(1):115–30. doi:10.1007/s00401-009-0501-8.
4. Wisniewski T, Haltia M, Ghiso J, Frangione B. Lewy bodies are immunoreactive with antibodies raised to gelsolin related amyloid-Finnish type. Am J Pathol. 1991;138(5):1077–83.
5. Bigio EH, Wu JY, Deng HX, Bit-Ivan EN, Mao Q, Ganti R, Peterson M, Siddique N, Geula C, Siddique T, Mesulam M. Inclusions in frontotemporal lobar degeneration with TDP-43 proteinopathy (FTLD-TDP) and amyotrophic lateral sclerosis (ALS), but not FTLD with FUS proteinopathy (FTLD-FUS), have properties of amyloid. Acta Neuropathol. 2013;125(3):463–5. doi:10.1007/s00401-013-1089-6.
6. Robinson JL, Geser F, Stieber A, Umoh M, Kwong LK, Van Deerlin VM, Lee VM, Trojanowski JQ. TDP-43 skeins show properties of amyloid in a subset of ALS cases. Acta Neuropathol. 2013;125(1):121–31. doi:10.1007/s00401-012-1055-8.
7. Fillenbaum GG, van Belle G, Morris JC, Mohs RC, Mirra SS, Davis PC, Tariot PN, Silverman JM, Clark CM, Welsh-Bohmer KA, Heyman A. Consortium to Establish a Registry for Alzheimer's Disease (CERAD): the first twenty years. Alzheimers Dement. 2008;4(2):96–109. doi:10.1016/j.jalz.2007.08.005.
8. Mirra SS, Heyman A, McKeel D, Sumi SM, Crain BJ, Brownlee LM, Vogel FS, Hughes JP, van Belle G, Berg L. The Consortium to Establish a Registry for Alzheimer's Disease (CERAD). Part II. Standardization

of the neuropathologic assessment of Alzheimer's disease. Neurology. 1991;41(4):479–86.

9. Galton CJ, Patterson K, Xuereb JH, Hodges JR. Atypical and typical presentations of Alzheimer's disease: a clinical, neuropsychological, neuroimaging and pathological study of 13 cases. Brain J Neurol. 2000;123(Pt 3):484–98.

10. Hof PR, Vogt BA, Bouras C, Morrison JH. Atypical form of Alzheimer's disease with prominent posterior cortical atrophy: a review of lesion distribution and circuit disconnection in cortical visual pathways. Vis Res. 1997;37(24):3609–25. doi:10.1016/S0042-6989(96)00240-4.

11. Mizutani T. Pathological diagnosis of Alzheimer-type dementia for old-old and oldest-old patients. Pathol Int. 1996;46(11):842–54.

12. Silver MH, Newell K, Brady C, Hedley-White ET, Perls TT. Distinguishing between neurodegenerative disease and disease-free aging: correlating neuropsychological evaluations and neuropathological studies in centenarians. Psychosom Med. 2002;64(3):493–501.

13. von Gunten A, Kovari E, Rivara CB, Bouras C, Hof PR, Giannakopoulos P. Stereologic analysis of hippocampal Alzheimer's disease pathology in the oldest-old: evidence for sparing of the entorhinal cortex and CA1 field. Exp Neurol. 2005;193(1):198–206. doi:10.1016/j.expneurol.2004.12.005.

14. Montine TJ, Phelps CH, Beach TG, Bigio EH, Cairns NJ, Dickson DW, Duyckaerts C, Frosch MP, Masliah E, Mirra SS, Nelson PT, Schneider JA, Thal DR, Trojanowski JQ, Vinters HV, Hyman BT, National Institute on A, Alzheimer's A. National Institute on Aging-Alzheimer's Association guidelines for the neuropathologic assessment of Alzheimer's disease: a practical approach. Acta Neuropathol. 2012;123(1):1–11. doi:10.1007/s00401-011-0910-3.

15. Lashley T, Revesz T, Plant G, Bandopadhyay R, Lees AJ, Frangione B, Wood NW, de Silva R, Ghiso J, Rostagno A, Holton JL. Expression of BRI2 mRNA and protein in normal human brain and familial British dementia: its relevance to the pathogenesis of disease. Neuropathol Appl Neurobiol. 2008;34(5):492–505. doi:10.1111/j.1365-2990.2008.00935.x.

16. Liberski PP. Amyloid plaques in transmissible spongiform encephalopathies. Folia Neuropathol. 2004;42(Suppl B):109–19.

17. Will RG, Ironside JW, Zeidler M, Cousens SN, Estibeiro K, Alperovitch A, Poser S, Pocchiari M, Hofman A, Smith PG. A new variant of Creutzfeldt-Jakob disease in the UK. Lancet. 1996;347(9006):921–5.

18. Budka H, Aguzzi A, Brown P, Brucher JM, Bugiani O, Collinge J, Diringer H, Gullotta F, Haltia M, Hauw JJ. Tissue handling in suspected Creutzfeldt-Jakob disease (CJD) and other human spongiform encephalopathies (prion diseases). Brain Pathol. 1995;5(3):319–22.

19. Bohl J, Storkel S, Steinmetz H. Involvement of the central nervous system and its coverings in different forms of amyloidosis. Prog Clin Biol Res. 1989;317:1007–19.

20. Ghiso J, Frangione B. Cerebral amyloidosis, amyloid angiopathy, and their relationship to stroke and dementia. J Alzheimers Dis. 2001;3(1):65–73.

21. Tian J, Shi J, Mann DM. Cerebral amyloid angiopathy and dementia. Panminerva Med. 2004;46(4):253–64.

22. Eisenberg D, Jucker M. The amyloid state of proteins in human diseases. Cell. 2012;148(6):1188–203. doi:10.1016/j.cell.2012.02.022.

23. Nagai A, Terashima M, Sheikh AM, Notsu Y, Shimode K, Yamaguchi S, Kobayashi S, Kim SU, Masuda J. Involvement of cystatin C in pathophysiology of CNS diseases. Front Biosci. 2008;13:3470–9.

24. Maury CP, Kere J, Tolvanen R, de la Chapelle A. Finnish hereditary amyloidosis is caused by a single nucleotide substitution in the gelsolin gene. FEBS Lett. 1990;276(1-2):75–7.

25. Araki S, Ando Y. Transthyretin-related familial amyloidotic polyneuropathy-progress in Kumamoto, Japan (1967-2010). Proc Jpn Acad Ser B Phys Biol Sci. 2010;86(7):694–706.

26. Nakagawa K, Sheikh SI, Snuderl M, Frosch MP, Greenberg SM. A new Thr49Pro transthyretin gene mutation associated with leptomeningeal amyloidosis. J Neurol Sci. 2008;272(1-2):186–90. doi:10.1016/j.jns.2008.05.014.

27. Scolding NJ, Joseph F, Kirby PA, Mazanti I, Gray F, Mikol J, Ellison D, Hilton DA, Williams TL, MacKenzie JM, Xuereb JH, Love S. Abeta-related angiitis: primary angiitis of the central nervous system associated with cerebral amyloid angiopathy. Brain J Neurol. 2005;128(Pt 3):500–15. doi:10.1093/brain/awh379.

28. Salvarani C, Hunder GG, Morris JM, Brown Jr RD, Christianson T, Giannini C. Abeta-related angiitis: comparison with CAA without inflammation and primary CNS vasculitis. Neurology. 2013;81(18):1596–603. doi:10.1212/WNL.0b013e3182a9f545.

29. Jansen C, Parchi P, Capellari S, Vermeij AJ, Corrado P, Baas F, Strammiello R, van Gool WA, van Swieten JC, Rozemuller AJ. Prion protein amyloidosis with divergent phenotype associated with two novel nonsense mutations in PRNP. Acta Neuropathol. 2010;119(2):189–97. doi:10.1007/s00401-009-0609-x.

30. Cohen M, Lanska D, Roessmann U, Karaman B, Ganz E, Whitehouse P, Gambetti P. Amyloidoma of the CNS. I. Clinical and pathologic study. Neurology. 1992;42(10):2019–23.

31. Laeng RH, Altermatt HJ, Scheithauer BW, Zimmermann DR. Amyloidomas of the nervous system: a monoclonal B-cell disorder with monotypic amyloid light chain lambda amyloid production. Cancer. 1998;82(2):362–74.

32. Vidal RG, Ghiso J, Gallo G, Cohen M, Gambetti PL, Frangione B. Amyloidoma of the CNS. II. Immunohistochemical and biochemical study. Neurology. 1992;42(10):2024–8.

33. Rodriguez FJ, Gamez JD, Vrana JA, Theis JD, Giannini C, Scheithauer BW, Parisi JE, Lucchinetti CF, Pendlebury WW, Bergen 3rd HR, Dogan A. Immunoglobulin derived depositions in the nervous

system: novel mass spectrometry application for protein characterization in formalin-fixed tissues. Lab Invest. 2008;88(10):1024–37. doi:10.1038/labinvest.2008.72.

34. Tu PH, Giannini C, Judkins AR, Schwalb JM, Burack R, O'Neill BP, Yachnis AT, Burger PC, Scheithauer BW, Perry A. Clinicopathologic and genetic profile of intracranial marginal zone lymphoma: a primary low-grade CNS lymphoma that mimics meningioma. J Clin Oncol. 2005;23(24):5718–27. doi:10.1200/JCO.2005.17.624.

35. Skardelly M, Pantazis G, Bisdas S, Feigl GC, Schuhmann MU, Tatagiba MS, Ritz R. Primary cerebral low-grade B-cell lymphoma, monoclonal immunoglobulin deposition disease, cerebral light chain deposition disease and "aggregoma": an update on classification and diagnosis. BMC Neurol. 2013;13:107. doi:10.1186/1471-2377-13-107.

36. Vital A, Ellie E, Loiseau H. A 61-year-old man with instability of gait and right hand clumsiness. Brain Pathol. 2010;20(1):273–4. doi:10.1111/j.1750-3639.2009.00349.x.

37. Fischer L, Korfel A, Stoltenburg-Didinger G, Ransco C, Thiel E. A 19-year-old male with generalized seizures, unconsciousness and a deviation of gaze. Brain Pathol. 2006;16(2):185–6. doi:10.1111/j.1750-3639.2006.00003_3.x. 187.

38. Menke JR, Jentoft ME, Dogan A, Avent JM, Miller DV, Giannini C. Periventricular white matter immunoglobulin lambda light chain deposition disease diagnosed by proteomic analysis. Acta Neuropathol. 2012;124(2):293–5. doi:10.1007/s00401-012-1008-2.

39. Pantazis G, Psaras T, Krope K, von Coelln R, Fend F, Bock T, Schittenhelm J, Melms A, Meyermann R, Bornemann A. Cerebral low-grade lymphoma and light chain deposition disease: exceedingly high IgG levels in the cerebrospinal fluid as a diagnostic clue. Clin Neuropathol. 2010;29(6):378–83.

40. Popovic M, Tavcar R, Glavac D, Volavsek M, Pirtosek Z, Vizjak A. Light chain deposition disease restricted to the brain: the first case report. Hum Pathol. 2007;38(1):179–84. doi:10.1016/j.humpath.2006.07.010.

41. Sasaki A, Iijima M, Yokoo H, Shoji M, Nakazato Y. Human choroid plexus is an uniquely involved area of the brain in amyloidosis: a histochemical, immunohistochemical and ultrastructural study. Brain Res. 1997;755(2):193–201.

42. Ishihara T, Nagasawa T, Yokota T, Gondo T, Takahashi M, Uchino F. Amyloid protein of vessels in leptomeninges, cortices, choroid plexuses, and pituitary glands from patients with systemic amyloidosis. Hum Path. 1989;20(9):891–5.

43. Schroder R, Deckert M, Linke RP. Novel isolated cerebral ALlambda amyloid angiopathy with widespread subcortical distribution and leukoencephalopathy due to atypical monoclonal plasma cell proliferation, and terminal systemic gammopathy. J Neuropathol Exp Neurol. 2009;68(3):286–99. doi:10.1097/NEN.0b013e31819a87f9.

44. Mawet J, Adam J, Errera MH, Oksenhendler E, Gray F, Massin P, Bousser MG, Vahedi K. Cerebral immunoglobulin light chain amyloid angiopathy-related hemorrhages. Rev Neurol. 2009;165(6-7):583–7. doi:10.1016/j.neurol.2008.10.009.

45. Ida CM, Yan X, Jentoft ME, Kip NS, Scheithauer BW, Morris JM, Dogan A, Parisi JE, Kovacs K. Pituicytoma with gelsolin amyloid deposition. Endocr Pathol. 2013;24(3):149–55. doi:10.1007/s12022-013-9254-y.

Differential Diagnosis of Amyloid in Surgical Pathology: Organized Deposits and Other Materials in the Differential Diagnosis of Amyloidosis

9

Guillermo A. Herrera and Elba A. Turbat-Herrera

Introduction

The Diagnosis of Amyloidosis: A Historical Account with Emphasis on Differentiating It from Other Diseases with Organized Deposits

Although there are comprehensive chapters in the book addressing the use of stains in the diagnosis of amyloidosis (indications, pitfalls, and expectations), a few historical events are worthwhile to recapitulate in this chapter to understand how the field has evolved over the years and to gain a better understanding of how diseases with organized deposits were recognized and characterized, as our ability to separate them into specific entities increased, and reproducible criteria were created.

In 1854, Virchow used a rather simple approach to diagnose amyloid. He coated the unfixed affected organs with alcoholic iodine (Lugol solution) resulting in a mahogany brown color that turned Prussian blue with the addition

of diluted sulfuric acid [1, 2]. This was akin to how cellulose reacted and, thus, he coined the term amyloid (a term we have proudly kept) to indicate that this material was starch-like. Because of the fact that carbohydrate moieties in amyloid are not the core material of amyloid fibers, not all amyloid stains with this method and some other materials that are not amyloid may stain. Although a crude diagnostic technique, it was useful at the time and this began the quest to begin to understand amyloid—totally unknown disease at the time—and how to detect it properly. Friedrich and Kekule recognized that amyloid was a proteinaceous material [3].

It is very interesting that the identification of Congo red as useful in the diagnosis of amyloidosis began, as not infrequently happens, with an astute observation by Bennhold in 1922 [4, 5]. While using Congo red dye for measuring blood volume in a patient, he realized that there was a rapid loss of the dye. This patient was diagnosed with amyloidosis at autopsy, and it was inferred that there was an attraction for Congo red to this patients' tissues where the Congo red dye likely disappeared. While this suspicion was confirmed, it took many adjustments to make the Congo red stain specific for amyloid detection in the histology laboratory.

One of the helpful additions to make amyloid detection using Congo red more specific was to introduce polarization of Congo red-stained tissue samples to confirm the presence of amyloid and rule out other non-amyloid material that may also

G.A. Herrera, MD (✉)
Department of Pathology, Louisiana State University Health Sciences Center, 1501 Kings Highway, 71103 Shreveport, LA, USA
e-mail: gherr1@lsuhsc.edu

E.A. Turbat-Herrera, MD
Departments of Pathology and Medicine, Louisiana State University, Shreveport, LA, USA
e-mail: eturb1@lsuhsc.edu

© Springer International Publishing Switzerland 2015
M.M. Picken et al. (eds.), Amyloid and Related Disorders, Current Clinical Pathology,
DOI 10.1007/978-3-319-19294-9_9

bind to the dye. This was introduced by Divry and Florkins in 1927 who recognized that apple green birefringence occurred when the Congo red-stained sections were polarized [6]. Their observations also helped to realize that amyloid had an internal structure and was not an amorphous material as thought to be due to its light microscopic appearance. The Congo red stain procedure went through a series of improvements during the next few years to help achieve specificity, reliability, and reproducibility. As a result, the Puchtler's alcoholic alkaline method to stain amyloid was established as the standard technique to detect amyloid in tissue sections and is used in laboratories around the globe [7]. Other metachromatic stains were introduced to aid in the detection of amyloid (i.e., crystal violet), but these were of limited value due to their nonspecificity for amyloid. However, other stains like thioflavin T or S, also nonspecific for amyloid, have retained significant applicability because of their ability to highlight very small amyloid deposits in situations when the Congo red stain does not provide a definitive answer and are very easy to perform [8]. As is the case with all techniques, there are expectations and pitfalls that need to be carefully considered when making the diagnosis of amyloidosis differentiating it from other organized deposits.

In 1977, Rosenmann and Eliakim reported a patient with nephrotic syndrome who had a peculiar material deposited in glomeruli that resembled amyloid in the hematoxylin and eosin sections, but did not show Congo red positivity [9]. The paper that ensued titled "Congo red-negative amyloidosis-like glomerulopathy: Report of a case" initiated the new field of amyloid-like organized deposits in renal biopsies. This manuscript was followed by other similar reports which clearly demonstrated that there were different types of amyloid-like deposits in renal biopsies that needed to be carefully scrutinized and properly characterized [10, 11]. In some cases, the structured deposits had a microtubular, rather than a fibrillary appearance, and originally it was thought that the spectrum of these diseases with Congo red negative deposits was quite broad and encompassed entities such as immunotactoid glomerulopathy [10–12]. As more work was done, it was realized that that was

not the case and that Congo red negative structured deposits belong to more than one category of renal diseases.

One group of such renal disorders with non-amyloid structured deposits is represented by cryo-globulinemic nephropathy. Cryoglobulinemia was first recognized in the early 1930s and in 1974 were classified into different types by Brouet et al. in a classical manuscript [13]. The renal manifestations in cryoglobulinemic nephropathy with the corresponding characterization of the structured deposits characteristic of cryoglobulins were recognized in the late 1970s and refined in the 1980s and early 1990s. Since the discovery of hepatitis C, most cases initially felt to represent idiopathic, or essential cryo-globulinemia are now linked to this disease.

The Different Entities in the Kidney and Extrarenal Manifestations Associated with Organized Deposits and Other Amyloid Look-Alike Conditions

These diseases should be conceptualized as specific clinicopathologic entities, not merely as pathologic entities, as their correct diagnosis is strengthened by the association with distinct clinical correlates [12]. The diagnosis of most of these diseases demands rather specific clinical management and therapeutic interventions and conveys in some cases important genetic and prognostic data. Among the conditions included in this category of renal diseases are amyloidosis, all types, fibrillary and immunotactoid, and cryo-globulinemic nephropathies. Other conditions that need to be considered include sclerotic/ hyalinized collagen and other hyaline deposits, most often vascular hyalinosis.

The Nature of the Problem: What Is in the Differential Diagnosis of Amyloidosis in the Kidney and Other Organs?

Our understanding of the diseases associated with organized deposits has advanced considerably in the last 25 years. Criteria for diagnosis are now reproducible, and clinicians have a much clearer understanding of the implications of the various disease processes for patients' management, treatment, and prognosis.

One of the most challenging problems in renal pathology is the differential diagnosis of organized deposits. In large renal practices, approximately 5–8 % of all biopsies represent amyloidosis, whereas all the other entities with organized deposits together generally account for less than 1 % of all biopsies, so this latter group of disorders is quite infrequent, bordering on rare [12, 14]. In some small nephropathology practices, a case with non-amyloid organized deposits may only occur every 2–3 years or even less often. This of course creates a lack of familiarity with diagnostic approaches and interpretation of findings. Proper characterization of these determines specific disease entities with important clinical connotations and dictates certain clinical approaches, including therapies [12]. This problem can also occur in virtually any other organ but much less commonly than in renal specimens.

Hematoxylin and eosin-stained sections alone are unable to resolve the differential diagnosis, as significant overlap in the appearances of the various organized deposits is the rule. They usually present as eosinophilic amorphous (hyaline) material. One very important differential diagnosis is simply the deposition of plasma proteins, as they create a "hyaline" appearance in the hematoxylin and eosin sections that could be confused with other organized deposits, most importantly amyloid. This is commonly seen in the vasculature and probably represents one of the main challenges in non-renal specimens [12]. While books from 30 years ago would have listed only amyloidosis and cryoglobulins as the only types of organized deposits of any significance, the list has grown considerably in more recent years further complicating the differential diagnosis.

The characterization of these disorders can be performed using a variety of approaches. Renal diseases with organized deposits are divided in two categories by some: Congo red positive diseases—encompassing all of the amyloidoses—and those that are Congo red negative. This approach should carefully consider pitfalls asso-

ciated with Congo red staining, including the lack of staining when the amounts of amyloid are small or, if staining occurs, it is difficult to obtain the apple green birefringence (a requirement to make a definitive diagnosis of amyloidosis) by polarizing the specimen. Another situation where the Congo red stain is negative is in the so-called preamyloidotic situations where the precursor amyloid protein can be detected, but the deposits are Congo red negative [15]. An important point to remember is that different amyloids bind to Congo red with variable affinity resulting in different intensities of salmon pink staining. Tissue congophilia can also be artifactual and not indicative of amyloid deposits [16].

Another popular way to conceptualize these diseases is to separate them into those in which the deposits are composed of immunoglobulins, including truncated forms, and those that are not. With the exception of the category of non-AL amyloidosis, the majority of these disorders are immunoglobulin-related. To properly diagnose these conditions, electron microscopy is essential in some instances [12, 17–19].

The first and foremost manifestation of diseases with organized deposits in the kidneys is mesangial expansion. The deposits present in these conditions are generally extracellular. Whether there is replacement of the normal mesangial matrix or an increase of mesangial extracellular matrix proteins represents a good starting point for the renal pathologist to approach the morphologic diagnosis of these disorders [12]. Extracellular matrix proteins are generally positive with the silver methenamine stain resulting in an increase in mesangial argyrophilia. In contrast, loss of mesangial silver positivity is associated with the presence of material that has replaced the normal mesangial matrix [20] (Fig. 9.1a–c). Therefore, in the algorithmic approach to the evaluation of these diseases, the silver stain may play a crucial role in determining what diagnostic pathway to follow to characterize the disorder. Full characterization of these disorders is only possible at the ultrastructural level where the specific findings that characterize the various organized deposits can be appreciated. However, there are light microscopic and immunofluorescence

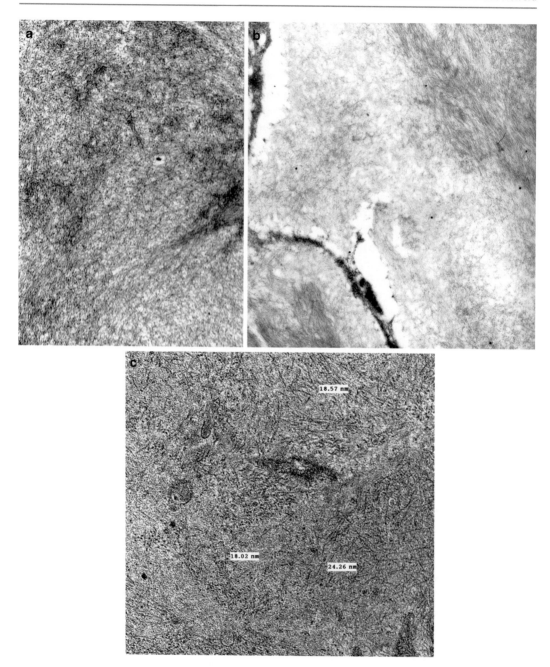

Fig. 9.1 (**a**) Amyloidosis, fibrils. (**b, c**) Fibrillary glomerulonephritis, fibrils. (**a, b, c**) Transmission electron microscopy. Uranyl acetate and lead citrate. **AX8500, BX8500. In both conditions (**a, b**), the fibrils are randomly distributed and non-branching. The only difference is that the diameter of the fibrils in amyloidosis generally ranges from 8 to 12 nm in diameter, whereas in fibrillary glomerulonephritis they typically range from 15 to 25 nm in diameter clearly evident on (**c**)

features that are important in some of these conditions and may, in some cases, be quite characteristic and virtually pathognomonic of the disease entity (i.e., fibrillary and cryoglobulinemia glomerulopathies).

Fibrillary Glomerulonephritis (Nephropathy)

Renal

This entity, as previously mentioned, first recognized in 1977 remains of uncertain etiology. Alpers coined the term fibrillary glomerulonephritis 10 years later to refer to this entity. Fibrillary glomerulonephritis is characterized by the deposition of randomly disposed fibrils that are Congo red, thioflavin T and S negative, and are thicker than amyloid fibrils with a diameter generally ranging from 15 to 25 nm [21–24] (Fig. 9.1a–c), thicker than those in amyloidosis (Fig. 9.1c). The fibrils are not only predominantly seen in the mesangium, but also frequently present along peripheral capillary walls. Interestingly,

amyloid P protein has been shown to be associated with these fibrils [25].

The morphologic glomerular expressions of this disease are indeed heterogeneous. The earliest light microscopic appearance is the expansion of mesangial areas with replacement of the mesangial matrix by amorphous and eosinophilic material noticeable in the hematoxylin and eosin stains (Fig. 9.2a). Amyloidosis is in the differential diagnosis because of the overlap in the light microscopic appearance (Fig. 9.2b). A small percentage of patients with this condition exhibit crescents, though the percentage of glomeruli with crescents is generally small.

The accumulation of these fibrils results in variable mesangial expansion sometimes associated with mesangial nodularity, and the deposition of fibrils along peripheral capillary walls results in recognizable wall thickening, which may bring up diabetic nephropathy as a differential diagnostic consideration. Silver stain may be useful in this situation as it is typically positive in the expanded mesangium in diabetes and weak to negative in cases of fibrillary glomerulonephritis and also in amyloidosis (Fig. 9.3).

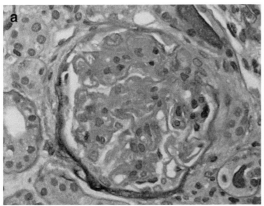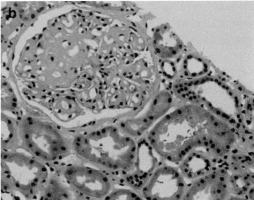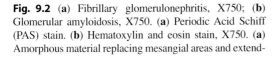

Fig. 9.2 (**a**) Fibrillary glomerulonephritis, X750; (**b**) Glomerular amyloidosis, X750. (**a**) Periodic Acid Schiff (PAS) stain. (**b**) Hematoxylin and eosin stain, X750. (**a**) Amorphous material replacing mesangial areas and extend-

ing to some peripheral capillary walls (**b**). By light microscopy, similar material as in (**a**) (eosinophilic and amorphous—"hyaline"), replacing significant portions of a glomerulus with a somewhat nodular pattern of deposition

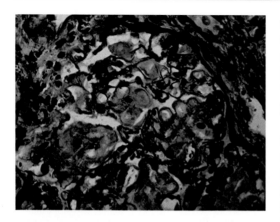

Fig. 9.3 Glomerular amyloidosis. Silver methenamine stain, X500. Mesangial matrix is replaced by silver negative material. The normal mesangial argyrophilia due to the mesangial matrix is lost

The largest series of cases with fibrillary glomerulonephritis with the longest follow-up published in 2011 highlighted characteristic clinicopathologic features of this disease and emphasized the importance of careful immunomorphologic evaluation to make this diagnosis accurate [26].

An important diagnosis to rule out is diabetic fibrillosis [27, 28] because of the morphologic ultrastructural similarity of the fibrils in this entity with those of fibrillary glomerulonephritis [12]. However, they lack the typical immunofluorescence staining pattern that is associated with fibrillary glomerulonephritis (and described below). In contrast, in these cases, the staining observed is characteristically associated with diabetic nephropathy (i.e., linear staining for albumin and IgG along peripheral capillary walls in glomeruli).

In some selected cases, light chain monoclonality has been demonstrated, most typically kappa, in fibrillary glomerulonephritis [21, 29]. By immunofluorescence, a ribbon-like pattern is characteristically seen for IgG (IgG4 subclass), C3, kappa, and lambda light chains (Fig. 9.4a, b). However, there are cases with a more "granular" immunofluorescence appearance and because of the distribution along peripheral capillary walls in glomeruli it may be confused with membranous nephropathy [30, 31].

Fibrillary deposits can also be found in the kidney outside the glomeruli. In a study of 1,266 renal biopsies, nine biopsies from eight patients with fibrillary glomerulonephritis were studied carefully ultrastructurally. Extraglomerular fibrillary deposits were seen in 60 % of the cases [32]. Therefore, a better name for this condition is probably fibrillary nephropathy.

Clinically, the manifestations are nonspecific and these patients typically present with proteinuria, sometimes with full blown nephrotic syndrome. Some of these patients exhibit rapidly progressive renal dysfunction and renal prognosis is poor, although remission may occur [26]. The condition is associated with poor prognosis in term of renal function, and renal deterioration occurs rather rapidly. A small percentage of these cases is associated with an underlying plasma cell dyscrasia [26, 29], but most have no associated systemic disorder.

Extrarenal

Fibrillary glomerulonephritis, as its name implies, is primarily a renal (glomerular) disorder. In contrast to amyloidosis, which is a recognized systemic disorder, it is much less common to find reports of extrarenal fibril deposition in this condition.

A few cases of pulmonary hemorrhage in patients with fibrillary glomerulonephritis and similar fibrillary deposits to those seen in the kidney were found in the lung—along alveolar capillary basement membranes [33, 34], including one case occurring in a patient's post-renal transplantation [35]. In addition, in a patient with fibrillary glomerulonephritis, typical fibrils were demonstrated in the skin associated with leukocytoclastic vasculitis [33].

An autopsy case reported in the literature described massive fibrillary deposits in the liver and bone marrow of a patient with apparent fibrillary glomerulopathy and a concomitant monoclonal gammopathy [36], and another report showed widespread splenic involvement [37]. The previously mentioned study [32] included a case with an autopsy. During the postmortem examination, fibrillary deposits were documented in the pancreas, spleen, lungs, and liver.

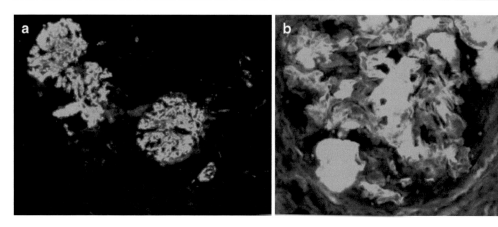

Fig. 9.4 Fibrillary glomerulonephritis. ** (**a**, **b**) Direct fluorescence; fluorescein stain for IgG. AX350, BX750. Strong smudgy staining of peripheral capillary walls and mesangium

The finding of extrarenal involvement in a significant number of patients with fibrillary glomerulonephritis has clearly demonstrated the systemic nature of this condition. However, since this diagnosis requires ultrastructural evaluation for confirmation, it is very likely that extrarenal manifestations in fibrillary glomerulonephritis are underdiagnosed.

Pathogenesis

The pathogenesis of this disorder has been debated for years. Some early reports considered it in the same spectrum with immunotactoid glomerulopathy as one entity [17, 18, 38, 39]. However, a number of publications and case series have clearly and conclusively documented that these are two different diseases each with unique clinicopathologic features [40–44].

The predominant association of these fibrillary deposits with IgG4 has led to the hypothesis that this subtype of IgG has a unique propensity to form fibrils [22]. At one point, it was suggested that these fibrils were unusual morphologic manifestations of cryoglobulins, but this idea has essentially been abandoned, as no sound support has been found for this hypothesis. What we know is that the distribution of the deposits and their composition are consistent with this entity likely representing an immune complex-mediated process [42], which is supported by the finding of

a cryoprecipitate in one of the patients with fibrillary glomerulonephritis containing immunoglobulin–fibronectin complexes consistent with immune complexes [45]. This is also supported by a few cases of lupus nephritis that are associated with fibrillary deposits indistinguishable from those seen in fibrillary glomerulonephritis in one way or another. A case of de novo fibrillary glomerulonephritis has been reported arising in a cadaveric renal allograft of a patient who required transplantation because of end-stage lupus nephritis [46], further suggesting that a fibrillary glomerulonephritis represents part of the spectrum of immune complex-mediated renal diseases.

Fibrillary glomerulonephritis is also seen in a small subset of patients with an underlying neoplastic lymphoplasmacytic disorder which suggests that polymerization of monoclonal light chains into fibrils may occur [14, 29, 47].

Mass spectroscopy studies of deposits in fibrillary glomerulonephritis have shown midspectra numbers of apolipoprotein E and Igλ-1 chain C region and complement proteins for the classic and terminal pathways [48, 49].

Cryoglobulinemic Nephropathy

The recognition of renal disease in patients with cryoglobulinemia dates back to the mid-1950s [50]. However, more recently, this condition has significantly increased in incidence, and its recognition by renal pathologists has also improved considerably. The increase in cryoglobulinemic nephropathy parallels the discovery and spread of hepatitis C in the general population.

These patients typically present with a nephrotic syndrome but may also come to seek medical attention because of hematuria, proteinuria, or nephritic syndrome. Important laboratory clues for the diagnosis of cryoglobulinemia include markedly decreased complement levels, sometimes undetectable (most commonly C4), and a very high rheumatoid factor [50]. Systemic manifestations such as purpura, arthralgias, and vasculitis can be seen. Exacerbations and remissions are common components of this disease process. Only rarely these patients progress to end-stage renal disease.

There are several distinct varieties of cryoglobulins and depending on which is the one involved, the immunomorphologic renal manifestations may vary. Some of these cryoglobulins may be monoclonal, but most are polyclonal. Mixed cryoglobulinemia, type II, monoclonal IgM, and polyclonal IgG subtypes represent the most common types of the spectrum of these diseases [50–54]. By immunofluorescence, monoclonality can be detected in the monoclonal cryoglobulinemic nephropathy. Cryoglobulin deposits are most commonly seen in thrombi, subendothelial, or mesangial areas, but can be seen in other glomerular locations and in extraglomerular renal vasculature.

Currently, the majority of these cases are associated with hepatitis C, but cryoglobulinemia has also been shown to occur associated with fibrillary and immunotactoid nephropathies [55]. The development of cryoglobulinemic nephropathy has been linked in these cases to an antigen-driven rheumatoid factor response to chronic hepatitis C infection. Other diseases that are associated with cryoglobulinemia include systemic lupus erythematosus, any chronic liver diseases, infections, other collagen vascular diseases, and lymphoproliferative disorders. Relatively, few cases remain in the category of "idiopathic" or "essential cryoglobulinemia."

The ultrastructural characteristics of the cryoglobulinemic deposits are quite variable which

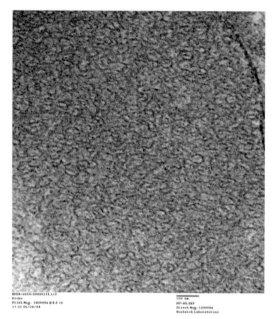

Fig. 9.5 Cryoglobulinemic nephropathy. Transmission electron microscopy. Uranyl acetate and citrate X. Paired microtubular structures characteristic of cryoglobulins

makes diagnosis a challenge in a significant number of instances. A recent publication analyzing 47 cases of cryoglobulinemic nephropathy focused on the ultrastructural findings (i.e., substructure of electron dense deposits) [56]. The most typical appearance and the one easiest to recognize is represented by deposits with a microtubular substructure with slightly curved pairs of microtubules or cylinders, in various glomerular locations, including in capillary thrombi and in thrombi in arterioles and small arteries in rare cases (Fig. 9.5). The cylinders are each about 25 nm in diameter, and in cross sections the cylinders appear as a hollow center around which 9–12 spokes project [56–61]. The cryoglobulin deposits associated with monoclonal IgG cryoglobulinemia type I, uncommonly associated with renal disease, have been described as composed of either straight structures forming bundles 80-nm wide, which on cross section appear crosshatched or as tubular structures with a fingerprint-like array [50]. Unfortunately, cryoglobulin deposits may have variable ultrastructural appearances [55], which on occasions may not be characteristic enough for proper identification. Also, deposits with the appearance of immune complexes may be seen in

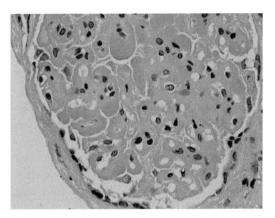

Fig. 9.6 Cryoglobulinemic nephropathy. Hematoxylin and eosin stain, AX750. Hyaline thrombi in capillary spaces, exudative changes, and cellular proliferation with accentuation of the electron microscopy

cryoglobulinemic nephropathy [56]. The deposits within thrombi are generally the ones that display the most characteristic findings [56]. These cryoglobulins have not been morphologically altered by cellular processes, and they essentially represent aggregates of pristine microtubular aggregates occluding vessels. Ultrastructural identification of cryoglobulin deposits remains crucial for establishing an unequivocal diagnosis.

The most common microscopic appearance seen in renal biopsies is that of membranoproliferative type I pattern with an exudative component and, in some cases, hyaline thrombi in glomerular capillaries are conspicuous (Fig. 9.6). Monocytes may be detected in glomerular capillaries. Rarely an inflammatory vasculitis is seen in the renal vasculature away from glomeruli [57–61]. How often this vasculitis occurs in cryoglobulinemic nephropathy depends on the series of cases studied [50, 56].

Extrarenal

One of the most important clues to suspect the presence of circulating cryoglobulins is the finding of intravascular hyaline thrombi. These can be seen in any organ. The challenge is to properly identify them as containing cryoglobulins. The

thrombi are eosinophilic in the hematoxylin and eosin stains (hyaline) and amorphous, and do not exhibit the fibrillary substructure which is typical of fibrin thrombi; these fibrin thrombi represent the main differential diagnosis. In renal biopsies, immune complexes can also be seen in the form of hyaline intravascular deposits in glomerular capillaries, most often in lupus nephritis. Clinical information and other light, immunofluorescence, and ultrastructural findings can be used to establish a definitive diagnosis. One complication is the fact that deposits with cryoglobulins can coexist with otherwise typical lupus nephritis.

Immunofluorescence evaluation may detect the presence of polyclonal or monoclonal immunoglobulin components associated with the thrombi, but proper tissue is not procured for immunofluorescence in the great majority of these specimens, as the diagnosis may not be suspected. In renal biopsies, the situation is different as routine immunofluorescence and ultrastructural evaluations are carried out, permitting a much more complete assessment. In some cases, where obtaining the tissue is not too invasive, a repeat biopsy with tissue collected for immunofluorescence and electron microscopy in proper fixatives should be recommended to clarify a differential diagnosis.

One of the fundamental problems associated with this diagnosis is that clinical confirmation with detection of cryoglobulins in the serum is difficult and only possible in a relatively small percentage of these cases. The currently available test for detecting cryoglobulins in the serum appears to be very insensitive to detect all cryoglobulins capable to deposit in organized microtubular structures in various organs where the tissue microenvironment makes their organization into recognizable deposits possible. The different cryoglobulins require variable amounts of time (some are quite slow) to precipitate in order to be detected in the serum, and the test only calls for 4 hours of precipitation [48]. In addition, the serum collected from the patients should be kept cold until tested. Otherwise, cryoglobulins can be missed.

Pathogenesis

The main pathology that is seen results from the aggregation of cryoglobulins in the vasculature leading to varying degrees of vascular luminal compromise, including complete occlusion and associated ischemic complications. In rare cases, even infarcts of the affected organs occur. The disappearance of the thrombi from the vasculature may lead to complete reestablishment of function, and this happens with frequency explaining how the renal dysfunction that may be seen in these patients is cyclical. Reducing the amounts of circulating cryoglobulins represents a key therapeutic maneuver to resolve a clinical crisis.

Immunotactoid Glomerulopathy

This even more unusual (very rare) renal condition is characterized by the finding of organized deposits in the glomeruli composed of hollow or cylindrical, microtubular structures with a diameter ranging from 30 to 90 nm predominantly, or at least focally, in a parallel arrangement or displaying intersectioning bundles. These structures can be found in small aggregates, predominantly in the mesangium, replacing mesangial matrix or may arrange forming quite complex structures. These microtubular aggregates resemble cryoglobulins. They are generally not only thicker but also longer than cryoglobulins. By light microscopy, a mesangial proliferative (mesangiopathic) pattern is the most commonly recognized, but other morphologic expressions have also been documented, including a more proliferative pattern akin to membranoproliferative glomerulonephritis. In some cases, expansion of mesangial matrix predominates and in others the appearance mimics a membranous nephropathy. Crescents may be present. Hyalin thrombi are rarely noted in glomerular capillaries. By immunofluorescence, coarse deposits containing predominantly IgG and C3, either in mesangial or peripheral capillary walls, represent the most common finding and often exhibit light chain restriction but mostly IgGκ. These patients generally present with proteinuria/nephrotic syndrome and/or hematuria [12, 18, 19]. There is an important relationship with underlying lymphoproliferative disorders and, in some cases, Sjögren's syndrome in patients with this disorder. In the series published by Bridoux et al., 7 of the 14 cases reported had chronic lymphocytic leukemia, small lymphocytic B cell lymphoma, and three patients had monoclonal gammopathies of uncertain significance [44]. In contrast to fibrillary glomerulonephritis, renal function tends to remain rather well preserved with mild renal insufficiency remaining for many years. In the more recent series of cases with immunotactoid glomerulopathy, Nasr et al. reported M serum protein spikes in 10 of 16 cases and in 8 of 15 patients tested in the urine. Hematologic malignancies were confirmed in 6 of the patients (38 %) with 5 exhibiting chronic lymphocytic leukemia, small lymphocytic lymphoma, and myeloma in two additional patients [62].

Even though this disease entity has predominantly been documented in the great majority of the cases in the kidney (not extrarenally), it needs to be addressed because it participates in the differential diagnosis of fibrillary and cryoglobulinemic nephropathies, and there are some important conceptual ideas that need to be considered in this comprehensive chapter of diseases with organized deposits mimicking amyloidosis.

Extrarenal Manifestations

Rare cases of systemic immunotactoid disease have been reported in the literature. Perineural deposits with microtubular aggregates similar to those detected in glomeruli have been demonstrated in one patient with clinical mononeuritis multiplex [44]. A case of leukocytoclastic vasculitis in the skin associated with immunotactoid glomerulopathy has been published; however, it is not clear whether this case is indeed an example of immunotactoid or fibrillary disease [63]. An additional case reported 4 years later clearly documents cutaneous vasculitis in a patient with immunotactoid glomerulopathy [64]. More interesting is the report of immunotactoid keratopathy in a patient with a paraproteinemia which suggests that similar structures to those seen in immunotactoid glomerulopathy can be present in rare patients with corneal disease [65]. The failure to recognize this entity outside of the kidney is very likely due to the absolute need for ultrastructural evaluation for proper diagnosis combined with the decreased use to the point of almost complete disappearance of this diagnostic technique in diagnostic pathology, except in fields such as renal pathology.

Pathogenesis

The strong association with lymphoproliferative disorders led to the hypothesis that this disease occurs as a consequence of a peculiar polymerization of monotypical light chains into microtubular structures. Specific physicochemical characteristics of certain light chains involved may predispose them to polymerize in this unusual fashion.

There has been recent speculation that immunotactoid glomerulopathy may be closely associated with cryoglobulinemic nephropathy with some authors suggesting that these two entities are part of a spectrum [66]. Though detection of circulating cryoglobulins in cases of immunotactoid glomerulopathy has only been sporadic, it is a common practice that the detection of cryoglobulins in the serum has been an immediate exclusion for making a diagnosis of ITG. A similar experience has occurred in patients diagnosed as cryoglobulinemic nephropathy where detection of serum cryoglobulins is only possible in about 30 % of the patients attesting to the fact that current laboratory methods of detection of serum cryoglobulins are rather insensitive. One study demonstrated that a serum cryoprecipitate and glomerular deposits were identical biochemically in one ITG case [67] lending support to this hypothesis.

Laser microdissection and mass spectroscopy-based proteomic analysis have been performed in three ITG cases. The profile detected is consistent with the immunofluorescence findings and showed accumulation of complement factors of the classical and terminal pathways and is similar to that seen in cryoglobulinemic nephropathy.

Unexpectedly, the three cases also revealed peptides associated with amyloidosis such as amyloid P-component (SAP), apolipoprotein E, and clusterin [54, 55, 62].

Hyalinosis

Some cases with prominent vascular hyalinosis [68, 69] can be confused with amyloidosis, especially since vascular amyloid deposition is common in systemic amyloidosis. Since the vascular deposits are also hyaline and amorphous, like amyloid, it is sometimes difficult to separate these (Figs. 9.7 and 9.8a, b). Careful morphological analysis, Congo red/thioflavin T stains, and evaluation of the clinical situation are all that are needed in the great majority of the cases, but in selected situations other ancillary techniques, such as electron microscopy, are needed to clarify the diagnostic dilemma. This is particularly true when the results of the above-mentioned stains become equivocal or in cases where clinical suspicion for amyloidosis is significant and the amount of possible amyloid appears to be small and possibly beyond the expected accurate recognition by the stains normally used. A rare variant of renal amyloidosis is characterized by vascular involvement and rather unremarkable glomerular and interstitial compartments [13, 70]. The ultrastructural features of hyalinosis are pathognomonic and allow to differentiate it from other possibilities with certainty (Fig. 9.8c).

Pathogenesis

Vascular hyalinosis results from the exudation of plasma proteins into vessel walls resulting from increased permeability and leakage. Conditions such as diabetes mellitus exacerbate the leakage of plasma proteins sometimes creating spectacular hyalinotic vascular lesions, which are also commonly seen associated with benign hypertension and may be seen in virtually every vessel in the body, but tend to be quite prominent in the renal parenchyma.

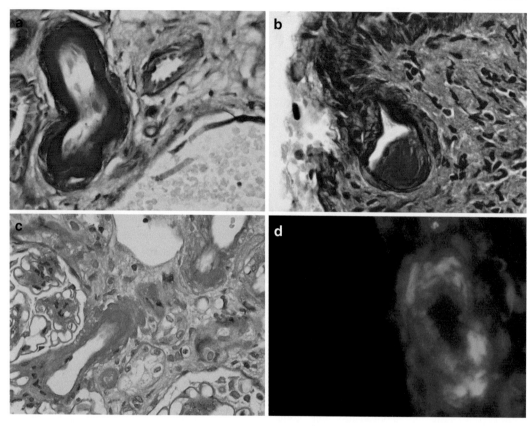

Fig. 9.7 Vascular hyalinosis mimicking amyloidosis and amyloid deposits in vessel wall for comparison. (**a, b**) X500-PAS stain. C X500-Hematoxylin and eosin stain. (**d**) X750-Thioflavin T fluorescence stain. Compare vascular hyalinosis (**a, b**) with amyloid deposits in vessel walls (**c**) which fluoresce with Thioflavin T (**d**)

Hyalinized Collagen

Hyalinized collagen is also amorphous and "hyaline" in appearance, making differentiation from amyloid difficult in some situations (Fig. 9.9a). Again, Congo red and thioflavin T or S stains solve the majority of the diagnostic challenges, but in some instances the stains reveal equivocal results. Before making a diagnosis of amyloidosis or ruling it out when the situation is not clear, it is highly recommended that additional studies be performed. If preservation is adequate, ultrastructural evaluation may settle the issue easily and satisfactorily (Fig. 9.9b). Additional samples should be requested to perform immunofluorescence and ultrastructural studies to reach a definitife diagnosis if needed.

Pathogenesis

Hyalinized collagen results from alterations in the biochemical composition of collagen. It was suggested years ago that an increase in hydroxyproline in the collagen resulted in the "hyalinized" appearance [70].

Other Nonspecific Fibrils that Are Confused with Amyloid

This is perhaps most significant when ultrastructural studies have been ordered and fibrils resembling amyloid are encountered [18, 19]. In this case, the differential diagnosis may include nonspecific fibrils seen in association with sclerotic tissue [71], precollagen fibers, or other forms of

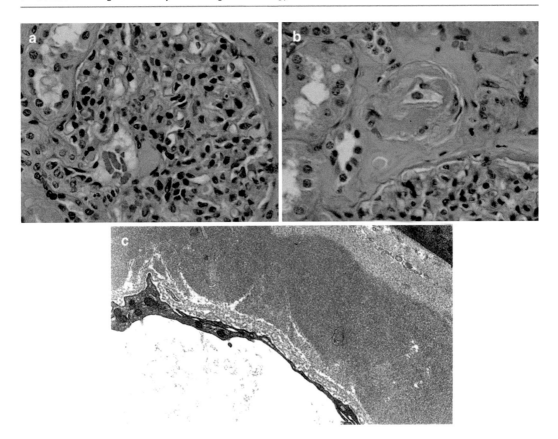

Fig. 9.8 Vascular hyalinosis in the wall of an afferent/efferent arteriole in a glomerulus mimicking amyloid deposition. (**a, b**) Hematoxylin and eosin stain. (**c**) Transmission electron microscopy. Uranyl acetate and lead citrate, X8500. (**a, b**) Eosinophilic, amorphous material in the wall of arterioles mimicking amyloid. (**c**) Electron dense material in arteriolar wall represents hyalinosis. Note the absence of fibrillary internal appearance in area with hyalinosis

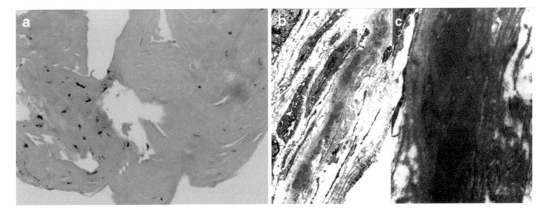

Fig. 9.9 (**a**). Hematoxylin a eosin stain ×350: Hyalinized collagen. (**b–c**) Transmission electron microscopy. Uranyl acetate and lead citrate, (**b**) X9500, (**c**) X12500 Hyaline area representing sclerotic collagen (**a**). There are identifiable collagen fibers adjacent to the hyalinized collagenous tissue (**b, c**)

altered collagen represented by fibrils lacking the typical collagen periodicity of collagen fibers [18, 19].

A Logical Approach to the Differential Diagnosis with Emphasis on Type of Specimens Required

One of the key issues here is proper specimen preservation for accurate diagnosis and what is required depends on the technique to be used. The differentiation of structured deposits can be difficult and generally requires specimens to be evaluated that have been well fixed and adequately processed. Artifacts can be a source of confusion and must be avoided at all cost. In some cases to obtain the material for electron microscopy that can be interpreted with accuracy will require obtaining a new specimen and fixing it correctly. There should be no hesitation to do this as the final diagnosis must be a solid one. In other instances, immunofluorescence evaluation is very valuable and although there are methods to do fluorescence in paraffin-embedded tissues,

these are not reproducible and should be avoided in addressing this type of differential diagnosis.

Fortunately, the light microscopic, tinctorial, and ultrastructural (Fig. 9.10a, b) features of generic amyloid are quite specific [72, 73]; thus, this diagnosis can generally be made with certainty when in the differential diagnosis. However, pitfalls that may be associated with the diagnosis of amyloidosis must be kept in mind [14–16, 74, 75]. Furthermore, while it is imperative to characterize the amyloid if identified, performing stains for the precursor proteins may be associated with some difficulties. While in some cases, immunohistochemistry suffices to characterize the amyloid type (Fig. 9.11a–d), this is not always the case. Unfortunately, immunohistochemical stains for light and heavy chains result in too much background staining for proper interpretation in a significant number of cases. In contrast, a properly handled specimen stained using direct fluorescence techniques can provide unequivocal diagnostic information avoiding problems and is always much preferred [76].

Techniques such as immunolabeling at the ultrastructural level may be of unique value in characterizing the type of amyloid present [76],

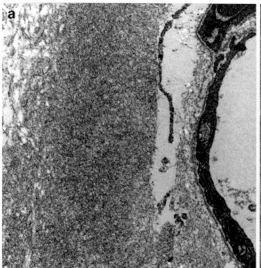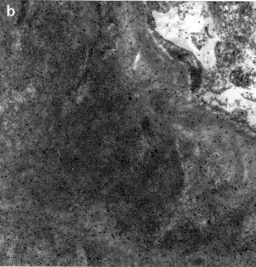

Fig. 9.10 Vascular amyloidosis. (**a**) Transmission electron microscopy. (**b**) Immunogold labeling for lambda light chains. Uranyl acetate and lead citrate, AX 30500; BX 30500. (**a**) Typical appearance of amyloid fibrils in vessel wall. (**b**) Gold particles labeling the fibrils indicating that the amyloid is associated with monoclonal lambda light chains (precursor protein). No labeling noted for kappa light chains

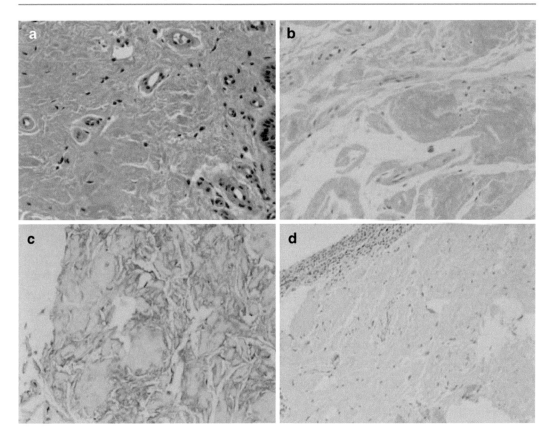

Fig. 9.11 Amyloidosis in urethra. (**a**) Hematoxylin and eosin stain; (**b**) Congo red stain; (**c**) Immunohistochemical stain for kappa light chains; (**d**) Immunohistochemical stain for lambda light chains. (**a**) Eosinophilic, amorphous (hyaline) deposits underneath the surface epithelium in urethra. (**b**) The material deposited is Congo red positive. (**c** and **d**) Amyloid stains for kappa (**c**) but not for lambda light chains (**d**)

and may sometimes support a diagnosis of amyloidosis made by identifying unequivocally the precursor protein associated with the fibrillary material (Fig. 9.10b). This technique can also exclude such a diagnosis in a doubtful case. Immunolabeling amalgamates immunomorphologic data in an elegant fashion. There are requirements for achieving good, reproducible results [77].

Another consideration is to use mass spectroscopy to characterize deposited proteins in difficult cases using paraffin-embedded tissue, thus permitting a definitive diagnosis [54, 55, 78]. This is covered in detail in a separate chapter.

An additional specimen may be needed to be able to make a definitive assessment. Immunohistochemical stains depend much on how tissue is processed and can vary significantly from one laboratory to another. While a particular laboratory may realize the challenges involved in the various techniques, when a specimen is submitted to another laboratory for workup, these challenges are often totally ignored which may lead to poor results that should not be used for interpretation and rendering a final diagnosis.

In diseases such as systemic lupus erythematosus, determination of type of organized deposit present may be challenging even in properly fixed tissue examined ultrastructurally [79].

Conclusions

It is imperative that organized deposits be accurately identified and separated from amyloid. How far the diagnostic workup should be taken depends on the specific case. The intelligent use of the proper stains can be very helpful in assessing these deposits and suggesting, if not confirming, a given diagnosis. However, it appears that in a significant number of the cases electron microscopy may be very helpful, needed, or absolutely essential to make an accurate assessment. This can be challenging as proper preservation of the tissue for ultrastructural evaluation is needed so that the subtle differences among the different organized deposits can be appreciated to make a precise diagnosis.

References

1. Rokitansky MH. Virchow and, Heschl on the problem of amyloidosis [German]. Zentrablatt fur Allgeneine Pathologie and Pathologische Anatomie (Jena). 1968;111:103–7.
2. Aterman K. A historical note on the iodine-sulphuric acid reaction of amyloid. Histochemistry. 1976;49: 131–43.
3. Ruske W. August Kekule and the development of the theory of chemical structure [German]. Naturwissenschaften. 1965;52:485–9.
4. Kallee E. The 110th birthday of Hans Hermann Bennhold [German]. Dtsch Med Wochenschr. 1993; 118:1336–8.
5. Elghetany MT, Saleen A, Barr K. The Congo red stain revisited. Ann Clin Lab Sci. 1989;19:190–5.
6. Reznik M. Paul Divry: the discovery of cerebral amyloidosis [French]. Acta Neurol Belg. 1989;89: 168–78.
7. Puchtler H, Waldrop FS, McPolan SN. A review of light, polarization and fluorescence microscopic methods for amyloid. Appl Pathol. 1985;3:5–17.
8. Hobbs JR, Morgan AD. Fluorescence microscopy with thioflavin-T in the diagnosis of amyloid. J Pathol Bacteriol. 1963;86:437–42.
9. Rosenmann E, Eliakim M. Nephrotic syndrome associated with amyloid-like glomerular deposits. Nephron. 1977;18:301–8.
10. Duffy JL, Khurana E, Susin M, Gomez-Leon G. Fibrillary renal deposits and nephritis. Am J Pathol. 1983;113:279–90.
11. Olesnicky L, Doty SB, Bertani T, Pirani CL. Tubular microfibrils in the glomeruli of membranous nephropathy. Arch Pathol Lab Med. 1984;108:902–5.
12. Herrera GA, Turbat-Herrera EA. Renal diseases with organized deposits: an algorithmic approach to classification and diagnosis. Arch Pathol Lab Med. 2010;134:512–31.
13. Brouet JC, Clauvel JP, Danon F, et al. Biologic and clinical significance of cryoglobulins: a report of 86 cases. Am J Med. 1974;57:775–8.
14. Herrera GA, Gu X. Lesions associated with plasma cell dyscrasias in renal biopsies: a 10 year retrospective study (abstract). Lab Invest. 2006;86:A262.
15. Koike H, Misu K, Sugiura M, et al. Pathology of early-vs late-onset TTR Met30 familial amyloid polyneuropathy. Neurology. 2004;63:129–38.
16. Carson FL, Kingsley WB. Non-amyloid green birefringence following Congo red staining. Arch Pathol Lab Med. 1980;104:333–5.
17. Korbet SM, Schwartz MM, Lewis EJ. The fibrillary glomerulopathies. Am J Kidney Dis. 1994;23: 751–65.
18. Iskandar SS, Herrera GA. Glomerulopathies with organized deposits. Semin Diagn Pathol. 2002;19: 116–32.
19. Howell D, Gu X, Herrera GA. Organized deposits and look-alikes. Ultrastruct Pathol. 2003;27:295–312.
20. Herrera GA, Lott RL. Silver stains in diagnostic renal pathology. J Histotechnol. 1996;19:219–23.
21. Alpers CE, Rennke HG, Hopper J, et al. Fibrillary glomerulonephritis: an entity with unusual immunofluorescence features. Kidney Int. 1987;31:781–9.
22. Iskandar SS, Falk RJ, Jennette C. Clinical and pathologic features of fibrillary glomerulonephritis. Kidney Int. 1992;42:1401–7.
23. D'Agati V, Sacchi G, Truong L, et al. Fibrillary glomerulopathy: defining the disease spectrum (abstract). J Am Soc Nephrol. 1991;2:591.
24. Nasr SH, Valeri AM, Cornell LD, et al. Fibrillary glomerulonephritis: a report of 66 cases from a single institution. Clin J Am Soc Nephrol. 2011;6:775–84.
25. Yang GCH, Nieto R, Stachura I, Gallo GR. Ultrastructural immunohistochemical localization of polyclonal IgG, C3, and amyloid P component on the Congo red-negative amyloid-like fibrils of fibrillary glomerulopathy. Am J Pathol. 1992;141: 409–19.
26. Nasr SH, Valeri AM, Cornell LD, et al. Fibrillary glomerulonephritis: a report of 66 cases from a single institution. Clin J Am Soc Nephrol. 2011;6: 775–84.
27. Sohar E, Ravid M, Ben-Shaul Y, Reshef T, Gafni J. Diabetic fibrillosis. Am J Med. 1970;49:64–9.
28. Gonul II, Gough J, Jim K, Benediktsson H. Glomerular mesangial fibrillary deposits in a patient with diabetes mellitus. Int Urol Nephrol. 2006;38:767–72.
29. Sanders PW, Herrera GA, Kirk KA, Old CW, Galla JH. The spectrum of glomerular and tubulointerstitial renal lesions associated with monotypical immunoglobulin light chain deposition. Lab Invest. 1991;64:527–37.
30. Müller-Höcker J, Weiss M, Sitter T, et al. Fibrillary glomerulonephritis mimicking membranous nephropathy—A diagnostic pitfall. Pathol Res Pract. 2009;205:265–71.
31. Rosenmann E, Brisson M-L, Bercovitch DD, Rosenberg A. Atypical membranous glomerulonephritis with fibrillary subepithelial deposits in a patient with malignant lymphoma. Nephron. 1988;48:226–30.

32. Hvala A, Ferluga D, Vizjak A, et al. Fibrillary non-congophilic renal and extrarenal deposits: a report on 10 cases. Ultrastruct Pathol. 2003;27:341–7.
33. Masson RG, Rennke HG, Gotlieb MN. Pulmonary hemorrhage in a patient with fibrillary glomerulonephritis. N Eng J Med. 1992;326:36–9.
34. Rovin BH, Bou-Khalil P, Sedmak D. Pulmonary renal syndrome in a patient with fibrillary glomerulonephritis. Am J Kidney Dis. 1993;22:713–6.
35. Calls GJ, Torras A, Ricart MJ, et al. Fibrillary glomerulonephritis and pulmonary hemorrhage in a patient with renal transplantation. Clin Nephrol. 1995;43:180–3.
36. Strom EH, Hurwitz N, Mayr AC, et al. Immunotactoidlike glomerulopathy with fibrillary deposits in liver and bone marrow gammopathy. Am J Nephrol. 1996;16(52):3–8.
37. Satoskar A, Calomeni E, Nadasdy G, et al. Fibrillary glomerulonephritis with splenic involvement: a detailed autopsy study. Ultrastruct Pathol. 2008;32:113–21.
38. Korbet SM, Schwartz MM, Lewis EJ. Immunotactoid glomerulopathy (Fibrillary glomerulonephritis). Clin J Am Soc Nephrol. 2006;1:1351–56.
39. Schwartz MM, Korbet SM, Lewis EJ. Immunotactoid glomerulopathy. J Am Soc Nephrol. 2002;13:1390–7.
40. Alpers C, Kowalewska J. Fibrillary glomerulonephritis and immunotactoid glomerulopathy. J Am Soc Nephrol. 2008;19:34–7.
41. Alpers C. Fibrillary glomerulonephritis and immunotactoid glomerulopathy: two entities, not one. Am J Kidney Dis. 1993;22:448–51.
42. Fogo A, Qureshi N, Horn RG. Morphologic and clinical features of fibrillary glomerulonephritis versus immunotactoid glomerulopathy. Am J Kidney Dis. 1993;22:367–77.
43. Rosenstock JL, Markowitz GS, Valeri AM, et al. Fibrillary and immunotactoid glomerulonephritis: distinct entities with different clinical and pathologic features. Kidney Int. 2003;63:1450–61.
44. Bridoux F, Hugue V, Coldefy O, et al. Fibrillary glomerulonephritis and immunotactoid (microtubular) glomerulopathy are associated with distinct immunologic features. Kidney Int. 2002;62:1764–75.
45. Rostagno A, Kumar VR, Chuba J, et al. Fibrillary glomerulonephritis related to serum fibrillar immunoglobulin-fibronectin complexes. Am J Kidney Dis. 1996;28:676–84.
46. Isaac J, Herrera GA, Shihab FS. De-novo fibrillary glomerulopathy in the renal allograft of a patient with systemic lupus erythematosus. Nephron. 2001;87:365–8.
47. Sundaram S, Mainali R, Norfolk ER, et al. Fibrillary glomerulopathy secondary to light chain deposition disease in a patient with monoclonal gammopathy. Ann Clin Lab Sci. 2007;37:370–4.
48. Sethi S, Theis JD, Vrana JA, et al. Laser microdissection and proteomic analysis of amyloidosis, cryoglobulinemic GN, fibrillary GN and immunotactoid glomerulopathy. Clin J Am Soc Nephrol. 2013; 8:915–21.
49. Sethi S, Vrana J, Theis JD, Dogan A. Mass spectrometry based proteomics in the diagnosis of kidney disease. Curr Opin Nephrol Hypertens. 2013;22:273–80.
50. Dispenzieri A, Gorevic PD. Cryoglobulinemia. Hematol Oncol Clin North Am. 1999;13:1315–49.
51. Porush JG, Grishman E, Alter AA, et al. Paraproteinemia and cryoglobulinemia associated with atypical glomerulonephritis and the nephrotic syndrome. Am J Med. 1969;47:957–64.
52. Karras A, Noel L-H, Droz D, et al. Renal involvement in monoclonal (type I) cryoglobulinemia: two cases associated with IgG3κ cryoglobulin. Am J Kidney Dis. 2002;40:1091–6.
53. D'Amico G. Renal involvement in human hepatitis C infection: cryoglobulinemic glomerulonephritis. Kidney Int. 1998;54:650–71.
54. Golde D, Epstein W. Mixed cryoglobulins and glomerulonephritis. Ann Intern Med. 1956;69:1221–7.
55. Markowitz GS, Cheng J-T, Colvin RB, Trbbin WM, D'Agati VD. Hepatitis C infection is associated with fibrillary glomerulonephritis and immunotactoid glomerulopathy. J Am Soc Nephrol. 1998;9:2244–52.
56. Ojemakinde K, Turbat-Herrera EA, Zeng X, Gu, X, Herrera GA: The many faces of cryoglobulinemic nephropathy: a clinico-apthologic study with emphasis on the value of electron microscopy. Ultrastruct Pathol 2014;38:367–76.
57. Pais B, Panadés MJ, Ramos J, Montoliu J. Glomerular involvement in type I monoclonal cryoglobulinaemia. Nephrol Dial Transplant. 1995;10:130–2.
58. Verroust P, Mery JP, Morel-Maroger L, et al. Glomerular lesions in monoclonal gammopathies and mixed essential cryoglobulinemias IgG-IgM. Adv Nephrol Necker Hosp. 1871;1:161–94.
59. Feiner H, Gallo G. Ultrastructure in glomerulonephritis associated with cryoglobulinemia. Am J Pathol. 1977;88:145–55.
60. Ogihara T, Saruta T, Saito I, Abe S, Ozawa Y, Kato E, Sakaguchi H. Finger print deposits of the kidney in pure monoclonal IgG kappa cryoglobulinemia. Clin Nephrol. 1979;12:186–90.
61. Cordonnier D, Martin H, Groslambert P, Micouin C. Mixed IgG-IgM cryoglobulinemia with glomerulonephritis. Am J Med. 1975;59:867–72.
62. Nasr SH, Fidler ME, Cornell LD, et al. Immunotactoid glomerulopathy: clinicopathologic and proteomic study. Nephrol Dial Transplant. 2012;27:4137–46.
63. Schifferli JA, Merot Y, Cruchaud A, Chatenat F. Immunotactoid glomerulopathy with leukocytoclastic skin vasculitis and hypocomplementemia: a case report. Clin Nephrol. 1987;27:151–5.
64. Orfila C, Meeus F, Bernadet P, et al. Immunotactoid glomerulopathy and cutaneous vasculitis. Am J Nephrol. 1991;11:67–72.
65. Garibaldi DC, Gottsch J, de la Cruz Z, Haas M, Green R. Immunotactoid keratopathy: a clinicopathologic case review and review of reports of corneal involvement in paraproteinemias. Surv Ophthalmol. 2005;1:61–80.
66. Herrera GA, Ojemakinde K, Gu X, Iskandar S. Immunotactoid glomerulopathy and cryoglobulinemic

nephropathy: two entities with many similarities. A unified conceptual approach. Ultrastruct Pathol. 2015.

67. Rostagno A, Vidal R, Kumar A, et al. Fibrillary glomerulonephritis related to serum fibrillar immunoglobulin fibronectin complexes. Am J Kidney Dis. 1996;28:675–84.

68. Saltykov BB, Malkina LA. Vascular hyalinosis in diabetic microangiopathy. Ann Pathol. 1975;37:38–44.

69. Kubo M, Kiyohara Y, Kato I, et al. Risk factors for renal glomerular and vascular changes in an autopsy-based population survey: the Hisayama Study. Kidney Int. 2003;63:1508–15.

70. Denduchis B, Gonzalez N, Mancini RE. Concentration of hydroxyproline in testes of hypophysectomized patients before and after treatment with gonadotropins and testosterone. J Reprod Fertil. 1972;31:111–4.

71. Kronz JD, Neu AM, Nadasdy T. When noncongophilic glomerular fibrils do not represent fibrillary glomerulonephritis: nonspecific mesangial fibrils in sclerosing glomeruli. Clin Nephrol. 1998;50:218–23.

72. Shirahama T, Cohen AS. Fine structure of the glomerulus in human and experimental amyloidosis. Am J Pathol. 1973;73:97–114.

73. Linke RP. Congo red staining of amyloid: improvements and practical guide for a more precise diagnosis of amyloid and the different amyloidoses. In: Uversky VN, Fink AL, editors. Protein misfolding, aggregation, and conformational diseases, Protein reviews (Atassi MZ, editor), vol. 4. New York, NY: Springer; 2006. p. 239–76. Chapter 11.

74. Klastskin G. Non-specific green birefringence in Congo-red stained tissues. Am J Pathol. 1969;56:1–13.

75. Picken MM, Herrera GA. The burden of "sticky" amyloid. Arch Pathol Lab Med. 2007;131:850–1.

76. Satoskar AA, Burdge K, Cowden DJ, Nadasdy GM, Hebert LA, Nadasdy T. Typing of amyloidosis in renal biopsies. Diagnostic pitfalls. Arch Pathol Lab Med. 2007;131:917–23.

77. Herrera GA, Richard P, Turbat EA, et al. Ultrastructural immunolabeling in the diagnosis of light chain related renal disease. Pathol Immunopathol Res. 1986;5:170–87.

78. Murphy CL, Eulitz M, Hrncic R, et al. Chemical typing of amyloid protein contained in formalin-fixed paraffin-embedded biopsy specimens. Am J Clin Pathol. 2001;116:135–42.

79. Hvala A, Kobenter T, Fergula D. Fingerprint and other organized deposits in lupus nephritis. Wien Klin Wochenschr. 2000;112:711–5.

Light/Heavy Chain Deposition Disease as a Systemic Disorder

10

Guillermo A. Herrera and Elba A. Turbat-Herrera

Introduction

While the great majority of these patients have an underlying plasma cell disorder, some may be associated with other diseases where there is a lymphoplasmacytic process producing the abnormal light or heavy chains. These include Waldenström's macroglobulinemia, chronic lymphocytic leukemia/lymphoma, and nodal marginal cell lymphoma. Criteria for a diagnosis of myeloma are present in approximately 50 % of patients with LCDD or light and heavy chain deposition disease (LHCDD) and only in approximately 25 % of patients with HCDD. LHCDD, generally diagnosed in the kidney, is often the presenting disease that eventually leads to the discovery of the underlying plasma cell dyscrasia. In a smaller subset of patients, LCDD appears in patients with treated myeloma after relapse, and may be the result of the emergence of a mutated clone of plasma cells that occurs after the use of certain chemotherapeutic agents such as Melphalan.

G.A. Herrera, MD (✉)
Department of Pathology, Louisiana State University
Health Sciences Center, 1501 Kings Highway,
71103 Shreveport, LA, USA
e-mail: gherr1@lsuhsc.edu

E.A. Turbat-Herrera, MD
Departments of Pathology and Medicine,
Louisiana State University, Shreveport, LA, USA
e-mail: eturb1@lsuhsc.edu

LHCDD may occur in the absence of detectable underlying systemic neoplastic lymphoproliferative processes, even after prolonged follow-up for more than 10 years. In these instances, LCDD may be associated with a local clone of plasma cells at the site of the light chain deposits (extramedullary plasmacytomas).

LHCDDs are rare conditions. They are most common in the sixth decade but have been described in the literature in patients with a wide age range (from 22 to 94 years) and display a male predominance [1–8]. In autopsy series of patients with myeloma, it has been found that only 5 % of these patients exhibit LCDD [8, 9].

Heavy chain diseases manifest as lymphoplasmacytic proliferative disorders [1]. The alpha variant, also referred to as Mediterranean lymphoma, is the most common. It typically occurs between ages 10 and 30 and is geographically concentrated in the Middle East. Most of these patients present with abdominal lymphoma and malabsorption. It is conceptualized as a form of mucosa-associated lymphoid tissue (MALT) lymphoma and it is also known as immunoproliferative small intestinal disease (IPSID), Mediterranean lymphoma, or Seligmann's disease. In contrast, IgG (γ) is primarily found in elderly men and IgM (μ) in adults over 50 years of age. While γ-HCD (Franklin's disease) is generally an aggressive malignant lymphoma, μ-HCD resembles small cell lymphocytic lymphoma/chronic lymphocytic leukemia and

© Springer International Publishing Switzerland 2015
M.M. Picken et al. (eds.), *Amyloid and Related Disorders*, Current Clinical Pathology,
DOI 10.1007/978-3-319-19294-9_10

exhibits a protracted clinical course [1]. Interestingly, HCDD appears to be a peculiar and unusual manifestation of HCD due to the fact that tissue deposition of heavy chains is restricted to only certain heavy chains. When the structures of heavy chains in HCDD and HCD are compared, the variable regions are found to be partially or entirely deleted in HCD which impedes tissue deposition [10, 11]. In HCDD, the preserved variable regions contain unusual amino acid substitutions in the complementarity-determining and framework regions, but they exhibit no significant structural abnormalities or deletions in the variable domain. The amino acid substitutions result in alterations in the physico-chemical characteristics of the heavy chains with changes in hydrophobicity and charge responsible for their propensity to deposit in tissues. Similar variable domain mutations have been described in LCDD [12, 13].

Some of the patients with HCDD are hypo-complementemic, especially if they secrete IgG1 and 3 subclasses. These IgG subclasses have the greatest ability to fix complement, which is dependent on intact CH2 constant domains in the heavy chains [14]. Complement consumption results through activation of IgG1 or 3 heavy chain deposits.

Deposition of abnormal light and heavy chains in tissues results in certain morphologic manifestations that can suggest to the pathologist that such has happened. These alterations, however, are not necessarily specific for these disorders and demonstrating the presence of the pathologic light/heavy chains is essential for a definitive diagnosis. In the case of amyloidosis, the amyloid replaces normal tissues and deposits as amorphous, eosinophilic areas that can be detected with the hematoxylin and eosin stain and with the aid of the proper stains can be identified generically (as amyloid), and the demonstration of the particular precursor protein allows a final characterization. The situation in LHCDD is somewhat more difficult. The deposits of monoclonal light or heavy chains generally result in a fibrogenic response (Fig. 10.1a), and the deposited proteinaceous material is found admixed with the abnormal precursor proteins

(Fig. 10.1b). The abundance of extracellular matrix may make the detection of abnormal light or heavy chains a challenge or make it appear as sclerotic tissue and be missed. Morphologically speaking, the material deposited is also eosinophilic and amorphous when viewed with the hematoxylin and eosin stain and can be readily seen if it deposits in significant amounts (Fig. 10.2a). The challenge for the pathologist is to actually identify the abnormal light and/or heavy chains buried in the sclerotic tissue to render a diagnosis.

Ultrastructurally, light and heavy chain deposits may not only appear as organized material with 8–12 nm in diameter fibrils which disposes randomly and are non-branching (characteristics that can be clearly seen by electron microscopy) in the case of AL/AH amyloidosis, but also as non-organized, punctate to powdery, electron-dense material in LHCDD [15, 16] (Fig. 10.2b). While P-component is an invariable constituent of amyloid, it is not found in association with LHCDD [17].

The systemic nature of amyloidosis has been recognized for more than a century with involvement of any organ and the same is true of LHCDD, but not as well documented and/or recognized. The use of the Congo red and Thioflavin T stains is very helpful in the detection of amyloid deposits, but demonstrating the presence of monoclonal light/heavy chains to make a diagnosis of LHCDD is more difficult.

Immunohistochemistry is successful in occasional cases (Fig. 10.1b). These stains depend heavily on fixation and proper handling of the specimens and are frequently difficult to read due to background staining resulting in difficulties to document unequivocal monoclonality (i.e., staining for only one of the light or heavy chains) in association with deposits, a crucial requirement for confirming the diagnosis of LHCDD.

In contrast, immunofluorescence evaluation is a rather clean and sensitive technique for demonstrating light/heavy chain monoclonality in tissues (Fig. 10.3), but in the great majority of the cases, no tissue is preserved for this technique. An additional biopsy for this purpose may not be possible or may be rather cumbersome.

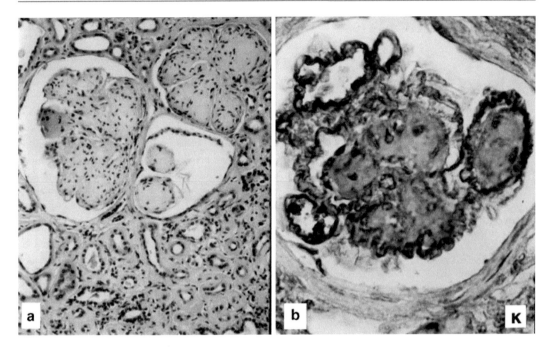

Fig. 10.1 Nodular glomerulosclerosis secondary to κ-LCDD. (**a**) X500 and (**b**) X750. (**a**) Hematoxylin and eosin and (**b**) immunohistochemical stain for κ-light chains. (**a**) The glomerulus displays the typical nodularity—nodular glomerulosclerosis—that is characteristic of the advanced stage of this lesion. (**b**) κ light chains are noted to be predominantly in subendothelial zones and are difficult to see clearly in the mesangial nodules as the sclerotic mesangial tissue makes it difficult to detect

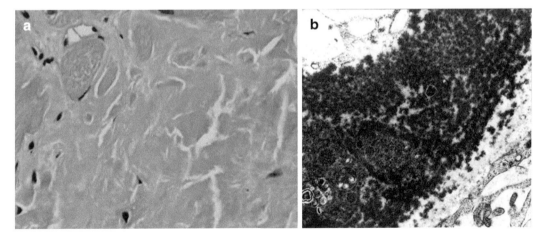

Fig. 10.2 κ-LCDD. Light chain deposits in heart. (**a**) X500—Hematoxylin and eosin stain. (**b**) X35,000—Transmission electron microscopy. Uranyl acetate and lead citrate stain. (**a**) Eosinophilic, amorphous material deposited in myocardium corresponding to light chain deposits. (**b**) Punctate, markedly electron-dense material corresponding to the deposits of light chain material. This is the typical appearance of light chain deposits when they are in high concentration and display a contrasting electron density. Not all light chain deposits are so easy to recognize

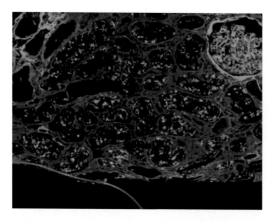

Fig. 10.3 Nodular glomerulosclerosis secondary to κ-LCDD. X500—Direct immunofluorescence for κ light chains. Fluorescein stain (FITC). Staining along peripheral capillary walls and also staining in mesangial areas in glomerulus and along tubular basement membranes (*top, right*). Also granular staining in proximal tubular cells and linear staining along tubular basement membranes

Electron microscopy remains a powerful tool to detect these non-organized light chain deposits and should be used whenever such diagnosis is suspected. While formalin-fixed, paraffin-embedded tissues are adequate for many of these cases, there are situations where specimen handling may cause such tissue damage that the key ultrastructural details are lost, making it impossible to make a definitive assessment. Of course, it is much better to properly fix tissue for electron microscopy to assure a proper ultrastructural evaluation.

Therefore, it is highly recommended that when it is known prior to obtaining samples that these entities are in the differential diagnosis, that tissue be procured and properly placed in fixatives/tissue transport media that will permit the most precise evaluations using both immunofluorescence and electron microscopy. Because many laboratories lack the ability to perform these diagnostic techniques, it may be necessary to send the specimens to a regional laboratory properly equipped to handle these cases. Otherwise, there is a risk of making an incorrect diagnosis.

Historical Perspective

Antonovych recognized the presence of monoclonal light chains associated with glomerular lesions in patients with myeloma [18]. Light chain deposition disease (LCDD) was first recognized as a specific entity in 1976 by Randall and associates [19], who reported two patients with renal failure and clinical manifestations involving multiple organ systems. In both cases, autopsies were performed and they showed that deposition of monoclonal light chains occurred in many organs, to highlight which the term systemic LCDD was coined. Light chain deposits were confirmed in the kidneys, liver, pancreas, heart, central and peripheral nervous system, skin, muscle, thyroid, and gastrointestinal tract. Extrarenal deposits appear to be less common in HCDD, but they have been reported in the heart [20], synovial tissues [20, 21], skin [22], striated muscles [22], thyroid [23], pancreas [23], and the liver [23].

In spite of the clear systemic nature of this disorder, most of the studies that followed focused on the recognition of this disease and understanding of its pathogenesis as a renal disorder. In the kidney, all three renal compartments have been demonstrated to be involved in most (but not all) cases. It has been shown that the glomerulopathic light chains associated with LCDD interact with a purported receptor on mesangial cells eliciting a cascade of pathological alterations anchored by the activation of transforming growth factor-β and resulting in increased matrix, rich in tenascin.

HCDD was first recognized in 1993 by Aucouturier et al. [23]. HCDD is a disease characterized by deletions in the heavy chains. A deletion in the constant domain of the γ gamma (IgG) heavy chain—CH1—predominates in these patients, but there are published cases with deletions in the hinge and CH2 domains of the heavy chains involved. In HC disease, the variable domain is also partially or completely deleted and this may be a factor in promoting tissue precipitation. Structural studies of HCDD have shown physicochemical abnormalities with unusual amino acid substitutions in the VH region which generally alter charge and hydrophobicity. The deletion in the heavy chains is likely to be necessary for abnormal light chains to be able to be secreted from the neoplastic plasma cells. Normal heavy chains must associate posttranslationally with heavy chain binding protein (BiP) in the endoplasmic reticulum [24], later assembling with heavy chains and eventually delivered to the Golgi complex where additional packaging and processing occur. When a mutant heavy chain lacks one of the key domains (especially CH1), it fails to properly associate with the BiP and may be prematurely secreted into the circulation.

The morphologic characteristics of HCDD are similar to those of LCDD. Light and electron microscopic features are identical. Research in HCDD has been rather limited and certainly the in vitro mesangial cell-oriented studies that have been conducted in LCDD to understand pathogenesis and progressive development of this disease have not taken place. However, it is assumed that HCDD shares rather similar pathogenetic pathways (as those shown to occur in LCDD).

This chapter focuses on the systemic manifestations of LCDD (with only a short but necessary incursion into kidneys) in an effort to increase exposure of this entity to surgical pathologists and, hopefully, maximize its detection.

Kidneys

In the advanced stage of LHCDD, a nodular glomerulopathy (Fig. 10.1a) that mimics the classical lesion that has been described in diabetic nephropathy—nodular glomerulosclerosis with so-called Kimmelstiel-Wilson nodules—is identified in the kidneys [25–28]. However, a number of other morphologic manifestations are seen prior to this more classically recognized pattern and may be the source of diagnostic confusion [27, 28]. Immunofluorescence and electron microscopy are of crucial value to identify these variants. The reader is referred to a number of excellent publications which describe this disease as a renal disorder in detail, emphasizing its pathogenesis, clinical presentation, treatment,

and prognosis [2–7, 25–28]. The criteria for diagnosis in tissues other than in kidneys have emanated from the renal studies.

Extrarenal Manifestations of Light/ Heavy Chain Deposition Disease

Isolated reports of the involvement of various organs have been published in the literature. However, these reports have generally been descriptive and have emphasized diagnostic criteria and suggested workup for appropriate diagnosis. The most complete reports are those emanating from autopsies with ample sampling to study the extent of multiorgan involvement [19]. It is very likely that systemic deposits in LHCDD are not detected or even misdiagnosed in surgical material. The question remains as to how aggressive clinicians are in documenting extrarenal disease in these patients and, therefore, this figure may not be at all accurate.

Liver and cardiac involvement is most common and has been documented to occur in approximately 25 % of patients with LCDD or LHCDD [29] but appears to occur less commonly in patients with HCDD.

Liver

Mild hepatic dysfunction is commonly noted. Liver deposits are often found in the hepatic sinusoids (Figs. 10.4a, b and 10.5a) and basement membranes of biliary ducts without associated parenchymal alterations [30]. In fact, liver deposits of monoclonal light chains are found in virtually every patient with LCDD whose liver is examined [31–33]. The material may be deposited in a similar fashion as amyloid. Amyloid seems to involve blood vessel walls with much greater frequency than LHCDD, and this can be used to favor one entity over the other. Nevertheless, It remains essential to rule OUT amyloidosis using the appropriate stains such as Congo red and Thioflavin T and/or ultrastructural criteria (Fig. 10.5a). Immunohistochemical stains can be used to demonstrate the presence of

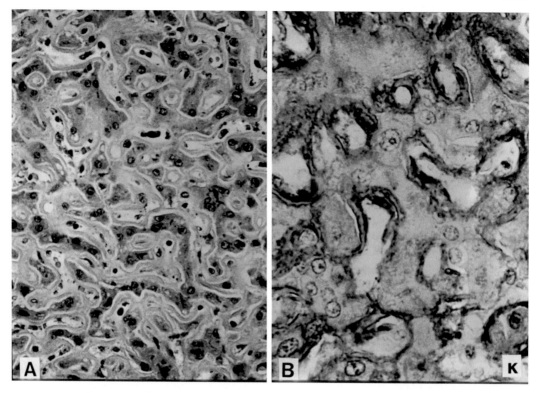

Fig. 10.4 LCDD in liver. (**a**) X500 and (**b**) X750. (**a**) Hematoxylin and eosin stain. (**b**) Immunohistochemical stain for κ light chains. (**a**) Eosinophilic material filling up the hepatic sinusoids. (**b**) This material stains for κ and not λ light chains

monoclonal light chains (Fig. 10.4b) in eosinophilic material filling sinusoids. Immunogold labeling at the ultrastructural level can confirm monoclonality (Fig. 10.5b, c). In a few instances, there may be destruction of the liver parenchyma creating an appearance reminiscent of peliosis hepatis [34].

Clinically, hepatomegaly is usually seen and alterations of liver function may be rather mild. Some patients present with altered liver enzymes and a liver biopsy is performed to diagnose the liver ailment. In a few cases, portal hypertension or hepatic failure has been reported.

Heart

Cardiac involvement in LHCDD is life-threatening and tends to occur commonly in the advanced stages of the disease process. The incidence of car-diac manifestation is difficult to be determined and varies from approximately 19–80 % depending on the series [3, 6]. Congestive heart failure is frequently seen in these patients resulting in severe cardiac failure in the advanced stages of the disease [35]. Cardiomegaly is a common finding in patients with cardiac involvement. Conduction disturbances with arrhythmias represent a common clinical presentation [36]. Varying degrees of restrictive cardiac failure may also be detected depending on the amount of light/heavy chain parenchymal deposition. Echocardiography and catheterization studies have demonstrated diastolic dysfunction and reduction in myocardial compliance similar to cases with cardiac amyloidosis. Deposition of light chains in cardiac vessels and perivascular areas is always identified in autopsies of patients with LHCDD [34], but can also be seen in biopsy specimens from patients with these conditions (Fig. 10.2a, b).

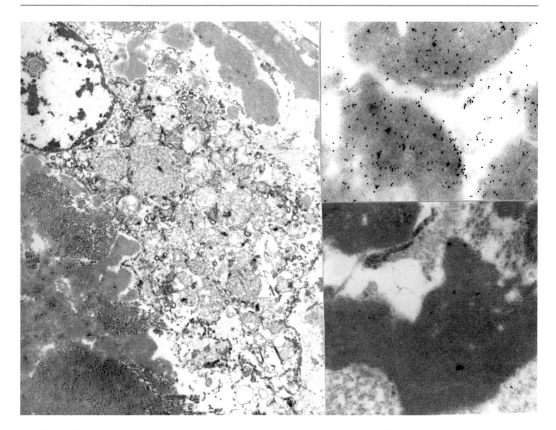

Fig. 10.5 Light chain deposits in hepatic sinusoids. (**a** and **b**) Transmission electron microscopy. Uranyl acetate and lead citrate stain. (**b,c**) Immunogold labeling for κ light chains. (**a**) Light chain deposits appear as punctate, electron-dense material. (**b**) Gold particles clearly label the sinusoidal deposits detecting the presence of κ light chain in them (**c**). No label for λ light chains

Peripheral and Central Nervous System Involvement

Peripheral neuropathy related to LHCDD has been documented in approximately 20 % of the reported cases. Light chain deposits may be in the endoneurium. In cases of LCDD, peripheral nerve involvement has been reported occasionally with patients presenting clinically with a polyneuropathy.

Deposits of light chains in the choroid plexus represent a common finding in these patients. A couple of case reports of LCDD restricted to the brain appeared in 2006 and 2007 by Fisher et al. and Popovic et al., respectively [37, 38]. The concept that has prevailed is that the blood–brain barrier protected the central nervous system from the circulating and sometimes misfolded monoclonal light chains, preventing both AL amyloidosis and pristine light chains from reaching and producing pathologic changes in the brain. Thus, it is not difficult to understand why the periventricular white matter is the most common site for the deposits of these monoclonal proteins, either in LCDD or amyloidosis.

Lungs

Deposition of light chains in the lungs of patients with LCDD has been documented in case reports and small series [39–49]. The first case report was published in 1988 [39]. Less than 30 cases of LCDD involving the lungs have been reported. The major clinical manifestation is dyspnea on exertion. The clinical and immunopathologic findings have been summarized in one of the publications referenced [40].

While in most cases the lesions are in the pulmonary parenchyma itself, cases with endobronchial lesions have also been documented. Two different histologic patterns have been reported: diffuse and nodular, similar to what has been observed in AL amyloidosis with pulmonary involvement [41–47]. The diffuse form appears to have a more ominous prognosis than the nodular form. Approximately 50 % of patients with the nodular form will have an identifiable lymphoproliferative disorder at the time of diagnosis, and also evidence of renal involvement, generally in the form of renal failure. One case was associated with extensive cystic changes in the pulmonary parenchyma [43].

The light chain deposits are usually punctate and electron dense, but may also infrequently acquire a needle-shaped electron-dense crystalline appearance [40]. Interstitial fibrosis generally accompanies and surrounds the light chain deposits.

The differential diagnosis of light chain deposition in the lung includes several conditions. One of the most common manifestations of LCDD in the lung is the presence of amyloid-like nodules which fail to stain with Congo red and Thioflavin T, thus essentially ruling out amyloidosis. In cases with nodules, hyalinizing and infectious granulomata and old sarcoid nodules are conditions that should be considered as part of the differential diagnosis [40, 45].

It appears that pulmonary nodules similar to those seen in LCDD can be found in a small subset of patients as a manifestation of localized LCDD without systemic involvement [46–48]. Three patients with nodules mimicking amyloidosis were found without demonstrable systemic LCDD [45]. Three additional similar patients have been reported in the literature by Morinaga, Piard, and Stokes, respectively [47–49]. Interestingly, one of these patients showed a combination of amyloid and light chain deposits with both lambda and kappa light chain specificity, respectively [49]. However, such conclusion (the absence of a systemic process) can only be definitely confirmed after a careful and extensive diagnostic workup is performed and at least several years of follow-up, as local manifestations

may precede overt generalized disease quite sometime. Nevertheless, there is no doubt that in some of these cases, localized monoclonal light chain production by a clone of plasma cells located at the site where the paraprotein deposits are present is responsible for the disease process (extramedullary plasmacytomas). The diffuse form must be distinguished from interstitial fibrosis and dense scars, as the light chains elicit much fibrosis and can be easily missed.

Gastrointestinal

Diarrhea is often a complaint of patients with LCDD affecting the gastrointestinal (GI) tract. However, findings in the GI tract appear to be infrequent and only approximately 20 % of the cases reported address gastrointestinal symptoms (present or absent), while less than 10 % of the patients afflicted with these disorders manifest clinical and/or pathological gastrointestinal manifestations [6]. This data suggests that only approximately 10 % of patients with LCDD have symptomatic gastrointestinal light chain deposition [6]. The light chain deposits are typically found in the vasculature and surrounding areas [3] (Fig. 10.6).

Heavy chain disease can be an enteric disease and it is in the majority of the cases of alpha-heavy chain disease. The usual clinical presentation is diarrhea and abdominal pain, vomiting, weight

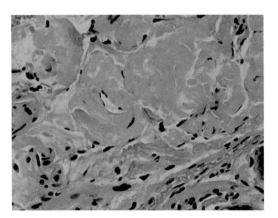

Fig. 10.6 Light chain deposits in the lamina propria of the stomach in patients with LHCDD. X750—Hematoxylin and eosin stain. The light chain deposits appear as eosinophilic, amorphous material closely resembling amyloid

loss, and evidence of malabsorption. Morphologic studies usually reveal an infiltrative plasmacytic or lymphoplasmacytic disorder localized to the GI tract, in some cases involving the lamina propria of the whole length of the small intestine and often associated with variable villous atrophy. However, there is no data documenting heavy chain deposits in the GI tract of patients with HCDD.

Pancreas

Deposition in the pancreas of monotypical light chains can be associated with destruction of the islets and development of diabetes mellitus [23].

Skin

Although skin deposits of light chains may occur [19], they appear rather infrequently, precluding the use of skin biopsy in lieu of invasive sampling of deep organs for diagnostic purposes [6]. A case of HCDD with skin deposits of IgG gamma chains (IgG-gamma) has been documented in the literature. Deposits were detected in the papillary and reticular dermis and in arteriolar walls [22].

Muscle

Deposition of paraproteins in striated muscles is rare. One patient with LCDD presented with chronic myopathic symptoms and another with acute rhabdomyolysis [6, 22], suggesting that there may be cases where the muscle is selectively affected. The same patient noted above with HCDD revealed heavy chain deposits in a skeletal muscle biopsy in endomysium, vessel walls, and perimysium.

Other Organs

In all organs, perivascular deposition is generally common and the earliest noticeable change, but parenchymal deposition is seen invariably in the more advanced stages of the disease process

leading to replacement of the normal structures. Deposition of light chains in patients with these diseases has also been documented in synovial tissues [20, 21], adrenal glands, submandibular glands, and abdominal vessels. Deposition of light/heavy chains in the thyroid may result in hypothyroidism [23].

Diagnostic Criteria/Pitfalls

Light/heavy chain deposits appear as eosinophilic, amorphous materials on hematoxylin and eosin sections, and amyloid is very much in the differential diagnosis in the majority of the cases, regardless of the organ involved. Negative Congo red and Thioflavin T stains can be used to rule out amyloidosis. To confirm LHCDD, monoclonality for light or heavy chains needs to be demonstrated and/or definitive ultrastructural evidence to support the diagnosis should be present. Ideally, both should be used to confirm the diagnosis unequivocally.

The main problem is that when using immunohistochemistry on paraffin-embedded tissues, there may be nonspecific staining for the nonpertinent light or heavy chains making a definitive interpretation impossible or equivocal. However, in some cases it turns out to be a definitive way to make a diagnosis (Figs. 10.1b and 10.4b). The results depend much on tissue fixation and processing, and it is virtually impossible to predict when the results would be satisfactory. Unquestionably, immunofluorescence provides a much more specific and reproducible ancillary diagnostic technique to make a diagnosis.

Ultrastructurally, the light and heavy chain deposits can be quite characteristic; however, that is not always the case. They exhibit a punctate to flocculent electron-dense appearance and are not fibrillary. The electron density of the deposits is variable with the more electron-dense deposits representing the most typical and diagnostic. The electron density depends on the amount of light/heavy chain deposited and also the physicochemical characteristics of the same (Fig. 10.7). In some instances, the electron-dense material is barely electron dense and could be easily missed. These deposited

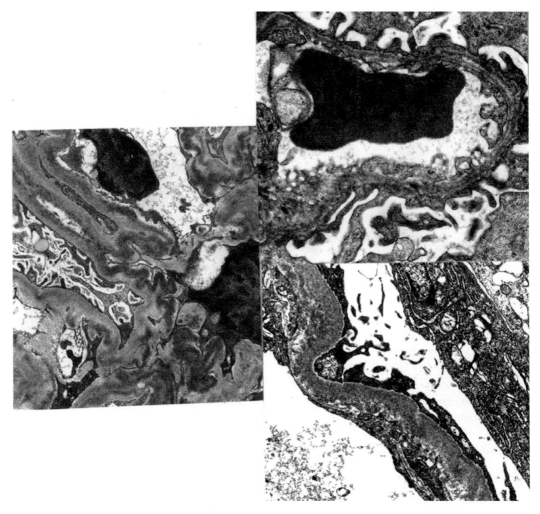

Fig. 10.7 Light chain deposits along subendothelial aspect in peripheral capillary walls. Transmission electron microscopy. Uranyl acetate and lead citrate stain. Note variable electron density associated with the light chain deposits depending on amount deposited and characteristics of the light chains. Some of the light chain deposits may be easily missed

pristine light and heavy chains can be seen by electron microscopy even in poorly fixed tissues or in paraffin-embedded materials reprocessed for ultrastructural evaluation (Fig. 10.8). Ultrastructural labeling may help in recognizing these (Fig. 10.9), as the specific light/heavy chain can be definitely localized to the deposits. However, this technique is only available at a few selected diagnostic laboratories.

Mechanisms Associated with Organ Pathology

Renal research has provided useful information regarding the pathologic events that take place as monoclonal light chains interact with renal compartments and lead to pathological consequences. In the case of LHCDD, the mesangium is the

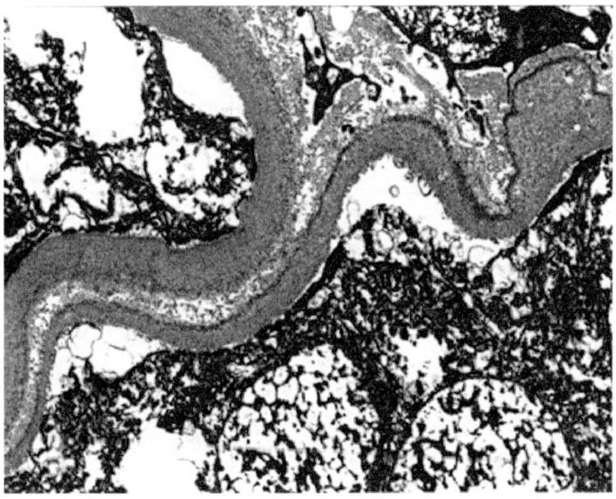

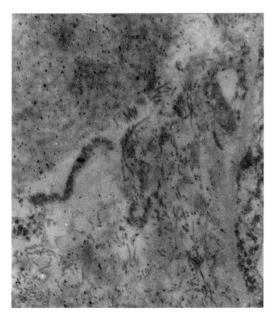

Fig. 10.8 Light chain deposits on the external aspect of renal tubular basement membranes. Tissue fixed in formalin, embedded in paraffin, and reprocessed for electron microscopy. In spite of the poor tissue preservation, the light chain deposits are easily identifiable

Fig. 10.9 Light chain deposits in heart. Transmission electron microscopy. Uranyl acetate and lead citrate stain. Immunogold labeling for lambda light chains. Light chain deposits are barely electron dense but clearly delineated with the gold particles labeling λ light chains. No labeling for κ light chains

primary target for pathological events to occur. The light chains interact with specific receptors on the surface of mesangial cells, activating effector molecules such as NF-kB and c-myc that produce downstream activation of a number of molecules,

including some crucial growth factors [50]. Initially there is activation of PDGF-β resulting in increased cellularity. Essential to the pathogenesis of these disorders is the activation of transforming growth factor-β which results in stimulation of mesangial cells to form matrix rich in tenascin (Fig. 10.10). PDGF-β and TGF-β act independently but in a coordinated fashion [51–53]. Amyloidogenic and LCDD light chains interact with the mesangial cells in a similar fashion, sharing the same receptors on mesangial cells, but follow different intracellular pathways and induce divergent phenotypic differentiation in the mesangial cells [54]. The sequence of events that takes place when LCDD glomerulopathic light chains and the mesangium interact is summarized in reference [55].

Likely a similar pathogenetic mechanism is involved when other cell types (such as fibroblasts) engage in interactions with pathogenic light chains in a number of different sites to as they engage in interactions with pathogenic light chains. While this may be an attractive hypothesis, work performed analyzing how cardiac fibroblasts interact with amyloidogenic light chains has shown that internalization occurs like in mesangial cells, but fibroblasts appear to process the light chains in a different manner than mesangial cells [56]. Nothing is known about how fibroblasts handle non-amyloidogenic (LCDD-associated) light chains. In essence, some of the information that has emerged from the in vitro and in vivo mesangial cell/LCDD light chain experimental work [51–55], but most likely not all, may be extrapolated to other organs to understand the pathologic events eventually leading to increased extracellular protein production (fibrogenic response) [53].

Physicochemical Characteristics of Pathologic Light/Heavy Chains Associated with LHCDD

A crucial element in the pathogenesis of LHCDD is the biochemical composition of the monotypical light or heavy chains associated with the pathologic process. Several studies have been conducted analyzing structural features of pathogenic light/heavy chains. The first such

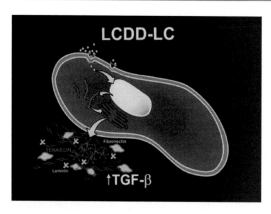

Fig. 10.10 Schematic representation of monoclonal light chain interactions with mesangial cells. Light chains interact with a receptor present at the surface of mesangial cells activating cellular effectors such as c-myc and NF-kB which produce downstream activities leading to enhanced production of extracellular matrix rich in tenascin

biochemical analysis by Picken et al. in 1989 used tissue obtained from a patient with systemic LCDD and cardiac deposits [57].

The light chain deposits from myocardium were extracted in 6 M guanidine–HCl under reducing conditions, partially purified by column chromatography, and analyzed by immunoblotting and amino-terminal sequencing. The extracted material contained four main bands reactive with anti-kappa antibody: intact kappa light chain (MW, 28 kDa), under reducing conditions, and three fragments (MW, 20, 16, and 15 kDa). As revealed by the amino-terminal sequencing performed on three of the four bands, the intact light chain molecule and two fragments belonged to the kappa I subgroup. Thus, similar to light chain amyloid (AL), the deposits in LCDD were derived from both intact light chain and fragments. Unlike in AL, amyloid P component was not detected in the deposits of this patient or those examined previously.

Other studies have focused on the biochemical characterization of monoclonal light chains in the bone marrow, urine, and those deposited in glomeruli in patients with LHCDD. Though there are no specific amino acid sequences in these glomerulopathic light chains that are associated with LHCDD, there are some similarities in their physicochemical characteristics. These light chains typically belong to V Kappa I and IV subtypes, although a few truncated V kappa III have also been detected. Proteins produced from the B3 gene (KIV) have received much attention as being over represented among LCDD-associated light chains [23, 58–60]. A general review of light chain diversification and pathological outcomes can be found in reference [60].

The structure of a few heavy chains associated with HCDD have also been biochemically analyzed [10, 23]. γ heavy chains are the ones most commonly involved in HCDD with γ1, γ3, and γ4 having been documented in the literature.

Conclusions

The deposition of pathologic monoclonal light and heavy chains leading to pathologic alterations can virtually occur in any organ. While the kidneys are preferentially affected, other organs can also show evidence of dysfunction, and biopsies from these organs may present a challenge to diagnostic pathologists who are only exposed sporadically to these rather rare disorders. The pathologic manifestations may be subtle or overt, but regardless a high index of suspicion is needed to identify and properly characterize the pathologic findings using the appropriate set of ancillary diagnostic techniques. This chapter has highlighted the most salient facts associated with the extrarenal diagnosis of these disorders with emphasis on how to separate them from amyloidosis and other confusing pathology. Finally, it should be pointed out that LHCDD and AL amyloidosis coexist in rare instances, further complicating the diagnostic process [34, 49, 61].

References

1. Fernand J-P, Brouet J-C. Heavy-chain diseases. Hematol Oncol Clin N Am. 1999;13:1281–94.
2. Ronco P, Plaisier E, Mougenot B, Aucouturier P. Immunoglobulin light (heavy)-chain deposition disease: from molecular medicine to pathophysiology-driven therapy. Clin J Am Soc Nephrol. 2006;1:1342–50.
3. Ronco PM, Alyanakian M-A, Mougenot B, et al. Light chain deposition disease: a model of

glomerulosclerosis defined at the molecular level. J Am Soc Nephrol. 2001;12:1558–65.

4. Kambham N, Markowitz GS, Appel GB, et al. Heavy chain deposition disease: the disease spectrum. Am J Kidney Dis. 1999;33:954–62.

5. Buxbaum J, Gallo G. Nonamyloidotic monoclonal immunoglobulin deposition diseases. Hematol Oncol Clin North Am. 1999;13:1235–48.

6. Lin J, Markowitz GS, Valeri AM, Kambham N, et al. Renal monoclonal immunoglobulin deposition disease: the disease spectrum. J Am Soc Nephrol. 2001;12:1482–92.

7. Herrera GA, Joseph L, Gu X, et al. Renal pathologic spectrum in an autopsy series of patients with plasma cell dyscrasias. Arch Pathol Lab Med. 2004;128; 875–9.

8. Nasr SH, Valeri AM, Cornell LD, Fidler ME, et al. Renal monoclonal immunoglobulin deposition disease: A report of 64 patients from a single institution. Clin J Am Soc Nephrol. 2012;7:231–9.

9. Ivanyi B. Frequency of light chain nephropathy relative to renal amyloidosis and Bence Jones cast nephropathy in a necropsy study of patients with myeloma. Arch Pathol Lab Med. 1990;114:986–7.

10. Khamlichi AA, Aucouturier P, Preud'Homme JL, Cogne M, et al. Structure of abnormal heavy chains in human heavy-chain deposition disease. Eur J Biochem. 1995;229:54–60.

11. Cogne M, Silvain C, Khamlichi AS, et al. Structurally abnormal immunoglobulins in human lymphoproliferative disorders. Blood. 1992;79:2181–95.

12. Preud'homme JL, Aucouturiere P, Touchard G, et al. Monoclonal immunoglobulin deposition disease: a review of immunoglobulin chain alterations. Int J Immunopharmacol. 1994;16:425–31.

13. Khamlichi AA, Rocca A, Touchard G, et al. Role of light chain variable region in myeloma with light chain deposition disease: evidence from experimental model. Blood. 1995;86:3655–9.

14. Turner M. Molecules which recognize antigen. In: Roitt IM, Brostoff J, Male DK, editors. Immunology. St Louis, MO: Mosby; 1989. p. 5.1–5.11.

15. Santostefano M, Zanchelli F, Zaccaria A, et al. The ultrastructural basis of renal pathology in monoclonal gammopathies. J Nephrol. 2005;18:659–75.

16. Herrera GA. The contributions of electron microscopy to the understanding and diagnosis of plasma cell dyscrasia-related renal lesions. Med Electron Microsc. 2001;34:1–18.

17. Gallo G, Picken MM, Buxbaum J, et al. Deposits in monoclonal immunoglobulin deposition disease lack amyloid P component. Mod Pathol. 1988;1:453–6.

18. Antonovych TT, Lin RC, Parrish E. Light chain deposits in multiple myeloma. 7th Annual Meeting of the American Society of Nephrology, 173 (Abstract #3). Lab Invest. 1974; 30: 370A.

19. Randall RE, Williamson WC, Mullinax F, et al. Manifestations of systemic light chain deposition. Am J Med. 1976;60:293–9.

20. Husby G, Blichfeld P, Brinch L, et al. Chronic arthritis and gamma heavy chain disease: coincidence or pathogenic link? Scand J Rheumatol. 1998;27:257–64.

21. Husby G. Is there a pathogenetic link between gamma heavy chain disease and chronic arthritis? Curr Opin Rheumatol. 2000;12:65–70.

22. Rott T, Vizjak A, Lindic J, et al. IgG heavy-chain deposition disease affecting both kidneys, skin, and skeletal muscle. Nephrol Dial Transplant. 1998;13:1825–8.

23. Aucouturier P, Khamlichi AA, Touchard G, et al. Brief report: heavy chain deposition disease. N Engl J Med. 1993;329:1389–93.

24. Hendershot I, Bole D, Kearney JF. Assembly and secretion of heavy chains that do not associate posttranslationally with immunoglobulin heavy chain binding protein. J Cell Biol. 1987;104:761–7.

25. Cohen JJ. Case records of the Massachusetts General Hospital. Weekly clinicopathologic exercises. Case 1–1981. N Engl J Med. 1981;304:33–43.

26. Linder J, Croker BP, Vollmer RT, et al. Systemic kappa light-chain deposition. An ultrastructural study. Am J Surg Pathol. 1983;7:85–93.

27. Herrera GA. Renal manifestations in plasma cell dyscrasias: an appraisal from the patients' bedside to the research laboratory. Ann Diagn Pathol. 2000;4:174–200.

28. Herrera GA. Renal lesions associated with plasma cell dyscrasias: practical approach to diagnosis, new concepts, and challenges. Arch Pathol Lab Med. 2009;133:249–67.

29. Ganeval D, Mignon F, Preud'homme JL, et al. Visceral deposition of monoclonal light chains and immunoglobulins: a study of renal and immunopathologic abnormalities. Adv Nephrol Necker Hosp. 1982;11:25.

30. Herrera GA, Turbat-Herrera EA, Viale G, et al. Ultrastructural immunolabeling in renal diseases: past, present and future expectations. Pathol Immunopathol Res. 1987;6:51–63.

31. Girelli CM, Lodi G, Rocca F. K Light chain deposition disease of the liver. Eur J Gastroenterol Hepatol. 1998;10:429–30.

32. Katz A, Zent R, Bargman JM. IgG heavy-chain deposition disease. Mod Pathol. 1994;7:874.

33. Droz D, Noel LH, Carnot F, et al. Liver involvement in nonamyloid light chain deposition disease. Lab Invest. 1984;50:683–9.

34. Ganeval D, Noel LH, Preud'homme JL, et al. Light chain deposition disease: Its relation to AL-type amyloidosis. Kidney Int. 1984;26:1–9.

35. Jego P, Paillard F, Ramée MP, Grosbois B. Congestive heart failure: revealing light chain deposition disease. Eur J Intern Med. 2000;11:101–3.

36. Fabbian F, Stabellini N, Sartori S, et al. Light chain deposition disease presenting as paroxysmal atrial fibrillation: a case report. J Med Case Rep. 2007;1:187–93.

37. Fisher L, Korfel A, Stoltenburg-Didinger G, et al. A 19-year-old male with generalized seizures, unconsciousness and a deviation of gaze. Brain Pathol. 2006;16:185–6.

38. Popovic M, Tavcar R, Glavac D, et al. Light chain deposition disease restricted to the brain: the firs case report. Hum Pathol. 2007;38:179–84.

39. Kijner CH, Yousem SA. Systemic light chain deposition disease presenting as multiple pulmonary nodules. A case report and review of the literature. Am J Surg Pathol. 1988;12:401–13.

40. Bhargava P, Rushin JM, Rusnok EJ, et al. Pulmonary light chain deposition disease. Report of five cases and review of the literature. Am J Surg Pathol. 2007;31:267–76.

41. Chen KT. Amyloidosis presenting in the respiratory tract. Pathol Ann. 1989;24:253–73.

42. Colby T, Kos MN, Travis WD. Tumors of lower respiratory tract. Atlas of tumor pathology. Washington, DC: American Registry of Pathology; 1995. p. 495–501.

43. Colombat M, Stern M, Groussard O, et al. Pulmonary cystic disease related to light chain deposition disease. Am J Respir Crit Care Med. 2006;173:777–80.

44. Morinaga S, Watanabe H, Gemma A, et al. Plasmacytoma of the lung associated with nodular deposits of immunoglobulins. Am J Surg Pathol. 1987;11:989–9995.

45. Warfel K, Benson MD, Hull MT, et al. Pulmonary nodules and pleural plaques in systemic light chain deposition disease (LCDD). Lab Invest. 1987;500:84a.

46. Khoor A, Myers JL, Tazelaar HD, et al. Amyloid-like pulmonary nodules, including localized light chain deposition: clinicopathologic analysis of three cases. Am J Clin Pathol. 2004;121:200–4.

47. Morigana S, Watanabe H, Gemma A, et al. Plasmacytoma of the lung with nodular deposits of immunoglobulin. Am J Surg Pathol. 1987;11:989–95.

48. Piard F, Yaziji N, Jarry O, et al. Solitary plasmacytoma of the lung with light chain extracellular deposits: a case report and review of the literature. Histopathology. 1998;32:356–61.

49. Stokes MB, Jagirdar J, Burchstin O, et al. Nodular pulmonary immunoglobulin light chain deposits with coexistent amyloid and non-amyloid features in an HIV-infected patient. Mod Pathol. 1997;10:1059–65.

50. Russell WJ, Cardelli J, Harris E, et al. Monoclonal light chain-mesangial cell interactions: early signaling events and subsequent pathologic effects. Lab Invest. 2001;81:689–703.

51. Zhu L, Herrera GA, Murphy-Ullrich JE, et al. Pathogenesis of glomerulosclerosis in light chain deposition disease. Am J Pathol. 1995;147:375–85.

52. Keeling J, Herrera GA. An in vitro model of light chain deposition disease. Kidney Int. 2009;75:634–45.

53. Teng J, Zhang PL, Russell WJ, et al. Insights into mechanisms responsible for mesangial alterations associated with fibrogenic glomerulopathic light chains. Nephron Physiol. 2003;94:28–38.

54. Keeling J, Teng J, Herrera GA. AL-amyloidosis and light chain deposition disease light chains induce divergent phenotypic transformations of human mesangial cells. Lab Invest. 2004;84:1322–38.

55. Ronco P, Plaisier E, Aucouturier P. Monoclonal immunoglobulin light and heavy chain deposition diseases: molecular models of common diseases. In: Ronco C, editor, Herrera G, editor. Experimental models of renal diseases Pathogenesis and diagnosis contributions to nephrology. Basel: Karger; 2011. p. 220–31.

56. Trinkaus-Randall V, Walsh MT, Steeves S, et al. Cellular response of cardiac fibroblasts to amyloidogenic light chains. Am J Pathol. 2005;106:197–208.

57. Picken MM, Frangione B, Barlogie B, Luna M, Gallo G. Light chain deposition disease derived from the kappa I light chain subgroup. Biochemical characterization. Am J Pathol. 1989;134:749–54.

58. Rocca A, Khamlichi AA, Noël L-H, et al. Primary structure of a variable region of the VκI subgroup (ISE) in light chain deposition disease. Clin Exp Immunol. 1993;91:506–9.

59. Decourt C, Cogne M, Rocca A. Structural peculiarities of a truncated VκIII immunoglobulin light chain in myeloma with light chain deposition disease. Clin Exp Immunol. 1996;106:357–61.

60. Gu M, Wilton R, Stevens FJ. Diversity and diversification of light chains in myeloma: the specter of amyloidogenesis by proxy. In: Herrera GA, editor. The kidney in plasma cell dyscrasias, Contributions to Nephrology series. S Karger AG: Basel; 2007. p. 156–81.

61. Jacquot C, Saint-Andre JP, Touchard G, et al. Association of systemic light chain deposition disease and amyloidosis: a report of 3 patients with renal involvement. Clin Nephrol. 1985;24:93–8.

Non-Randall Glomerulonephritis with Non-Organized Monoclonal Ig Deposits

11

Pierre Ronco, Alexandre Karras, and Emmanuelle Plaisier

In the past 10 years, the spectrum of glomerular diseases associated with multiple myeloma and myeloma-related disorders has expanded with the use of appropriate reagents including highly specific anti-light chain (LC) and anti-heavy chain (HC) subclass antibodies, and electron microscopy. For a long time, since the identification of the variable region of a circulating Ig LC in amyloid fibrils by Glenner and associates [1], AL amyloid was considered the only cause of glomerular involvement in myeloma and related disorders. Then, the description of non-amyloid light chain deposition disease (LCDD) by

P. Ronco, MD, PhD (✉)
Sorbonne Universités, UPMC Univ Paris 06,
UMR_S 1155, Paris 75005, France

Department of Nephrology and Dialysis,
AP-HP, Hôpital Tenon, Paris 75020, France

UMR_S 1155, Batiment Recherche, Hôpital Tenon,
4 rue de la Chine, Paris 75020, France
e-mail: pierreronco@yahoo.fr

A. Karras, MD
Department of Nephrology, AP-HP, University Paris
Descartes, Hôpital Européen Georges Pompidou,
Paris, France

E. Plaisier, MD, PhD
Sorbonne Universités, UPMC Univ Paris 06,
UMR_S 1155, Paris 75005, France

Department of Nephrology and Dialysis,
AP-HP, Hôpital Tenon, Paris 75020, France

Randall and associates [2] opened up new perspectives in plasma cell-related glomerular pathology, although the nodular glomerulosclerosis characteristic of the disease was constantly associated with LC deposits along renal tubules. Together with myeloma cast nephropathy, AL amyloidosis and LCDD are the most common complications of plasma cell-related disorders [3], thus indicating that the majority of these disorders are caused by Ig LC deposition in renal parenchyma.

Deposition of monoclonal Ig containing both heavy and light chains is far less common and may manifest as type-I cryoglobulinemic GN [4], Randall-type light and heavy chain deposition disease [5], immunotactoid GN [6–8], and light and heavy chain amyloidosis [9, 10] (Table 11.1).

In type 1 cryoglobulinemia, a membranoproliferative glomerulonephritis (MPGN) with macrophage infiltration is the most characteristic histologic pattern and the deposits are typically, but not invariably, organized into fibrillary or microtubular structures at the ultrastructural level. The hallmark of immunotactoid glomerulonephritis is the presence of highly organized non-amyloidotic microtubular deposits, usually of >30 nm in diameter, with hollow cores and parallel stacking, although thinner tubules can be observed [6]. Light and heavy chain amyloidosis is extremely rare and, similar to AL amyloidosis, is characterized by the pres-

Table 11.1 Glomerulonephritis (GN) with deposits of monoclonal Ig light and heavy chains

Organized deposits	Non-organized deposits
Type-1 cryoglobulinemic GN	Light and heavy chain deposition disease (LHCDD)
Immunotactoid GN	Proliferative GN with monoclonal Ig deposits(PGNMID)
Light and heavy chain amyloidosis (Fibrillary GN)	Nonproliferative GN with monoclonal Ig deposits

ence of Congo red-positive deposits composed of haphazardly oriented fibrils that measure 8–14 nm in diameter. Among diseases with non-organized deposits, LHCDD is characterized by the presence of nodular sclerosing glomerulopathy by light microscopy, linear staining of glomerular and tubular basement membranes for a single heavy and light chain by immunofluorescence, and non-fibrillar, granular electron-dense deposits involving glomerular and tubular basement membranes by electron microscopy. Recently, a second entity has emerged, which is characterized by non-Randall-type and non-organized glomerular Ig deposition that does not conform to any of the previous categories [11–14]. In most cases reviewed by Nasr in 2004 [15] and 2009 [16], lesions were those of MPGN. The authors coined the term proliferative glomerulonephritis with monoclonal IgG deposits (PGNMID) to call this new entity. In other rarer cases, lesions were those of atypical membranous nephropathy (MN) [13, 15, 17–19]. Although the clinicopathological presentation of these patients is shared with common cases of MPGN and MN, specificity is provided by the monoclonal Ig deposits which should lead to adapted diagnostic procedure and therapeutic strategy.

In this chapter, we revisit the spectrum of non-organized monoclonal Ig deposits. We will discuss important diagnostic issues including demonstration of monoclonality of the deposits and search for underlying lymphocyte and/or plasma cell proliferation, as well as the treatment options in the light of recent pathophysiologic and therapeutic advances.

Proliferative GN with Non-Organized Monoclonal Ig Deposits

Alpers et al. [11] first described six patients with an MPGN pattern of GN, including mesangial hypercellularity, increased mesangial matrix and mesangial interposition, and monoclonal IgGκ and C3 staining. Granular subendothelial and mesangial deposits were seen by electron microscopy. None of these six patients had detectable serum or urine monoclonal Ig, and bone marrow examination in four patients was normal. The authors pointed out the female predominance (five of the six patients), the young age of onset (31 years old or less in three patients), and the absence of overt plasma cell dyscrasia.

Bridoux et al. [13] reported the cases of five patients manifesting glomerulopathy with non-organized, non-Randall-type monoclonal Ig deposits; two of these patients being described in detail by Touchard [12]. The mean age was 54 ± 17 years. All patients presented with microhematuria and renal failure; four of five had a nephrotic syndrome. Kidney biopsy revealed atypical membranous, endocapillary proliferative, and membranoproliferative patterns. By immunofluorescence, the glomerular capillary wall deposits consisted of IgG3κ in two patients, IgG3λ in one, IgG2κ in one, and isolated λLC in one. Corresponding monoclonal proteins were detected in serum or urine in three patients.

In 2004, Nasr et al. [15] reported the first extensive description of PGNMID in a series of 10 patients, and recently enlarged this series to 37 cases [16], thus allowing a thorough description of the disease

Epidemiology Nasr et al. [15] reported a biopsy incidence of 0.21 % of a total of 4650 native biopsies referred to the Renal Pathology Laboratory of Columbia University College of Physicians and Surgeons from January 2000 to February 2003. By comparison, the biopsy incidences of AL amyloidosis and Randall-type MIDD were 1.66 and 0.52 % over the same time period, respectively. In Japan, Masai et al. [20] identified four patients with PGNMID after reviewing 5443 kidney biopsies (biopsy incidence of 0.07 %).

Clinical Features In Nasr et al.'s largest series, the majority of patients were white (81 %) and female (62 %). All patients were adults and had a mean age of 55 years (range 20–81). At presentation, all patients had proteinuria. Proteinuria was in the nephrotic range in 69 % of patients, and 49 % developed full nephrotic syndrome. Microhematuria was documented in 77 % of patients. Two-thirds of patients had renal insufficiency, including three who were on hemodialysis. None of the patients had significant extra-renal symptoms. A case where crescentic glomerulonephritis was superimposed to PGNMID was recently reported with autoimmune hemolytic anemia, thus widening the spectrum of PGNMID [21]. Two cases with a rapidly favorable outcome were associated with Parvovirus B19 infection, suggesting that virus infection-associated immune disorders could be implicated in the pathogenesis of PGNMID [22].

Pathologic Findings Four histologic patterns were observed. The most common seen in 57 % of cases was MPGN, often associated with endocapillary hypercellularity including focal macrophage infiltration. The second most common pattern, seen in 35 %, was predominantly endocapillary proliferative GN. The third histologic pattern, seen in 5 % of cases, was predominantly membranous GN but with focal endocapillary hypercellularity and segmental membranoproliferative features. The fourth and rarest pattern was pure mesangial proliferative GN. Crescents were present in 32 % of cases. Interstitial inflammation was predominantly focal and associated with a variable degree of tubular atrophy and arteriosclerosis.

Results of immunofluorescence staining with anti-LC isotype and anti-Ig subclass antibodies obtained in three different series [13, 16, 20] are shown in Table 11.2. Deposits were identified exclusively in the glomeruli. They were mostly granular and localized to the glomerular capillary wall and mesangium. IgG was the only Ig deposited, with the exception of a case where only λLC was detected [13] and another case with exclusive

Table 11.2 Glomerular immunofluorescence staining in patients with PGNMID

Parameter	No. of patients	Percentage of patients
IgG	45/46	97.8
IgG1κ	7/39	17.9
IgG1λ	2/39	5.1
IgG2κ	1/39	2.6
IgG2λ	2/39	5.1
IgG3κ	22/39	56.4
IgG3λ	5/39	12.8
C3	40/41	97.6
C1q	27/40	67.5

Series from Nasr et al. [16], Bridoux et al. [13], and Masai et al. [20]

IgM κ deposits [23]. All cases showed LC isotype restriction, including 30 cases (76.9 %) with sole positivity for κ. Ig subclass analysis showed a huge predominance of IgG3 (69.2 % of cases), whereas IgG3 represents a minor subclass in healthy subjects (8 %) and myeloma patients (4 %) [24]. No case showed positivity for IgG4. On statistical analysis, IgG3 subtype correlated with the absence of M-spike, with only 2 of 21 patients with IgG3 deposits having a positive M-spike in Nasr et al.'s series [16]. Immunofluorescence studies using antibodies specific for γ-heavy chain, C_H1, C_h2, and C_H3 domains, and γ3 hinge did not show apparent deletion [16, 20].

In all cases, granular electron-dense deposits were confined to the glomerular compartment, while they were both glomerular and tubular in LHCDD. They were primarily subendothelial and mesangial, but subepithelial deposits were also seen. In Nasr et al.'s series [16], some patients showed rare ill-defined fibrils with focal lattice-like arrays although the deposits never formed well-organized structures as seen in fibrillary or immunotactoid GN.

Immunologic Data. Only 14 of 52 (27 %) patients had evidence of dysproteinemia by serum and/ or urine electrophoresis and immunofixation [11, 13, 16, 20]. Of the 26 of 37 patients reported by Nasr et al. [16] who had no detectable monoclonal component in serum or urine, four were tested with the serum free LC assay; of these, three were found to have normal κ:λ ratio, and one (who had glomerular monoclonal IgG3κ deposits) had an elevated κ:λ ratio.

Bone marrow examination, performed in 30 patients [11, 16, 20], showed marrow plasmacytosis in two patients and clear signs of myeloma in one patient. None of the patients had lymphadenopathy, hepatomegaly, or lymphoma.

Search for cryoglobulinemia was negative in all patients (performed repeatedly in many patients), and none of the patients had any systemic manifestations of cryoglobulinemia. Serum complement was decreased in 11 of 41 (27 %) patients [16, 20]. Of the 11 patients with hypocomplementemia, 8 had IgG3 glomerular deposits and 3 had IgG1 glomerular deposits.

Treatment Outcome In the largest series reported so far [16], 18 of 37 patients received immunosuppressive agents either with or without concurrent renin–angiotensin system (RAS) blockade. It is remarkable that 12 patients (37.5 %) developed complete ($n=4$) or partial ($n=8$) remission, whereas only two reached ESRD (Table 11.3).

Transplantation Because 20–25 % of PGNMID progress to ESRD [16], potential recurrence of the disease in the allograft is an important issue. Nasr et al. [25] reported recurrence of PGNMID in four Caucasians (three women and one man), although no patient had a detectable circulating monoclonal component or hematologic malignancy. Recurrence was first documented by biopsy performed at a mean of 3.8 months posttransplant because of renal insufficiency (four patients), proteinuria (three patients), and microhematuria (three patients). Histologic patterns in the allograft were endocapillary or mesangial GN.

Monoclonal IgG deposits (three IgG3κ and one IgG3λ) in the transplants had identical heavy and light chain isotypes as in the native kidneys. Recurrence was treated with combined high-dose prednisone plus rituximab ($n=3$) or plus cyclosporine ($n=1$). After a mean posttransplant follow-up of 43 months, all four patients achieved reduction in proteinuria and three had reduction in creatinine. Repeat biopsies showed reduced histologic activity after treatment.

Table 11.3 Clinical follow-up of patients with PGNMID

Parameter	Value
Duration of follow-up (mo; mean [range])	30.3 (1.0–114.0)
Treatment	
None	5 (15.6)
RAS blockade alone	9 (28.1)
Immunosuppressor agents	18 (56.3)
Steroids	11
Cyclophosphamide	3
Cyclosporine	2
Mycophenolate mofetil	5
Rituximab	4
Chlorambucil	1
Thalidomide	2
Bortezomib (velcade)	1
Outcome[a]	
CR	4 (12.5)
PR	8 (25.0)
PRD	12 (37.5)
Persistent hematuria (with normal creatinine and no proteinuria)	1 (3.1)
ESRD	7 (21.9)
Death	5 (15.6)

[a]CR: remission of proteinuria to <500 mg/day with normal renal function; PR: reduction in proteinuria by at least 50 % and to <2 g/day with stable renal function (no more than a 20 % increase in serum creatinine); PRD: failure to meet criteria for either CR or PR but not reaching ESRD, including patients with unremitting proteinuria, or progressive chronic kidney disease. From Nasr et al. [16], with permission

Posttransplant PGNMID has also been reported by other authors [26–28], either as a recurrence of a pre-transplant PGNMID or as a de novo glomerulopathy, in patients having reached ESRD for other reasons, such as polycystic disease or type-1 diabetes mellitus. These observations confirm the severity of the disease and the poor renal outcome despite non-rituximab immunosuppressive regimens.

Nonproliferative GN with Non-Organized Monoclonal Ig Deposits

Next to PGNMID, isolated case reports and small series suggested that some patients developed GNMID with no or minimal glomerular cell proliferation. One of the patients reported by Bridoux et al. [13] and described in detail by Touchard [12] had nephrotic syndrome related to thickened glomerular capillary walls with IgG3λ and complement deposits. Immunoblotting revealed the presence of monoclonal IgG3λ. Evans et al. [18] described a patient with follicular B-cell lymphoma who developed nephrotic syndrome related to subepithelial granular IgG1κ deposits. One patient in Nasr et al.'s series [15] of PGNMID had a pattern of MN, however, with segmental membranoproliferative features and IgG1κ deposits.

Komatsuda et al. [19] reviewed 5,443 kidney biopsies from their own department in Akita (Japan) and identified three patients with monoclonal immunoglobulin deposition disease associated with membranous features. All patients had proteinuria, and one patient developed nephrotic syndrome. Renal insufficiency was not observed. Cryoglobulin or monoclonal protein in serum and urine was not detected. A renal biopsy showed thickening of the glomerular capillary walls and spike formation. Tubulointerstitial and vascular alterations were mild or absent. Immunofluorescence studies revealed granular IgG3κ deposits in two patients and IgG1κ deposits in one patient, along the glomerular capillary walls. Significant deposition along the tubular basement membranes was not observed in any patient. Immunofluorescence studies using antibodies specific for γ-heavy chain Fab containing C_H1 domain, C_H2 domain, and C_H3 domain did not show any apparent deletion. On confocal microscopy, glomerular colocalization of light and heavy chains was observed. Electron microscopy showed predominant subepithelial granular deposits without distinct ultrastructural organization. All patients were treated with steroids, and good effects were observed. A follow-up renal biopsy performed in one patient showed histological improvement. No patient developed myeloma or other hematological malignancy during the course of follow-up (mean 44 months).

Revisiting the Disease Spectrum of GN with Monoclonal Ig Deposits

To get further insight into the glomerulopathies with monoclonal Ig deposits, we recently reviewed the cases of 26 patients with non-cryoglobulinemic GN and monoclonal Ig deposits referred to three nephrology departments in Paris between 1980 and 2008 [17]. We found that there were more patients with MN ($n = 14$) than with MPGN ($n = 12$) (Fig. 11.1). In five of the MN patients, the glomerular lesions were, however, atypical with mesangial hypertrophy and increased mesangial cellularity (Fig. 11.1a). Overall, extracapillary proliferation with crescents was observed in 13 cases (4 of 14 MN, 9 of 12 MPGN), whereas glomerular necrotic lesions were present in only six biopsies. Interstitial inflammation with infiltration by neutrophils and nonmalignant lymphocytes was noted in 17 patients (65 %). Interstitial fibrosis with tubular atrophy ranged from absent or mild (57 %) to moderate (27 %) and severe (16 %). Vascular lesions were frequent, mainly arteriolar hyalinosis (15/26) and arteriosclerosis (19/26).

Demographic, clinical, and biological characteristics of these patients are shown in Table 11.4. At presentation, all patients had glomerular proteinuria >1 g/24 h and most (85 %) of the patients presented with nephrotic syndrome. Mean serum creatinine level at presentation was 211 µmol/l (eGFR: 49.3 ± 34.6 ml/min/1.73 m²), and 14 of 26 (54 %) patients initially had significant renal dysfunction, including three patients who needed temporary hemodialysis. In eight cases (31 %), a circulating monoclonal IgG was detected by standard methods (serum and urine protein electrophoresis with immunofixation). In all of these cases, the serum monoclonal IgG had the same light and heavy chain isotype as the monoclonal compound identified in the glomerular deposits, on the renal biopsy. Hypocomplementemia was observed in 8 of 22 patients (36 %) with available data, showing either isolated C4 or combined C3 and C4 consumption. Low serum

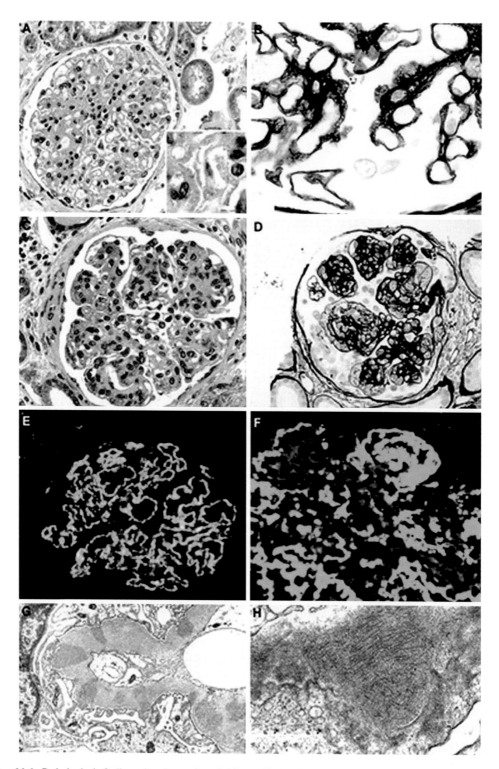

Fig. 11.1 Pathological findings in glomerulonephritis with monoclonal Ig deposits. Light microscopy findings in *MN* membranous nephropathy, showing immune deposits on the external side of the glomerular basement membrane, with frequent mesangial hypertrophy (**a**, Masson's trichrome stain); the deposits have irregular size (*inset* **a**) and are embedded in basement membrane expansions (**b**, JMS stain). In patients with membranoproliferative pattern, light microscopy shows proliferation of mesangial cells (**c**, Masson's trichrome stain) and double contours (**d**, JMS stain). By immunofluorescence, parietal granular IgG deposits in MN (**e**) are different from the more diffuse pattern seen in the MPGN (**f**). Ultrastuctural studies found that most patients have granular, non-organized deposits in the subepithelial (**g**) or subendothelial spaces, whereas in some cases, the deposits show microtubular substructure (**h**), as previously described in immunotactoid glomerulonephritis. From Guiard et al. [17], with permission

Table 11.4 Demographic, clinical, and biological characteristics at presentation of patients with non-cryoglobulinemic GN with monoclonal Ig deposits

Characteristics	Value
Female/male, n (%)	16/10 (61/39)
Age, years (mean ± SD) (range)	52 ± 16 (29–77)
40 years, n (%)	20 (77)
<40 years, n (%)	3 (23)
Ethnicity, n (%)	
Caucasian	22 (85)
Other	4(15)
Proteinuria, g/24 h, (mean ± SD) (range)	5.3 ± 4.6 (1.4–10)
Serum albumin, g/L, (mean ± SD) (range)	26 ± 7 (13–46)
Total serum protein, g/L, (mean ± SD) (range)	55.1 ± 6.1 (46–65)
Nephrotic syndrome, n (%)	22 (85)
Hematuria, n (%)	21 of 24 (87.5)
Serum creatinine, μmol/L, (mean ± SD) (range)	211 ± 90 (45–814)
eGFR, ml/min/1.73 m², (mean ± SD) (range)	49.3 ± 34.6 (10–130)
Renal dysfunction, n (%)	14 (54)
Hypertension, n (%)	16 of 24 (66.7)
Dysproteinemia, n (%)	8 (30.7)
Serum paraprotein only	6 (23)
Serum and urine paraprotein	2 (7.7)
Hematological malignancy, n (%)	9 of 26 (34.6)
Low C3, n (%)	1 of 22 (4.5)
Low C4, n (%)	3 of 22 (13.6)
Low C3 and C4, n (%)	4 of 22 (18.1)
Adenopathy, n (%)	2 (7.7)
Hepatosplenomegaly, n (%)	1 (3.8)

From Guiard et al. [17], with permission

complement concentration was equally observed among patients with either MPGN or MN and independently of the monoclonal IgG isotype. Serum cryoglobulin, hepatitis C, hepatitis B, and HIV serology were negative in all patients.

Bone marrow examination and blood lymphocyte phenotype were performed in 22 of 26 patients and a hematological malignancy was identified in nine of them: two had multiple myeloma (MM), four had chronic lymphocytic leukemia (CLL), and three non-Hodgkin's lymphoma (NHL). Five of the patients with malignancy had detectable serum monoclonal IgG. The hematological disease was revealed by the nephropathy in four of nine patients, whereas four patients had a long-standing history of hemopathy when GN was detected (mean delay was 32 months [3–89]). One patient, who was initially diagnosed with monoclonal gammopathy of undetermined significance, converted to overt MM 81 months after the onset of renal disease. A positron emission tomography (PET) scan was performed in three patients with no proven hematological malignancy and found no tumoral mass.

Although a circulating monoclonal IgG was detected in less than a third of the patients even by sensitive techniques, all patients did have monoclonal Ig glomerular deposits. Light chain isotype restriction was found in all patients with positivity for κ light chain in 80 % of patients. The subclasses of IgG deposits were determined for 21 patients: deposits stained for γ1 in eight patients (6 IgG1κ and 2 IgG1λ), γ2 in two patients (IgG2κ), γ3 in ten patients (9 IgG3κ and 1 IgG3λ), and γ4 in one patient (IgG4κ). IgG subclass distribution was different according to the observed glomerular pattern: IgG3 deposits were identified in 80 % of cases in MPGN (seven of eight, IgG3k; one of eight, IgG3λ), whereas only 18 % of MN had IgG3 deposits ($p = 0.0021$). On the other hand, IgG1 deposits were present in 64 % of MN (four of seven, IgG1k; three of seven, IgGλ, whereas only 10 % of MPGN had IgG1 deposits ($p = 0.014$). In most of the examined patients (11 of 14), ultrastructural study showed that immune deposits were not organized. EM demonstrated large, granular deposits that were subepithelial in eight patients (with associated mesangial deposits in two of them) and subendothelial in three patients (Fig. 11.1g, h). Three patients had immunotactoid GN, with organized subepithelial deposits with microtubular substructure (Fig. 11.1h). The diameter of the microtubular structures was 25–40 nm. Of note, these three patients had CLL.

MPGN was also reported with IgM-secreting monoclonal proliferations in the absence of cryoglobulinemia [10].

Pathophysiological Considerations

One of the important points shown by the immunofluorescence studies is the striking correspondence between the localization of the IgG deposits, defining either MPGN or MN histological patterns, and the subclass of the monoclonal IgG found in the deposits. IgG3 is the predominant subclass in proliferative GN with monoclonal IgG deposits, as it is in type-1 cryoglobulinemia [4, 9, 16, 17]. Classic MPGN is triggered by deposition of immune complexes in the mesangium and the glomerular capillaries, activating the complement cascade and recruiting inflammatory cells such as macrophages and lymphocytes. In monoclonal IgG3-associated MPGN, there is no evidence for an antigen–antibody immune complex, either circulating or formed in situ. This rather uncommon serum subclass of human IgG (mean normal adult level, 0.42 mg/ml; range 0.18–0.80 mg/ml) is the most nephritogenic because of its ability to aggregate in the glomerular capillary via a specific Fc–Fc interaction. IgG3 is also the most positively charged human IgG, favoring its affinity towards the anionic sites of the glomerular membrane [29, 30]. This high avidity of IgG3 for the glomeruli may explain the fact that monoclonal components can remain undetectable in the serum of patients with proven monoclonal IgG3 kidney deposits. Last but not least, IgG3 has the greatest complement-fixing capacity, which in turn could activate downstream inflammatory mediators that promote glomerular leukocyte infiltration and proliferation. Interestingly, IgG3 is the predominant Ig subclass in monoclonal components observed in immunodeficiency states, including aging and treatment with anti-calcineurin inhibitors [31]. This observation suggests that PGNMID occurs in an unusual immunological setting that requires further investigation.

On the other hand, most (64 %) cases of monoclonal MN are due to IgG1 deposits, while IgG3 is rarely observed [17, 19, 32, 33]. These data confirm the observations of Bridoux et al. who found that five of ten patients with atypical MN due to monotypic Ig deposits had IgG1 subclass deposited in their glomeruli [6]. The one patient from Nasr et al.'s series with membranous features also had IgG1 deposits. Interestingly, IgG4 was not found in our series, although this subclass is the most prominent in idiopathic MN [34]. However, it is difficult to draw definitive conclusions about the propensity of IgG1 subclass for membranous deposits, because it is the most frequent Ig subclass found in monoclonal gammopathies [35]. Nevertheless, one of our previous reports supports the hypothesis that, in contrast to classic MN [36], the deposited immunoglobulin may, in some cases, not be directed against a local antigen, but rather precipitates, because of peculiar physicochemical properties [33]. In a patient with a membranous pattern of GN, the circulating monoclonal IgG1λ showed unusual in vitro aggregation properties, including dependence on low ionic strength and neutral pH, suggesting that electrostatic interactions had a role in the precipitation process. We speculate that in vivo precipitation is facilitated by the local concentration of the protein in glomerular basement membrane and the ionic properties of the negatively charged local milieu. Interestingly, the IgG precipitated from serum had a non-organized ultrastructure similar to that of kidney deposits [33]. On the other hand, we recently reported a very particular case of recurrent MN, occurring 13 days after kidney transplantation. The graft biopsy specimen showed granular staining for complement and monoclonal IgG3k and electron microscopy revealed subepithelial non-organized deposits. A search for hematologic disorders was negative. Retrospective evaluation of a biopsy sample from the native kidney revealed a similar pattern: monotypic IgG3k deposits together with C3, C1q, and C5b-9. Glomerular deposits contained PLA2R in both the graft and the native kidney, suggesting that the recurrence was the result of circulating monoclonal anti-PLA2R antibodies binding to PLA2R antigen expressed on donor podocytes. Confocal analysis of anti-PLA2R and anti-human IgG3 showed colocalization, and the patient had IgG3k-restricted circulating anti-PLA2R antibodies [37]. This case reveals that the occurrence of monoclonal MN should lead to systematic testing of anti-PLA2R antibodies.

A unique case of hypocomplementemic MPGN associated with monoclonal λ light chain dimers, isolated from the serum and urine, has also been reported [14]. The dimers formed a miniautoantibody against complement factor H and thus activated the alternative pathway of complement. Several cases of GN with isolated renal C3 deposits and circulating monoclonal gammopathy have been recently reported [38, 39]. These cases might represent an unusual complication of plasma cell dyscrasia, related to complement activation through an autoantibody activity of the monoclonal Ig against a complement alternative pathway regulator protein such as complement factor H, as it has been shown for one patient reported by Bridoux et al. [38]. Whether this can occur also in GN with monoclonal Ig deposits remains to be established, but several patients, both in Nasr's series [16] and in our study [17], showed isolated C3 consumption and deposition in glomeruli, without involvement of C1q or low peripheral C4 levels, suggesting that complement activation in this setting can probably be mediated by the alternative pathway.

Diagnostic Considerations

Monoclonal gammopathy should be considered as an important and common cause of MPGN. The Mayo Clinic recently reviewed the case of 68 patients with MPGN who were negative for hepatitis B and C and were evaluated for gammopathies, during the period of 2001 through 2006 [40]. Twenty-eight (41.1 %) had serum and/or urine electrophoresis studies positive for monoclonal gammopathy. Sixteen patients had so-called MGUS (this term is usually not employed in the presence of visceral complications), while 12 patients had various lymphoplasmacytic cell proliferations including multiple myeloma (six patients), low-grade B-cell lymphoma (three patients), CLL (two patients), and lymphoplasmacytic lymphoma (LPL)/Waldenström's macroglobulinemia (one patient). Ten of 28 patients had circulating monoclonal IgMk. Data of immunofluorescence microscopy of kidney biopsies correlated with immunofixation results.

Therefore, all patients with a diagnosis of MPGN should be evaluated for an underlying monoclonal gammopathy. A careful analysis of the biopsy with anti-LC isotype antibodies is the first step of the workup. If light chain isotype restriction is found, then the biopsy should be analyzed with anti-γHC subclass antibodies to confirm monoclonality. The same analysis should be done for the patients with MN.

Irrespective of the histological pattern, MPGN or MN, the finding of monoclonal deposits should lead to analyze the organization of deposits by EM, and to search for cryoglobulinemia, circulating monoclonal component by highly sensitive techniques, and signs of a lymphoplasmacytic cell proliferation by bone marrow examination, blood lymphocyte phenotyping, and CT or PET scan.

In cases of endocapillary proliferative or MPGN in which the deposits stain for a single γHC subclass and a single LC, diagnostic considerations would include PGNMID, type-1 cryoglobulinemia GN, and immunotactoid GN (Table 11.5). Two points should be emphasized. First, the distinction with type-1 cryoglobulinemia may be difficult because the characteristic feature of thrombi with annular structure of deposits by EM is not always found. Second, EM may not be available or the results delayed and, therefore, the distinction with immunotactoid GN may be impossible for some time. However, from a therapeutic point of view, the key point is the presence of monoclonal Ig deposits which should lead to a detailed workup for a lymphoplasmacytic cell disorder and to appropriate treatment against the overt or low-grade incipience proliferation.

Therapeutic Considerations

All patients who present with a well-defined hematological malignancy, such as multiple myeloma and high-grade NHL associated with a monoclonal compound, must be treated according to the standard chemotherapy protocols, including newly introduced drugs such as thalidomide, bortezomib, or rituximab in addition to inhibitors of

Table 11.5 Clinical and pathologic differences among PGNMID, type-1 cryoglobulinemic glomerulonephritis, and immunotactoid glomerulonephritis

Parameter	PGNMID	Type-1 cryoglobulinemic glomerulonephritis	Immunotactoid glomerulonephritis
Hypocomplementemia	27 %	58 %	33 %
Evidence of serum or urine monoclonal protein	30 %	76 %	67 %
Underlying MM	Very rare	Very rare	Very rare
Underlying lymphoma/leukemia	Very rare	33 %	17 %
Renal insufficiency at presentation	60 %	76 %	83 %
Nephrotic syndrome	53 %	38 %	50 %
Intracapillary monocyte infiltration	+	++	+
Intracapillary protein thrombi	No	Yes	No
Most common IgG subclass	IgG3	IgG3	IgG1
Texture of deposits on EM	Granular	Focal annular–tubular or fibrillar	Microtubular with a diameter of 30–50 nm and hollow centers in parallel stacks

From Nasr et al. [16], with permission

the RAS. If the treatment permits sustained hematological remission and suppression of the circulating monoclonal IgG, then the renal disease can disappear. In nonmalignant cases with a low-tumoral mass plasma cell dyscrasia or a low-grade lymphoproliferative disease, nephrologists have to convince hematologists that, as in AL amyloidosis, the treatment of the otherwise "benign" neoplasm is mandatory to hamper the renal disease. These last years, the term of *Monoclonal Gammopathy of Renal Significance* (MGRS) has emerged to describe those patients with monoclonal Ig-related renal disease, such as AL amyloidosis, MICDD, or PGNMID, and an hematological disorder which is more consistent with MGUS than with multiple myeloma [41]. In contrast with typical MGUS, for which treatment is not recommended, the identification of a MGRS must lead to a rapid therapeutic intervention, in order to preserve or restore kidney function but also to avoid recurrence of renal disease after kidney transplantation [42].

In our recent series [17], complete remission of the nephrotic syndrome was obtained in 13 patients (54 %). In all of these patients, remission of nephropathy was reached only after the disappearance of the circulating M-spike. Absence of renal remission was mainly observed among patients who were diagnosed at a late stage of chronic kidney disease, with elevated serum creatinine levels and presence of extensive fibrosis on the renal biopsy. The presence of an identified hematological malignancy was not associated with a worse renal outcome, and complete remission of nephropathy could be obtained in five of nine patients with myeloma, CLL, or lymphoma. Patients with MPGN or MN had the same prognosis. Complete or partial remission was obtained in 6 of 12 patients with MPGN and 8 of 14 patients with MN. Response to treatment was not associated with any clinical or laboratory feature, such as age, presence of malignancy, and level of proteinuria. The only nonstatistically significant differences between responders and nonresponders were the initial glomerular filtration rate.

For patients without overt malignancy, rituximab may be the optimal therapeutic choice. Indeed, our study confirms previously published data, showing that treatment with RAS inhibitors or corticosteroids alone is not sufficient to achieve long-term remission [17]. Rituximab has a very favorable benefit-to-tolerance ratio in this subgroup of patients. In the series reported by Nasr et al. [16], two of four patients with MPGN and monoclonal IgG deposits who received this B-cell depleting drug experienced partial remission. Three other reports on monoclonal MPGN or immunotactoid GN [40, 43, 44] also suggest that rituximab can be beneficial in this setting.

In our series, five of seven patients with either MPGN or MN showed complete remission and two experienced a good-quality partial remission, with no major side effects. In the case of the monoclonal MN associated with IgG3-restricted antiPLA2R antibodies, rituximab permitted remission of the nephrotic syndrome and stabilization of serum creatinine [37]. Further studies are necessary to define which patients should be treated with this drug and what should be the best therapeutic scheme.

In conclusion, GNs with non-Randall-type, non-organized monoclonal Ig deposits are a new evolving entity whose diagnosis relies on a careful examination of the kidney biopsy with specific anti-LC isotype and anti-IgG subclass antibodies. Therefore, recognition of this entity mainly relies on the pathologist. The diagnosis of these diseases has two main consequences. The first is a detailed workup in search of a lymphoplasmacytic disorder. The second regards therapeutic strategy aimed at annihilating the underlying B-cell proliferation and improving the associated kidney disease.

References

1. Glenner GG, Terry W, Harada M, et al. Amyloid fibril proteins: proof of homology with immunoglobulin light chains by sequence analyses. Science. 1971;172:1150–1.
2. Randall RE, Williamson Jr WC, Mullinax F, et al. Manifestations of systemic light chain deposition. Am J Med. 1976;60:293–9.
3. Ivanyi B. Frequency of light chain deposition nephropathy relative to renal amyloidosis and Bence Jones cast nephropathy in a necropsy study of patients with myeloma. Arch Pathol Lab Med. 1990;114:986–7.
4. Karras A, Noel LH, Droz D, et al. Renal involvement in monoclonal (type I) cryoglobulinemia: two cases associated with IgG3 kappa cryoglobulin. Am J Kidney Dis. 2002;40:1091–6.
5. Lin J, Markowitz GS, Valeri AM, et al. Renal monoclonal immunoglobulin deposition disease: the disease spectrum. J Am Soc Nephrol. 2001;12:1482–92.
6. Bridoux F, Hugue V, Coldefy O, et al. Fibrillary glomerulonephritis and immunotactoid (microtubular) glomerulopathy are associated with distinct immunologic features. Kidney Int. 2002;62:1764–75.
7. Rosenstock JL, Markowitz GS, Valeri AM, et al. Fibrillary and immunotactoid glomerulonephritis:

8. distinct entities with different clinical and pathologic features. Kidney Int. 2003;63:1450–61.
8. Nasr SH, Valeri AM, Cornell LD, et al. Fibrillary glomerulonephritis: a report of 66 cases from a single institution. Clin J Am Soc Nephrol. 2011;6:775–84.
9. Nasr SH, Colvin R, Markowitz GS. IgG1 lambda light and heavy chain renal amyloidosis. Kidney Int. 2006;70:7.
10. Audard V, Georges B, Vanhille P, et al. Renal lesions associated with IgM-secreting monoclonal proliferations: revisiting the disease spectrum. Clin J Am Soc Nephrol. 2008;3:1339–49.
11. Alpers CE, Tu WH, Hopper Jr J, Biava CG. Single light chain subclass (kappa chain) immunoglobulin deposition in glomerulonephritis. Hum Pathol. 1985;16:294–304.
12. Touchard G. Ultrastructural pattern and classification of renal monoclonal immunoglobulin deposits. In: Touchard G, Aucouturier P, Hermine O, Ronco P, editors. Monoclonal gammopathies and the kidney. Dordrecht: Kluwer; 2003. p. 95–117.
13. Bridoux F, Zanetta G, Vanhille P, Goujon JM, Vanhille P, Bauwens M, Chevet D, Ronco P, Preud'homme JL, Touchard G. Glomerulopathy with non-organized and non-Randall type monoclonal immunoglobulin deposits: a rare entity [abstract]. J Am Soc Nephrol. 2001;12:94A.
14. Jokiranta TS, Solomon A, Pangburn MK, et al. Nephritogenic lambda light chain dimer: a unique human miniautoantibody against complement factor H. J Immunol. 1999;15(163):4590–6.
15. Nasr SH, Markowitz GS, Stokes MB, et al. Proliferative glomerulonephritis with monoclonal IgG deposits: a distinct entity mimicking immune-complex glomerulonephritis. Kidney Int. 2004;65:85–96.
16. Nasr SH, Satoskar A, Markowitz GS, et al. Proliferative glomerulonephritis with monoclonal IgG deposits. J Am Soc Nephrol. 2009;20:2055–64.
17. Guiard E, Karras A, Plaisier E, et al. Patterns of non-cryoglobulinemic glomerulonephritis with monoclonal Ig deposits: correlation with IgG subclass and response to rituximab. Clin J Am Soc Nephrol. 2011;6:1609–16.
18. Evans DJ, Macanovic M, Dunn MJ, et al. Membranous glomerulonephritis associated with follicular B-cell lymphoma and subepithelial deposition of IgG1-kappa paraprotein. Nephron Clin Pract. 2003;93:c112.
19. Komatsuda A, Masai R, Ohtani H, et al. Monoclonal immunoglobulin deposition disease associated with membranous features. Nephrol Dial Transplant. 2008;23:3888–94.
20. Masai R, Wakui H, Komatsuda A, Togashi M, Maki N, Ohtani H, Oyama Y, Sawada K. Characteristics of proliferative glomerulonephritis with monoclonal IgG deposits associated with membranoproliferative features. Clin Nephrol. 2009;72:46–54.
21. Fujiwara T, Komatsuda A, Ohtani H, Togashi M, Sawada K, Wakui H. Proliferative glomerulonephritis with monoclonal IgG deposits in a patient with

autoimmune hemolytic anemia. Clin Nephrol. 2013; 79(6):494–8.

22. Fujita E, Shimizu A, Kaneko T, Masuda Y, Ishihara C, Mii A, Higo S, Kajimoto Y, Kanzaki G, Nagasaka S, Iino Y, Katayama Y, Fukuda Y. Proliferative glomerulonephritis with monoclonal immunoglobulin G3κ deposits in association with parvovirus B19 infection. Hum Pathol. 2012;43(12):2326–33.

23. Yahata M, Nakaya I, Takahashi S, Sakuma T, Sato H, Soma J. Proliferative glomerulonephritis with monoclonal IgM deposits without Waldenström's macroglobulinemia: case report and review of the literature. Clin Nephrol. 2012;77(3):254–60.

24. Aucouturier P, Preud'Homme JL. Subclass distribution of human myeloma proteins as determined with monoclonal antibodies. Immunol Lett. 1987;16:55–7.

25. Nasr SH, Sethi S, Cornell LD, Fidler ME, Boelkins M, Fervenza FC, Cosio FG, D'Agati VD. Proliferative glomerulonephritis with monoclonal IgG deposits recurs in the allograft. Clin J Am Soc Nephrol. 2011;6(1):122–32.

26. Albawardi A, Satoskar A, Von Visger J, Brodsky S, Nadasdy G, Nadasdy T. Proliferative glomerulonephritis with monoclonal IgG deposits recurs or may develop de novo in kidney allografts. Am J Kidney Dis. 2011;58(2):276–81.

27. Sumida K, Ubara Y, Marui Y, Nakamura M, Takaichi K, Tomikawa S, Fujii T, Ohashi K. Recurrent proliferative glomerulonephritis with monoclonal IgG deposits of IgG2lambda subtype in a transplanted kidney: a case report. Am J Kidney Dis. 2013;62(3):587–90.

28. Batal I, Bijol V, Schlossman RL, Rennke HG. Proliferative glomerulonephritis with monoclonal immunoglobulin deposits in a kidney allograft. Am J Kidney Dis. 2014;63(2):318–23.

29. Capra JD, Kunkel HG. Aggregation of gamma-G3 proteins: relevance to the hyperviscosity syndrome. J Clin Invest. 1970;49:610–21.

30. Abdelmoula M, Spertini F, Shibata T, Gyotoku Y, Luzuy S, Lambert PH, Izui S. IgG3 is the major source of cryoglobulins in mice. J Immunol. 1989; 143:526–32.

31. Aucouturier P, Bremard-Oury C, Clauvel JP, Debré M, Griscelli C, Seligmann M, Preud'homme JL. Serum IgG subclass levels in primary and acquired immunodeficiency. Monogr Allergy. 1986;20:62–74.

32. Moulin B, Ronco PM, Mougenot B, Francois A, Fillastre JP, Mignon F. Glomerulonephritis in chronic lymphocytic leukemia and related B-cell lymphomas. Kidney Int. 1992;42:127–35.

33. de Seigneux S, Bindi P, Debiec H, Alyanakian MA, Aymard B, Callard P, Ronco P, Aucouturier P. Immunoglobulin deposition disease with a membranous pattern and a circulating monoclonal immunoglobulin G with charge-dependent aggregation properties. Am J Kidney Dis. 2010;56:117–21.

34. Oliveira DB. Membranous nephropathy: an IgG4-mediated disease. Lancet. 1998;351:670–1.

35. Aucouturier P, Mounir S, Preud'homme JL. Distribution of IgG subclass levels in normal adult sera as determined by a competitive enzyme immunoassay using monoclonal antibodies. Diagn Immunol. 1985;3:191–6.

36. Ronco P, Debiec H. Advances in membranous nephropathy: success stories of a long journey. Clin Exp Pharmacol Physiol. 2011;38:410–6.

37. Debiec H, Hanoy M, Francois A, Guerrot D, Ferlicot S, Johanet C, Aucouturier P, Godin M, Ronco P. Recurrent membranous nephropathy in an allograft caused by IgG3k targeting the PLA2 receptor. J Am Soc Nephrol. 2012;23(12):1949–54.

38. Bridoux F, Desport E, Frémeaux-Bacchi V, Chong CF, Gombert JM, Lacombe C, Quellard N, Touchard G. Glomerulonephritis with isolated C3 deposits and monoclonal gammopathy: a fortuitous association? Clin J Am Soc Nephrol. 2011;6:2165–74.

39. Sethi S, Sukov WR, Zhang Y, Fervenza FC, Lager DJ, Miller DV, Cornell LD, Krishnan SG, Smith RJ. Dense deposit disease associated with monoclonal gammopathy of undetermined significance. Am J Kidney Dis. 2010;56:977–82.

40. Sethi S, Zand L, Leung N, Smith RJ, Jevremonic D, Herrmann SS, Fervenza FC. Membranoproliferative glomerulonephritis secondary to monoclonal gammopathy. Clin J Am Soc Nephrol. 2010;5:770–82.

41. Leung N, Bridoux F, Hutchison CA, Nasr SH, Cockwell P, Fermand JP, Dispenzieri A, Song KW, Kyle RA, International Kidney and Monoclonal Gammopathy Research Group. Monoclonal gammopathy of renal significance: when MGUS is no longer undetermined or insignificant. Blood. 2012; 120(22):4292–5.

42. Fermand JP, Bridoux F, Kyle RA, Kastritis E, Weiss BM, Cook MA, Drayson MT, Dispenzieri A, Leung N, International Kidney and Monoclonal Gammopathy Research Group. How I treat monoclonal gammopathy of renal significance (MGRS). Blood. 2013; 122(22):3583–90.

43. Bhat P, Weiss S, Appel GB, Radhakrishnan J. Rituximab treatment of dysproteinemias affecting the kidney: a review of three cases. Am J Kidney Dis. 2007;50:641–4.

44. Vilayur E, Trevillian P, Walsh M. Monoclonal gammopathy and glomerulopathy associated with chronic lymphocytic leukemia. Nat Clin Pract Nephrol. 2009;5:54–8.

Pathologies of Renal and Systemic Intracellular Paraprotein Storage: Crystalopathies and Beyond

12

Maria M. Picken and Ahmet Dogan

In prior chapters of this section, various organized and non-organized extracellular deposits were discussed, some of which are associated with paraproteins, but all of which are in the differential diagnosis of amyloid, in particular AL, since they can either mimic or coexist with it. Moreover, there are indications that some of these entities may share a similar pathogenesis (incomplete proteolytic digestion, amino acid substitutions) and several may be associated with a low tumor burden. This chapter provides a brief overview of pathologies that are associated with intracellular paraproteins, both renal and systemic. The expanding spectrum of intracellular immunoglobulin storage pathologies, including both organized deposits (crystalline or rarely fibrillar) and non-organized deposits, will be addressed [1, 2]. In crystalopathies, various compounds form intra- or extracellular tissue deposits. While some crystalopathies may be associated with drugs, toxins, or circulating soluble metabolites that may crystallize in tissues, crystal deposition can also be seen in association with plasma cell disorders (PCD)/B-cell lymphoplasmacytic disorders, and this is the focus of this chapter [1–3].

Kidney Pathology Associated with Intracellular Paraprotein Storage: Light Chain Proximal Tubulopathy and Renal Crystal-Storing Histiocytosis

The overwhelming majority of paraproteins consist of monoclonal light chains and are nephrotoxic, leading to frequent renal involvement. Thus, PCD/B-cell lymphoplasmacytic disorders can be associated with a wide range of renal pathologies that include light chain cast nephropathy, light and heavy chain amyloidosis, monoclonal immunoglobulin deposition disease, cryoglobulin- and crystal globulin-induced nephropathy, immunotactoid glomerulopathy, various glomerulopathies with non-organized monoclonal immunoglobulin deposits (proliferative, nonproliferative), and proximal tubulopathy; in addition, tubulointerstitial nephritis may accompany many of these entities (at least focally), may precede development of the respective full-blown pathologies, or even, potentially, may be seen by itself (Table 12.1; [1, 2, 4, 5]).

While pathology associated with light chain cast nephropathy affecting distal tubules is

M.M. Picken, MD, PhD (✉)
Department of Pathology, Loyola University Medical Center, Loyola University Chicago, Building 110, Room 2242, 2160 South First Avenue, Maywood, IL 60153, USA
e-mail: mpicken@luc.edu; MMPicken@aol.com

A. Dogan, MD, PhD
Departments of Pathology and Laboratory Medicine, Memorial Sloan Kettering Cancer Center, 1275 York Avenue, New York, NY 10065, USA
e-mail: dogana@mskcc.org

© Springer International Publishing Switzerland 2015
M.M. Picken et al. (eds.), *Amyloid and Related Disorders*, Current Clinical Pathology,
DOI 10.1007/978-3-319-19294-9_12

Table 12.1 Paraprotein-associated pathologies; renal and extrarenal

Pathology	Extracellular	Intracellular	Intra-vascular	Organized	Non-organized	Renal	Extrarenal
Light chain cast nephropathy	+[a]				Amorphous	+	–
AL/AH amyloid	+			Fibrillar Congo red (+)		+	S/L
MIDD	+				Powdery	+	S
LCPT		+		Crystalline	Noncrystalline	+	–
CSH/ISH		+		Crystalline	Noncrystalline	+	S/L
Cryoglobulinemia	+/–		+	Focally[b]		+	Skin/S?
Waldenström macroglobulinemia	+		+			+	Skin/S?
Crystalglobulinemia			+			+	Skin/S?
GN with monoclonal deposits	+				Electron dense	+	?
Immunotactoid GN	+			Microtubules		+	?S
Paraprotein-associated tubulointerstitial GN[c]	+/–?	+/–?	+/–?	+/–?	+/–?	+	?

S systemic, *L* localized, *MIDD* monoclonal immunoglobulin deposition disease, *CSH/ISH* crystal/immunoglobulin-storing histiocytosis, *GN* glomerulonephritis

[a] Intratubular casts

[b] Paracrystalline arrays

[c] Cellular reaction to circulating paraprotein, may precede or accompany other pathologies which may be subtle and/or focal

frequent and a well-known complication of para-proteinemia, proximal tubule injury is less frequently reported, less well known, and, most likely, underreported. Currently, only approximately 110 cases have been reported that deal with this subject. The most frequently used terms include adult Fanconi syndrome (FS), light chain Fanconi syndrome (LCFS), crystalopathies, and/or light chain proximal tubulopathy (LCPT) [1, 2, 6–11] (see Figs. 12.1, 12.2, 12.3); proximal tubular pathology may be associated with renal interstitial and/or systemic crystal-storing histiocytosis ([12–14], see also below).

Since 1954, it has been known that adult patients may develop acquired FS in association with PCD as a consequence of acquired proximal tubular injury [6]. In 1975, Maldonado et al. reviewed the first large series of 17 (new and previously published) cases of FS with Bence Jones proteinuria and myeloma or amyloidosis [7]. In most cases, the diagnosis of FS preceded the development of myeloma or amyloidosis, but not the reverse, while, in some patients, the diagnosis of FS and multiple myeloma or amyloidosis was established simultaneously. There was a relatively indolent renal dysfunction, Bence Jones proteinuria of κ-type, and, in some cases, osteomalacia resulting from chronic hypophosphatemia. Kidney biopsy showed prominent crystals in proximal tubular epithelium and similar crystals were also seen in the bone marrow in many patients. No myeloma casts were seen in the distal tubules. The authors could not demonstrate serum protein monoclonal abnormalities. Based on this initial series, it was proposed that patients with Fanconi syndrome and Bence Jones proteinuria have a distinct type of plasma cell disorder or a variant of the monoclonal gammopathies, termed LCFS, characterized by slow progression of the tumor and an early phase dominated by the metabolic complications of renal proximal tubular dysfunction.

In 1993, Aucouturier et al. sequenced the κ-cDNA from a patient with LCFS and demonstrated that it belonged to the VK1 subgroup and was characterized by resistance to complete proteolysis and the ability to form crystals [8]. In contrast, the light chains from 12 patients with

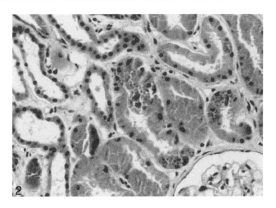

Fig. 12.1 Paraffin section showing rare crystals in the proximal tubular epithelial cells. There is also a striking granularity of the cytoplasm (hematoxylin–eosin, original magnification×200)

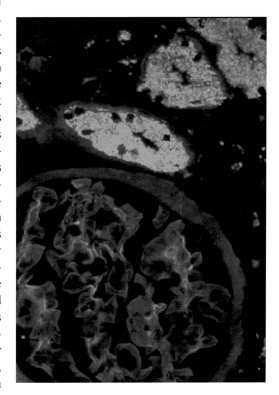

Fig. 12.2 Immunofluorescence stain for kappa light chain limited to the proximal tubular epithelium. No deposits are detectable by immunofluorescence in the adjacent glomerulus. Stains for lambda light chains, immunoglobulin (Ig) G, IgA, IgM, and complements were negative (not shown) (original magnification×400)

myeloma cast nephropathy were susceptible to proteolytic digestion. The propensity of light chains in LCFS to form crystals that precipitate

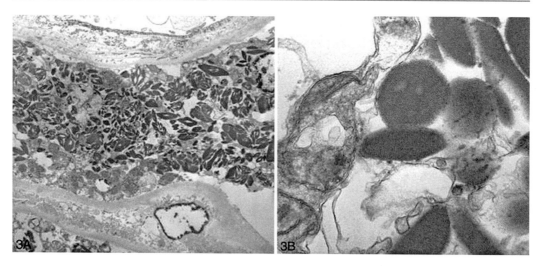

Fig. 12.3 (a) Electron micrograph showing abundant rhomboid crystals within the proximal tubular epithelium (uranyl acetate stain, original magnification×3000). (b) Electron micrograph showing the lattice-like structure of the rhomboid crystals (uranyl acetate stain, original magnification×50,000)

within the cytoplasm of proximal tubules appears to be determined by changes in their amino acid sequences. The circulating light chains are filtered through the glomerular capillary wall and bind to the luminal surface of the proximal tubular epithelial cells; subsequently, the light chains are incorporated into endosomes, which fuse with lysosomes, where they are then degraded into amino acids and returned to the circulation. While the "non-pathogenic" light chains are completely degraded, in FS there is incomplete proteolysis, which leads to the accumulation of protease-resistant fragments that constitute a nidus for crystal formation. Thus, the development of LCFS appears to be associated with the common origin of the fragments—from the light chain VK1 subgroup—and their primary sequence peculiarities, which lead to partial resistance to proteolysis with the formation of a truncated NH_2-terminal fragment with a propensity to crystallize. In 2006, Sirac et al. published a transgenic murine model of LCFS, which supported the above-proposed pathogenesis of this condition [9]. Subsequent research by El Hamel et al. [14] and Toly-Ndour et al. [15] extended the molecular studies, further supporting the evidence that amino acid substitutions, including distinct hydrophobic residues, favor the formation of crystals. Specific impairment of proximal tubular cell proliferation by a monoclonal κ-light chain responsible for FS was

demonstrated by El-Hammel et al. in 2012 [16]. However, the mechanism(s) leading to FS (glycosuria, phosphaturia, aminoaciduria) is/are poorly understood and, indeed, some patients may have only partial FS or no FS (reviewed by Sirac et al. [17–19]).

With subsequent publications, the clinical picture associated with injury to the proximal tubular epithelium was expanded and the associated pathologic spectrum was increased to include non-organized intracellular paraprotein deposits as well [11, 20]. In 2007, the authors (MMP et al.) published a report of five cases of light chain proximal tubulopathy and broadened its definition to include three cases in which electron microscopy revealed only prominent phagolysosomes within tubular epithelia; by immunoelectron microscopy, these phagolysosomes contained a single light chain, kappa or lambda [11] Thus, the authors concluded that some patients with PCD may have more subtle evidence of proximal tubular injury not associated with crystals but only with lysosomal light chain restriction. This restriction can be detected by immunofluorescence as well as by immunoEM. The light microscopic morphology may be quite subtle and only suggestive of acute tubular injury. To encompass this expanded definition, the authors proposed the term "light chain proximal tubulopathy" (LCPT) [11] (Fig. 12.4).

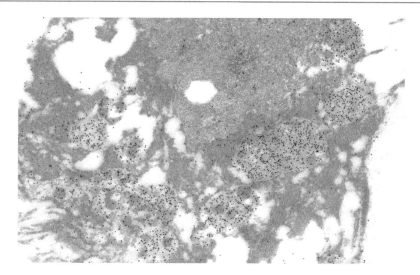

Fig. 12.4 Immunogold stain for lambda light chain, which is positive within phagolysosomes in the proximal tubular epithelium. The stain for kappa light chain was negative (not shown) (original magnification×12,000). (Figures 12.1–12.4. reprinted with permission from Kapur U, Barton K, Fresco R, Leehey DJ, Picken MM. Expanding the pathologic spectrum of immunoglobulin light chain proximal tubulopathy. Arch Pathol Lab Med. 2007 Sep;131(9):1368–72)

Subsequent studies suggested that LCPT not associated with crystals was more frequent than LCPT with crystals. In 2011, Larsen et al. reported ten cases of LCPT without crystals, which constituted 3.1 % of their light chain-related diseases, while, in their material, only three cases (0.9 %) had crystals [20]. Similar results were reported by others [21–23]. In Herrera's series of 57 cases with proximal tubulopathies, only four biopsies showed crystalline inclusions [23]. At the molecular level, the absence of crystals is often associated with normal sensitivity to proteolysis, suggesting that reabsorption of monoclonal light chains might also interfere with proximal tubule function through a direct toxic effect [17]. To this end, it is postulated that excessive endocytosis of the light chains promotes apoptosis and tubular damage.

In previous years, most cases of LCPT have been reported with kappa light chain, while only rare cases of LCPT were associated with λ-light chains (with or without crystals) [1, 2, 6–8, 10–31]. However, more recent reports indicate that lambda light chains may be more often associated with LCPT than kappa light chains [11, 20, 21]. While kappa light chains are preferentially associated with crystals, lambda light chains are typically associated with noncrystal-line LCPT. Thus, in Larsen's series, nine out of ten biopsies with LCPT without crystals showed λ-light chain restriction [20].

The prognosis is variable and largely depends on the tumor burden [11, 32]. However, the diagnosis of LCPT is of critical importance since this condition is often associated with previously unrecognized myeloma/PCD/B-cell lymphoplasmacytic disorder [11, 20, 23, 33]. Moreover, tubular injury progresses over time leading to renal failure.

Pathology

Light microscopic findings are largely nonspecific and suggestive of acute proximal tubular injury and/or chronic tubulointerstitial nephropathy [11–31]. Rare tubular epithelial cells may contain pale needle-shaped crystals that are mainly visible at high magnification [11, 23, 33] (Fig. 12.1). These crystals are PAS negative and may stain red or green with trichrome stain. At times, in cases where no crystals are discernible by light microscopy, there may be a diffuse proximal clear cell transformation resulting in a pseudo-osmotic nephrosis pattern [33, 34]. Some cells exhibit only prominent cytoplasmic granularity, or a glassy appearance, vacuolization, cellular enlargement ("hypertrophy"), loss of brush border, and sloughing, resulting in an acute tubular necrosis-like picture [11, 14, 23, 33, 34].

Based on morphology, Herrera recently subdivided LCPT into four categories including (1) proximal tubulopathy without cytoplasmic inclusions, (2) tubulopathy associated with interstitial inflammatory reaction, (3) proximal tubulopathy with cytoplasmic inclusions, and (4) proximal tubulopathy with lysosomal indigestion/constipation; each category was represented by 22, 28, 4, and 3 cases, respectively, in his series of 57 patients [23].

Crystal deposition in the mesangial cells [35] or in podocytes with glomerular dysfunction [36] and isotypic light chain cast nephropathy has also been reported [13, 37]. In one recently reported case, histiocytes with lysosomal accumulation of λ-light chain and absence of κ-light chain were seen within the glomerular capillaries [38]; segmental endocapillary proliferative glomerulonephritis was also visible.

In some patients, infiltration by mononuclear cells with interstitial fibrosis may dominate the light microscopic pathology. The presence of intracytoplasmic crystals in the proximal tubular epithelium may be associated with the presence of crystals in the interstitial macrophages in the kidney and/or of the bone marrow and/or other organs (termed crystal-storing histiocytosis; see below and [13, 14, 39]).

By immunofluorescence, in most (but not all) cases, there is light chain restriction, either for kappa or lambda light chain, which is limited to proximal tubular epithelium [11, 20, 23] (Fig. 12.2). Interestingly, in rare cases, crystals were negative by standard immunofluorescence performed on frozen tissue, while immunofluorescence on formalin-fixed, paraffin-embedded, pronase-digested tissue showed positivity for a single light chain [33]. It is proposed that, with pronase digestion, a denaturing effect on cell membranes is achieved, which may facilitate access of the antibody to the lysosome-bound crystals and, possibly thereby, unmask sequestered antigenic sites.

By electron microscopy, abundant crystals of varying sizes and shapes are seen [11, 20, 23,

33] (Fig. 12.3a and b). These crystals may be rectangular, rhomboid, round, or needle-shaped and are surrounded by a single membrane, most likely of lysosomal origin. Similar crystals in the urinary sediment have also been reported [14]. Interestingly, there is a certain range of ultrastructural morphology of crystals, including hexagonal or diamond-shaped crystals with a lattice-like structure in some, and needle-shaped, rectangular, and rhomboid patterns in others. El-Hammel et al. suggested that these differences may result from distinct structures of monoclonal light chains [14]. Moreover, in one of their patients with Fanconi syndrome, crystals showed a fibrillar amyloid-like organization, which, by immuno-electron microscopy, strongly reacted with anti-kappa light chain antibody [14]. A microtubular or fibrillary amyloid-like structure of inclusions was also reported earlier by Taneda et al. [40] and Herlitz et al. [33], Yao et al. [41], and Corbett et al. [42]. In Herrera's series, among four cases of LCPT with inclusions, in one case electron microscopy demonstrated a fibrillary rather than a crystalline appearance [23]. However, the authors provided no information as to whether these inclusions were Congo red positive and birefringent when viewed under polarized light, which would fully qualify them as intracellular amyloid. However, in 2012, two reports of an apparent amyloid proximal tubulopathy were published [43, 44]. In both cases, rare proximal tubular cells showed a distinct Congo red-positive inclusion, which were birefringent under polarized light (Fig. 12.5). In case reported by Hemminger et al., intracellular amyloid formation was associated with concomitant phenotypic changes, suggestive of histiocytic differentiation of tubular epithelial cells [44].

In biopsies without crystals, there are abundant and often enlarged and bizarre phagolysosomes, which show light chain restriction by immuno-electron microscopy and/or immunofluorescence [11, 20, 23] (Fig. 12.4). In some patients, such lysosomal inclusions in the proximal tubular epithelium have been associated with crystal-bearing histiocytes infiltrating the renal interstitium [14].

Clinical picture. While an underlying PCD is largely unsuspected prior to kidney biopsy,

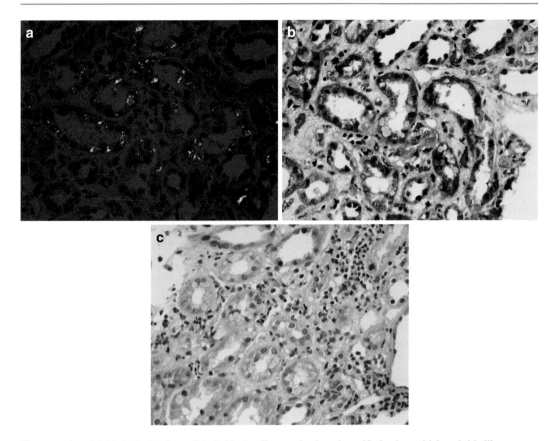

Fig. 12.5 Amyloid LCPT: (**a**) Several individual cells show apple-green birefringence. Congo red-stained slide viewed under polarized light, (**b** and **c**) Focal intracytoplasmic, round, and homogeneous inclusions are pale blue in trichrome-stained section (**b**) and amphophilic in H&E- stained sections. Notice interstitial nephritis-like component with lymphocytes and occasional eosinophils (slides courtesy of C. Larsen, photographed and published with permission)

following the diagnosis of LCPT, virtually all patients are found to have some form of PCD, including MGUS, multiple myeloma ("smoldering multiple myeloma"), or, less commonly, isotypic amyloidosis; some patients may have lymphoplasmacytic lymphoma [7, 10–36]. The clinical picture may be subtle and diverse, depending on tumor burden [7, 11, 18, 20–23, 32]. Nevertheless, even in cases associated with low tumor burden and a seemingly indolent clinical course, kidney failure develops [11]. Interestingly, kidney failure can be reversed upon elimination of the abnormal protein ([33, 39], Picken—unpublished observation). Reversibility of LCPT has also been supported by animal studies [9]. If untreated, LCPT can recur in kidney transplant patients [11]. Given that LCPT leads to

renal failure, this suggests that it should be treated to suppress the production of nephrotoxic monoclonal light chains [39, 45]. Some preliminary studies suggest that novel immunomodulating agents, as well as direct removal of the light chains by plasma exchange or intensive dialysis using high cutoff membranes, may improve renal prognosis in LCPT ([39, 45, 46], Picken—unpublished observation).

Thus, adult patients with Fanconi syndrome should be carefully investigated for plasmacytic dyscrasia/B-cell lymphoproliferative disorder; similarly, a pathologic diagnosis of LCPT should prompt a thorough hematologic workup. LCPT may be underdiagnosed because of limited awareness of the entity. In Herrera's series, which is largest to date, the 57 cases of proximal tubulopathy represented approximately 1.5 % of all patients. However, among lesions related to PCD, proximal tubulopathies were diagnosed in approximately 46 % of all cases [23].

Extrarenal Pathology Associated with Intracellular Paraprotein Storage: Crystal-Storing Histiocytosis (CSH) and Beyond

CSH is a reactive histiocytic hyperplasia in which the histiocytes contain intralysosomal prominent, crystalline, cytoplasmic, immunoglobulin inclusions [12, 14, 47–66]. CSH occurs in plasma cell/B-cell lymphoproliferative disorders. The neoplastic plasma/B-cells may also contain prominent immunoglobulin inclusions and show predominantly kappa light chain restriction. Most reported cases of CSH are associated with multiple myeloma and other PCD or low-grade B-cell lymphomas such as lymphoplasmacytic lymphoma, and marginal zone B-cell lymphoma (typically extranodal, associated with mucosa-associated lymphoid tissue, MALT lymphoma), some of which arise in association with reactive conditions such as Sjögren's syndrome [55]. Rarely, CSH was reported in apparently inflammatory-reactive processes. However, in these latter cases, the possibility of an undiagnosed low-grade lymphoproliferative process could not be excluded [3, 56, 57]. The crystal deposition can be localized at the site of lymphoplasmacellular proliferation or may be systemic. In systemic CSH, the reticuloendothelial system is involved, with extramedullary sites.

Crystals can be seen either in histiocytes in soft tissues or parenchymal cells. The presence of intracytoplasmic crystals in the macrophages of the bone marrow may be coincident with the presence of similar crystals in renal interstitial macrophages and/or in the proximal tubular epithelium. The crystals usually accumulate within lymphoid cells and hematopoietic tissues (bone marrow, lymph nodes, spleen, thymus) or within epithelial cells and connective tissue stroma of the kidney, lungs, pleural effusion, thyroid, parotid gland, eye structures (cornea, orbital fat,

lacrimal gland, eyelid, conjunctiva), skin, subcutaneous fat, heart, testes, tongue, liver, stomach, adrenals, or skull and even brain parenchyma [12, 14, 47–62, 67–80]. Initial presentation largely depends on the localization: some patients present with a soft-tissue mass with abundant histiocytes and fibroblasts containing crystals.

The mechanism of crystal formation and their storage in the histiocytes appears to be similar to that occurring in proximal tubular epithelium [12, 14]. Thus, similar to LCPT, in most reported cases of CSH, kappa light chain was involved, though lambda light chain-associated cases have also occasionally been described; there is no relationship between the types of heavy chains [12, 14, 47, 75, 81]. A single case of plasmacytoma with crystal-storing histiocytosis exhibiting FGFR3 and IgH translocation has recently been published [76].

Thus far only single cases of CSH were examined by laser microdissection (LMD)-tandem mass spectrometry (MS/MS) including three cases of CNS (2 cases [77], 1 case [75]) and two cases of gastric and a single case of nodal CSH [78]. In one case of CNS CSH, associated with monotypic κ-plasma cells by in situ hybridization, LC-MS/MS demonstrated k-light chain. In a second case, IgG was identified by LC-MS/MS [77], while IHC showed reactivity with IgG and λ- light chain. In a third case, LM-MS/MS confirmed the presence of κ-light chain and an IgA constant region [75]. Interestingly, there was an especially high signal for the somatically mutated variable domain fragment of the immunoglobulin κ-light chain [75]. In two cases of gastric CSH, LC-MS/MS demonstrated fragments of the variable domain (V-2) of IgG in one case and fragments of the variable domains (V-1, V-3) of kappa light chain in the second case. In one case of nodal CSH, fragments of variable (V-3) and constant regions of kappa were detected. Variable regions V-1 and V-3 of kappa and the variable region (V-2) of the immunoglobulin heavy chain appeared to have selective representation. These proteomic findings indicate that the crystals are formed by a cleavage product of the immunoglobulin molecule, representing a unique variable region rather than the whole immunoglobulin.

Thus, similar to LCPT, sequence abnormalities at specific sites in the light chain, especially in the kappa light chain, may be responsible for crystal formation as a consequence of defects leading to the loss of a proteolytic site(s) and the generation of fragments with a high intrinsic stability, which then form a nidus for crystallization. Thus, crystallization occurs after endocytosis and proteolysis within the endolysosomal compartment of histiocytes (or epithelial cells in LCPT).

Although abnormalities in the light chain are the most likely cause of CSH, overproduction of the paraprotein should also be critical for pathogenesis. To this end, crystals may also be seen in plasma cells, where they are present in the rough endoplasmic reticulum; this suggests that their crystallization takes place at the site of production. Furthermore, it is postulated that the formation of intracellular crystals may be toxic to cell function and affect cellular growth potential; hence, many of these cases are associated with low tumor burden and slow progression, but, in some patients, rapid progression may be seen (reviewed in [12, 17, 45]).

Pathology

CSH may be associated with a mass composed predominantly of sheets of macrophages (CD-68-positive cells), which may be spindle shaped and resemble striated muscle cells, and scattered aggregates of atypical lymphoid cells at the periphery of the tumor (Figs. 12.6, 12.7). The latter frequently show prominent plasmacytoid differentiation with monotypic expression of immunoglobulin. The histiocytes may contain rodlike and/or rectangular crystals in their cytoplasm. On H&E-stained sections the crystals may be at times inconspicuous and seen only focally; negative images of crystalline immunoglobulin have also been reported [62]. Therefore, the differential diagnosis may include (a) an infectious process caused by persistent intracytoplasmic organisms, (b) a storage disease associated with a benign reactive lymphoid infiltrate, (c) hemophagocytosis, (d) a lymphoid neoplasm, and (e) a mesenchymal lesion (in particular striated muscle neoplasm). Thus, mycobacteria, fungi, Whipple's disease, and various other bacteria should be ruled out. A subset of infectious microorganisms can persist within the cells, owing to either a specialized capsule or acquired adaptations that either enable them to escape the lysosomal enzymes or inhibit the fusion of lysosomes and phagosomes. Mycobacteria, in particular M. avium complex, can induce the accumulation of macrophages without formation of typical epithelioid granulomas. Negative images of crystalline immunoglobulin in cytology smears mimicking mycobacteria have also been reported [62]. Other bacteria causing the accumulation of macrophages include Listeria and Bartonella species and Tropheryma whipplei. Malakoplakia and various storage diseases should also be considered in the differential diagnosis. To this end, macrophages in CSH may resemble Gaucher's disease, Weber–Christian disease, or other forms of histiocytosis or pseudo-Gaucher's cells seen in chronic myelogenous leukemia [10, 82, 83]. For this reason, macrophages in CSH are at times referred as "pseudo-pseudo-Gaucher's cells" [14, 83, 84]. Difficulties in the diagnosis of an underlying lymphoproliferative disorder may arise, especially in cases showing an excessive accumulation of crystal-laden histiocytes, which obliterate the underlying neoplastic lymphoproliferative process. In breast lesions, fine needle aspiration biopsy may be confused with fat necrosis [51]. Indeed, there seems to be a predilection of crystal-containing mononuclear cells for subcutaneous fat tissue [14, 52, 59]. Thus, awareness of the association of CSH with an underlying plasma cell dyscrasia/B-cell lymphoproliferative disorder is important in order to perform clonality studies and avoid misdiagnosis. In particular. immunoglobulin light chain staining to establish the clonal nature of the plasma cells is very helpful. Virtually in all cases of CSH lesional plasma cells are light chain restricted (predominantly kappa). The intensity of staining is often much stronger in plasma cells than in the immunoglobulin crystals of histiocytes which can be entirely negative. This is likely to be caused by epitope loss in the crystals, which are thought to be composed mostly

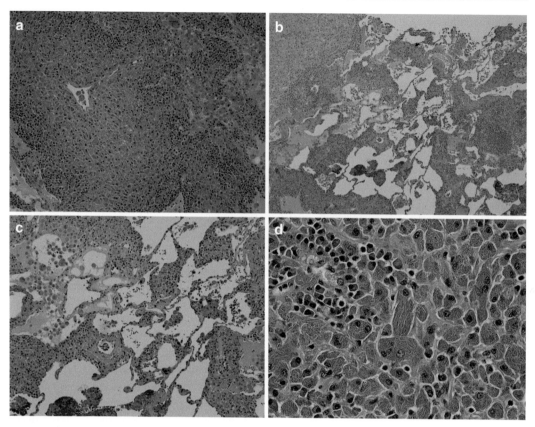

Fig. 12.6 Pulmonary CSH. (**a**). Mass-forming sheet of macrophages surrounded by lymphoplasmacytic cells at the periphery. Crystalline texture of the histiocytic cytoplasm is not readily apparent. (**b** and **c**). Histiocytes also permeate the pulmonary septa. (**d**) At higher magnifica-tion (viewed with condenser removed to increase contrast), the distinctly crystalline texture of the cytoplasm can be appreciated. (slide courtesy of SH Swerdlow, photographed and published with permission)

of immunoglobulin variable region products, whereas most antibodies used to detect immu-noglobulins by immunohistochemistry bind to constant region epitopes.

More recent reports indicate that, similar to LCPT, the extrarenal pathology associated with intracellular immunoglobulin storage is expand-ing. Thus, in 2007, Chantranuwat [51] reported a 52-year-old man, with a known case of multiple myeloma, who developed chronic bilateral pul-monary infiltration. Open lung biopsy displayed a desquamated interstitial pneumonia-like pat-tern, characterized by a diffuse patchy intra-alveolar accumulation of unusual macrophages, containing abundant round intracytoplasmic eosinophilic globular structures that were 1–7 μm in size. The globules showed restriction for kappa light chain by immunoperoxidase stain. Electron microscopic examination revealed amorphous material without a crystalline shape or a fine ultrastructure of lattice or linear parallel configu-ration, indicating storage of noncrystallized immunoglobulin. This report documented, for the first time, the noncrystallized form of immunoglobulin-storing histiocytosis, causing an unusual pulmonary pathology in a patient with multiple myeloma. More recently, Kurabayashi et al. [55] reported a similar noncrystallized immunoglobulin-storing histiocytosis with abun-dant eosinophilic globular, IgG-kappa-restricted inclusions in the histiocytic cytoplasm. Thus, in view of these reports, the term CSH should be replaced by immunoglobulin-storing histiocyto-sis (IgSH).

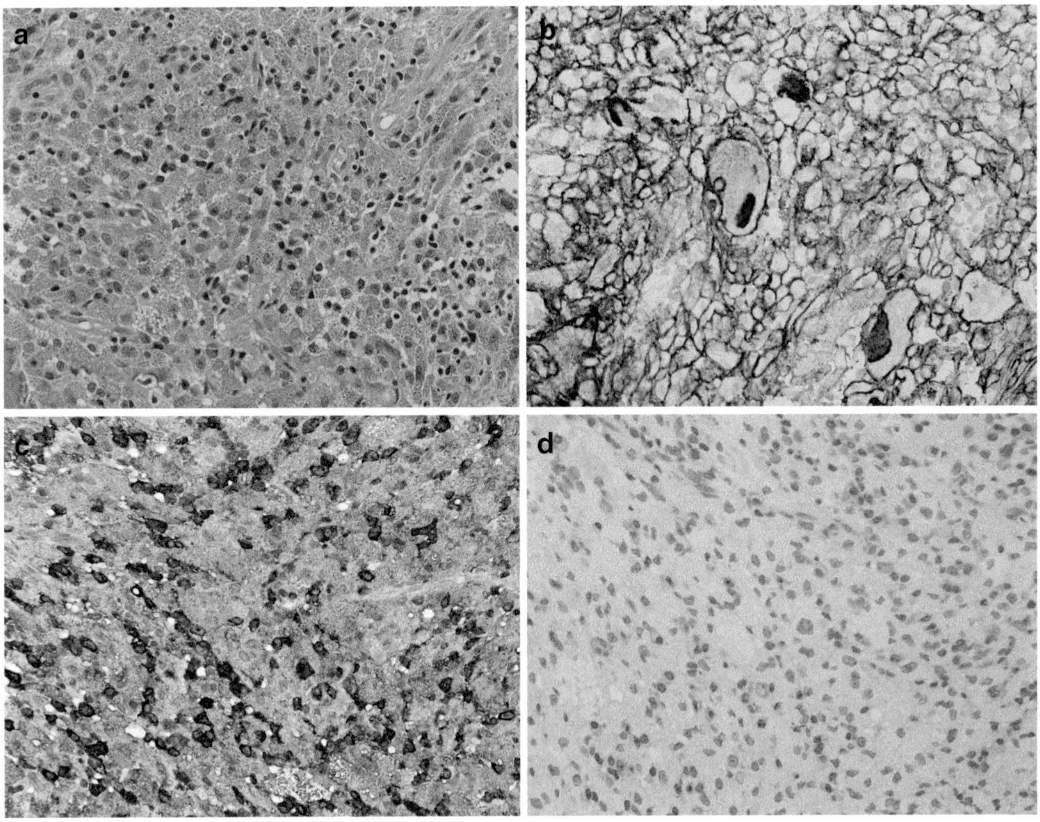

Fig. 12.7 Bone lesion. A, B—numerous histiocytes with discrete intracytoplasmic inclusions dominate the picture. (**a**). H&E-stained section, (**b**). Immunostain with CD11c—highlighting the histiocytes. (**c** and **d**) demonstrating light chain restriction with strong positivity for kappa light chain (**c**) while stain for lambda light chain (**d**) is negative. Note that the light chain staining is much weaker in the histiocytes compared to plasma cells due to epitope loss (see the corresponding comment in the chapter)

Interestingly, similar large noncrystalline inclusions were also recently reported by Li et al. in a case of extranodal B-cell lymphoma [61]. The patient presented with a soft-tissue mass causing enlargement of the shoulder (Fig. 12.8).

The excised tumor was composed of large, rhabdoid cells in a diffuse pattern, suggestive of adult rhabdomyoma (Fig. 12.9). However, subsequent studies demonstrated a B-cell lineage and immunoglobulin heavy chain-specific and immunoglobulin light chain kappa-specific rearrangement. Electron microscopy showed pools of homogeneous, electron-dense material in dilated rough endoplasmic reticulum. While occasional, intracellular, intranuclear, or other crystalline structures are not unusual in B-cell disorders, their presence, in abundance, may mimic other conditions and cause diagnostic difficulties.

Similar to AL amyloidosis, CSH can be localized or systemic. While treatment strategies are evolving, both surgical and/or radiotherapy techniques have been applied in the case of localized disease; however, for systemic processes, various combinations of chemotherapy, immunomodulatory drugs, and even bone marrow transplantation have been used [39, 46, 84, 85].

In summary, the spectrum of intracellular paraprotein storage disorders is expanding and includes organized as well as non-organized intracellular deposits, which may be seen in histiocytes, stromal and epithelial cells, and cells with B-cell lineage. In another chapter, Ronco et al. extend the discussion of paraproteins further to

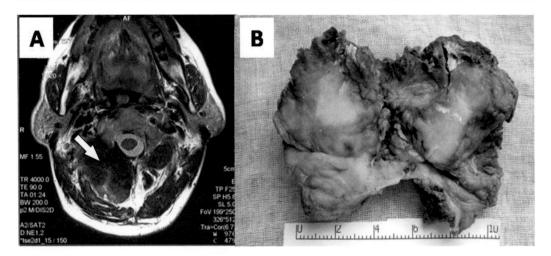

Fig. 12.8 Views of the tissue mass. (**a**) Magnetic resonance imaging scan. A soft-tissue mass is seen in the right shoulder (*white arrow*). (**b**) Gross morphology. (Figure 12.8 reprinted with permission from [61])

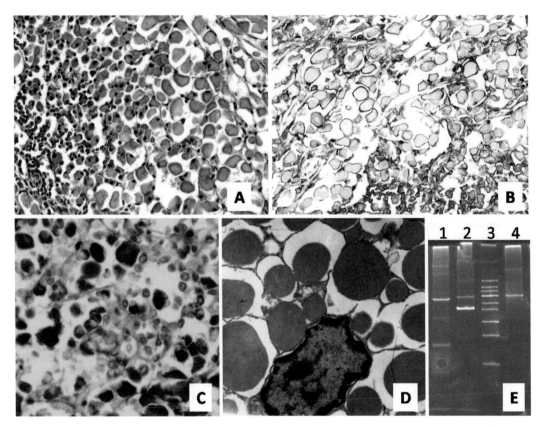

Fig. 12.9 (**a**) Hematoxylin and eosin staining (original magnification, ×400). (**b**) Immunohistochemical detection of CD79a (original magnification, ×400). (**c**). Double staining with periodic acid–Schiff stain (histochemistry) and paired box protein 5 (PAX5) (immunohistochemistry). (**d**). Electron micrograph of inclusion (original magnification, ×7250). (**e**). Lane 1 is immunoglobulin heavy chain (IGH) rearrangements, lane 4 is immunoglobulin light chain kappa (IGκ) rearrangements, and lane 3 is a 50 bp ladder. (Figure 12.9 reprinted with permission from [61])

include non-organized extracellular deposits. Although the lesions discussed in this and the prior chapter are relatively rare, collectively, they may represent an ever-increasing proportion of pathologies associated with underlying plasma cell dyscrasia/B-cell lymphoproliferative disorders. Therefore, awareness of these lesions is important since they represent a useful clue that can facilitate the early diagnosis of an underlying plasma cell dyscrasia/lymphoproliferative process. A further significance lies in the fact that these lesions mimic other conditions. While, in many instances, the clinical course may be indolent, significant target organ damage occurs over time. Although there is no consensus regarding the best treatment options, elimination of the involved clone is associated with reversal of target organ injury. Therefore, efforts to design effective treatments for these "small but dangerous" clones should continue. In this regard, the new generation of immunomodulatory treatments may offer hope for the prevention of injury to target organs.

References

1. Picken MM. Monoclonal gammopathies: glomerular and tubular injuries. In: McManus LM, Mitchell RN, editors. Pathobiology of human disease. A dynamic encyclopedia of disease mechanisms. Oxford: Elsevier; 2014.
2. Herrera GA, Picken MM. Renal diseases associated with plasma cell dyscrasias, Waldenstrom macroglobulinemia and cryoglobulinemic nephropathies. In: Jennette JC, Olson JL, Schwartz MM, Silva FG, editors. Heptinstall's pathology of the kidney. 7th ed. Philadelphia, PA: Lippincott Williams & Wilkins; 2014. p. 951–1014.
3. Dogan S, Barnes L, Cruz-Vetrano WP. Crystal-storing histiocytosis: report of a case, review of the literature (80 cases) and a proposed classification. Head Neck Pathol. 2012;6(1):111–20. Epub 2012 Mar 20.
4. Gupta V, El Ters M, Kashani K, Leung N, Nasr SH. Crystalglobulin-induced nephropathy. J Am Soc Nephrol. 2015;26(3):525–9. doi:10.1681/ASN.2014050509. Epub 2014 Sep 4.
5. Sicard A, Karras A, Goujon JM, Sirac C, Bender S, Labatut D, Callard P, Sarkozy C, Essig M, Vanhille P, Provot F, Nony A, Nochy D, Ronco P, Bridoux F, Touchard G. Light chain deposition disease without glomerular proteinuria: a diagnostic challenge for the nephrologist. Nephrol Dial Transplant. 2014;29(10):1894–902. Epub 2014 Mar 11.
6. Sirota JH, Hamerman D. Renal function studies in an adult subject with the Fanconi syndrome. Am J Med. 1954;16:138.
7. Maldonado JE, Velosa JA, Kyle RA, et al. Fanconi syndrome in adults. A manifestation of a latent form of myeloma. Am J Med. 1975;58:354.
8. Aucouturier P, Bauwens M, Khamlichi AA, et al. Monoclonal Ig L chain and L chain V domain fragment crystallization in myeloma-associated Fanconi's syndrome. J Immunol. 1993;150:3561.
9. Sirac C, Bridoux F, Carrion C, et al. Role of the monoclonal kappa chain V domain and reversibility of renal damage in a transgenic model of acquired Fanconi syndrome. Blood. 2006;108:536.
10. Messiaen T, Deret S, Mougenot B, et al. Adult Fanconi syndrome secondary to light chain gammopathy: clinicopathologic heterogeneity and unusual features in 11 patients. Medicine. 2000;79:135.
11. Kapur U, Barton K, Fresco R, Leehey DJ, Picken MM. Expanding the pathologic spectrum of immunoglobulin light chain proximal tubulopathy. Arch Pathol Lab Med. 2007;131(9):1368–72.
12. Lebeau A, Zeindl-Eberhart E, Muller EC, Muller-Hocker J, Jungblut PR, Emmerich B, Lohrs U. Generalized crystal-storing histiocytosis associated with monoclonal gammopathy: molecular analysis of a disorder with rapid clinical course and review of the literature. Blood. 2002;200(5):1817–27.
13. Stokes MB, Aronoff B, Siegel D, D'Agati VD. Dysproteinemia-related nephropathy associated with crystal-storing histiocytosis. Kidney Int. 2006; 70:597–602.
14. El Hamel C, Thierry A, Trouillas P, Bridoux F, Carrion C, Quellard N, Goujon JM, Aldigier JC, Gombert JM, Cogne M, Touchard G. Crystal-storing histiocytosis with renal Fanconi syndrome: pathological and molecular characteristics compared with classical myeloma-associated Fanconi syndrome. Nephrol Dial Transplant. 2010;25:2982.
15. Toly-Ndour C, Peltier J, Piedagnel R, Coppo P, Sachon E, Ronco P, Rondeau E, Callard P, Aucouturier P. Acute renal failure with lambda light chain-derived crystals in a patient with IgD myeloma. Nephrol Dial Transplant 2011;26(9):3057–9. doi:10.1093/ndt/gfr377. Epub 2011 Jul 7.
16. El Hamel C, Aldigier JC, Oblet C, Laffleur B, Bridoux F, Cogné M. Specific impairment of proximal tubular cell proliferation by a monoclonal κ light chain responsible for Fanconi syndrome. Nephrol Dial Transplant. 2012;27(12):4368–77. doi:10.1093/ndt/gfs261. Epub 2012 Sep 28.
17. Sirac C, Bridoux F, Essig M, Devuyst O, Touchard G, Cogné M. Toward understanding renal Fanconi syndrome: step by step advances through experimental models. Contrib Nephrol. 2011;169:247–61. Epub 2011 Jan 20.

18. Elliott MR, Cortese C, Moreno-Aspitia A, Dwyer JP. Plasma cell dyscrasia causing light chain tubulopathy without Fanconi syndrome. Am J Kid Diseases. 2010;55(6):1136–41.

19. Sanders PW. Mechanisms of light chain injury along the tubular nephron. J Am Soc Nephrol. 2012;23:1777–81. doi:10.1681/ASN.2012040388.

20. Larsen CP, Bell JM, Harris AA, Messias NC, Wang YH, Walker PD. The morphologic spectrum and clinical significance of light chain proximal tubulopathy with and without crystal formation. Mod Pathol. 2011;24(11):1462–9. doi:10.1038/modpathol.2011.104. Epub 2011 Jun 24.

21. Sharma SG, Bonsib SM, Portilla D, Shukla A, Woodruff AB, Gokden N. Light chain proximal tubulopathy: expanding the pathologic spectrum with and without deposition of crystalline inclusions. ISRN Pathol. 2012;2012:1–6; Article ID 541075, 6 pp., doi:10.5402/2012/541075.

22. Rane S, Rana S, Sachdeva M, Joshi K. Light chain proximal tubulopathy without crystals in a case of burkitt lymphoma presenting with acute kidney injury. Am J Kid Diseases. 2013;62(3):638–41.

23. Herrera GA. Proximal tubulopathies associated with monoclonal light chains: the spectrum of clinicopathologic manifestations and molecular pathogenesis. Arch Pathol Lab Med. 2014;138(10):1365–80.

24. Deret S, Denoroy L, Lamarine M, et al. Kappa light chain-associated Fanconi's syndrome: molecular analysis of monoclonal immunoglobulin light chains from patients with and without intracellular crystals. Protein Eng. 1999;12:363.

25. Bridoux F, Sirac C, Hugue V, et al. Fanconi's syndrome induced by a monoclonal Vkappa3 light chain in Waldenstrom's macroglobulinemia. Am J Kidney Dis. 2005;45:749–57.

26. Lajoie G, Leung R, Bargman JM. Clinical, biochemical, and pathological features in a patient with plasma cell dyscrasia and Fanconi's syndrome. Ultrastruct Pathol. 2000;24:221–6.

27. Decourt C, Bridoux F, Touchard G, et al. A monoclonal V kappa l light chain responsible for incomplete proximal tubulopathy. Am J Kidney Dis. 2003;41:497.

28. Gu X, Barrios R, Cartwright J, et al. Light chain crystal deposition as a manifestation of plasma cell dyscrasias: the role of immunoelectron microscopy. Hum Pathol. 2003;34:270–7.

29. Cai G, Sidhu GS, Wieczorek R, et al. Plasma cell dyscrasia with kappa light- chain crystals in proximal tubular cells: a histological, immunofluorescent, and ultrastructural study. Ultrastruct Pathol. 2006;30:315–9.

30. Thorner PS, Bedard YC, Fernandes BJ. Lambda-light-chain nephropathy with Fanconi's syndrome. Arch Pathol Lab Med. 1983;107:654–7.

31. Noguchi K, Munemura C, Maeda S, et al. Myeloma-associated Fanconi syndrome due to λ-light chain crystal deposition. Yonago Acta Medica. 2004;47:91–6.

32. Ma CX, Lacy MQ, Rompala JF, et al. Acquired Fanconi syndrome is an indolent disorder in the absence of overt multiple myeloma. Blood. 2004;104:40.

33. Herlitz LC, Roglieri J, Resta R, Bhagat G, Markowitz GS. Light chain proximal tubulopathy. Kidney Int. 2009;76:792–7.

34. Figueres M, Beaume J, Vuiblet V, Rabant M, Bassilios N, Herody M, Touchard G, Noël LH. Crystalline light chain proximal tubulopathy with chronic renal failure and silicone gel breast implants: 1 case report. Hum Path. 2015;46(1):165–8. Published Online: October 24, 2014.

35. Sethi S, Cuiffo BP, Pinkus GS, Rennke HG. Crystal-storing histiocytosis involving the kidney in a low-grade B-cell lymphoproliferative disorder. Am J Kidney Dis. 2002;39(1):183–8.

36. Tomika M, Ueki K, Nakahashi A, et al. Widespread crystalline inclusions affecting podocytes, tubular cells and interstitial histiocytes in the myeloma kidney. Clin Nephrol. 2003;62:229–33.

37. Akilesh S, Alem A, Nicosia RF. Combined crystalline podocytopathy and tubulopathy associated with multiple myeloma. Hum Pathol. 2014;45(4):875–9. Epub 2013 Oct 19.

38. Watanabe H, Osawa Y, Goto S, Habuka M, Imai N, Ito Y, Hirose T, Chou T, Ohashi R, Shimizu A, Ehara T, Shimotori T, Narita I. A case of endocapillary proliferative glomerulonephritis with macrophages phagocytosing monoclonal immunoglobulin lambda light chain. Pathol Int. 2015;65(1):38–42. doi:10.1111/pin.12229. Epub 2014 Nov 19.

39. Duquesne A, Werbrouck A, Fabiani B, Denoyer A, Cervera P, Verpont MC, Bender S, Piedagnel R, Brocheriou I, Ronco P, Boffa JJ, Aucouturier P, Garderet L. Complete remission of monoclonal gammopathy with ocular and periorbital crystal storing histiocytosis and Fanconi syndrome. Hum Pathol. 2013;44(5):927–33. Epub 2013 Jan 11.

40. Taneda S, Honda K, Horita S, et al. Proximal tubule cytoplasmic fibrillary inclusions following kidney transplantation in a patient with a paraproteinemia. Am J Kid Dis. 2009;53:715–8.

41. Yao Y, Wang S-X, Zhang Y-K, Wang Y, Liu L, Liu G. Acquired Fanconi syndrome with proximal tubular cytoplasmic fibrillary inclusions of λ light chain restriction. Intern Med. 2014;53:121–4.

42. Corbett RW, Cook HT, Duncan N, Moss J. Fibrillary inclusions in light chain proximal tubulopathy associated with myeloma. Clin Kidney J. 2012;5(1):75–6.

43. Larsen CP, Borrelli GS, Walker PD. Amyloid proximal tubulopathy: a novel form of light chain proximal tubulopathy. Clin Kidney J. 2012;5(2):130–2.

44. Hemminger J, Satoskar A, Brodsky SV, Calomeni E, Nadasdy GM, Kovach P, Hofmeister CC, Nadasdy T. Unique pattern of renal κ light chain amyloid deposition with histiocytic transdifferentiation of tubular epithelial cells. Am J Surg Pathol. 2012;36(8):1253–7.

45. Merlini G, Stone MJ. Dangerous small clones. Blood. 2006;108:2520–30.

46. Fermand JP, Bridoux F, Kyle RA, Kastritis E, Weiss BM, Cook MA, Drayson MT, Dispenzieri A, Leung N. International kidney and Monoclonal Gammopathy Research Group. How i treat Monoclonal Gammopathy of Renal Significance (MGRS). Blood. 2013; 122(22):3583–90. Epub 2013 Oct 9.

47. Jones D, Bhatia VK, Krausz T, Pinkus GS. Crystal storing histiocytosis: a disorder occurring in plasmacytic tumors expressing immunoglobulin kappa light chain. Hum Pathol. 1999;30(12):1441–8.

48. Sun Y, Tawfiqul B, Valderrama E, Kline G, Kahn LB. Pulmonary crystal-storing histiocytosis and extranodal marginal zone B-cell lymphoma associated with a fibroleiomyomatous hamartoma. Ann Diagn Pathol. 2003;7(1):47–53.

49. Galed-Placed I. Immunoglobulin crystal-storing histiocytosis in a pleural effusion from a woman with IgA κ multiple myeloma. Acta Cytol. 2006; 50:539–41.

50. Pock L, Stuchlik D, Hercegova J. Crystal storing histiocytosis of the skin associated with multiple myeloma. Int J Dermatol. 2006;45(12):1408–11.

51. Chantranuwat C. Noncrystallized form of immunoglobulin-storing histiocytosis as a cause of chronic lung infiltration in multiple myeloma. Ann Diagn Pathol. 2007;11(3):220–2.

52. Kusakabe T, Watanabe K, Mori T, Iida T, Suzuki T. Crystal-storing histiocytosis associated with MALT lymphoma of the ocular adnexa: a case report with review of literature. Virchows Arch. 2007;450(1):103–8. Epub 2006 Nov 17.

53. de Alba Campomanes AG, Rutar T, Crawford JB, Seiff S, Goodman D, Grenert J. Crystal-storing histiocytosis and crystalline keratopathy caused by monoclonal gammopathy of undetermined significance. Cornea. 2009;28(9):1081–4.

54. Sailey CJ, Alexiev BA, Gammie JS, Pinell-Salles P, Stafford JL, Burke A. Crystal-storing histiocytosis as a cause of symptomatic cardiac mass. Arch Pathol Lab Med. 2009;133:1861–4.

55. Kurabayashi A, Iguchi M, Matsumoto M, Hiroi M, Kume M, Furihata M. Thymic mucosa-associated lymphoid tissue lymphoma with immunoglobulin-storing histiocytosis in Sjögren's syndrome. Pathol Int. 2010;60(2):125–30.

56. Bosman C, Camassei FD, Boldrini R, Piro FR, Saponara M, Romeo R, Corsi A. Solitary crystal-storing histiocytosis of the tongue in a patient with rheumatoid arthritis and polyclonal hypergammaglobulinemia. Arch Pathol Lab Med. 1998; 122:920–4.

57. Lee WS, Kim SR, Moon H, Choe YH, Park SJ, Lee HB, Jin GY, Chung MJ, Lee YC. Pulmonary crystal-storing histiocytoma in a patient without a lymphoproliferative disorder. Am J Med Sci. 2009; 338(5):421–4.

58. Khurram SA, McPhadden A, Hislop WS, Hunter KD. Crystal storing histiocytosis of the tongue as the initial presentation of multiple myeloma. Oral Surg Oral Med Oral Pathol Oral Radiol Endocrinol. 2011;111(4):494–6.

59. Gao FF, Khalbuss WE, Austin RM, Monaco SE. Cytomorphology of crystal storing histiocytosis in the breast associated with lymphoma: a case report. Acta Cytol. 2011;55(3):302–6. Epub 2011 Apr 27.

60. Kaminsky IA, Wang AM, Olsen J, Schechter S, Wilson J, Olson R. Central nervous system crystal-storing histiocytosis: neuroimaging, neuropathology, and literature review. AJNR. 2011;32:E26–8.

61. Li Z, Li P, Wang Z, Huang G. Primary extranodal soft-tissue B-cell lymphoma with abundant immunoglobulin inclusions mimicking adult rhabdomyoma: a case report. J Med Case Rep. 2011;5:53. http://www.jmedicalcasereports.com/content/5/1/53.

62. Ko HM, da Cunha Santos G, Boerner SL, Bailey DJ, Geddie WR. Negative images of crystalline immunoglobulin in crystal storing histiocytosis: A potential cytologic mimic of mycobacteria in smears. Diagn Cytopathol. 2012;40(10):916–9. doi:10.1002/dc.21677. Epub 2011 May 4.

63. Saluja K, Thakral B, Goldschmidt RA. Crystal storing histiocytosis associated with marginal zone B-cell lymphoma: a rare initial clinical presentation diagnosed by fine-needle aspiration. Cytojournal. 2014;11:17. Published online Jun 12, 2014.

64. Tsuji T, Yamasaki H, Hirano T, Toyozumi Y, Arima N, Tsuda H. Crystal-storing histiocytosis complicating marginal zone B-cell lymphoma of mucosa-associated lymphoid tissue. Int J Hematol. 2014;100(6):519–20. Epub 2014 Sep 13.

65. Vaid A, Caradine KD, Lai KK, Rego R. Isolated gastric crystal-storing histiocytosis: a rare marker of occult lymphoproliferative disorders. J Clin Pathol. 2014;67(8):740–1. Epub 2014 May 9.

66. Tahara K, Miyajima K, Ono M, Sugio Y, Yamamoto I, Tamiya S. Crystal-storing histiocytosis associated with marginal-zone lymphoma. Jpn J Radiol. 2014;32(5):296–301. Epub 2014 Mar 16.

67. Li JJ, Henderson C. Cutaneous crystal storing histiocytosis: a report of two cases. J Cutan Pathol. 2015;42(2):136–43. doi:10.1111/cup.12413. Epub 2014 Nov 24.

68. Chaudhary S, Navarro M, Laser J, Berman E, Bhuiya T. Localized crystal-storing histiocytosis presenting as a breast nodule: an unusual presentation of a rare entity. Breast J. 2014;20(5):539–42. Epub 2014 Jul 17.

69. Kai K, Miyahara M, Tokuda Y, Kido S, Masuda M, Takase Y, Tokunaga O. A case of mucosa-associated lymphoid tissue lymphoma of the gastrointestinal tract showing extensive plasma cell differentiation with prominent Russell bodies. World J Clin Cases. 2013;1(5):176–80.

70. Johnson M, Mazariegos J, Lewis PJ, Pomakova D. Crystal storing histiocytosis presenting as a temporal lobe mass lesion. Surg Neurol Int. 2013;4:112.

71. Rossi G, De Rosa N, Cavazza A, Mengoli MC, Della Casa G, Nannini N, Colby TV. Localized pleuropul-

monary crystal-storing histiocytosis: 5 cases of a rare histiocytic disorder with variable clinicoradiologic features. Am J Surg Pathol. 2013;37(6):906–12.

72. da Cruz Perez DE, Silva-Sousa YT, de Andrade BA, Rizo VH, Almeida LY, León JE, de Almeida OP. Crystal-storing histiocytosis: a rare lesion in periapical pathology. Ann Diagn Pathol. 2012; 16(6):527–31. Epub 2011 Aug 16.

73. Rossi G, Morandi U, Nannini N, Fontana G, Pifferi M, Casali C. Crystal-storing histiocytosis presenting with pleural disease. Histopathology. 2010;56(3):403–5.

74. Todd WU, Drabick JJ, Benninghoff MG, Frauenhoffer EE, Zander DS. Pulmonary crystal-storing histiocytosis diagnosed by computed tomography-guided fine-needle aspiration. Diagn Cytopathol. 2010;38(4): 274–8.

75. Orr BA, Gallia GL, Dogan A, Rodriguez FJ. IgA/kappa-restricted crystal storing histiocytosis involving the central nervous system characterized by proteomic analysis. Clin Neuropathol. 2014;33(1):23–8.

76. Lv Y, Liu Y, Li X, Yan Q, Wang Z. Plasmacytoma with crystal-storing histiocytosis exhibiting FGFR3 and IgH translocation. Pathology. 2015;47(1):82–5. doi:10.1097/PAT.0000000000000200.

77. Rodriguez FJ, Gamez JD, Vrana JA, Theis JD, Giannini C, Scheithauer BW, Parisi JE, Lucchinetti CF, Pendlebury WW, Bergen 3rd HR, Dogan A. Immunoglobulin derived depositions in the nervous system: novel mass spectrometry application for protein characterization in formalin-fixed tissues. Lab Invest. 2008;88(10):1024–37. Epub 2008 Aug 18.

78. Shamanna RK, Xu-Monette ZY, Miranda RN, Zou D, Weber D, Dogan A, O'Malley DP, Bueso-Ramos C, Orlowski RZ, Medeiros LJ, Young KH. Clinicopathologic and molecular features of crystal (immunoglobulin) storing histiocytosis associated with lymphoplasmacytic neoplasms. Histopathology 2015, in press.

79. Magnano L, Fernández de Larrea C, Cibeira MT, Rozman M, Tovar N, Rovira M, Rosiñol L, Bladé J. Acquired Fanconi syndrome secondary to monoclonal gammopathies. Clin Lymphoma Myeloma Leuk. 2013;13(5):614–8. Epub 2013 Jun 15.

80. Thakral B, Courville E. Crystal-storing histiocytosis with IgD–κ associated plasma cell neoplasm. Blood. 2014;123:3540.

81. Lesesve JF, Bronowicki JP, Galed-Placed I. Crystal-storing histiocytosis in ascites from a patient with IgM kappa lymphoplasmacytic lymphoma. Cytopathology. 2011;22(3):207–8. Epub 2010 Nov 9.

82. Miura TE, Takihi IY, Maekawa YH, Chauffaille Mde L, Rizzatti EG, Sandes AF. Iron staining in gammopathy-related crystal-storing histiocytosis: a misleading feature to the differential diagnosis with Gaucher's disease. Mol Genet Metab. 2013; 110(3):414–5. Epub 2013 Aug 8.

83. Chan JK. The wonderful colors of the hematoxylin-eosin stain in diagnostic surgical pathology. Int J Surg Pathol. 2014;22(1):12–32. Epub 2014 Jan 9.

84. Kawano N, Beppu K, Oyama M, Himeji D, Yoshida S, Kuriyama T, Ono N, Masuyama H, Yamashita K, Yamaguchi K, Shimao Y, Oshima K, Ueda Y, Ueda A. Successful surgical treatment for pulmonary crystal-storing histiocytosis following the onset of gastric non-hodgkin lymphoma. J Clin Exp Hematop. 2013;53(3):241–5.

85. Hu X, Liu J, Bai C, Wang J, Song X. Bortezomib combined with thalidomide and dexamethasone is effective for patient with crystal-storing histiocytosis associated with monoclonal gammopathy of undermined significance. Eur J Haematol. 2012;89(2):183–4. Epub 2012 Jun 7.

Part III

Diagnosis

Diagnosis of Amyloid Using Congo Red

13

Alexander J. Howie

Amyloid and Congo Red: Historical and Technical Notes

Various methods have been used to detect amyloid. Until Hans Hermann Bennhold (1893–1976) found by chance and reported in 1922 that amyloid was stained by Congo red [1–3], the most popular methods were probably those using methyl violet or crystal violet to give a metachromatic reaction which was also given by other materials [4]. Before the metachromatic methods, amyloid was detected by the sulphuric acid and iodine stain which was difficult and inconsistent [5]. Congo red does not only stain amyloid, but the other materials that may be stained by a technically correct method can be distinguished from amyloid. Materials such as elastic laminae and eosinophils can be distinguished by their lack of some of the optical properties of amyloid stained by Congo red, and others such as cellulose in plant residues and casts in myelomatous light chain nephropathy can be distinguished by their appearance and position within tissues, even though they have similar optical properties to amyloid.

Congo red can be used as a pH indicator because it changes colour from red to blue in strongly acid conditions, changing in the pH range 3–5 [6]. For this reason, alkaline conditions are used in staining methods. Early methods required differentiation, meaning removal of stain from sections, which gave irregular reactions. The method of Puchtler et al. was an advance because it did not require differentiation, but the working solutions were unstable and had to be made shortly before use [7]. Stokes' method is a simple modification of this, is most useful in everyday practice and is described below (Section 'Stokes' Method for Congo Red Staining of Amyloid'). Gwen (Gwendolyn Mary) Stokes (1932–2009) was in the Surgical Pathology laboratory, St Thomas' Hospital, London, UK, when she published the method in 1976 [8].

Two technical points about Congo red staining of amyloid can be made. The first is that amyloid may be missed in thin sections, and sections at least 5 μm thick are better, with virtually no practical upper limit to the thickness of sections. The second point is that a method of distinguishing different types of amyloid by modification of Congo red staining is obsolete because it has been superseded by immunohistological and other methods. This modification is the pretreatment of sections with potassium permanganate [9].

A.J. Howie (✉)
Department of Pathology, University College London, London WC1E 6BT, UK
e-mail: a.j.howie@ucl.ac.uk

© Springer International Publishing Switzerland 2015
M.M. Picken et al. (eds.), *Amyloid and Related Disorders*, Current Clinical Pathology,
DOI 10.1007/978-3-319-19294-9_13

Stokes' Method for Congo Red Staining of Amyloid

The stock solution, which retains its properties for several months at room temperature, is 200 ml industrial methylated spirits, 50 ml distilled water and 0.5 g potassium hydroxide, to which 4 g Congo red is added to produce a saturated solution. This is left to stand overnight before first use.

Sections of the appropriate thickness of tissue fixed in formaldehyde, preferably 10 % formal saline, and embedded in paraffin wax, are rehydrated. A known case of amyloid should be included as a control. The Congo red solution is filtered into a staining jar, and the sections are put in this for 25 min. The sections are then washed thoroughly in distilled water and placed in running tap water for 5 min. A haematoxylin counterstain, such as Carazzi's haematoxylin, is then applied for 1 min followed by blueing in running tap water for 5 min. Sections are dehydrated, cleared in xylene and mounted.

Analysis of Congo Red Staining

On ordinary microscopy, technically satisfactory Congo red staining gives a red or pink or orange colour of various intensities in amyloid deposits, with blue nuclei and a faint blue or colourless background (Fig. 13.1).

Even with satisfactory staining by Congo red, there may be staining of normal structures such as elastic laminae in arteries, or there may be overstaining of the background, and more elaborate microscopy is usually used to confirm that positive staining identifies amyloid, or to exclude amyloid, which may be missed on ordinary microscopy. The special technique is polarisation microscopy. The findings of polarisation microscopy will be described before the relevant principles of optical physics, supported by experimental evidence, are used to explain the scientific basis of those findings (Section 'Principles of Polarisation Microscopy and Explanation of the Optical Properties of Amyloid Stained by Congo Red') [3, 10, 11].

Polarisation Microscopy of Amyloid Stained by Congo Red

Most microscopes can be fitted with a polarising filter between the light source and the condenser, called the polariser, and also another polarising filter between the objective lens and the eyepieces, called the analyser. These filters convert ordinary, unpolarised light into light which is only vibrating in one plane, and do not allow light to pass if it is polarised perpendicularly to the plane of the filter. When the planes of the polariser and analyser are perpendicular to each other, the filters are said to be crossed, and no linearly polarised light produced by the polariser can pass the analyser. The microscope field now appears its darkest. Often, when descriptions are given of the conditions needed to study Congo red-stained amyloid, the terms 'in polarised light' and 'on polarising microscopy' and so on are used, but these should be understood to mean examination of a section between polariser and analyser [11].

When amyloid stained by Congo red is examined between crossed polariser and analyser, some appears bright and coloured (Fig. 13.2). This is best looked for on a microscope using

Fig. 13.1 An artery containing amyloid stained by Congo red. In ordinary, unpolarised illumination, amyloid appears *red*

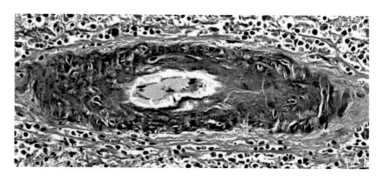

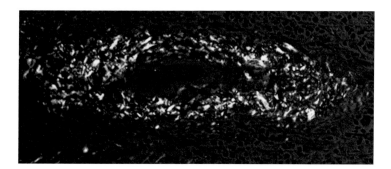

Fig. 13.2 The artery in Fig. 13.1 examined between accurately crossed polariser and analyser. The background is dark. Some parts of the amyloid appear bright and coloured, with combinations of anomalous colours that could appear *blue/green* and *yellow/green*, or *green* and *yellow*, or *blue* and *yellow*. The different colours are in areas roughly perpendicular to each other

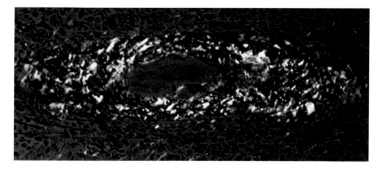

Fig. 13.3 The artery in Fig. 13.1 examined between accurately crossed polariser and analyser, with insertion of an elliptical compensator into the light path. Adjustment of the amount of compensation has nullified effects of strain birefringence in the optical system and has given a relatively *pure green* anomalous colour, with different amounts of brightness

maximum light intensity and minimum condenser aperture. If the section can be rotated on the microscope stage, the bright and dark areas in amyloid deposits will be seen to change positions, depending on their relation to the plane of the polariser.

The colour is almost always said to be green or apple green, often qualified with the words characteristic or typical [11]. A pure green colour may occasionally be seen on an ordinary microscope, but this is usually by chance, and to produce pure green may need either use of a microscope specifically designed for polarisation microscopy, or insertion into an ordinary microscope of a piece of equipment called a compensator (Fig. 13.3). The function of a compensator is explained later (Section 'Compensation').

More commonly, the colour is not pure green but a combination of colours. These, including green, are called anomalous colours. The combinations may appear blue/green and yellow/green, or green and yellow, or blue and yellow (Fig. 13.2). The different colours are seen in areas roughly perpendicular to each other, appear to rotate as the section is rotated and exchange positions when the stage is rotated by 90°. The colours are not always uniformly distributed across a section. Often, changing the objective lens to one of a different magnification changes the colours.

When either the polariser or the analyser is rotated from the position that gives the darkest background, the background becomes lighter, more of the amyloid stained by Congo red appears coloured and other anomalous colours appear. These are orange and light blue/green (Fig. 13.4), or purplish red and greenish white (Fig. 13.5), or other combinations. If these

Fig. 13.4 The artery in
Fig. 13.2 examined with
slight uncrossing of
polariser and analyser. The
background is lighter, and
the anomalous colours are
predominantly *orange* and
light blue/green

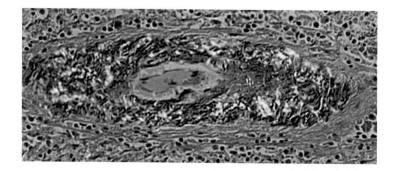

Fig. 13.5 The artery in
Fig. 13.2 examined with
slight uncrossing of
polariser and analyser in
the opposite direction to
that in Fig. 13.4. The
anomalous colours are now
purplish red and *faint
green*, almost *white*

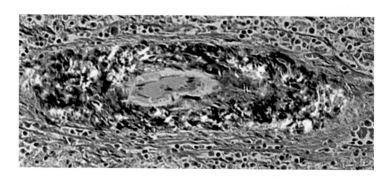

colours are seen when the polariser and analyser are supposedly crossed, this means that the polarising filters are not accurately crossed. In contrast, blue/green and yellow/green, or green and yellow, or blue and yellow may be seen with perfectly accurate crossing of the filters.

The orange and other anomalous colours change when the section is rotated or when the polariser or analyser is rotated either further in the same direction or in the opposite direction. Amyloid deposits pass through a mixed red and colourless appearance, and then, when the planes of the polariser and analyser are parallel, amyloid deposits appear red and virtually indistinguishable from the appearance in ordinary illumination. These changes in colour are a useful way to confirm amyloid.

Colours other than green are hardly ever reported in papers on Congo red-stained amyloid, even though they can be easily seen in published illustrations. Some figures show the colours produced by uncrossing the polariser and analyser, but the legends rarely mention this. Only 59 (31 %) of 191 published figures showed a pure green colour, including those given the benefit of doubt in equivocal cases. The others showed green and yellow or blue and yellow in

62 (32 %), green and red or green and a colour other than red or yellow in 38 (20 %), and various colours without any green or blue, either combinations or single colours, in 32 (17 %). In 127 (66 %) of these 191 figures, there was a discrepancy between the description of colours and their illustration, mostly because green alone was mentioned in descriptions, but green and other colours could be seen in figures, although the other colours were ignored. In 30 (24 %) of these 127, green was mentioned in descriptions, but there was no green at all visible in figures [11].

No paper blamed an inability to illustrate pure green, or to show any green, on failure of accurate reproduction of colours. Accordingly, the illustrated colours can be considered representative of what was seen and accepted by authors, reviewers and editors as diagnostic of amyloid [11]. One implication is that most people using Congo red to stain amyloid assume that green is essential for the diagnosis and that they should only report green, even if they do not see either green on its own or any green at all. The mention of green is considered sufficient for the diagnosis. Another implication is that any explanation of the optical properties of Congo red-stained amyloid must account for all the colours, and not just green.

All these optical properties arise from the orientation of Congo red molecules on amyloid fibrils and are identical in specimens in which Congo red is orientated in other ways, such as experimentally in smears of solutions of the stain. Congo red is orientated on cellulose in plant cell walls and sometimes on aggregated immunoglobulin light chains in casts in myeloma kidney, but these materials should be easily distinguishable from amyloid by their appearance and position within a section. Other things that commonly stain with Congo red, such as elastic laminae and eosinophils, do not align the molecules sufficiently to give anomalous colours.

Principles of Polarisation Microscopy and Explanation of the Optical Properties of Amyloid Stained by Congo Red

Birefringence

Parts of Congo red-stained amyloid appear bright and coloured between crossed polariser and analyser (Fig. 13.2). The brightness is because the orientation of Congo red molecules on amyloid fibrils makes the Congo red molecules birefringent. This means that they have an asymmetrical arrangement of components that affect the velocity of light as it passes through. The refractive index is the velocity of light in air or a vacuum compared with the velocity in a material. A birefringent material has two extremes of refractive index, because light passing through one axis travels more slowly, giving a higher refractive index, than light passing through the axis perpendicular to this. These are called the slow axis and the fast axis. The birefringence is measured as the difference between the refractive indices of the two axes.

When linearly polarised light passes through a birefringent material with its axes at 45° to the plane of the light, the light becomes elliptically polarised (Fig. 13.6). This means that an observer looking at the light source and able to detect just one light wave would see a change from a wave vibrating in one linear plane to a wave tracing an elliptical path. The size of the ellipse depends on the retardance, which is the birefringence multiplied by the thickness of the material. Thicker layers of a material give more pronounced birefringent effects. This is how thicker sections allow easier detection of these effects, and how the effects may not be detectable in thin sections. Some elliptically polarised light is able to pass the analyser because it is no longer only vibrating perpendicularly to the plane of the analyser, and the material appears bright against the dark background.

Elliptical polarisation occurs because a wave of polarised light entering a birefringent material with its axes at 45° to the plane of the light can be considered to be split into two vectors perpendicular to each other, one in the fast axis and the other in the slow axis. These take a different time to travel through the material. On leaving the material, the vectors recombine into one wave, but the tip of one vector lags behind the tip of the other vector in time and is vibrating in a different plane in space. The distance travelled in air by the tip of the vector in the fast axis before the tip of the vector in the slow axis emerges from the material is equal to the retardance, which can be measured.

Because the vectors are separated in time and space before recombining, the tip of their resultant combined wave is no longer vibrating only in the plane of the polariser, but appears to trace an elliptical path as it approaches the observer. This can be imagined to follow the shape of a corkscrew flattened from side to side, with either a clockwise or an anticlockwise helix (Fig. 13.6). Within the range of retardances that have ever been reported in Congo red-stained amyloid, the dimension of the ellipse in the plane of the analyser is proportional to the retardance. Larger retardances give a larger component in the plane of the analyser and potentially more transmittance of light by the analyser. For any particular retardance, the orientation of the fast and slow axes relative to the plane of the polariser determines the direction of rotation of the tip of the combined vector. This means that if the birefringent object is rotated by 90°, the ellipse has an opposite direction of rotation. Similarly, the direction of rotation is opposite in a part of the birefringent object with the fast and slow axes orientated at 90° to those elsewhere [3, 10].

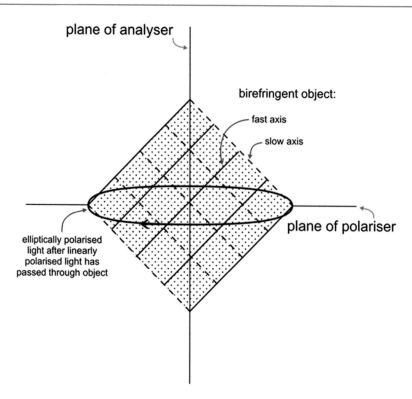

plane of analyser

birefringent object:

— fast axis

— slow axis

plane of polariser

elliptically polarised
light after linearly
polarised light has
passed through object

Fig. 13.6 Diagram showing production of elliptically polarised light from linearly polarised light, such as in orientated Congo red. When a light wave imagined to be coming towards the observer passes through a polariser and then through a birefringent material with its fast and slow axes at 45° to the plane of the polariser, there is a change from linear to elliptical polarisation. This allows transmittance of some light by a crossed analyser. For the retardances of Congo red, the retardance determines the size of the ellipse in the plane of the analyser and the orientation of the fast and slow axes determines the direction of rotation of the elliptically polarised light. Reproduced from Bull R C Path. October 2008;144:263–6 with permission

This production of elliptically polarised light is the mechanism that explains how some light can be transmitted by a crossed analyser, rather than other suggested mechanisms, which are insignificant in Congo red-stained amyloid. One erroneous suggestion was a change of the plane of linearly polarised light by optical rotation, also called optical activity, but this is too slight to have any detectable effect in sections, no matter how thick [3, 10].

Birefringent effects are most marked when the fast and slow axes of the material are orientated at 45° between the planes of the crossed polariser and analyser, and decline away from this position, if there is rotation of either the material or a polarising filter, for example. Birefringent effects disappear when the axes are parallel and perpendicular to the planes of polarisation (Fig. 13.7).

This is because the light can no longer be split into vectors in both the fast axis and the slow axis, and explains how only some parts of randomly orientated Congo red-stained amyloid appear bright between crossed polariser and analyser (Fig. 13.2).

A birefringent material that has no colour on ordinary microscopy, such as unstained collagen, usually appears bright white under these conditions, because all wavelengths of light are elliptically polarised to virtually the same extent and are transmitted equally by the analyser. A coloured birefringent material, such as Congo red-stained amyloid, appears coloured under these conditions, although the colours seen are usually different from those seen in ordinary illumination, and are called anomalous colours. These colours appear because there is a differ-

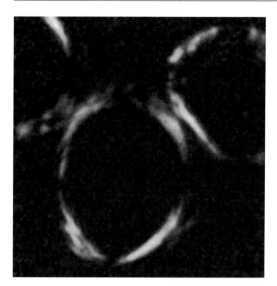

Fig. 13.7 Renal tubules stained by Congo red. Ordinary microscopy shows amyloid distributed uniformly in the circular basement membranes. When examined between accurately crossed polariser and analyser, as illustrated, an anomalous *green* colour with different amounts of brightness is seen, except at the four points on the circular objects that correspond with planes parallel and perpendicular to the planes of the polariser and analyser. *Pure green* is only seen in optically perfect conditions. Reproduced from Lab Invest. 2008;88:232–42 with permission

ence in how wavelengths of light are affected through the spectrum. There are two fundamental processes that interact to affect wavelengths transmitted by an analyser, which are absorption and anomalous dispersion of the refractive index, although another factor, compensation, is often a contributor to the final outcome.

Absorption

Absorption means a reduction in intensity of light. A coloured material has at least one absorption peak in the visible spectrum, and removal of the absorbed wavelengths from white light, or reduction of their transmittance, gives the observed colour in ordinary illumination. Congo red has an absorption peak at a wavelength of about 500 nm, which is in the blue/green part of the spectrum (Fig. 13.8). Removal of blue/green or green from white light gives red (Fig. 13.1).

Usually, absorption in a coloured material only occurs in one axis, and still occurs when that axis is at 45° to the plane of the polariser, although the amount of absorption is half that of the maximum absorption, when the axis is parallel to the polariser plane. When the absorbing axis is perpendicular to the polariser plane, the absorption is least. Variation of the amount of absorption depending on the plane of polarisation is called dichroism.

In linearly polarised light produced by use of either just a polariser or just an analyser, Congo red molecules orientated on amyloid fibrils have maximum absorption of light polarised parallel to fibrils, producing the deepest red colour, and minimum absorption of light polarised perpendicularly to fibrils, giving the weakest red colour, or even no colour. Although it is often difficult to see long, thick runs of parallel amyloid fibrils, because the fibrils are usually scattered randomly in tissues, if suitable parallel runs are present in a section that is examined with only a rotatable polariser or only a rotatable analyser, or when the section is rotated, the red colour of fibrils varies in intensity depending on the plane of polarised light. This dichroism of Congo red-stained sections is usually so weak that it is of no practical value in the study of amyloid [3, 10, 11].

Anomalous Dispersion of the Refractive Index

Birefringence has usually been postulated as the explanation of green in Congo red-stained amyloid between crossed polariser and analyser, and other colours have often been overlooked. Generally, either there has been no attempt to explain exactly how birefringence could give green or other colours, or attempts to explain this have been confused and scientifically unsatisfactory. For example, suggestions are wrong that interference colours are produced resembling those seen in soap bubbles. The retardance of Congo red-stained amyloid is too small to produce interference colours [3, 10].

The main reason for unsatisfactory explanations is a failure to realise the significance of

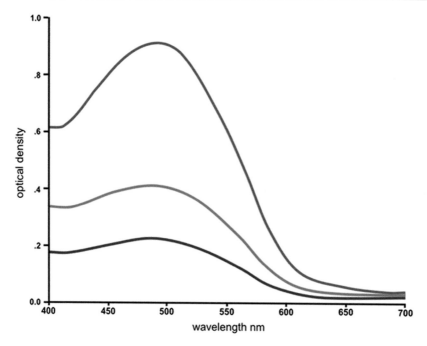

Fig. 13.8 Optical density of Congo red at different wavelengths and at various orientations. Optical density is a measure of absorption on a logarithmic scale. The *uppermost curve* is that of Congo red orientated parallel to the plane of polarised light, with most absorption at about 500 nm in the *blue/green* part of the spectrum, giving the *deepest red* colour. The *lowest curve* is that of Congo red orientated perpendicularly to the polarised light, giving the least absorption and the weakest colour. The *middle curve* is that of Congo red orientated at 45° to the polarised light, giving absorption and colour halfway between the maximum and the minimum. Reproduced from Lab Invest. 2008;88:232–42 with permission

anomalous dispersion of the refractive index. This process is related to the absorption peak. The refractive index of the absorbing axis of a coloured, birefringent material is not constant through the spectrum, but falls to a low value on the shortwave side of an absorption peak and rises to a high value on the longwave side, falling gradually after that. This is called anomalous dispersion of the refractive index. Meanwhile, the other axis which is not absorbing light has a relatively constant refractive index, between the lowest and highest values of the refractive index in the absorbing axis (Fig. 13.9).

Anomalous dispersion is a property of all materials that transmit light, including Congo red, although materials that are colourless are not absorbing in the visible spectrum and do not show anomalous dispersion in visible wavelengths. As a result of anomalous dispersion, the birefringence of orientated Congo red, which is the difference between the refractive indices of

the two axes, varies with wavelength (Fig. 13.10). The absolute difference is greatest around the absorption peak, approximately equally on both shortwave and longwave sides of the peak, and so the ellipses of light produced by birefringence are largest around the peak. If absorption did not occur, wavelengths on both sides around the absorption peak would be most transmitted by a crossed analyser. In fact, absorption does occur, as explained later in this section.

There is also a change in sign of birefringence. The sign is said to be positive if the higher refractive index, or slow axis, is parallel to a distinctive feature, in this case the orientation of the long axis of amyloid fibrils. If the higher refractive index is perpendicular to that feature, the birefringence is negative. At wavelengths above the absorption peak of Congo red, the higher refractive index is in the axis parallel to amyloid fibrils, which is the absorbing axis, and the birefringence is positive. At wavelengths below the peak, the

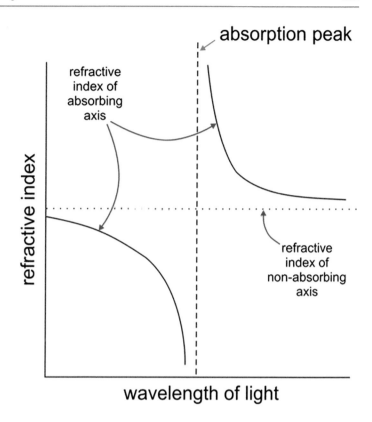

Fig. 13.9 Diagram showing anomalous dispersion of the refractive index around the absorption peak in the absorbing axis of a coloured, birefringent material, such as orientated Congo red, and the relatively constant refractive index of the non-absorbing axis. The birefringence is the absolute difference between the refractive indices of the two axes. This is maximum on both sides around the absorption peak, and also changes sign as the higher refractive index changes from one axis to the other. Reproduced from Bull R C Path. October 2008;144:263–6 with permission

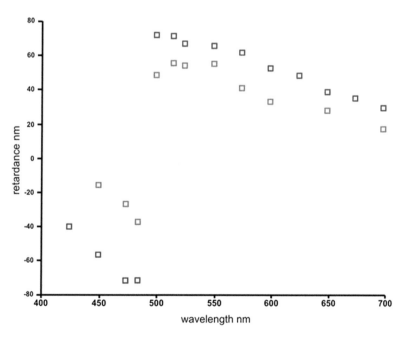

Fig. 13.10 Birefringence of orientated Congo red, expressed as retardance measured by use of an elliptical compensator, at various wavelengths of light. *Red boxes* are measurements on smears and *green boxes* are measurements on amyloid fibrils. Birefringence is maximum on both sides around the absorption peak, with a change of sign from negative at wavelengths below the peak to positive above the peak. Both signs of birefringence can transmit light through a crossed analyser. Reproduced from Lab Invest. 2008;88:232–42 with permission

axis with the higher refractive index is the non-absorbing axis, which is perpendicular to the amyloid fibrils, and the birefringence is negative (Figs. 13.9 and 13.10).

The change of sign means that without moving the section, the slow and fast axes exchange positions relative to the plane of the polariser, depending on the wavelength relative to the absorption peak. This is similar to the exchange of positions of the slow and fast axes relative to the plane of the polariser at any wavelength in any birefringent object when the section is rotated by 90°, although in that case the birefringence does not change sign. Because the orientation of the slow and fast axes in relation to the plane of the polariser affects the direction of rotation of elliptically polarised light (Section 'Birefringence'), the direction of rotation is opposite for wavelengths above and below the absorption peak. Both these directions of rotation of elliptically polarised light can be transmitted simultaneously and can be passed by a crossed analyser.

Contrary to a widespread opinion, the green that may be seen in Congo red-stained amyloid between crossed polariser and analyser is not produced by pure birefringence, without any other mechanism. Accordingly, 'green birefringence' is a misleading description of it, even when pure green is seen, which is uncommon [11]. This is because even when arranged at 45° to the polariser plane, orientated Congo red absorbs light, although only half the maximum amount (Fig. 13.8). Birefringence and absorption interact to produce the spectrum of wavelengths transmitted by a crossed analyser (Fig. 13.11). This observed spectrum is different from that expected from birefringence alone. Peaks of optical density, which is a measure of absorption and the inverse of transmittance, in violet wavelengths, around 400 nm, and red wavelengths, around 700 nm, give light which is perceived as green (Fig. 13.7).

The green light is produced by a mixture of yellow and blue light. Any green shade can be matched by an appropriate mixture of yellow and

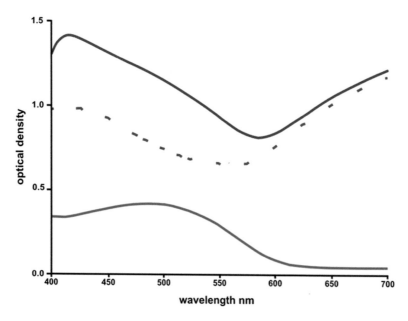

Fig. 13.11 The measured absorption curve of Congo red orientated at 45° to the polarised light between accurately crossed polariser and analyser (*uppermost line*). This corresponds to the observed *green* colour (Fig. 13.7), but does not resemble the curve expected from birefringent effects alone (*middle interrupted line*). This is because there is absorption of some wavelengths by Congo red (*lowest line*). Reproduced from Lab Invest. 2008;88:232–42 with permission

blue. In general, yellow is produced by absorption or non-transmittance of at least some violet or blue wavelengths. In the case of Congo red between crossed polariser and analyser, yellow is the net result of transmittance of wavelengths above the absorption peak, all with the same direction of rotation of elliptical polarisation produced by positive birefringence, but with different sizes of ellipses and modification by absorption. Similarly, in general, blue is produced by absorption of at least some yellow, orange or red wavelengths, and in the case of Congo red, blue is the net result of transmittance of wavelengths below the absorption peak to different extents, by the combination of negative birefringence and absorption.

The observer, able to see only one colour when blue and yellow are transmitted at the same point, and unable to distinguish directions of rotation of elliptically polarised light, blends the colours to see a shade of green (Fig. 13.7). The three colours, blue, yellow and green, are the outcome of interaction between birefringence and absorption, and only guesswork can give an idea of what shades they would be if just birefringence explained them, which is the only mechanism usually suggested.

Absorption or non-transmittance of wavelengths towards both ends of the spectrum is necessary to give green. This fact eliminates some suggested mechanisms of the production of green in Congo red-stained amyloid, such as the removal of only red wavelengths by interference between the slow and fast axes, which would give blue, even if it could happen in the way postulated [3].

Experimentally, thicker sections of Congo red-stained amyloid than are ever likely to be used in practice, perhaps more than 20 μm thick or so, can give a change of pure colour between crossed polariser and analyser from green to yellow, or even to orange or red, if sections are thick enough. This is from increasing dominance of absorption of blue and green wavelengths over birefringent effects at these wavelengths, leaving an increase in birefringent effects at longer wavelengths. The effect is unlikely to be noted in everyday microscopy,

although it may be the explanation of some pure colours other than green in illustrations [11]. Different thicknesses throughout a section are not the explanation that has been suggested for the green and yellow that may be seen simultaneously (Fig. 13.2). If this were so, the colours would not exchange positions as the section is rotated [3, 10].

In sections of usual thicknesses, orange and red cannot be produced by the combination of birefringent effects and absorption when there is accurate crossing of polariser and analyser. If this appears to have happened, these colours are never seen on their own, and are combined with shades of green inevitably lighter than when green is seen on its own. The explanation, given in detail later (Section 'Effect of Uncrossing of Polariser and Analyser'), is that the polariser and analyser are not in fact accurately crossed.

Compensation

Green is only seen in ideal conditions in Congo red-stained amyloid between crossed polariser and analyser (Fig. 13.7). Usually, there is more than one colour (Fig. 13.2). This is because some wavelengths are affected by the mechanism called compensation.

If elliptically polarised light of particular wavelengths with one direction of rotation interacts with elliptically polarised light of the same wavelengths but opposite direction of rotation, the ellipses are partially reduced or completely converted to linearly polarised light, depending on the relative size of the ellipses. The linearly polarised light is in the plane of the polariser, and so cannot be passed by a crossed analyser. This is compensation, which has the effect of reducing or abolishing the amount of light of the affected wavelengths that is transmitted by an analyser. Ellipses with opposite directions of rotation can only interact and produce compensation if they are of the same wavelengths. This is how wavelengths on opposite sides of the absorption peak do not compensate each other and can be transmitted simultaneously, even though their ellipses

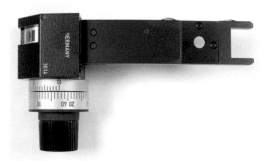

Fig. 13.12 An elliptical compensator. The long arm can be inserted in a slot on some microscopes between the objective lens and the analyser. The small round opening in this contains a transparent, colourless, birefringent plate that can be rotated in the light path using the knob, which has a graduated dial to show the angle and direction of rotation. Reproduced from Bull R C Path. October 2008;144:263–6 with permission

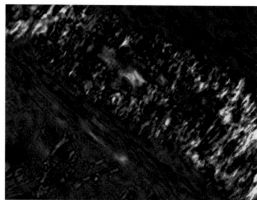

Fig. 13.13 A section of an artery containing amyloid stained by Congo red, between accurately crossed polariser and analyser, with insertion and adjustment of an elliptical compensator to give *yellow* and *blue*. These colours exchange positions either if the slide is rotated or when the compensator is rotated to the same extent the opposite way, in which case there is a stage during rotation of the compensator when *pure green* is seen. This shows that *yellow* and *blue* are both transmitted and blend to give *green*, as in Fig. 13.7, provided there is no additional birefringence in the light path that compensates the colours partially or completely. Reproduced from Bull R C Path. October 2008;144:263–6 with permission

have opposite directions of rotation (Section 'Anomalous Dispersion of the Refractive Index').

Anything transparent that introduces birefringence into the light path in a microscope may produce compensation. This could be introduced accidentally by birefringence called strain birefringence in stressed glass such as in glass slides, cover slips, condenser lenses and objective lenses. Most microscopes have strain birefringence in some optical components. Birefringence could also be introduced deliberately by use of the piece of optical apparatus mentioned earlier (Section 'Polarisation Microscopy of Amyloid Stained by Congo Red'), called a compensator (Fig. 13.3). One type of such equipment is an elliptical compensator, which has a colourless birefringent plate of known retardance (Fig. 13.12). This device can be fitted on some microscopes between the objective lens and the analyser, and can be adjusted by rotation of the birefringent plate to give polarised light of variable ellipticity and variable direction of rotation of the ellipse. An elliptical compensator can be used to measure the retardance of materials such as orientated Congo red, and to determine the sign of the birefringence (Fig. 13.10) [3, 10].

The anomalous pure green colour only appears in perfect optical conditions because there is uniform blending of blue and yellow light throughout the microscopic field. Anomalous colours other than green appear because additional birefringence in the light path, introduced either accidentally or deliberately, compensates the effects of the birefringence of Congo red, either partially or completely. The materials giving additional birefringence are usually colourless and so do not show anomalous dispersion within the visible spectrum (Section 'Anomalous Dispersion of the Refractive Index'). As a result, all wavelengths are converted by these materials to elliptically polarised light to virtually the same extent and with the same direction of rotation, and so any wavelength is potentially compensatable, depending on the size and direction of rotation of its ellipse.

The wavelengths giving blue light may be partially or completely compensated, allowing yellow to dominate to different extents. This gives yellowish green or yellow/green or even yellow. The opposite direction of elliptically polarised light produced by compensation allows blue to dominate, giving bluish green or blue/green or blue. Compensation cannot add colours that are not already being transmitted, but can only remove them to different extents (Fig. 13.13).

Effects of compensation of blue and yellow can be seen in a section at different sites, depending on the orientation of Congo red molecules and the orientation of the compensating birefringence, meaning the relative orientation of their fast and slow axes (Figs. 13.2 and 13.13). Different extents of the effects may be seen if compensation is not uniform across a microscopic field. Objective lenses may have different amounts of strain birefringence, which explains how changing the lens may change the colours.

The reason that the different colours are seen in areas roughly perpendicular to each other, appear to rotate as the section is rotated and exchange positions when the stage is rotated by 90° is because the elliptical light produced by either strain birefringence or birefringence of a compensator has a direction of rotation that at some positions of the orientated Congo red compensates the yellow light, and at other positions compensates the blue light (Figs. 13.2 and 13.13).

A pure green colour may occasionally be seen on an ordinary microscope if conditions happen to be ideal, but to produce pure green may need introduction and adjustment of a compensator (Fig. 13.3). This uses the compensator to counteract effects of strain birefringence and give balanced transmittance of yellow and blue seen as green, but this is unnecessary in everyday microscopy. Alternatively, but equally unnecessarily, if detection of pure green is considered essential, a microscope specifically designed for polarisation microscopy may be used with optical components free from strain birefringence, but even on this there may be strain birefringence in slides or cover slips.

This account of the optical physics explains how there is no need to see only green, or even any green if there are yellow and blue, to make a diagnosis of amyloid, because the various anomalous colours are themselves characteristic of amyloid stained by Congo red. The idea that green is essential for the diagnosis is not entirely correct. This is proved unintentionally by many authors in their illustrations in papers on Congo red [11].

Effect of Uncrossing of Polariser and Analyser

There are colour changes when either the polariser or the analyser is rotated from the crossed position (Figs. 13.4 and 13.5). These changes have been said to be related to the optical activity of Congo red, but this is wrong, as mentioned before (Section 'Birefringence') [3]. The explanation is that birefringent effects progressively weaken, more light is transmitted directly, the background lightens and the plane of polarisation is altered relative to the orientation of Congo red molecules, which for maximum birefringent effects are at 45° to the planes of the polariser and analyser (Section 'Birefringence'). The plane of polarisation moves closer to being parallel to the absorbing axis of some molecules, which absorb progressively more light, and so approach their deepest red colour (Fig. 13.8). As birefringent effects decline, the transmittance of yellow and blue declines, and these colours gradually mix with red until they are overpowered by it. The transmitted colour changes from green in ideal conditions through yellow and orange to red [10].

Elsewhere, the plane of polarisation becomes perpendicular to other Congo red molecules, which absorb less light and become more nearly colourless, while the transmittance of yellow and blue declines. The transmitted colour changes from green in ideal conditions through blue/green and bright white to colourless. When the polariser and analyser are parallel, there are no birefringent effects, but only dichroic effects, which can scarcely be detected (Section 'Absorption'). Detection of birefringent effects against a dark microscopic field is much easier than either detection of dichroic effects against a light background or detection of small amounts of amyloid on ordinary microscopy.

If compensation gives more than one colour between crossed polariser and analyser, modification of the colours by progressive uncrossing of polariser and analyser can produce a wide range of anomalous colours. These differ depending on whether the uncrossing is one way or the other, unlike the symmetrical effects that should be seen if there is initially just a pure green colour. Yellow/green or yellow passes through orange when uncrossing is one way, and through greenish white when uncrossing is the other way, while blue/green or blue passes through light blue/green when uncrossing is one way, and through purplish red when uncrossing is the other way, with various intermediate shades and other combinations (Figs. 13.4 and 13.5) [10]. Uncrossing of polariser and analyser explains many of the combinations of colours, including green and red, seen in illustrations. This emphasises that the insistence on green alone is not supported by theory or practice [11].

Description of the Effects Seen

Various anomalous colours other than the anomalous pure green are seen in Congo red-stained amyloid between crossed or partially uncrossed polariser and analyser (Figs. 13.2, 13.3, 13.4, 13.5, 13.7 and 13.13). These are just as typical of Congo red-stained amyloid as pure green, and the best way to describe the effects is to include the words anomalous colour or colours.

Simple ways to report the findings are to say that in the unusual event that green alone is seen there is an anomalous green colour between crossed polariser and analyser, or, which is more likely, that typical anomalous colours are seen between crossed polariser and analyser, or, as a less detailed term to cover study including uncrossing of polariser and analyser, which is almost always done in practice, that characteristic anomalous colours are seen on polarising microscopy.

As descriptions of these findings, the widely used terms 'green birefringence', 'apple green birefringence', 'green polarisation colour' and similar have uncertain origins, but are deeply embedded in the amyloid literature, apparently because of reinforcement by repetition and habit. A consequence is that many observers think that they must see and report what they expect to see and report, rather than what they actually see. Another consequence is that observers think that other colours are irrelevant and should be overlooked [11].

One investigator into Congo red staining of amyloid, representative of those who seem to have had a profound, indirect, misleading influence on others, was Hans-Peter Missmahl (1920–2008). In various papers and meetings, he insisted that only green should be seen, that an ordinary microscope with a polariser and an analyser was not suitable for this purpose and that the finding of any other colour was an error. This type of rigid idea of what should be found is widespread and is at least partly based on persistent misquotation of previous work. Missmahl and others claimed that some early papers reported green, although these papers did not mention a colour. In fact, the earliest paper to report any colour described yellow and green, but this was not mentioned by Missmahl, who quoted the paper [3]. Another instance of the lack of scientific rigour and consistency in Missmahl's rules is that even he did not show only green in illustrations of Congo red-stained amyloid [11, 12].

Missmahl's views appear to show an incomplete understanding of the optical physics. An example is that he did not seem familiar with anomalous dispersion of the refractive index and seemed unaware of the change of sign of birefringence around an absorption peak, which explains many of the otherwise inexplicable optical properties of Congo red (Figs. 13.9 and 13.10). Another example is that he asserted that absorption was undetectable and had no contribution to the colour seen between crossed polariser and analyser, although if this were true, a section of Congo red-stained amyloid would have no colour in ordinary illumination (Figs. 13.8 and 13.11). Additional objections to his views, and to those of others, are given above in various parts of the text, and there is further discussion of them elsewhere [3, 10, 11].

Summary of the Procedure to Diagnose Amyloid Using Congo Red

Sections of tissue preferably at least 5 μm thick should be stained by Stokes' method or a similar method, along with a control section known to contain amyloid [13]. On ordinary microscopy, amyloid appears red or a closely related colour (Fig. 13.1). If amyloid is suspected, or if exclusion of amyloid is required, a polariser and an analyser should be inserted into the light path of the microscope, and adjusted by rotation until they are accurately crossed, which is the point at which the background is darkest. The light intensity should now be increased to maximum, and the condenser aperture should be reduced to minimum.

On most microscopes, amyloid shows combinations of anomalous colours, namely, blue/green and yellow/green, or green and yellow, or blue and yellow, but sometimes pure green may be seen (Figs. 13.2 and 13.3). The colours appear to rotate and exchange positions if the section can be rotated on the microscope stage. If the polariser and analyser are then progressively uncrossed by rotation of one of them, the background becomes lighter and other combinations of anomalous colours appear, such as orange and light blue/green, which change with further rotation of the polariser or analyser, or when the polariser or analyser is rotated the opposite way, or if the section is rotated (Figs. 13.4 and 13.5). The colours progress to red and colourless.

The various anomalous colours are characteristic of orientated Congo red molecules such as in Congo red-stained amyloid, and can be explained by the principles of optical physics. They can be accepted as genuine, respectable and helpful findings, rather than artefacts or technical errors that should be ignored [3, 10, 11]. A routine microscope with a polariser and an analyser, one of which can be rotated, is all that is required for the everyday diagnosis of amyloid.

References

1. Bennhold H. Eine spezifische Amyloidfärbung mit Kongorot (a specific staining of amyloid with Congo red). Münch Med Woch. 1922;69:1537–8.
2. Bennhold H. Über die Ausscheidung intravenös einverleibten Kongorotes bei den verschiedensten Erkrangungen insbesondere bei Amyloidosis (on the elimination of intravenously absorbed Congo red in various diseases, in particular in amyloidosis). Deut Arch Klin Med. 1923;142:32–46.
3. Howie AJ, Brewer DB. Optical properties of amyloid stained by Congo red: history and mechanisms. Micron. 2009;40:285–301.
4. Aterman K. A pretty *a vista* reaction for tissues with amyloid degeneration. 1875: an important year for pathology. J Hist Med. 1976;31:431–47.
5. Aterman K. A historical note on the iodine-sulphuric acid reaction of amyloid. Histochemistry. 1976;49:131–43.
6. Horobin RW, Kiernan JA. Conn's biological stains. 10th ed. Oxford: BIOS Scientific; 2002. p. 132–4.
7. Puchtler H, Sweat F, Levine M. On the binding of Congo red by amyloid. J Histochem Cytochem. 1962;10:355–64.
8. Stokes G. An improved Congo red method for amyloid. Med Lab Sci. 1976;33:79–80.
9. Wright JR, Calkins E, Humphrey RL. Potassium permanganate reaction in amyloidosis: a histologic method to assist in differentiating forms of this disease. Lab Invest. 1977;36:274–81.
10. Howie AJ, Brewer DB, Howell D, Jones AP. Physical basis of colors seen in Congo red-stained amyloid in polarized light. Lab Invest. 2008;88:232–42.
11. Howie AJ, Owen-Casey MP. Discrepancies between descriptions and illustrations of colours in Congo red-stained amyloid, and explanation of discrepant colours. Amyloid. 2010;17:109–17.
12. Heller H, Missmahl HP, Sohar E, Gafni J. Amyloidosis: its differentiation into peri-reticulin and peri-collagen types. J Pathol Bacteriol. 1964;88:15–34.
13. Picken MM. Generic diagnosis of amyloid: a summary of current recommendations and the editorial comments on chapters 13–16. In: Picken MM, Herrera GA, Dogan A, editors. Amyloid and related disorders: surgical pathology and clinical correlations. New York: Springer; 2015.

Diagnosis of Minimal Amyloid Deposits by Congo Red Fluorescence and Amyloid Type-Specific Immunohistochemistry: A Review

14

Reinhold P. Linke

Introduction and Overview

Recent technical advances in the acquisition of biopsy material from almost every human organ have meant that pathologists are increasingly confronted by the need to quickly and accurately diagnose deposits of amyloid in tissues. Furthermore, significant improvements in the treatment of amyloidoses have increased the awareness of clinicians, and this has meant that the proportion of undiagnosed amyloidotic conditions has been declining in comparison to earlier times, when amyloid was considered an "untreatable disease." The ongoing discovery of novel amyloid diseases that are based on different amyloidotic proteins also seems to be important; currently, almost 30 pathogenetically different amyloid types have been distinguished on the basis of their individual amyloid proteins [1]. This necessarily implies that the amyloid protein type must be identified precisely in routine clinicopathologic practice. Amyloidosis cannot be diagnosed definitively based on risk factors such as blood constituents, genetic mutations, or preceding diseases: diagnosis must be based on

the examination of tissue. The examination of Congo red-stained sections under polarized light is the current "gold standard" for diagnosis of amyloid, and all other stains/techniques must be verified by comparison to this "gold standard." The purpose of this review is to show how *amyloid can be diagnosed reliably,* and *with high sensitivity,* using Bennhold's Congo red (CR) procedure [2] as modified by Puchtler et al. [3]. This has resulted in a considerable enhancement of the sensitivity of detection [4, 5] with attendant benefit for the patient [6]. It will be shown that the classical CR-staining method [3] can be quite insensitive in routine practice and that this shortcoming can be overcome by combining the CR stain with fluorescent illumination (CRF) and a second immunohistochemical staining, performed as an "overlay" technique and evaluated in bright-field illumination [4, 5]. This double stain enhances the specificity of the immunohistochemical typing of the amyloidoses [7, 8]; see also Chap. 17 of this book. The most important issues of this chapter are concerned with the pitfalls of the procedure, such as the role of quality of the biopsy and the phenomenon polarization shadow. Other problems, such as the role of sampling error in the assessment of tissue sections from patient biopsies, will also be discussed.

It should be emphasized that the *diagnosis of amyloid is not trivial, even when the additional and more sensitive enhancements of the CR method, described below, are incorporated.*

R.P. Linke, MD, PhD (✉)
Reference Center of Amyloid Diseases amYmed,
Innovation Center of Biotechnology,
Am Klopferspitz 19, Martinsried D-82152, Germany
e-mail: linke@amymed.de

© Springer International Publishing Switzerland 2015
M.M. Picken et al. (eds.), *Amyloid and Related Disorders*, Current Clinical Pathology,
DOI 10.1007/978-3-319-19294-9_14

Practical experience is the most important factor for successful diagnosis of amyloidosis. Moreover, since amyloidosis is only treatable successfully when diagnosed early, there is a need for rapid and reliable diagnosis by both the clinician and the pathologist.

Tissues and Congo Red Staining for the Diagnosis of Amyloid

Diagnosis of amyloid is based on the examination of tissue sections from biopsies or autopsies or smears from tissue aspirates. Clinicians who suspect amyloidosis typically obtain biopsy tissue from the heart, kidney, nerve, skin, and, most commonly, the gastrointestinal tract (minor salivary gland and in particular, the rectum, which is the most frequently biopsied site). Aspirates of subcutaneous abdominal fatty tissue are becoming increasingly common due to the ease of sampling and their proven diagnostic value. After routine processing, 4–8-μm-thick paraffin sections are collected onto charged slides, and the classical *CR-staining method* of Puchtler et al. [3] is strictly adhered to. Since the CR method is somewhat laborious, other stains and fluorochromes (i.e., Thioflavin S and T) have also been applied. Also, many other chemical stains used for diagnosing amyloid have been reviewed and discussed by Picken in this book (Chap. 16 and others). In addition to Puchtler's staining procedure, other modifications of Bennhold's method have been described by Highman [9], Romhányi [10], and Stokes [11].

Evaluation of Congo Red-Stained Sections and Pitfalls

CR-stained sections should be *evaluated by an experienced observer* and always using a positive control. An appropriate microscope, with a powerful light source, used in a dimmed room, is an essential requisite.

The classic CR method involves the evaluation of CR-stained sections under bright and polarized light; in this review, a more sensitive and enhanced version of the classic CR method,

involving immunohistochemistry and CR fluorescence, is described. The routine use of all three types of illumination, called "triple illumination" (bright-field, fluorescent, and polarized light) for the diagnosis of amyloid, has permitted the detection of even very minute deposits. Microscopic inspection of a positive control is used to check and adjust the light intensities used for triple illumination of the same amyloid deposits as shown in Fig. 14.1. In this figure, five different CR-stained tissues (A–E) are shown, each of which is presented in three different illuminations: (a) in bright light, (b) in fluorescent light, and (c) in polarized light.

In A (a), an autopsy tissue section of normal thickness (approximately 6 μm) displaying renal vascular amyloid is marked in red. In (b), the same frame is shown in CRF. Here, the entire amyloid-containing area shows bright orange-red fluorescence. In (c), the same frame is seen again under polarized light—here, the amyloid-containing areas only partially show the pathognomonic green birefringence (GB). Other sections of the amyloid-containing area are dark, show no birefringence, and are therefore said to be in the "polarization shadow," as indicated by the arrows in A(c) [7]. While in (a) and (c), this particular area, containing amyloid deposits, shows clear evidence of staining/fluorescence, it is partially obscured in (c). However, by rotating the slide table further, this area can also be shown to display GB [7].

In B (a), the rim of the subcutaneous fatty tissue aspirate (FTA) shows a somewhat reddish area suspicious for amyloid, which in (b) is clearly seen to produce very bright orange-red fluorescence by CRF. The diagnosis of amyloid is verified in (c) through GB, which is seen only in some parts of the amyloid deposits, while other parts are in the polarization shadow. Thus, in Fig. 14.1b, again *only CRF shows the full extent of the small amyloid deposits*. Under these conditions, smaller amyloid deposits could have been missed without CRF. CRF is particularly useful in specimens that contain very bright whitish collagen (such as FTA), which may mask the GB in polarized light (see Figs. 11.1–11.4 in [7]). When GB is not visible under such conditions (i.e.,

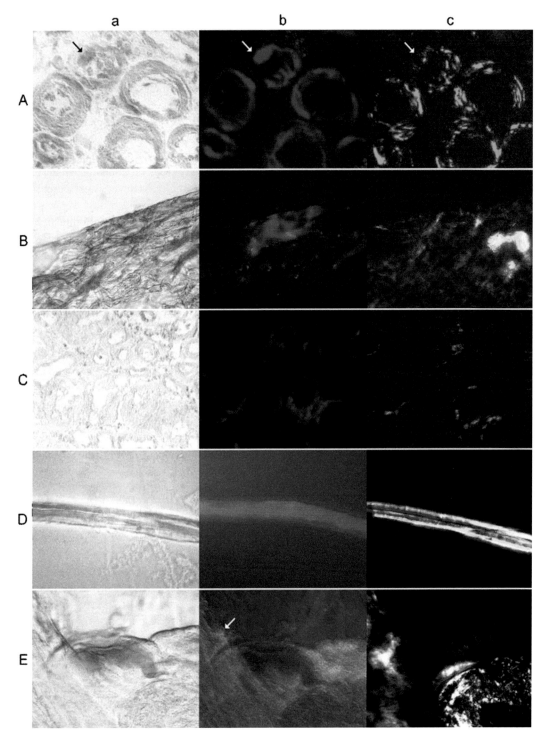

Fig. 14.1 Diagnosis of amyloid in fixed tissues after CR staining, as viewed under three different types of illumination ("triple illumination"), in order to demonstrate the detection of amyloid and the pitfalls that may be encountered therein. Five different tissues **A–E** were examined, and the same frame of each of the five was photographed under three different types of illumination: (a)–(c). **A** Diagnosis of renal amyloid in a normal renal tissue section (autopsy tissue). **B** Diagnosis of amyloid in a fatty tissue smear; the tissue is too thick. **C** Diagnosis of amyloid in a very thin section. **D** Fatty tissue smear with false-positive CRF. **E** Fatty tissue smear with a false-positive CR-stained section and a false-positive CRF. (a) Viewed in bright light for recognition of CR staining. (b) Viewed under CR fluorescent illumination (CRF). (c) Viewed *under* polarized light to show the presence of green birefringence (GB). The main point of this illustration is to show the diagnostic value of CRF in the diagnosis of amyloid with a high level of sensitivity and specificity and also for the exclusion of artifacts

when there is abundant bright collagen), amyloid cannot be *reliably* excluded. In contrast, since CRF can shine through moderately thick FTAs, a negative CRF result essentially excludes the presence of amyloid. Thus, CRF can add precision to the diagnosis of amyloid in tissue smears obtained from FTA or elsewhere.

C (a) shows renal biopsy tissue (of approximately 2 μm thickness) with very pale reddish amyloid that is hardly visible at all in bright light. Its full extent is only clearly visible through the application of CRF in (b) and is confirmed as amyloid by GB in (c). Here, again, amyloid deposits are only partially visualized by GB. Without CRF screening, smaller and, in particular, minute amyloid deposits can easily be overlooked.

D and E present FTAs that are prone to artifacts as a consequence of their thickness (such artifacts can also occur in tissue sections, but less frequently). Figure 14.1a–c shows that when CRF is negative, amyloid is, most likely, not present. However, when CRF is visible, it cannot be assumed that amyloid is present, unless its presence can be confirmed by GB. Thus, CRF must be verified by GB before the presence of amyloid is diagnosed. However, false-positive GB can also occur. In such instances, the concomitant absence of orange-red fluorescence by CRF (not shown in this report) is helpful. This underscores the central role of CRF for the precise diagnosis of amyloid in tissue sections.

In D (b), a bright, unidentified fiber displays an intense CRF signal but is not co-stained with CR in (a) and does not show GB in (c). Thus, the CRF result represents a false-positive signal.

Another artifact is seen in E (a), which shows a bright red deposit that, at the first glance, appears to resemble amyloid. However, since there is neither a CRF signal in (b) nor a GB signal in (c), the false positivity of the CR-stained section seen in bright light is apparent. In the left upper corner in E (b), there is a CRF signal, as indicated by a white arrow, which is false-positive since it yields neither a CR signal in bright light (a) nor a GB signal in polarized light (c). Summarizing the results obtained from Fig. 14.1, it can be concluded that CRF is very useful as a

screening method for the detection of amyloid deposits derived from all of the chemically different amyloids including artificial amyloids produced in vitro [5, 7]. An area that is identified as positive by CRF needs to be subsequently examined for the presence of amyloid using GB since the increased sensitivity of CRF also increases its lack of specificity (John H. Cooper, cited in [12]). The lack of specificity, however, is not a problem, since the artifacts can be identified as such and immediately excluded by triple illumination of the same frame in a tissue section. This is easily achieved by changing the light source while the same tissue frame remains in place. By this means, amyloid can easily be detected with high levels of both sensitivity and precision [5, 7].

Other problems can be encountered in sections that have been submitted for a second opinion or an "expert" opinion. Thus, sections may be very thin (as used in nephropathology) or (rarely) too thick or slashed due to an inappropriate biopsy technique. Sometimes, submitted, prestained tissue sections can appear overstained with Congo red, when the whole section will polarize green without discrimination. This situation arises, most probably, from a missed or inadequate differentiation step or the use of an inappropriate staining solution. More severe still is overstaining with hemalum on thicker sections: the hemalum can conceal the CR staining and GB. In these cases, CRF can be helpful since, to a certain extent, it can also "shine through" the overstained areas as a result of its very bright fluorescence (see above [7]).

It should be kept in mind that the pathognomonic GB seen by polarization microscopy (with appropriate equipment) can be demonstrated only in sections that are cut within standard thicknesses. When sections are below 1 μm in thickness, the anisotropy turns to bluish white, and when the thickness increases beyond the standard thickness, the green turns to yellow green and, with further increase, to yellow orange and finally red. All these colors are "specific for amyloid" [12]. Therefore, the pathognomonic characteristic of amyloid is most properly "colored anisotropy," while green birefringence is only a consequence of the standard thickness of paraffin sections as published by J. H. Cooper, reviewed in [7].

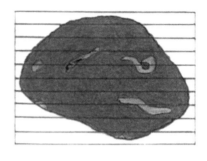

Sampling Error as a Major Pitfall

Sampling error is one of the most common pitfalls encountered in the diagnosis of amyloid and deserves a separate section since it remains largely unmentioned and underdiscussed. It is characterized by the perceived absence of amyloid in a biopsy tissue section in patients with amyloidosis . It occurs most often in small biopsies and, in particular, in the very early phases of amyloidosis, when amyloid is still sparse as a consequence of its uneven distribution in tissues and organs. Another important peculiarity that must be considered in the search for early amyloid deposits is that amyloid deposition may not begin at the same time in all organs or may not accumulate with equal speed and strength in all organs. This conclusion is based on the author's personal experience of experimental amyloidosis in mice. Since there is an organ preference in certain amyloid types, when abdominal fat (or other, "safer" sites used for screening) is negative for amyloid, one should consider obtaining biopsies from the most affected organs, such as heart, kidney, liver, etc. [13].

In the early stages of amyloidosis, the main question in small tissue sections that contain few amyloid deposits is as follows: *how representative is a single tissue section?* This situation is presented schematically in Fig. 14.2 where a small biopsy has been sectioned and the individual sections examined for amyloid. In Fig. 14.2, sections "Introduction and Overview," "Tissues and Congo Red Staining for the Diagnosis of Amyloid," "Minute Amounts of Missed Amyloids," "Identified and Classified," and "Take-Home Lessons" would yield a false-negative diagnosis. Also, in the absence of the increased sensitivity provided by CRF, the sparse amyloid deposits seen in sections "Evaluation of Congo Red-Stained Sections and Pitfalls" could be easily missed, possibly even during expert evaluation. It is also clear from Fig. 14.2 that the statement "no amyloid" without further qualifica-

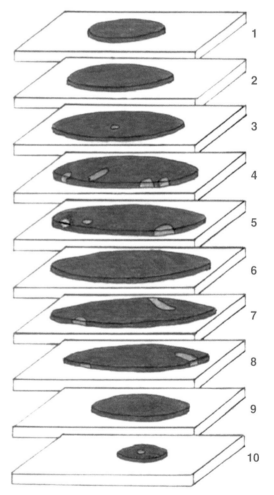

Fig. 14.2 Sampling error. A schematic illustration of how sampling error can occur in small biopsies with an uneven distribution of amyloid (seen most commonly in early amyloidosis). In this example, all sections of a small biopsy have been examined for amyloid (in *red color*) and presented in an enlarged view

tion is incomplete. Since *a negative amyloid diagnosis from a single tissue section can never be conclusive*, in cases where a single tissue section is found to be negative, ten or more additional sections from the biopsy should be examined [7, 13]. These examples should serve to raise awareness of the importance of sampling errors in general; sampling errors due to organ preference have also been reported [13]. Thus, a comment should be added that biopsies which contain a limited amount of amyloid may be subject to sampling error (as illustrated in Fig. 14.2).

Sampling error should also be considered when measuring the sensitivity of different methods for diagnosis of amyloid in tissue sections, and to avoid sampling errors, the same sections should always be evaluated when conducting interlaboratory comparisons (see Figs. 14.3, 14.4, 14.5, and 14.6). Finally, tissue sections that are prone to sampling errors, and which contain areas with variable amounts of amyloid, offer the possibility of measuring the sensitivity of various amyloid detection methods as shown in Fig. 14.5c (discussed below).

The Low Sensitivity of the Classical Congo Red Method and Possibilities for Improvements

The low sensitivity of the classical Congo red staining method in the diagnosis of amyloid has been shown in several different reports [7] and discussed in a retrospective study [4]. This low sensitivity of a method that is considered to be the "gold standard" for amyloid diagnosis represents yet another serious pitfall. The issue will be briefly illustrated here, showing how this fact was discovered and, most importantly, how the shortcomings can be overcome in certain clinical situations. As shown in Fig. 14.5c, the low sensitivity of the classic Congo red method can be overcome by the addition of CRF examination. In Fig. 14.3, the author would like to introduce the use of the double staining, i.e., of a combined Congo red stain and antibody immunohistochemistry (4) performed on the same section—also known as an "overlay technique." To illustrate this technique, a prior study by the author will be briefly summarized.

Prior to 1990, in central Europe, 2–5 % of children with juvenile rheumatoid arthritis succumbed to AA amyloidosis. Therefore, after proteinuria was diagnosed, frequent rectal biopsies were obtained in order to detect early amyloidosis. These rectal biopsies were examined by several nonspecialized laboratories (designated lab 1) using the classical CR-staining method. When proteinuria progressed and *rectal* biopsies were diagnosed as negative for amyloid by lab 1, *renal* biopsies were obtained and examined, also using the classical CR method; in addition, electron microscopic (EM) examination was performed in an expert laboratory (lab 2). Results showed that amyloid was rarely detected in rectal biopsies but was detected far more frequently in renal biopsies from the same patients.

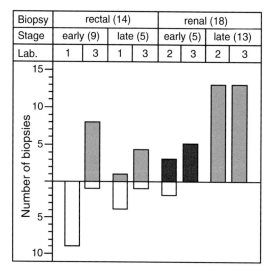

Fig. 14.3 Quality of diagnosis of amyloid (*shaded area*) shown by comparison of the results from three different laboratories using retrieved and reexamined biopsies of children with early amyloid who later developed full-blown amyloidosis [4, 6]. Lab 1 evaluated 14 rectal biopsies (unspecialized institutes of pathology using CR), lab 2 evaluated 18 renal biopsies (expert laboratory using EM), and lab 3 (reexamination of all 32 biopsies some years later) used CRIC (CR and immunohistochemistry double staining). Most of the rectal biopsies were early biopsies obtained at the beginning of the onset of systemic amyloidosis, and most of the renal biopsies were late biopsies. (Reproduced with written permission from Linke RP, Gärtner V, Michels H. High-sensitivity diagnosis of AA amyloidosis using Congo red and immunohistochemistry detects missed amyloid deposits. J Histochem Cytochem. 1995;43:863–9)

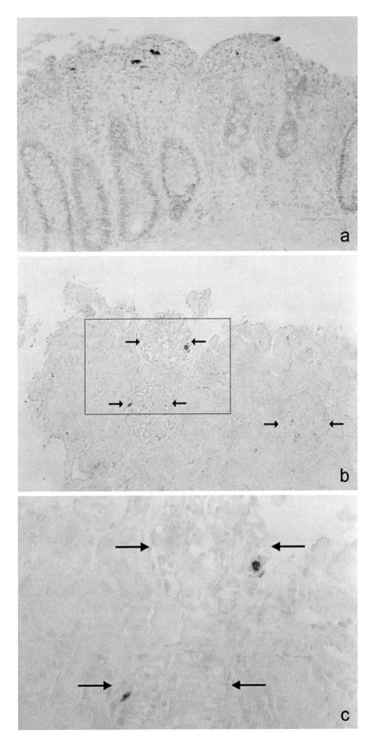

Fig. 14.4 High-sensitivity detection of early AA amyloid in children with rheumatoid arthritis, retrospective study using CRIC. This highly sensitive method identified extremely small amyloid deposits that were present in the early stages of AA amyloidosis that were originally missed at the time of biopsy (see text) since this CRIC method was developed only years later [4–6]. (**a**) Minute amyloid deposits of early amyloid detected by CRIC in the lamina propria of a rectal biopsy (*dark brown dots*). (**b**) Small glomerular amyloid deposits as detected by CRIC (low power, one glomerulus does not show amyloid). (**c**) The *boxed* area of (**b**) is magnified to better recognize the few amyloid spots and their site within the glomeruli (*glomeruli are indicated by arrows*). (Reproduced with written permission from Linke RP, Gärtner V, Michels H. High-sensitivity diagnosis of AA amyloidosis using Congo red and immunohistochemistry detects missed amyloid deposits. J Histochem Cytochem. 1995;43:863–9, modified)

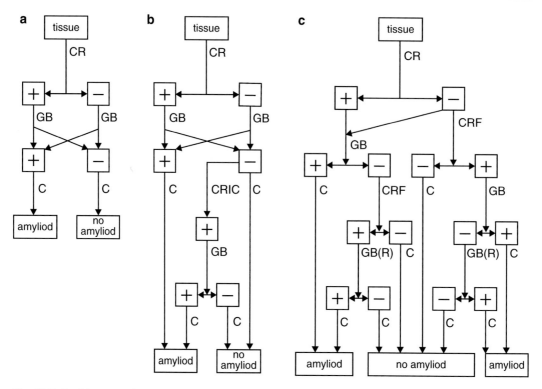

Fig. 14.5 Decision trees for the diagnosis of amyloid using the three different methods: CR in (**a**), CRIC in (**b**), and CRF in (**c**). The use of the trees is explained in the text. *CR* classic Congo red stain examined under bright light, *GB* green birefringence in Congo red stain exam- ined under polarized light, C final conclusion, *R* rotating slide table (Reproduced with written permission from Linke RP. Highly sensitive diagnosis of amyloid and vari- ous amyloid syndromes using Congo red fluorescence. Virchows Arch. 2000;436:439–48)

Noting this disparity, we obtained, from sev- eral different institutes, 14 rectal and 18 renal tis- sue blocks from 17 patients for reexamination in our laboratory (lab 3) years later. We used the classical CR method (performed previously by labs 1 and 2) as well as an enhanced technique where classical *CR* staining was combined with an immunohistochemical overlay (CRIC) using the murine monoclonal AA (mcl) antibody [7] on the same section.

As shown in Fig. 14.3, reexamination of the *rectal* biopsies using CRIC (lab 3) revealed amy- loid in 12 of 14 samples. In contrast, according to the medical records, amyloid was detected in only 1/14 rectal biopsies by lab 1 at the time of biopsy. In *renal* biopsies, reexamination using CRIC by lab three detected amyloid in *all* 18 samples, while, based on the medical records, by CR and EM (lab 2), amyloid was detected in 16

out of 18 samples. Both amyloids missed by CR and EM were from early amyloidosis.

Thus, CRIC, being the more sensitive assay, allowed a much earlier detection of amyloid than CR alone or CR combined with EM, and this time difference in the date of first detection could be measured retrospectively (in years). Examination using *CRIC in lab 3 detected amyloid 2–3 years earlier than CR alone in lab 1* [6]. The delayed diagnosis of amyloid in rectal biopsies by the classical CR method in lab 1 was also of con- siderable importance with respect to therapy and prognosis [6].

The conclusions from this retrospective study are as follows: (a) the CRIC method is far more sensitive when compared to the classical CR pro- cedure executed in nonspecialized labs (lab 1); (b) the high sensitivity of the EM technique did not counterbalance the low sensitivity of the

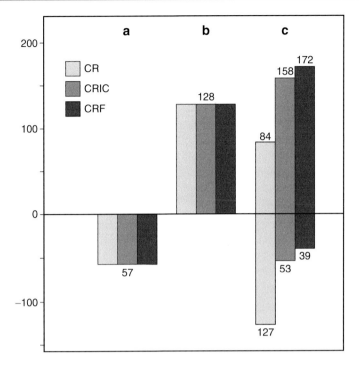

Fig. 14.6 Comparison of the sensitivity of the classical CR method (CR), CRIC, and CRF. Each method is marked with a different shading, as indicated in the inset. The columns above the zero line show the number of sections in which amyloid was detected, and the columns below the line show the number of sections without detection of amyloid using the respective method. (**a**) shows that the negative controls do not show amyloid with all three methods employed and (**b**) positive control shows that all three methods show amyloid. In (**c**), a tissue section with minute amounts of amyloid, and therefore prone to sampling error, has been examined with the three methods. The results differ according to the sensitivity of the method used. This comparison shows clearly that CRF is the method with the highest level of sensitivity for detecting amyloid and CR is the method with the lowest sensitivity (see text) (Reproduced with written permission from Linke RP. Highly sensitive diagnosis of amyloid and various amyloid syndromes using Congo red fluorescence. Virchows Arch. 2000;436:439–48)

classical CR method for detecting amyloid in two early renal biopsies; (c) CRIC is more sensitive than EM in early renal biopsies of patients with AA amyloidosis as a consequence of sampling error; (d) the two *expert laboratories* (labs 2 and 3) *seem to be far more precise than any of the unspecialized routine laboratories* (lab 1) using only the classical CR method; (e) examination using CRIC, in lab 3, detected amyloid deposits earlier; while (f) EM detected amyloid relatively late in the course of the disease, mainly due to sampling error in the early stages.

In summary, the CRIC method was able to detect the earliest amyloid deposits, and this occurred at the time of the first biopsy. As a consequence of this study [6], the routine early diagnosis of amyloid led to the early instigation of therapies employing anti-inflammatory and disease-modifying drugs and, as a result, no child subsequently developed fatal amyloidosis. Moreover, the belief that renal biopsies are more sensitive than rectal biopsies for the detection of amyloid and that, therefore, the former should be preferred was not supported by this study. The observed differences were not caused by the different sensitivities of the two types of biopsy but by the different times at which biopsies were taken. Thus, when similar high-sensitivity methods were compared in the detection of amyloid deposits in rectal versus renal biopsies, the differences were marginal [4]. In the study discussed above, in all cases where amyloidosis was missed initially, patients progressed to full-blown AA amyloidosis [6].

Minute Amounts of Missed Amyloids: Identified and Classified

The disadvantage of EM in the diagnosis of very early and tiny amyloid deposits is that only a very small tissue area can be screened for amyloid due to the *high level of magnification* employed. Even in cases where several tissue fragments are examined, this may not make up for the disadvantage imposed by the high magnification and the possible sampling error that this implies (see Fig. 14.2). In contrast, the advantage of CRIC lies in its ability to allow screening of the entire biopsy material (several sections) at *moderate magnification* and, thus, to detect all amyloid deposits present, no matter how minute. The sensitivity that can be achieved by CRIC in the detection of minute and early amyloid deposits is illustrated in Fig. 14.3. In an early *rectal* biopsy, amyloid was missed by lab 1, and in the corresponding early *renal* biopsy, amyloid was not diagnosed by an expert using EM (lab 2). Amyloid was detected in both biopsies by CRIC, as illustrated. In both cases, the patients progressed to full-blown AA amyloidosis [6].

The high sensitivity of this technique for detecting amyloid deposits, and the concomitant ability to classify even the smallest amount of amyloid with the highest level of sensitivity, is a major advantage of this method and has challenged the capabilities of mass spectrometry (see subsequent Chap. 17 on the typing of amyloidosis).

High-Sensitivity Diagnosis of Minute Amyloid Deposits with Congo Red Fluorescence

As shown in Fig. 14.3 above, in order to detect amyloid with increased sensitivity, the CRIC method requires a CR prestained tissue section with an immunohistochemical overlay stain [6]. Here, by definition, the amyloid type must be already known, or suspected, based on clinical grounds. This restriction does not apply when CR fluorescence (CRF) alone is being used [5]. The appearance of CRF is shown in Fig. 14.1 Ab–Eb,

illustrating the brilliant orange-red fluorescence that guarantees its high level of sensitivity. The fluorescence encompasses the whole area containing amyloid deposits. In contrast, GB highlights only a portion of the area containing amyloid at any given time (see "polarization shadow" above and in Fig. 14.1c) and, therefore, increases the possibility of missing small amyloidotic areas, unless the slide table is systematically rotated.

In order to determine the most sensitive method for detecting amyloid in tissue sections, three different techniques have been compared: the classical CR method, CRF, and CRIC, in that order [4, 5]. Using a large number of tissue sections, amyloid was diagnosed repeatedly, in double-blind studies, using decision trees for each of the different readings, as shown in Fig. 14.4. The number of tissue sections examined is shown in the columns of Fig. 14.5. After the classical CR staining, shown in Fig. 14.4a, only two steps are required: one detects the specific binding of CR to amyloid; the other is the verification of the presence of amyloid by GB, which is still the most common technique used in all laboratories. The initial step of the CRIC method (Fig. 14.4b) is like CR in Fig. 14.4a. However, in cases with negative GB (as in Fig. 14.4a), CRIC, with its much higher level of sensitivity, can detect areas which have been missed by CR alone. These areas are examined for amyloid by GB. In cases where areas of CR-stained sections fluoresce (showing CRF), as in Fig. 14.4c, the sections are then assessed for GB using polarized light, both with and without rotation (R) of the slide table.

The results obtained with the three different methods for diagnosing amyloid, as shown in Fig. 14.4a–c, are presented in Fig. 14.5 (the three different methods used are indicated by the three different shadings as shown by the inset of Fig. 14.5). In Fig. 14.5a the results on 57 sections without amyloid show that in no section amyloid could be detected regardless of the methods used (negative control). In addition, the 128 sections in Fig. 14.5b containing at least moderate amyloid deposits were all found to contain amyloid with all three methods employed (positive control).

When, however, 211 serial sections with very small to minute amyloid deposits that are prone to sampling error (see Fig. 14.2) were examined with the three methods, the results were quite different as compared to those of Fig. 14.5a, b. The differences between the three tests shown in Fig. 14.6c are obvious. They indicate a different cutoff at the edge of sensitivity characteristic for each method used (in Fig. 14.2, the amyloid in sections "Evaluation of Congo Red-Stained Sections and Pitfalls" and 10 could have been missed by CR alone). In these 211 sections, in Fig. 14.5c, the amount of amyloid was (different from the schematic view presented in Fig. 14.2) a continuum from no amyloid in 39 sections, with the most sensitive method CRF, to no amyloid in 127 sections with CR alone, the least sensitive method. Starting with the least sensitive method (in Fig. 14.5c), only 84 sections showed amyloid. An additional 74 cases were only detected by CRIC and CRF, and 14 further cases were only detected by CRF. These results demonstrate how insensitive the classical CR method really is and explains why the first biopsies in the earliest phase of AA amyloidosis had been missed in 90 % of cases [4]; see Fig. 14.3. It also demonstrates CRF as the most sensitive method to identify amyloid. The comparison of the sensitivity of all three combinations (CR-CRIC, CR-CRF, CRIC-CRF) was highly significant ($p < 0.001$). Therefore, based on this study, the ranking of the sensitivity of the detection methods for the diagnosis of amyloid is CR≪CRIC<CRF [5]. The full details are as follows: (a) CRIC is significantly more sensitive than CR, (b) CRF is significantly more sensitive than CR, and (c) CRF is significantly more sensitive than CRIC. The difference between CRF and GB is most probably caused by the relative inefficiency of GB on very small samples that are susceptible to the polarization shadow (see above), and in the case of CRIC, the immunohistochemistry overlay may reduce the level of GB [7]. Most importantly, CRF in Fig. 14.5c is the universal amyloid marker due to its higher sensitivity ($p < 0.001$ against CRIC) for the diagnosis of amyloid [5]. These results are consistent with the notion that amyloid can best be quantified by CRF [7]. CRF

illumination has also been used successfully for microdissection prior to mass spectrometry for amyloid typing [14].

Report for the Clinician

After diagnosing the presence of amyloid (and classifying the protein type; see Chap. 17 on amyloid typing), the clinician should receive a report comprising some, or all, of the following information:

1. The results obtained should be presented, and a note concerning the reliability of the technique(s), including the controls used, should be added.
2. The quality of the biopsy should be commented upon since this has a major impact on the quality of the diagnosis, e.g., in a rectal biopsy, was there a sufficient number of submucosal blood vessels?
3. Problems that could not be overcome should be mentioned.
4. Since a negative diagnosis can never be conclusive, a comment regarding the issue of *sampling error must be included*, stating whether additional sections were examined and, if so, their number.
5. The level of sensitivity of the method used for detecting amyloid should be mentioned. It should also be stated whether a high-sensitivity method was used to exclude sampling error caused by low-sensitivity detection methods. Chap. 20 provides a comprehensive overview of electron microscopy immunohistochemistry. In addition, several other chapters in this book use EM in the diagnosis of amyloid.

Take-Home Lessons

1. Amyloid can only be diagnosed by the identification of amyloid deposits in "tissues." Tissue sections of 4–8 μm (micrometer) thickness are best for diagnosing amyloid. Paraffin

sections are preferred due to ease of handling and long-term storage issues.

2. The identification of amyloid after use of a stringent CR-staining method is not trivial due to various possible pitfalls. Therefore, evaluation is best performed by expert laboratories. In case of difficulty, a second opinion, from another expert laboratory, should be obtained.

3. A negative amyloid diagnosis obtained from a single examined section can never be conclusive. Several measures need to be taken in such a case: (a) the sensitivity of detection of amyloid must be increased by the use of fluorescence microscopy using CRF or by using immunohistochemistry (when the type of amyloid is known) and (b) the number of examined sections must be increased to ten (or more) in order to exclude sampling errors.

4. Clinical information, including blood constituents, genetic mutations, or characteristic syndromes (carpal tunnel syndrome, macroglossia, cardiopathy, renal problems) can only be helpful in suspecting amyloidosis but cannot, in themselves, be conclusive as a diagnosis of amyloid.

5. High-sensitivity diagnosis of amyloid has now reached a level of sophistication where amyloid can be detected at its most incipient (and even preclinical) stages before severe organ damage has ensued.

6. This type of early detection is the most desirable time point for the initiation of causal therapy, when progression of the disease can best be avoided and even regression of an otherwise fatal disease can be observed.

7. Every amyloid deposit detected now needs to be typed at once for therapeutic considerations and prognostic information by the most reliable techniques available (see Chap. 18 on the typing of amyloid).

Acknowledgments For technical assistance, I thank Mrs. A. Meinel; for secretarial help, Mrs. A. Feix, both Martinsried/Germany; and for artwork, I thank Ms. A.K.M. Linke, Essen/Germany.

References

1. Sipe JD, Benson MD, Buxbaum JN, Ikeda S, Merlini G, Saraiva MJ, Westermark P. Amyloid fibril protein nomenclature: 2010 recommendations from the nomenclature committee of the International Society of Amyloidosis. Amyloid. 2010;17:101–4.
2. Bennhold H. Eine spezifische Amyloidfärbung mit Kongorot. Münchn Med Wochenschr. 1922;69:1537–8.
3. Puchtler H, Sweat F, Levine M. On the binding of Congo red by amyloid. J Histochem Cytochem. 1962;10:355–64.
4. Linke RP, Gärtner V, Michels H. High-sensitivity diagnosis of AA-amyloidosis using Congo red and immunohistochemistry detects missed amyloid deposits. J Histochem Cytochem. 1995;43:863–9.
5. Linke RP. Highly sensitive diagnosis of amyloid and various amyloid syndromes using Congo red fluorescence. Virchows Arch. 2000;436:439–48.
6. Michels H, Linke RP. Clinical benefits of diagnosing incipient AA amyloidosis in pediatric rheumatic diseases as estimated from a retrospective study. Amyloid. 1998;5:200–7.
7. Linke RP. Congo red staining of amyloid. Improvements and practical guide for a more precise diagnosis of amyloid and the different amyloidoses. In: Uversky VN, Fink AL, editors. Protein misfolding, aggregation and conformational diseases, Protein reviews (Atassi MZ, editor), vol. 4. New York, NY: Springer; 2006. p. 239–76. Chapter 11.1.
8. Linke RP. On typing amyloidosis using immunohistochemistry. Detailed illustrations, review and a note on mass spectrometry. Prog Histochem Cytochem. 2012; 47:61–132.
9. Highman B. Improved method for demonstrating amyloid in paraffin sections. Arch Pathol. 1964;41:559–62.
10. Romhányi G. Selective differentiation between amyloid and connective tissue structures based on the collagen-specific topo-optical staining reaction with Congo red. Virchows Arch Pathol Anat. 1971;354:209–22.
11. Stokes G. An improved Congo red method for amyloid. Med Lab Sci. 1976;33:79–80.
12. Cooper JH. Selective amyloid staining as a function of amyloid composition and structure. Histochemical analysis of the alkaline Congo red, standardized toluidine blue and iodine methods. Lab Invest. 1974;31:232–8.
13. Bandmann M, Linke RP. The diagnosis of amyloidosis may be hindered by the sampling error, and how to prevent it. In: Skinner M, Berk JL, Conners LH, Sheldon DC, editors. XIth International symposium on amyloidosis. Boca Raton, FL: CRC Press; 2007. p. 347–9.
14. Vrana JA, Gamez JD, Madden BJ, Theis JD, Bergen 3rd HR, Dogan A. Classification of amyloidosis by laser microdissection and mass spectrometry based proteomic analysis in clinical biopsy specimens. Blood. 2009;114(24):4957–9.

Thioflavin T Stain: An Easier and More Sensitive Method for Amyloid Detection

15

Maria M. Picken and Guillermo A. Herrera

Congo red, an erstwhile fabric dye, has been in use for the histological detection of amyloid since the early twentieth century. As presented in the preceding chapters, the Congo red staining procedure requires expertise and the use of polarized light microscopy; additionally, the dye's diagnostic "apple green birefringence" may be difficult to visualize and therefore show low sensitivity. Congo red is a direct dye with different affinities for fibrillar and nonfibrillar materials. The staining protocol involves staining followed by washing, which may lead to significant levels of background staining and lower reproducibility. In contrast, fluorogenic compounds become highly fluorescent only when they are bound to a particular molecular entity [1]. The examination of Congo red stains by fluorescence microscopy using a tetramethylrhodamine isothiocyanate (TRITC)/Texas red filter significantly enhances the detection of amyloid, especially small amounts [2–4]. Although this technique was

reported in the literature many years ago [5], it is still not routinely used.

In 1959, Vassar and Culling [6] described the use of the fluorochrome dye thioflavin T as a potent fluorescent marker of amyloid in histology. They noted that this dye selectively localized to amyloid deposits, thereupon exhibiting a dramatic increase in fluorescent brightness. They demonstrated that, upon binding to fibrils, thioflavin T displayed a dramatic shift of its excitation maximum (from 385 to 450 nm) and emission maximum (from 445 to 482 nm) and that thioflavin T fluorescence originated only from the dye bound to amyloid fibrils. The substantial enhancement of its fluorescence emission upon binding to fibrils makes thioflavin a particularly powerful and convenient tool. It has subsequently been shown that binding of the dye is linked to the presence of cross-β structure in the fibrils (recently reviewed in [1]). Since their first description, the thioflavins, in particular thioflavin T, have become among the most widely used compounds for staining amyloid fibrils, both in vivo and in vitro [1, 6–8]. The ability of thioflavin T and its derivatives to specifically recognize and bind to amyloid has served as a starting point for further derivatization and the elaboration of a number of alternative amyloid stains and clinical reagents, including some that are being tested for use in the medical imaging of amyloid in living patients [1]. Similar to Congo red stain, thioflavin T

M.M. Picken, MD, PhD (✉)
Department of Pathology, Loyola University Medical Center, Loyola University Chicago, Building 110, Room 2242, 2160 South First Avenue, Maywood, IL 60153, USA
e-mail: mpicken@luc.edu; MMPicken@aol.com

G.A. Herrera, MD
Department of Pathology, Louisiana State University Health Sciences Center, 1501 Kings Highway, 71103 Shreveport, LA, USA
e-mail: gherr1@lsuhsc.edu

© Springer International Publishing Switzerland 2015
M.M. Picken et al. (eds.), *Amyloid and Related Disorders*, Current Clinical Pathology,
DOI 10.1007/978-3-319-19294-9_15

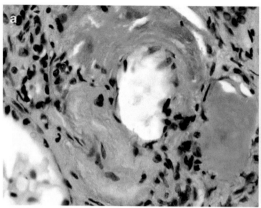

Fig. 15.1 (**a**) Vessel wall, with deposits of amyloid, in renal AL amyloidosis. Congophilia (*salmon-pink color*) is noted in the vessel wall, corresponding to amyloid deposits. *Congo red* stain, bright field. Magnification ×750. (**b**) Vessel wall with deposits of amyloid in renal AL amyloidosis. A distinct *bright yellow-green* fluorescence highlights the entire amyloid-containing area in the arteriolar wall; no equivalent to "polarization shadow" is seen (see Chap. 14). Thioflavin T stain viewed under fluorescein gate using a standard immunofluorescence microscope. Magnification ×700

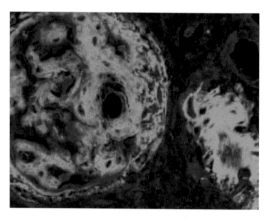

Fig. 15.2 Glomerulus with extensive amyloid deposition detected by strong fluorescence with thioflavin T stain. Note, also, staining of adjacent arteriolar wall. Thioflavin T stain viewed under fluorescent light. Magnification ×750

it detects even very small amounts of amyloid, where Congo red stain may be doubtful or negative (due in part at least to "polarization shadow" [[see Linke in Chap. 14]). Thioflavin stains, however, are not entirely specific for amyloid and stain other structures as well (including fibrin, keratin, intestinal muciphages, Paneth cells, zymogen granules, juxtaglomerular apparatus); hence, positive results obtained with thioflavin can be confirmed by either electron microscopy or the Congo red stain itself [5]. It should also be pointed out that false positive Congo red stains do occur (mostly congophilia alone without clear-cut apple green birefringence by polarization) due to red blood cells, thyroid colloid, and poorly cellular fibrous tissue [2], among others. Therefore, Thioflavin T and Congo red stains are best viewed as complementary of one another.

Thioflavin T Stain for Amyloid

A working solution of 0.5 % of thioflavin T in 0.1 N HCl (mixed well and filtered before use, aliquoted, and stored frozen as needed) is used. The sections are deparaffinized and rehydrated. Using a hydrophobic marker, the specimen section and an adjacent positive control section are

stains can be performed on both paraffin-embedded and frozen tissues but, unlike Congo red, thioflavin stains are not permanent, although faded sections can be restrained if necessary. Unlike Congo red stain, however, which can be tricky, the thioflavin stain is very easy to perform and the results are predictable, as well as being much easier to interpret. In the presence of amyloid, thioflavin T shows a bright yellow-green fluorescence (Figs. 15.1, 15.2, and 15.3). Another advantage of the thioflavin stain is that

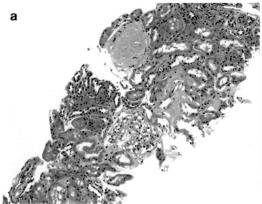

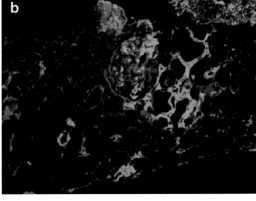

Fig. 15.3 (**a**) Eosinophilic, amorphous (hyaline) material corresponding to areas with amyloid deposition noted in the three renal compartments: glomerulus, interstitium, and extraglomerular vessels. Hematoxylin and eosin stain, original magnification ×350. (**b**) Distinct fluorescence highlighting amyloid deposits in the three renal compartments: glomerulus, interstitium, and extraglomerular vessels. Thioflavin T stain, original magnification ×350

encircled on the top of the slides. A drop of the working solution of thioflavin T is placed on the slides, which are subsequently kept in a humidity chamber for 15 min. The slides are rinsed in deionized water (for 5 min) and kept in deionized water while coverslipping with Aquamount. The frozen sections are rinsed two times in PBS (for 10 min each) prior to incubation with thioflavin T and, thereafter, rinsed sequentially in PBS and deionized water (for 5 min each) and coverslipped. Thioflavin stain is viewed under a fluorescein gate using a standard immunofluorescence microscope. Thioflavin T fluoresces only when bound to amyloid fibrils, where it shows a bright yellow-green fluorescence. In contrast, in the absence of amyloid deposits, the dye fluoresces faintly.

For amyloid diagnosis, ultimately, each pathology group should use the procedure(s) which work(s) best for them, that is, the histology laboratory is able to perform the stain(s) consistently and the pathologists know how to interpret it/them. Given the ease of staining, the predictability of stain outcome, and the ease of interpretation, adding thioflavin stain to the staining repertoire may be a welcome solution to problems that may arise from the use of Congo red stain in the clinical diagnosis of amyloid.

References

1. Biancalana M, Koide S. Molecular mechanism of Thioflavin-T binding to amyloid fibrils. Biochim Biophys Acta. 1804;2010:1405–12. Epub 2010 Apr 22.
2. Linke RP. Highly sensitive diagnosis of amyloid and various amyloid syndromes using Congo red fluorescence. Virchows Arch. 2000;436:439–48.
3. Picken MM. Modern approaches to the treatment of amyloidosis—the critical importance of early detection in surgical pathology. Adv Anat Pathol. 2013;20(6):424–39.
4. Clement CG, Truong LD. An evaluation of Congo red fluorescence for the diagnosis of amyloidosis. Hum Pathol. 2014;45:1766–72.
5. Puchtler H, Sweat F. Congo red as a stain for fluorescence microscopy of amyloid. J Histochem Cytochem. 1962;10:355–64.
6. Vassar PS, Culling CF. Fluorescent stains, with special reference to amyloid and connective tissues. Arch Pathol. 1959;68:487–98.
7. Hobbs JR, Morgan AD. Fluorescence microscopy with thioflavin-t in the diagnosis of amyloid. J Pathol Bacteriol. 1963;86:437–42.
8. Puchtler H, Waldrop FS, McPolan SN. A review of light, polarization and fluorescence microscopic methods for amyloid. Appl Pathol. 1985;3:5–17.

Fat Tissue Analysis in the Management of Patients with Systemic Amyloidosis

Johan Bijzet, Ingrid I. van Gameren, and Bouke P.C. Hazenberg

Introduction

About 100 years ago, Schilder observed amyloid to be frequently present in subcutaneous fat tissue in patients with amyloid A (AA) amyloidosis [1]. Forty years ago, Westermark and Stenkvist serendipitously used this knowledge for introducing the fine-needle biopsy of abdominal subcutaneous fat as an elegant and minimally invasive procedure to detect the presence of systemic AA amyloidosis [2–4]. Ten years later, the Boston group showed a similar high yield of amyloid detection (88 %) in patients with proven other types, i.e., immunoglobulin light chain (AL) and transthyretin-related (ATTR) types of systemic amyloidosis [5]. From that moment, the position of the abdominal subcutaneous fat tissue aspiration was established: it was advocated the simplest tissue biopsy technique—easily obtained at the bedside using readily available materials—with high sensitivity.

Aspiration Versus Biopsy

Initially aspiration was the method of choice to obtain fat tissue. However, the amount of fat tissue collected with the thin needle technique was usually very small and the material not suitable for standard histopathology. Therefore, it is not surprising that biopsy techniques were introduced, such as the Tru-Cut biopsy needle technique, producing much more fat tissue including blood vessels and allowing standard (immuno) histology to be performed [6]. A clear advantage of a biopsy over an aspirate is the preservation of the microarchitecture of the fat tissue visible in subsequent slices. Westermark introduced surgical (small knife) biopsies [7–9]. With this technique about 1 cm^3 of subcutaneous fat tissue is removed that can be used for (immuno)chemical analysis. However, biopsy techniques did not become popular and aspiration remained standard technique. The issue of too little material also became less important: adequate quantities of fat tissue (wet weight median 120 mg, ranging from 60 to 450 mg) can easily be obtained if a 16-gauge needle is used for aspiration instead of the narrower 18–23 gauge needles [10].

J. Bijzet • I.I. van Gameren • B.P.C. Hazenberg (✉)
Department of Rheumatology & Clinical Immunology, University Medical Center Groningen, University of Groningen, Hanzeplein 1, Groningen 9700 RB, The Netherlands
e-mail: j.bijzet@umcg.nl; i.i.van.gameren@umcg.nl; b.p.c.hazenberg@umcg.nl

© Springer International Publishing Switzerland 2015
M.M. Picken et al. (eds.), *Amyloid and Related Disorders*, Current Clinical Pathology,
DOI 10.1007/978-3-319-19294-9_16

Detection of Amyloid Using Congo Red-Stained Fat Tissue Specimens

The classic alkaline Congo red stain of Puchtler is a reliable standard staining technique of amyloid with low probability of false-positive results [11]. A positive Congo red stain with apple-green birefringence in polarized light continues to be the gold standard for detection of amyloid deposits in tissue [12]. Fluorescence microscopy may improve detection of minute Congo red-stained amyloid particles, which nevertheless must show apple-green birefringence [13]. In one publication, phenol Congo red staining enhanced the diagnostic value in a small number of patients, but this observation still needs confirmation [14]. Table 16.1 shows the sensitivity, specificity, positive predictive value (PPV), and negative predictive value (NPV) of Congo red-stained fat tissue specimens in 12 studies [6, 15–25]. Numbers of amyloid patients and controls vary considerably among the respective studies. The general picture, however, is clear. Specificity is high and reaches almost 100 % in experienced hands. False positivity is sometimes caused by overstaining and underdecolorization [17], sometimes by misinterpretation of collagen [17, 26], and sometimes obscured by ill-defined disease controls [20, 23, 25, 27]. Therefore, it is important to realize that if only minute amyloid deposits are found, supportive evidence should be sought before the patient is committed to a regimen with potentially high toxicity [17, 25, 27]. Sensitivity is highly variable (54–93 %) and depends on the adequacy of the tissue specimens, the quality of staining, the number of glass slides, the number of observers, and the time used for conscientious observation [24]. Pooled observations of the 623 controls and 417 patients with amyloidosis in all 12 studies yield a sensitivity of 79 % (95 % confidence interval (CI) 75–83 %) and a specificity of 97 % (95 % CI 95–98 %). Both the positive (94 %; 95 % CI 91–96 %) and negative (87 %; 95 % CI 85–90 %) predictive values are quite high.

In a group of 450 patients with peripheral polyneuropathy, Congo red-stained fat tissue helps to detect amyloid only in patients with a monoclonal protein, a family history, or other clinical findings associated with amyloidosis and it is useless in patients without such a characteristic [28].

In patients with long-standing (more than 5 years duration) inflammatory diseases, such as rheumatoid arthritis and ankylosing spondylitis, abdominal fat aspiration may help to detect AA amyloidosis in a presymptomatic state or associated with only minor symptoms in 5–10 % [29–35] and sometimes in even 25–30 % of the patients [36, 37]. However, the clinical relevance

Table 16.1 Sensitivity and specificity of amyloid detection using Congo red-stained fat tissue specimens

Year	Reference	Type of amyloid	Controls	Amyloid patients	Sensitivity (%)	Specificity (%)	PPV (%)	NPV (%)
1986	[15]	A, L, TTR	12	12	83	100	100	86
1987	[16]	A	81	65	82	100	100	87
1988	[17]	L	72	82	72	99	98	76
1988	[18]	A	80	44	75	100	100	88
1989	[19]	A, L, TTR	10	7	57	100	100	77
1989	[6]	A	18	26	54	100	100	60
1995	[20]	A, L	96	4	75	87	20	99
1997	[21]	A, L, TTR	89	11	82	100	100	98
2001	[22]	A, L	28	12	58	100	100	85
2004	[23]	A, L	62	20	75	92	75	92
2006	[24]	A, L, TTR	45	120	93	100	100	83
2007	[25]	A, L	30	14	78	93	84	90
	Total		623	417	79	97	94	87

PPV positive predictive value, *NPV* negative predictive value, *A* AA amyloid, *L* AL amyloid, *TTR* ATTR amyloid

of presymptomatic AA amyloidosis is not clear. Well-documented long-term (10–20 years) follow-up studies of such patients are lacking.

A recent study showed that the yield of a fat aspirate in diagnosing wild-type ATTR amyloid cardiomyopathy (84 patients) appears to be disappointedly low, i.e., sensitivity of 14 % [38]. Sensitivity can be increased to 73 % (8 of 11 patients), however, by careful looking for amyloid in the deep layer of surgically obtained subcutaneous fat tissue, where amyloid appears to be deposited in a patchy distribution [39]. Amyloid in blood vessel walls of fat tissue is seen more frequently in amyloid cardiomyopathy in AL amyloidosis than in ATTR amyloidosis in a small study of 14 patients [40].

There are only rare and incomplete data published about detection in fat tissue of types of systemic amyloidosis other than AA, AL, and ATTR [41], such as AApoAI (apolipoprotein AI) [42, 43], $A\beta_2M$ (β_2-microglobulin) that is frequently absent or infrequently present as small deposits [44–47], AFib (fibrinogen α-chain) [48], AGel (gelsolin) [49–51], and ALys (lysozyme) amyloidosis [51]. Amyloid was easily detected in fat tissue of all three patients with AGel amyloidosis, we recently saw at our outpatient clinics (unpublished observation). We are currently not aware of any published data about amyloid in fat tissue of patients with AApoAII (apolipoprotein AII), AH (immunoglobulin heavy chain), and ALect2 (leukocyte chemotactic factor 2) amyloidosis. In this respect, it is important to mention AIns (insulin) amyloidosis. This rare localized type of nodular amyloidosis is an iatrogenic type of amyloid in which insulin-derived amyloid is deposited in abdominal fat tissue after long periods of repeated insulin injections in that particular site [52, 53]. A constant feature of this type of amyloid seems to be a negative immunohistochemical staining of serum amyloid P component (SAP) [53]. This insulin-derived amyloid is a potential pitfall in the diagnosis of systemic amyloidosis using aspirated fat tissue. Because long-standing diabetics can have hypertrophic cardiomyopathy, proteinuria, peripheral polyneuropathy, and autonomic neuropathy, symptoms and signs can be mistaken for systemic amyloi-

dosis. Presence of monoclonal gammopathy may even confound the situation [54]. Therefore, in a patient with insulin-dependent diabetes mellitus, a Congo red-positive fat biopsy should always be treated with caution: either by making insulin-derived amyloid unlikely (e.g., by proteomics or immunohistochemistry) or by seeking additional conformation of systemic amyloidosis.

Typing of Amyloid

Antibody-Based Detection

Immunohistochemical staining of tissue biopsies is a standard technique used for typing amyloid. Orfila et al. used the immunofluorescence technique on abdominal fat tissue aspirates and detected five of nine samples with AA amyloid deposits [55] and Halloush et al. detected with immunoperoxidase technique three of five samples with AL and ATTR amyloid deposits [56]. Immunohistochemical staining of subcutaneous fat tissue, however, is fairly difficult due to non-specific reactions [7]. Therefore, Westermark developed different immunochemical methods for typing amyloid in fat tissue. The initial method was a double immunodiffusion method that satisfactorily identified some patients with AA amyloidosis [4, 7]. Later his group developed an enzyme-linked immunosorbent assay (ELISA) that was useful for typing AA, AL, and ATTR amyloidosis in 14 of 15 cases [8]. Recently he described a method based on Western blot analysis combined with specific amyloid fibril antibodies that was successful in typing 32 of 35 patients with AA, AL, and ATTR amyloidosis [49] and all of 33 patients with ATTR amyloidosis [57]. Kaplan et al. also used immunochemical methods to type amyloid successfully in three of four patients with AL-kappa, in five of six patients with AL-lambda, and in one patient with AA amyloid [58].

Because of unsatisfactory typing of amyloid in fat aspirates using immunohistochemistry, Arbustini et al. developed immunoelectron microscopy for typing amyloid of patients with cardiac amyloidosis. This appeared to be a promising technique, because in all 15 patients the amyloid types involved were identified: eight samples with AL-lambda, two with AL-kappa, three with ATTR, two with AApoAI, and none with AA amyloid [42]. In a recent study of this group, immunoelectron microscopy was used for typing amyloid in abdominal fat tissue in 423 patients. The specific type of amyloidosis was correctly identified in 99 % of the cases. An abstract of this study has been presented at the XIVth International Symposium on Amyloidosis in Indianapolis in April 2014 [59, 60].

Antibody-Based Quantification of Amyloid Proteins

Our group in Groningen also developed and used immunochemical methods for measuring the concentrations in fat tissue of the four major amyloid proteins, i.e., amyloid A protein, TTR, light chain kappa, and light chain lambda. See Table 16.2 for the panel of cutoff values we use for fat aspiration samples in our center. An ELISA was used to measure the concentration of amyloid A protein in fat tissue in a group of 24 patients with AA amyloidosis and a group of 72 controls, including 25 patients with AL or ATTR amyloidosis and 25 patients with chronic inflammation. The upper limit of the 99 % CI of controls (11.6 ng/mg tissue) was chosen as cutoff

Table 16.2 Immunochemical quantification of the four major amyloid proteins in subcutaneous abdominal fat tissue: cutoff values (Groningen), sensitivity, and specificity

	AA	ATTR	AL-κ	AL-λ
Cutoff value				
Amyloid A protein (ng/mg fat)	>11.6			
TTR (ng/mg fat)		>4.36		
κ/λ ratio			>5.86	<0.49
Patients (number)	154	49	23	84
Controls (number)	354	204	95	95
Specificity (%)	99	99	97	97
Sensitivity (%)	84	71	78	70

level [10]. In a large collaborative international study, this method was validated and identified 129 of 154 patients with AA amyloidosis, whereas only 3 of 354 controls (87 AL, 30 ATTR, and 27 localized amyloidosis and 210 non-amyloidosis patients) were identified incorrectly [61]. Thus, in this study the sensitivity of detecting AA amyloidosis was 84 % (95 % CI 77–89 %), specificity was 99 % (95 % CI 98–100 %), PPV was 98 % (95 % CI 94–100 %), and NPV was 93 % (95 % CI 90–96 %). Men had lower amyloid A protein concentrations in fat than women (Fig. 16.1a). Patients with familial Mediterranean fever (FMF) had lower values than patients with arthritis or other inflammatory diseases (Fig. 16.1b). The low yield of fat tissue aspirates for the detection of AA amyloidosis in patients with FMF was already observed and discussed by Tishler et al. in 1988: they even did not detect amyloid in any of the 15 FMF patients studied [62]. However, Congo red-positive amyloid deposits were detected in 20 fat tissue samples (80 %) and the amyloid A protein concentration was elevated in 13 samples (about 50 %) of the 25 FMF patients we studied [61]. In a study of Egyptian patients with long-standing rheumatoid arthritis, quantification of the amyloid A protein concentration in fat tissue appeared to be a useful screening tool for the detection of AA amyloidosis [32]. Subcutaneous fat tissue is a major source of the acute-phase reactant serum amyloid A protein (SAA), the protein precursor of AA protein [63]. Extensive washing of fat tissue, however, was effective to prevent unwanted contamination and retention of SAA from blood in fat tissue extracts of controls. Although indeed a positive correlation between the SAA concentration in blood and amyloid A protein concentration in fat tissue was present in controls, the magnitude of the effect was very small, resulting in maximum amyloid A protein concentrations in fat tissue largely within the reference range of controls [61].

An ELISA is also used in our center to measure the concentration of TTR in fat tissue. The upper limit of the 99 % CI of controls is 4.36 ng/mg fat tissue and this value has been chosen as cutoff value. Quantification of free light chains

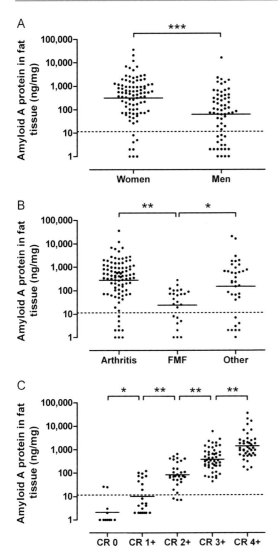

Fig. 16.1 Amyloid A protein concentration in fat tissue of patients with clinical AA amyloidosis. The *dotted line* marks the upper reference limit of controls (11.6 ng/mg fat). Asterisks (*), (**), and (***) represent $p < 0.05$, $p < 0.001$, and $p < 0.0001$, respectively. The *horizontal lines* denote the means of the log-transformed values. (**a**) Men ($N = 63$) and women ($N = 91$). (**b**) Patients with chronic arthritis ($N = 93$), patients with FMF ($N = 25$), and patients with other diseases or more than one disease ($N = 36$). (**c**) Congo red (CR) stain scores of fat tissue: CR negative ($N = 14$), CR 1+ ($N = 25$), CR 2+ ($N = 34$), CR 3+ ($N = 55$), and CR 4+ ($N = 45$) (Reproduced with permission of Informa UK Ltd. [61])

by nephelometry is used to measure light chain kappa (95 % CI upper limit 24.4 ng/mg fat tissue), light chain lambda (95 % CI upper limit

10.6 ng/mg fat tissue), and the resulting κ/λ ratio (95 % CI reference range 0.49–5.86). See also Table 16.2 [64, 65].

Advantages and Disadvantages of Antibody-Based Typing

Antibody-based detection of amyloid has the advantage of fast, inexpensive, and specific detection and amplification of minute amounts of a particular protein in an enormous background ocean of other proteins and tissue components. However, disadvantages are sometimes considerable: limited reactivity with commercial antibodies (false-negative), "contamination" by serum proteins (false-positive), the increasing number of other types of amyloidosis that are recognized, the issue of combined deposits (more than one type of amyloid protein present), and finally, experience and principles in the interpretation of results [66]. The consequences of mistyping amyloid may lead to a wrong choice of treatment and may be harmful for the patient. This is the main reason we wanted to develop in our center typing methods with high specificity (≥99 %) resulting in a high PPV. If a particular type is then successfully identified in a sample, the result should be virtually beyond doubt. The practical consequence of very high specificity on the other hand is relatively low sensitivity with corresponding low NPV. However, it is our opinion that it is easier to manage cases in which typing is not successful: these inconclusive or negative cases should be diagnosed as such and considered for evaluation by reference laboratories that have experience in amyloid typing using a wider antibody panel as well as the capacity to apply methods that are more sophisticated [66].

Proteomics-Based Detection

Typing of amyloid should be performed with confidence [67]: amyloid typing should result in certainty of both presence of a particular type of amyloid and absence of all other (relevant) types of amyloid. Chemical typing of the amino acid sequence of the amyloid protein involved has been the gold standard for a long time. Until recently, macropurification techniques were needed for isolation of these proteins from large amounts of tissue obtained at necropsy or after surgery, at least 10–30 g of amyloid-rich tissue [68, 69]. With some modifications, Westermark et al. were able to determine the amino acid sequence of the amyloid protein isolated from only 1 g of amyloid-rich fat tissue [70, 71] and 10 years later from an even lower amount of fat tissue [72].

New methodological approaches, including the search for appropriate extraction solvents and separation strategies, have been developed and tested in order to design efficient procedures for small scale isolation and purification of these amyloid proteins [73–75]. Kaplan et al. were among the first to investigate these micropurification techniques and they found that the strategy for small scale purification of amyloid proteins depends largely on the type of tissue sample (fresh or formalin fixed), sample size, amyloid content of the tissue, and its chemical nature [75]. Abdominal fat tissue aspirates were among the tissues they studied [58]. These techniques were further improved using different mass spectroscopic techniques in the following years [51, 76–79]. Vrana et al. introduced laser microdissection to concentrate the amyloid content in extracts from tissue samples of patients with AA, ATTR, AL-kappa, and AL-lambda amyloidosis [79]. Her group recently applied mass spectrometry-based proteomics to type amyloidosis in fat aspirates [51]. In the validation study, the presence of amyloid was detected with high sensitivity (88 %) and specificity (96 %). In 366 Congo red-positive cases, mass spectrometry analysis successfully identified an amyloid subtype in 330 cases, yielding a sensitivity of 90 %. The specific diagnoses were AL-lambda (58 %), AL-kappa (16 %), ATTR (12 %), AA (1 %), AGel (1 %), AIns (1 %), and ALys (1 %). A universal amyloid proteome signature (i.e., the universal presence of apoAIV, ApoE, and SAP) was identified with high sensitivity and specificity, similar to that of Congo red staining [51].

Lavatelli et al. developed a proteomics methodology utilizing two-dimensional (2D) polyacrylamide gel electrophoresis followed by matrix-assisted laser desorption/ionization mass spectrometry and peptide mass fingerprinting to directly characterize amyloid deposits in abdominal subcutaneous fat obtained by fine needle aspiration from seven patients with AL amyloidosis, two with ATTR amyloidosis, and seven controls. Striking differences in the 2D gel proteomes of adipose tissue were observed between controls and patients and between the two types of patients with distinct, additional spots present in the patient specimens that could be assigned as the amyloidogenic proteins in full-length and truncated forms [80]. The 2D-tandem MS technique was further developed (called Multidimensional Protein Identification Technology or shortly MudPIT) and was used to identify reliably 26 patients with the most common (AL, AA, and ATTR) types of amyloidosis who had grade 3+ or 4+ amyloid in fat tissue [81]. In another study of 30 patients with systemic amyloidosis, comprehensive protein profiles of human amyloid-affected adipose tissue from patients and its control (nonamyloid affected) counterpart were acquired. In particular, extracellular matrix (ECM), protein folding, lipid metabolism, and mitochondrial functions were among the most affected structural/functional pathways [82]. These proteomic techniques have great potential to diagnose and type amyloid, but also to clarify all kind of molecular mechanisms involved in amyloidosis [82–84].

Semiquantitative Assessment of Amyloid in Fat Tissue

Amyloid deposition in tissue is the result of the balance between accumulation and breakdown of amyloid. Progressive deposition of amyloid in a vital organ or tissue generally leads to loss of function of that organ or tissue. The mechanism behind this loss of function is not satisfactorily explained and both mere physical hindrance and toxic effects may play a role. Regression of amyloid deposition sometimes results in (partial) recovery of function of the organ or tissue involved. It is generally believed that continuous and massive supply of available amyloid protein precursors leads to accumulation of amyloid, whereas complete lack of supply of these precursors may facilitate endogenous breakdown of amyloid leading to regression of amyloid. Monitoring the intensity of amyloid deposition in tissue might help to understand more about the balance between accumulation and breakdown of the total amyloid load of the body. Screening of subcutaneous abdominal fat tissue seems to be a suitable tool for this purpose because this tissue is easily available by aspiration, amyloid can almost always be found if present, and aspiration can be repeated at intervals during the course of the disease. This was the background of our ambition to develop tools for measuring the intensity of amyloid deposition in fat tissue. A scoring system was developed that semiquantitatively graded the amount of amyloid in fat on a scale of 0 to 3+ [10, 32]. Severity was assessed by visual estimation of the percentage of the smear surface area affected by deposition of amyloid recognized in polarized light [32]. Later we widened the scale from 0 to 4+ and validated this scale (Fig. 16.1c) using AA protein quantification in a large group of patients with AA amyloidosis [61]. Figure 16.2 shows typical examples of this semiquantitative grading system: 0 (negative, no apple-green birefringence detectable), 1+ (minute, <1 % of surface area), 2+ (little, between 1 % and 10 %), 3+ (moderate, between 10 % and 60 %), 4+ (abundant, >60 %). Kimmich et al. demonstrate how this technique reliably can be introduced and implemented with confidence in another center [85].

Gómez-Casanovas et al. introduced in 2001 a comparable semiquantitative scoring system of Congo red-stained specimens and graded them as 3+ (marked), 2+ (moderate), and 1+ (mild) according to the amount of amyloid deposits. Marked refers to massive amyloid deposition in >25 % of the tissue fragments sampled and/or linear deposits in >75 % of fragments, moderate refers to massive amyloid deposits in <25 % of fragments or linear deposition in >25 % of fragments, and mild refers to linear deposits in <25 % of fragments. Very small and isolated Congo red-positive deposits were considered inconclusive and were classified as negative. Marked amyloid deposits were found more frequently in patients with clinical amyloidosis than in those whose amyloidosis remained subclinical [86].

In this respect, it is interesting to mention the study of Bardarov et al. who describe the development of a generally available computer-assisted image analysis of Congo red-stained amyloid deposits in abdominal fat tissue biopsies [87]. Further improvement of such techniques will make it easier and less subjective not only to detect amyloid but also to (semi)quantify the amount of amyloid present.

Quantification of Amyloid in Fat Tissue for Diagnosing and Typing Amyloid

Semiquantitative grading of amyloid in fat tissue may be helpful in diagnosing amyloidosis with confidence. Dhingra et al. propose that patients with grade 1+ of amyloid in fat tissue should not undergo a toxic therapeutic regimen on the basis of only this result. In this situation, they advise histologic confirmation of visceral amyloid deposition in deeper tissue [25].

Grading the amount of amyloid in fat tissue may be helpful in typing amyloidosis with confidence. All patients with grade 3+ or 4+ and 90 % of patients with grade 2+ AA amyloid (as shown in Fig. 16.1c) have an elevated amyloid A protein concentration in fat tissue [61]. This is true for only half of the patients with grade 1+ amyloid. Comparable results have been observed in patients with ATTR and AL amyloidosis [64, 65]. All patients with grade 3+ and 4+ ATTR amyloid had an elevated TTR concentration in fat tissue, whereas this was true for only half of the patients with grade 2+ and almost none of the patients with grade 1+. All patients with grade $\geq 2+$ AL-kappa amyloid had an elevated κ/λ ratio in fat tissue, whereas only 58, 78, and 90 % of the patients with grade 2+, 3+, and 4+ AL-lambda amyloid, respectively, had a decreased κ/λ ratio in fat tissue. We conclude that in nearly all patients

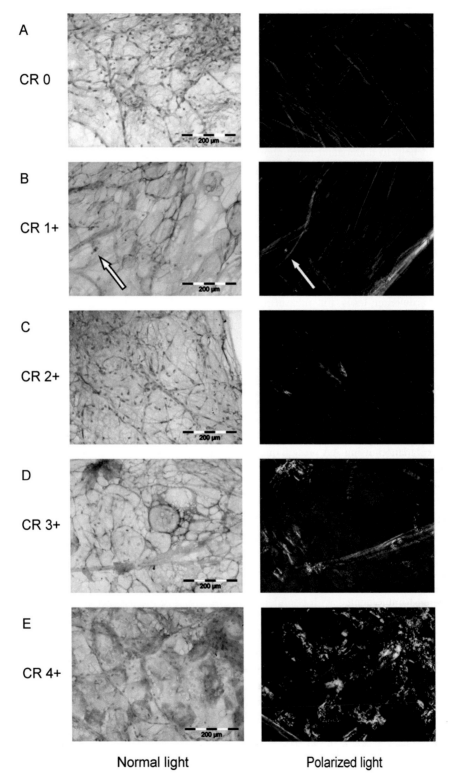

Normal light   **Polarized light**

Fig. 16.2 *Congo red*-based grading system of intensity of amyloid deposition in fat tissue (Reproduced with permission of Informa UK Ltd. [61])

with grade 3+ and 4+ amyloid in fat tissue immunochemical quantification enabled us to type AA, ATTR, AL-kappa, and AL-lambda with confidence. The chance of reliable typing of patients with grade 2+ amyloid is much lower (about 50 %) and in only a minority of patients with grade 1+ (about 10 %) immunochemical typing will be successful.

Amyloid Quantity in Fat Tissue and Clinical Characteristics

In patients with AA amyloidosis, amyloid was detected in fat tissue in 95 % of women and in 90 % of men [61]. Although this difference was not statistically significant, the grade of amyloid was higher in women (median 3+) than in men (median 2+). As stated earlier (Fig. 16.1a), the concentration of amyloid A protein in fat tissue was higher in women (geometric mean 315 ng/mg) than in men (geometric mean 63 ng/mg). This difference of amyloid quantity in fat tissue between men and women was confirmed in another study of 220 patients concerning all major types of systemic amyloidosis [88]. A satisfactory explanation of this increased deposition in women or decreased deposition in men of all types of amyloid in fat tissue is lacking. Amyloid grade in fat tissue was associated with the number of major organs involved and was a predictor

of decreased survival (Fig. 16.3), independent of other predictors such as heart involvement, the number of organs involved, type of amyloid, and age [88]. These data support the notion that, at least at group level, the amount of amyloid in subcutaneous fat tissue in systemic amyloidosis reflects disease severity.

Amyloid Quantity in Fat Tissue and Follow-Up

If the amount of amyloid in fat tissue indeed reflects disease severity, it may be interesting to study the effect of treatment on amyloid deposition in fat tissue. Only a few follow-up studies of amyloid in fat tissue have been published. In one study of patients with ATTR amyloidosis, fat tissue was monitored in nine patients before liver transplantation and in 11 patients thereafter [89]. When a change of at least two grades of amyloid in fat tissue was used as marker of significant progression or regression, no regression was seen whereas progression was seen in two of three patients followed for at least 7 years without transplantation. After transplantation, none of the patients showed progression and only one showed regression of amyloid in fat tissue. The numbers in the study were too small to draw any firm conclusion, but one may conclude that without liver transplantation some progression can be detected

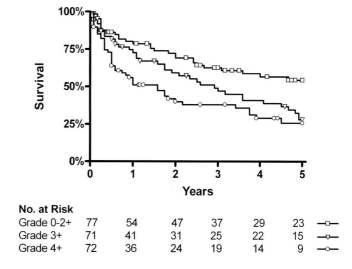

Fig. 16.3 Kaplan-Meier survival *curves* of equally sized groups for grades of amyloid in fat tissue (Reproduced with permission of John Wiley and Sons [88])

No. at Risk						
Grade 0-2+	77	54	47	37	29	23
Grade 3+	71	41	31	25	22	15
Grade 4+	72	36	24	19	14	9

after 7 years and that significant improvement following transplantation does not occur in most patients within 5 years. However, significant improvement may occur more than 10 years after transplantation as shown in one study of six ATTR patients in whom amyloid (almost) completely regressed in fat tissue [90].

Not only the quantity, but also the composition of ATTR-V30M amyloid in fat tissue of patients with a TTR-Val30Met mutation, is clinically relevant as has been shown in some studies before and after liver transplantation [57, 90–92]. Fibrils composed of only full-length TTR were associated with early age at onset, no clinical cardiac involvement and a strong affinity for Congo red. In contrast, the presence of TTR fragments in the amyloid was associated with late age at onset, signs of cardiac involvement and weak Congo red staining [57]. In a study of 63 patients carrying 29 different TTR non-V30M mutations a fibril composition with fragmented ATTR appears to be very common in ATTR amyloidosis, and suggests that fibrils composed of only full-length ATTR is an exception found only in a subset of patients [93]. In another study of 44 patients with ATTR amyloidosis without liver transplantation, proteomic analysis showed that the percentage of wild-type TTR, i.e., nonmutated TTR, was higher in patients older than 50 years than in patients younger than 50 years, i.e., 51 % vs. 31 %, respectively [91]. Wild-type TTR may be more strongly amyloidogenic than previously considered because it is detectable even in amyloid of young ATTR patients. The percentage of wild-type TTR in amyloid in fat tissue samples increased significantly to 90–100 % after liver transplantation compared to pretransplantation values of 35–60 % [90, 92]. Fat tissue was analyzed in 32 other patients with ATTR amyloidosis of whom 20 had received a liver transplant [91]. In pretransplant patients, it was found that cardiac amyloid more easily incorporated wild-type TTR than fat tissue amyloid, offering a potential explanation for the vulnerability of cardiac tissue for continued amyloidosis after liver transplantation. In fat tissue, a rapid increase in wild-type TTR proportion after liver transplantation indicates that a rather fast turnover of the deposits occurs. Some difference in wild-type TTR proportion between full-length TTR and fragmented TTR fibril types was seen after transplantation but not pretransplantation, possibly caused by differences in turnover rate [92].

In a follow-up study of 51 selected patients with AL amyloidosis of whom at least two fat tissue aspirates were available for analysis, significant improvement of amyloid deposition in fat tissue was exclusively seen after normalization of serum-free light chain: reduction of two grades of amyloid deposition in fat tissue was seen in 50 % of these patients after 2.4 years and in 80 % after 3.2 years (Fig. 16.4). This rapid significant regression of amyloid deposition in fat tissue was accompanied by stabilization or improvement of organ responses [94]. Systematic follow-up studies of amyloid in fat tissue in patients with AA amyloidosis have not been published yet.

Future Perspectives

A positive Congo red stain with apple-green birefringence in polarized light still is the gold standard for detection of amyloid deposits in tissue [12]. However, both staining and scoring of the slides can only yield reliable results by trained observers with good equipment. This is also true for electron microscopy. Therefore, there is a need for new staining methods using other microscopic techniques. Sjölander et al. introduced a new staining method using oligothiophene (hFTAA) fluorescence in which positively stained amyloid can be detected by using spectral imaging microscopy [95]. In a study of fat tissue, this group compares the results with Congo red-stained specimens showing concordant results of semiquantitative grading of the amount of amyloid and higher sensitivity, but lower specificity [96]. This new staining technique is really promising for amyloid screening if the authors succeed to increase the specificity in fat tissue.

Measuring the amyloid A protein and TTR concentrations in fat tissue by ELISA shows high accuracy for detection and typing of AA and

Fig. 16.4 Kaplan-Meier *curves* of patients with *CR* complete response, *PR* partial response, and *NR* no response of serum free light chain. Endpoint is a significant decrease of two grades of amyloid in fat tissue. The numbers of patients at start and later who had the potential to reflect such a decrease are shown at the bottom; *$p < 0.05$ (Reproduced with permission of The Ferrara Storti Foundation [94])

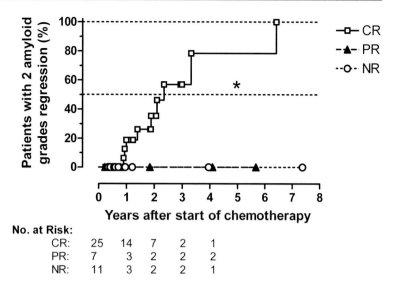

No. at Risk:

CR:	25	14	7	2	1
PR:	7	3	2	2	2
NR:	11	3	2	2	1

ATTR amyloidosis in samples with ample amyloid present (2+ or more) and has been introduced in our center for daily clinical practice. Immunochemical quantification of the amyloid proteins kappa and lambda using nephelometry shows acceptable results for detection and typing of AL amyloidosis, although we are still looking for opportunities to further improve sensitivity and specificity. Immunochemical quantification of other amyloid constituents such as SAP, laminin, entactin, collagen IV, apolipoprotein E, and glycosaminoglycans (GAGs) may be interesting too. In this respect, one should always keep in mind that the extraction procedure of proteins from amyloid fibrils, e.g., with guanidine, may induce conformational changes of some of the epitopes that will result in decreased antigen recognition by the antibodies used. Fortunately proteomics techniques, such as 2D blotting and various mass spectrometric techniques, have become available for this kind of research [51, 70–84]. As has been described above, application of these techniques to fat tissue has proven its utility and may become even more promising for detection of changes of amino acid sequence and composition, specific mutations and variants, and the assessment of relative amounts of mutations versus wild-type proteins. The first aim of all proteomic studies should still be to detect and diagnose a particular type of amyloid with confidence and to exclude all other possible types with similar confidence [67]. A second aim may be the unraveling of the role of wild-type protein, subtypes, variants, and mutated proteins, the role of enzymatic cleavage and other modifications of precursor proteins, and the role of other amyloid constituents such as SAP, laminin, entactin, collagen IV, and GAGs in amyloid fibril formation and deposition [51, 82].

Fat tissue analysis has great potential to enable dynamic studies of local tissue factors involved both in deposition and in removal of amyloid in vivo. As shown above, fat tissue can easily be obtained for analysis at regular intervals to monitor the actual course of amyloid deposition at tissue level. This monitoring of fat tissue may be useful especially in AL and ATTR amyloidosis because fat tissue in these diseases does not seem to be actively involved in the production of the precursor protein. Fat tissue in AA amyloidosis, however, may behave differently in this respect because of active production of SAA by adipocytes in fat tissue [63, 97, 98]. An in vitro monocyte culture system of amyloidogenesis has been developed in the mouse [99, 100]. A fully humanized cell culture model of amyloidogenesis, however, has recently been developed [101, 102]. Adipocyte cultures may provide a means to further elucidate the regulation of SAA synthesis, the processing of SAA into AA amyloid fibrils in a human system, the mechanisms of fibril deposition, amyloid toxicity in tissue, and the role of other amyloid components such as SAP, laminin, entactin, collagen IV, and GAGs.

In conclusion, subcutaneous abdominal fat tissue carries huge potential for early diagnosis, typing with confidence, monitoring the course of disease, and better understanding of disease behavior in tissue of patients with systemic amyloidosis. Some possibilities are already implemented in daily clinical practice, some are obvious improvements that may be used routinely in the near future, but it is a challenge to detect the possibilities that are still waiting to be discovered.

Appendix: Fat Aspiration Technique and Tissue Analysis Currently Practiced in Groningen

Fat Aspiration Technique

Stepwise Description of the Procedure

Aspiration of abdominal subcutaneous fat tissue is a simple outpatient procedure and a modification of the procedure was described by Gertz [17]. It should be noted that it takes at least 10–15 min to avoid unnecessary pain and bruising and to get adequate material. The patient should be told that bruising might occur. For a description and instruction video of the fat aspiration procedure one can visit our website www.amyloid.nl [103]. Alternative procedures have been described, such as by Kettwich et al. [104] and also for preparing and performing electron microscopy on fat tissue [105, 106].

See Table 16.3 for the equipment we use. A syringe of 10 ml is connected by a valve system to a 16-gauge needle (Fig. 16.5a). After closing the valve, the plunger is pulled out, fixed transiently between squeezed thumb and finger, the cap of the lidocaine needle is reused elegantly by positioning it upside-down inside the plunger (Tarek's trick) to fix firmly and definitely the position of the plunger, and thus maintaining negative pressure in the syringe during aspiration (Fig. 16.5b). The skin of the patient is marked and cleansed (e.g., with chloorhexidine) at both sides of the umbilicus at about 7–10 cm distance.

Table 16.3 Equipment for the fat aspiration

Number	Material	Aim
1 1 1	10 ml ampoule lidocaine (10 mg/ml) 5 ml syringe 22 Gauge needle	Local anesthesia, about 2 ml each side; intracutaneous at the puncture site and subcutaneous in three directions
2 2 2	10 ml syringe Valve system 16 Gauge needle	The syringe is connected by the valve system to the needle; then the valve is closed and the plunger fixed
1 2 1	Chloorhexidine solution for skin cleaning Small band-aids and gauzes Pair of protective gloves	

Check first that the patient is not allergic to lidocaine. Skin and subcutaneous tissue (three directions, see below) are then anesthetized with lidocaine (each side 2 ml = 20 mg).

After inserting the needle beneath the skin, the valve is opened to start aspiration of fat tissue (Fig. 16.6a). The needle can be moved into three directions (Northeast, East, and Southeast) at the left side of the abdomen and mirror-wise at the right side. The aspiration procedure should be performed slowly and gently into each of the three directions, going to and fro with some axial rotation, and one should realize that it will take some time before the needle will be filled with fat tissue and the first fat can be seen passing the valve and entering the top of the syringe. This should be continued at both sides of the umbilicus until at least 60 mg of fat tissue has been collected (Fig. 16.6b). After the procedure has been finished, the puncture site should be covered with a band aid and pressed for a while to prevent substantial bruising.

The next step may be as simple as this: Seal the syringe, keep it cool (4 °C) until shipment, and send it at room temperature to a diagnostic center (e.g., UMC Groningen) for analysis as soon as possible, but at the latest arriving there within 1 week after the procedure.

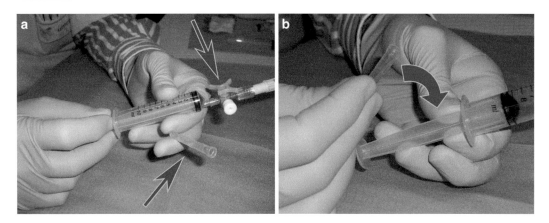

Fig. 16.5 (**a**) The closed valve; reusing the needle cap. (**b**) Pull and fix the plunger and position the needle cap

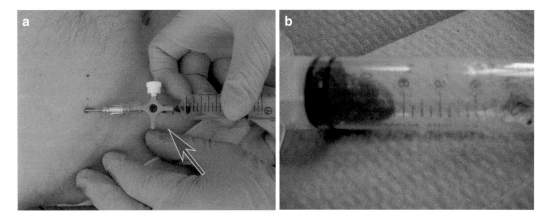

Fig. 16.6 (**a**) Insert the needle beneath the skin and open the valve. (**b**) Yield: about 60 mg of fat tissue

Frequently Encountered Problems During the Procedure

Two technical problems can be encountered during aspiration: no tissue at all or too much blood entering the syringe.

If no fat appears in the syringe or the aspiration has stopped completely for some time, the needle may have become obstructed. The simplest way to check this is to pull the needle out of the patient. Normally, fat tissue present in the needle is then directly and audibly forced into the syringe because of negative pressure. If this is not the case and fat tissue obstructs the needle completely, tissue in the needle can be removed by using positive pressure in the syringe. This may result in a rather explosive evacuation (firing fat tissue) and should therefore be carried out carefully. The needle is introduced into a clean container (e.g., sputum or urine) or empty syringe: tissue is then evacuated into this container or syringe, while fixing the needle firmly to the syringe to prevent the needle leaving the syringe (firing needles).

If much arterial or venous blood enters the syringe by accident, the needle should be removed out of the body. The puncture site should be pressed for at least 1 min, and the procedure can be repeated into a different direction or at a different site. Pain is infrequent, localized, and seldom a real problem necessitating the use of more lidocaine. If bruising is suspected to be present at the end of the procedure, the patient him/herself may press the puncture site for a couple of minutes before rising from the supine position. At the end of the procedure, after sealing the two syringes, both puncture sites should be inspected for the development of significant bruising. If these safety precautions are taken routinely, the chance of severe bleeding or infections is very small. In about 2,000 procedures in our hospital, we observed twice a bleeding complication necessitating surgical assistance to find and stop the bleeding locus and once a local infection of the abdominal wall necessitating surgical drainage after incision combined with antibiotic treatment.

Congo Red Stain and Grading of Amyloid in Fat Tissue

Preparing Slides for Microscopy

After extracting the plunger, fat tissue can be collected from the syringe on an empty glass slide to separate fat tissue from accidentally obtained blood. At least four visible fragments of fat tissue (not fat droplets!) should be put on each of three glass slides (preferably with a frosted edge, which can be used to write on it with a pencil). These fragments are crushed into a single layer by squeezing a second slide placed perpendicularly to the first ones (Fig. 16.7a, b). It is important to press in the middle of the glass slides to prevent breaking of glass. The resulting six smears are marked for identification, dried in the air at room temperature for 1 h, and subsequently fixed with acetone for 10 min. After drying and fixation, all slides can be stored at room temperature until shipped to a reference laboratory for staining with Congo red and further study if positive for amyloid. Fat tissue should not be frozen before slides have been made: freezing of fresh and unfixed tissue may affect the quality of the tissue.

Congo Red Stain, Microscopy, and Amyloid Grading

Staining with alkaline Congo red should be performed according to the classic method described by Puchtler [11]. See Table 16.4 for a short summary. Commercial kits for Congo red stain are also available and have been used successfully, in particular in the US (MM Picken, personal communication).

The affinity of tissue for Congo red can be analyzed by the apple-green birefringence in polarized light using a good microscope. In our institution, we use the Olympus BX 50 microscope and a strong (100 W) light source. Two investigators score the slides blinded to the clinical data and in a semiquantitative grading system (Fig. 16.2): 0 (negative, no apple-green birefringence detectable), 1+ (minute, <1 % of surface area), 2+ (little, between 1 % and 10 %), 3+ (moderate, between 10 % and 60 %), 4+ (abundant, >60 %). Because some deposits may be tiny and hardly visible in daylight conditions, the slides, ideally, should be read in the dark. Kimmich et al. show nicely how this technique reliably can be introduced and successfully implemented in another center [85].

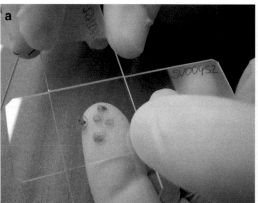 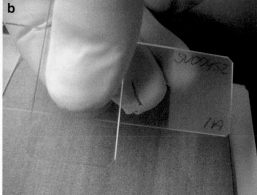

Fig. 16.7 (**a**) Perpendicularly positioned glass slides. (**b**) Squeezing in the middle of the glass slides

Table 16.4 Alkaline Congo red stain according to Puchtler [11]

Working solutions prepared from stock before use	Stock solution I: saturated solution of NaCl in 80 % ethanol
	Stock solution II: saturated solution of NaCl and Congo red in 80 % ethanol
	Working solutions I and II prepared by adding NaOH (final concentration 0.01 %) just before use and then filter
Sequence of staining steps	1. Stain for 30 s with Mayer's hematoxylin
	2. Rinse in running tap water for 10 min
	3. Stain for 30 min in freshly filtered working solution I
	4. Stain for 30 min in freshly filtered working solution II
	5. Rinse briefly in ethanol (100 %) 2×
	6. Rinse briefly in demineralized water 2×
	7. Cover the slides with Kaiser's glycerol gelatin and a covering glass

Immunochemical Quantification of Amyloid Proteins in Fat Tissue Extracts

Aim of the fat aspiration procedure is to obtain first an adequate quantity for microscopic analysis (3×4 lumps with total weight about 30 mg) and further at least 30 mg of fat tissue for immunochemical quantification of the amyloid proteins. After extracting the plunger, fat tissue is collected from the syringe on an empty glass slide to separate fat tissue from accidentally obtained blood and the 12 lumps of fat are used for the smears (vide supra). Before quantification, the amount of fat is weighed to get the "wet weight." The material is then first washed 3× in a Tris buffer supplemented with calcium to remove possible remnants of blood still present. Subsequently SAP is extracted from this solution by incubation for 24 h with a Tris buffer supplemented with EDTA and the SAP concentration can be measured in this extract by ELISA [107].

The washed fat tissue is then extracted in a solution of 6 M guanidine hydrochloride and 0.1 M Tris–HCl, pH 8.0, mixed thoroughly, and shaken overnight. The suspension is centrifuged at $10,000 \times g$ for 10 min and the supernatant fat tissue extract collected. Microtiter plates are coated with the IgG fraction of the SAA-reactive mouse monoclonal capture antibody Reu.86.5 (Hycult Biotechnology, Uden, The Netherlands). The plates are washed, followed by incubation of the samples. The plates are washed again, followed by incubation with the IgG fraction of the SAA1-reactive mouse monoclonal detection antibody Reu.86.1 (Hycult Biotechnology) coupled to horseradish peroxidase. After washing, the plates are incubated with the chromogen $3'3'5'5'$ tetramethylbenzidin (TMB, Carl Roth, Karlsruhe, Germany) dissolved in acetate buffer until the reaction is stopped by adding H_2SO_4. The absorption at 450–575 nm is read in a Versamax microplate reader and amyloid A protein concentrations are calculated by SOFTmax® PRO software (Molecular Devices, Sunnyvale, USA) according to a standard curve of purified SAA. The intra-assay and interassay coefficients of variation are both less than 10 % and the lower limit of detection of the amyloid A protein in fat extract is 1.6 ng/ml extraction fluid. Amyloid A protein concentration reference range of patients without AA amyloidosis is <11.6 ng/mg fat tissue [10, 61]. Recently Hycult has introduced a commercial SAA ELISA kit [108].

In a similar way, concentrations of other important amyloid proteins such as TTR and immunoglobulin light chains kappa and lambda can be measured using ELISA and nephelometry, respectively [64, 65]. Table 16.2 shows the cutoff values that were found in all four assays for the main amyloid types. However, after using the assays for a couple of years the new data have been analyzed to adapt the cutoff values for optimum prediction in daily practice (see Fig. 16.8). PPVs and NPVs have been based on 1886 routine fat tissue samples for AA, 742 samples for ATTR and 596 samples for AL-lambda and kappa immunochemical typing. Finally, 194 routine fat tissue samples have been used to test the assay. No amyloid was found in 34 samples and the remaining 160 amyloid-containing samples were analyzed for all four types. Typing was successful

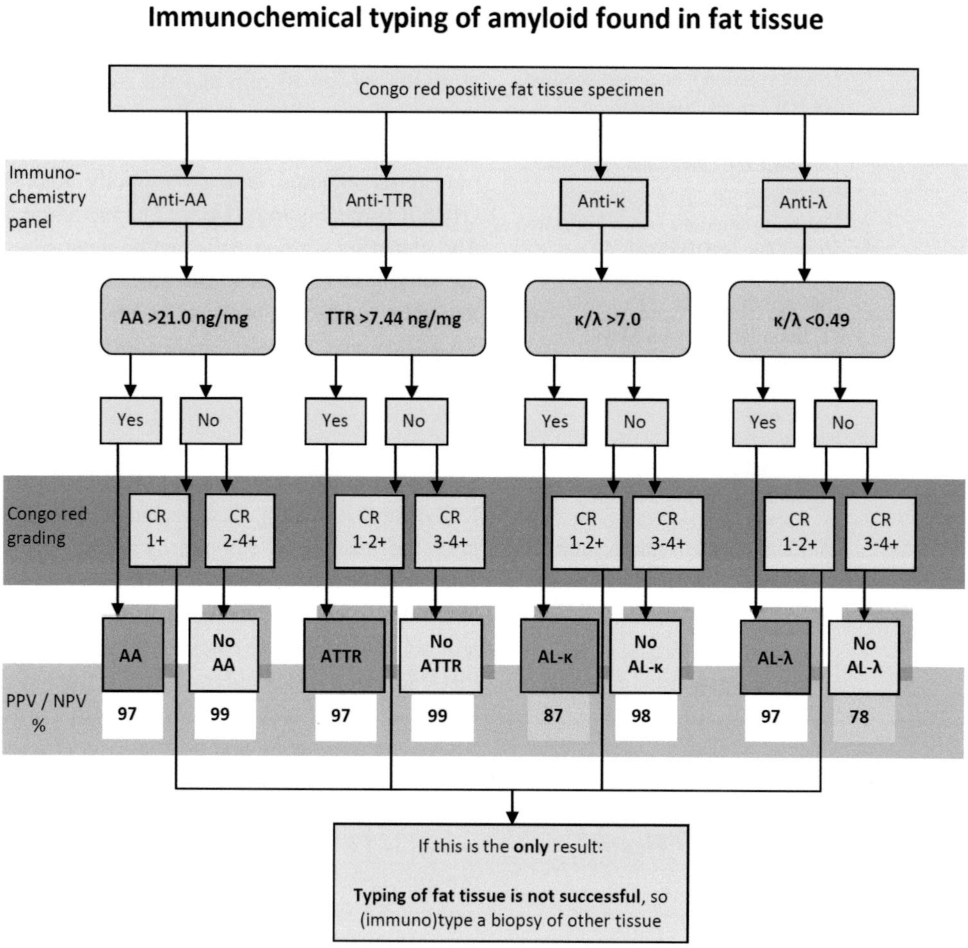
Immunochemical typing of amyloid found in fat tissue
Congo red positive fat tissue specimen
Immuno-chemistry panel
Anti-AA
Anti-TTR
Anti-κ
Anti-λ
AA >21.0 ng/mg
TTR >7.44 ng/mg
κ/λ >7.0
κ/λ <0.49
Yes
No
Yes
No
Yes
No
Yes
No
Congo red grading
CR 1+
CR 2-4+
CR 1-2+
CR 3-4+
CR 1-2+
CR 3-4+
CR 1-2+
CR 3-4+
AA
No AA
ATTR
No ATTR
AL-κ
No AL-κ
AL-λ
No AL-λ
PPV / NPV %
97
99
97
99
87
98
97
78
If this is the only result:
Typing of fat tissue is not successful, so (immuno)type a biopsy of other tissue

GUARD practice-oriented recommendations:

- If one of the four major types is positive and the other three are negative or unclear: choose the positive one as the type of amyloid involved, but only if it is compatible with the clinical picture (check especially in case of AL-κ)
- If two of the four major types are positive: choose the highest one, but only if the other is slightly positive, or AL-κ, and if the chosen type is compatible with the clinical picture (Note: two major types of amyloid present at the same time is extremely rare)
- If none of the four major types is positive: try to type other tissue. If that is not successful consider proteomics in a reference centre (e.g. Rochester, USA, or Pavia, Italy, or Kiel, Germany) or look for rarer types using DNA analysis of genes that might be involved
- If all four major types are actually excluded and therefore probably not present (though less sure in case of AL-λ), look for rarer types

Fig. 16.8 Cutoff values of the concentration of AA, TTR, and kappa/lambda light chain ratios in fat tissue for optimum prediction of the type of amyloid as being used in our center in Groningen (GUARD) in daily practice. PPV is positive predictive value, NPV is negative predictive value, and CR is *Congo red*-stained severity grading 1+ to 4+

in 58 of 59 CR4+ samples (98 %), 39 of 45 CR3+ samples (87 %), 5 of 25 CR2+ samples (20 %) and 4 of 32 CR1+ samples (13 %). Figure 16.8 shows the decision tree currently used in Groningen for immunochemical typing of amyloid found in fat tissue.

References

1. Schilder P. Über die amyloide Entartung der Haut. Frankfurt Z Pathol. 1909;3:782–94.
2. Westermark P, Stenkvist B. Diagnosis of secondary generalized amyloidosis by fine needle biopsy of the skin. Acta Med Scand. 1971;190:453–4.
3. Westermark P, Stenkvist B. A new method for the diagnosis of systemic amyloidosis. Arch Intern Med. 1973;132:522–3.
4. Westermark P, Stenkvist B, Natvig JB, et al. Demonstration of protein AA in subcutaneous fat tissue obtained by fine needle biopsy. Ann Rheum Dis. 1979;38:68–71.
5. Libbey CA, Skinner M, Cohen AS. Use of abdominal fat tissue aspirate in the diagnosis of systemic amyloidosis. Arch Intern Med. 1983;143:1549–52.
6. Breedveld FC, Markusse HM, MacFarlane JD. Subcutaneous fat biopsy in the diagnosis of amyloidosis secondary to chronic arthritis. Clin Exp Rheumatol. 1989;7:407–10.
7. Westermark P. Diagnosis and characterization of systemic amyloidosis by biopsy of subcutaneous abdominal fat tissue. Intern Med Specialist. 1984; 5:154–60.
8. Olsen KE, Sletten K, Westermark P. The use of subcutaneous fat tissue for amyloid typing by enzyme-linked immunosorbent assay. Am J Clin Pathol. 1999;111:355–62.
9. Westermark P. Subcutaneous adipose tissue biopsy for amyloid protein studies. Methods Mol Biol. 2012;849:363–71.
10. Hazenberg BP, Limburg PC, Bijzet J, van Rijswijk MH. A quantitative method for detecting deposits of amyloid A protein in aspirated fat tissue of patients with arthritis. Ann Rheum Dis. 1999;58:96–102.
11. Puchtler H, Sweat F, Levine M. On the binding of Congo red by amyloid. J Histochem Cytochem. 1962;10:355–63.
12. Picken MM. Amyloidosis-where are we now and where are we heading? Arch Pathol Lab Med. 2010;134:545–51.
13. Giorgadze TA, Shiina N, Baloch ZW, Tomaszewski JE, Gupta PK. Improved detection of amyloid in fat pad aspiration: an evaluation of Congo red stain by fluorescent microscopy. Diagn Cytopathol. 2004; 31:300–6.
14. Ishii W, Matsuda M, Nakamura N, et al. Phenol Congo red staining enhances the diagnostic value of

abdominal fat aspiration biopsy in reactive AA amyloidosis secondary to rheumatoid arthritis. Intern Med. 2003;42:400–5.
15. Ponce P, Carvalho F, Coelho A. Valeur de la ponction-aspiration de la graisse sous-cutanée dans le diagnostic de l'amylose. Nephrologie. 1986; 7:25–7.
16. Klemi PJ, Sorsa S, Happonen RP. Fine-needle aspiration biopsy from subcutaneous fat. An easy way to diagnose secondary amyloidosis. Scand J Rheumatol. 1987;16:429–31.
17. Gertz MA, Li CY, Shirahama T, Kyle RA. Utility of subcutaneous fat aspiration for the diagnosis of systemic amyloidosis (immunoglobulin light chain). Arch Intern Med. 1988;148:929–33.
18. Sorsa S, Happonen RP, Klemi P. Oral biopsy and fine needle aspiration biopsy from subcutaneous fat in diagnosis of secondary amyloidosis. Int J Oral Maxillofac Surg. 1988;17:14–6.
19. Duston MA, Skinner M, Meenan RF, Cohen AS. Sensitivity, specificity, and predictive value of abdominal fat aspiration for the diagnosis of amyloidosis. Arthritis Rheum. 1989;32:82–5.
20. Dupond JL, de Wazières B, Saile R, et al. L'amylose systémique du sujet âgé: valeur diagnostique de l'examen de la graisse sous-cutanée abdominale et des glandes salivaires accessoires. Étude prospective chez 100 patients âgés. Rev Med Interne. 1995; 16:314–7.
21. Masouye I. Diagnostic screening of systemic amyloidosis by abdominal fat aspiration: an analysis of 100 cases. Am J Dermatopathol. 1997;19:41–5.
22. Guy CD, Jones CK. Abdominal fat pad aspiration biopsy for tissue confirmation of systemic amyloidosis: specificity, positive predictive value, and diagnostic pitfalls. Diagn Cytopathol. 2001;24:181–5.
23. Ansari-Lari MA, Ali SZ. Fine-needle aspiration of abdominal fat pad for amyloid detection: a clinically useful test? Diagn Cytopathol. 2004;30:178–81.
24. van Gameren II, Hazenberg BP, Bijzet J, van Rijswijk MH. Diagnostic accuracy of subcutaneous abdominal fat tissue aspiration for detecting systemic amyloidosis and its utility in clinical practice. Arthritis Rheum. 2006;54:2015–21.
25. Dhingra S, Krishnani N, Kumari N, Pandey R. Evaluation of abdominal fat pad aspiration cytology and grading for detection in systemic amyloidosis. Acta Cytol. 2007;51:860–4.
26. Blumenfeld W, Hildebrandt RH. Fine needle aspiration of abdominal fat for the diagnosis of amyloidosis. Acta Cytol. 1993;37:170–4.
27. Lipschutz JH, Miller T, Yen TS, Vartanian RK, Graber ML, Damon L. Unreliability of the abdominal fat pad biopsy in the evaluation of nephrosis: report of 3 consecutive cases. Am J Nephrol. 1995;15:431–5.
28. Andrews TR, Colon-Otero G, Calamia KT, Menke DM, Boylan KB, Kyle RA. Utility of subcutaneous fat aspiration for diagnosing amyloidosis in patients

with isolated peripheral neuropathy. Mayo Clin Proc. 2002;77:1287–90.

29. Päi S, Helin H, Isomäki H. Frequency of amyloidosis in Estonian patients with rheumatoid arthritis. Scand J Rheumatol. 1993;22:248–9.

30. Tiitinen S, Kaarela K, Helin H, Kautiainen H, Isomäki H. Amyloidosis–incidence and early risk factors in patients with rheumatoid arthritis. Scand J Rheumatol. 1993;22:158–61.

31. Gratacos J, Orellana C, Sanmarti R, et al. Secondary amyloidosis in ankylosing spondylitis. A systematic survey of 137 patients using abdominal fat aspiration. J Rheumatol. 1997;24:912–5.

32. El Mansoury TM, Hazenberg BP, El Badawy SA, et al. Screening for amyloid in subcutaneous fat tissue of Egyptian patients with rheumatoid arthritis: clinical and laboratory characteristics. Ann Rheum Dis. 2002;61:42–7.

33. Ishii W, Matsuda M, Nakamura A, Nakamura N, Suzuki A, Ikeda S. Abdominal fat aspiration biopsy and genotyping of serum amyloid A contribute to early diagnosis of reactive AA amyloidosis secondary to rheumatoid arthritis. Intern Med. 2003; 42:800–5.

34. Alishiri GH, Salimzadeh A, Owlia MB, Forghanizadeh J, Setarehshenas R, Shayanfar N. Prevalence of amyloid deposition in long standing rheumatoid arthritis in Iranian patients by abdominal subcutaneous fat biopsy and assessment of clinical and laboratory characteristics. BMC Musculoskelet Disord. 2006;7:43.

35. Singh G, Kumari N, Aggarwal A, Krishnani N, Misra R. Prevalence of subclinical amyloidosis in ankylosing spondylitis. J Rheumatol. 2007;34:371–3.

36. Wakhlu A, Krisnani N, Hissaria P, Aggarwal A, Misra R. Prevalence of secondary amyloidosis in Asian North Indian patients with rheumatoid arthritis. J Rheumatol. 2003;30:948–51.

37. Wiland P, Wojtala R, Goodacre J, Szechinski J. The prevalence of subclinical amyloidosis in Polish patients with rheumatoid arthritis. Clin Rheumatol. 2004;23:193–8.

38. Fine NM, Arruda-Olson AM, Dispenzieri A, et al. Yield of noncardiac biopsy for the diagnosis of transthyretin cardiac amyloidosis. Am J Cardiol. 2014;113:1723–7.

39. Ikeda S, Sekijima Y, Tojo K, Koyama J. Diagnostic value of abdominal wall fat pad biopsy in senile systemic amyloidosis. Amyloid. 2011;18:211–5.

40. Takashio S, Izumiya Y, Jinnin M, et al. Diagnostic and prognostic value of subcutaneous tissue biopsy in patients with cardiac amyloidosis. Am J Cardiol. 2012;110:1507–11.

41. Sipe JD, Benson MD, Buxbaum JN, et al. Amyloid fibril protein nomenclature: 2012 recommendations from the Nomenclature Committee of the International Society of Amyloidosis. Amyloid. 2012;19:167–70.

42. Arbustini E, Verga L, Concardi M, Palladini G, Obici L, Merlini G. Electron and immuno-electron microscopy of abdominal fat identifies and characterizes amyloid fibrils in suspected cardiac amyloidosis. Amyloid. 2002;9:108–14.

43. Hazenberg AJ, Dikkers FG, Hawkins PN, et al. Laryngeal presentation of systemic AApoAI amyloidosis in patients with apolipoprotein AI variants Leu174Ser and Leu178Pro. Laryngoscope. 2009; 119:608–15.

44. Varga J, Idelson BA, Felson D, Skinner M, Cohen AS. Lack of amyloid in abdominal fat aspirates from patients undergoing long-term hemodialysis. Arch Intern Med. 1987;147:1455–7.

45. Orfila C, Goffinet F, Goudable C, et al. Unsuitable value of abdominal fat tissue aspirate examination for the diagnosis of amyloidosis in long-term hemodialysis patients. Am J Nephrol. 1988;8:454–6.

46. Solé Arqués M, Campistol JM, Muñoz-Gómez J. Abdominal fat aspiration biopsy in dialysis-related amyloidosis. Arch Intern Med. 1988;148:988.

47. Sethi D, Cary NR, Brown EA, Woodrow DF, Gower PE. Dialysis-associated amyloid: systemic or local? Nephrol Dial Transplant. 1989;4:1054–9.

48. Uemichi T, Liepnieks JJ, Gertz MA, Benson MD. Fibrinogen A alpha chain Leu 554: an African-American kindred with late onset renal amyloidosis. Amyloid. 1998;5:188–92.

49. Westermark P, Davey E, Lindbom K, Enqvist S. Subcutaneous fat tissue for diagnosis and studies of systemic amyloidosis. Acta Histochem. 2006; 108:209–13.

50. Kiuru S. Gelsolin-related familial amyloidosis, Finnish type (FAF), and its variants found worldwide. Amyloid. 1998;5:55–66.

51. Vrana JA, Theis JD, Dasari S, Mereuta OM, Dispenzieri A, Zeldenrust SR, Gertz MA, Kurtin PJ, Grogg KL, Dogan A. Clinical diagnosis and typing of systemic amyloidosis in subcutaneous fat aspirates by mass spectrometry-based. Haematologica. 2014;99:1239–47.

52. Sie MP, van der Wiel HE, Smedts FM, de Boer AC. Human recombinant insulin and amyloidosis: an unexpected association. Neth J Med. 2010;68: 138–40.

53. Shikama Y, Kitazawa J, Yagihashi N, et al. Localized amyloidosis at the site of repeated insulin injection in a diabetic patient. Intern Med. 2010;49:397–401.

54. D'Souza A, Theis JD, Vrana JA, Buadi F, Dispenzieri A, Dogan A. Localized insulin-derived amyloidosis: a potential pitfall in the diagnosis of systemic amyloidosis by fat aspirate. Am J Hematol. 2012;87: E131–2.

55. Orfila C, Giraud P, Modesto A, Suc JM. Abdominal fat tissue aspirate in human amyloidosis: light, electron, and immunofluorescence microscopic studies. Hum Pathol. 1986;17:366–9.

56. Halloush RA, Lavrovskaya E, Mody DR, Lager D, Truong L. Diagnosis and typing of systemic amyloidosis: the role of abdominal fat pad fine needle aspiration biopsy. Cytojournal. 2010;6:24.

57. Ihse E, Ybo A, Suhr O, Lindqvist P, Backman C, Westermark P. Amyloid fibril composition is related to the phenotype of hereditary transthyretin V30M amyloidosis. J Pathol. 2008;216:253–61.
58. Kaplan B, Vidal R, Kumar A, Ghiso J, Gallo G. Immunochemical microanalysis of amyloid proteins in fine-needle aspirates of abdominal fat. Am J Clin Pathol. 1999;112:403–7.
59. De Larrea CF, Verga L, Morbini P, et al. Immuno-electron microscopy in the classification of systemic amyloidosis: experience in 423 patients from a single institution. XIVth International symposium on amyloidosis 2014 "Amyloid: Insoluble, but solvable". Indianapolis, 2014; Abstract OP-15, p. 32–3.
60. Fernández de Larrea C, Verga L, Morbini P, et al. A practical approach to the diagnosis of systemic amyloidoses. Blood. 2015;125:2239–44.
61. Hazenberg BP, Bijzet J, Limburg PC, et al. Diagnostic performance of amyloid A protein quantification in fat tissue of patients with clinical AA amyloidosis. Amyloid. 2007;14:133–40.
62. Tishler M, Pras M, Yaron M. Abdominal fat tissue aspirate in amyloidosis of familial Mediterranean fever. Clin Exp Rheumatol. 1988;6:395–7.
63. Sjöholm K, Palming J, Olofsson LE, et al. A microarray search for genes predominantly expressed in human omental adipocytes: adipose tissue as a major production site of serum amyloid A. J Clin Endocrinol Metab. 2005;90:2233–9.
64. Bijzet J, de Boer L, Haagsma EB, Hazenberg BP. An indirect ELISA for transthyretin quantification in fat tissue of patients with ATTR amyloidosis. In: Hazenberg BP, Bijzet J, editors. XIIIth International symposium on amyloidosis 2012 "From misfolded proteins to well-designed treatment". Groningen: GUARD; 2013. p. 168–70.
65. Bijzet J, van Gameren II, Limburg PC, Bos R, Vellenga E, Hazenberg BP. Diagnostic performance of measuring free light chains in fat tissue of patients with AL amyloidosis. Amyloid. 2011;18 Suppl 1:71–2.
66. Picken MM, Herrera GA. The burden of "sticky" amyloid: typing challenges. Arch Pathol Lab Med. 2007;131:850–1.
67. Picken MM. New insights into systemic amyloidosis: the importance of diagnosis of specific type. Curr Opin Nephrol Hypertens. 2007;16:196–203.
68. Pras M, Schubert M, Zucker-Franklin D, et al. The characterization of soluble amyloid prepared in water. J Clin Invest. 1968;47:924–33.
69. Glenner GG, Wong CW. Alzheimer's disease: initial report of the purification and characterization of a novel cerebrovascular amyloid protein. Biochem Biophys Res Commun. 1984;120:885–90.
70. Westermark P, Benson L, Juul J, Sletten K. Use of subcutaneous abdominal fat biopsy specimen for detailed typing of amyloid fibril protein-AL by amino acid sequence analysis. J Clin Pathol. 1989;42:817–9.
71. Forsberg AH, Sletten K, Benson L, et al. Abdominal fat biopsy for characterization of the major amyloid fibril proteins by amino acid sequence. In: Natvig JB, Forre O, Husby G, editors. Amyloid and amyloidosis 1990. Norwell, MA: Kluver Academic; 1990. p. 797–800.
72. Olsen KE, Sletten K, Westermark P. Extended analysis of AL-amyloid protein from abdominal wall subcutaneous fat biopsy: kappa IV immunoglobulin light chain. Biochem Biophys Res Commun. 1998;245:713–6.
73. Kaplan B, Hrncic R, Murphy CL, Gallo G, Weiss DT, Solomon A. Microextraction and purification techniques applicable to chemical characterization of amyloid proteins in minute amounts of tissue. Methods Enzymol. 1999;309:67–81.
74. Kaplan B, Murphy CL, Ratner V, Pras M, Weiss DT, Solomon A. Micro-method to isolate and purify amyloid proteins for chemical characterization. Amyloid. 2001;8:22–9.
75. Kaplan B, Shtrasburg S, Pras M. Micropurification techniques in the analysis of amyloid proteins. J Clin Pathol. 2003;56:86–90.
76. Murphy CL, Eulitz M, Hrncic R, et al. Chemical typing of amyloid protein contained in formalin-fixed paraffin-embedded biopsy specimens. Am J Clin Pathol. 2001;116:135–42.
77. Kaplan B, Martin BM, Livneh A, Pras M, Gallo GR. Biochemical subtyping of amyloid in formalin-fixed tissue samples confirms and supplements immunohistologic data. Am J Clin Pathol. 2004; 121:794–800.
78. Murphy CL, Wang S, Williams T, Weiss DT, Solomon A. Characterization of systemic amyloid deposits by mass spectrometry. Methods Enzymol. 2006;412:48–62.
79. Vrana JA, Gamez JD, Madden BJ, Theis JD, Bergen 3rd HR, Dogan A. Classification of amyloidosis by laser microdissection and mass spectrometry-based proteomic analysis in clinical biopsy specimens. Blood. 2009;114:4957–9.
80. Lavatelli F, Perlman DH, Spencer B, et al. Amyloidogenic and associated proteins in systemic amyloidosis proteome of adipose tissue. Mol Cell Proteomics. 2008;7:1570–83.
81. Brambilla F, Lavatelli F, Di Silvestre D, et al. Reliable typing of systemic amyloidoses through proteomic analysis of subcutaneous adipose tissue. Blood. 2012;119:1844–7.
82. Brambilla F, Lavatelli F, Di Silvestre D, et al. Shotgun protein profile of human adipose tissue and its changes in relation to systemic amyloidoses. J Proteome Res. 2013;12:5642–55.
83. Lavatelli F, Vrana JA. Proteomic typing of amyloid deposits in systemic amyloidoses. Amyloid. 2011;18:177–82.
84. Westermark P. Amyloid diagnosis, subcutaneous adipose tissue, immunohistochemistry and mass spectrometry. Amyloid. 2011;18:175–6.

85. Kimmich C, Hegenbart U, Schönland SO, Bijzet J, Hazenberg BP. Introduction of fat aspiration at a tertiary institution to diagnose systemic amyloidosis. In: Benson MD, Kluve-Beckerman B, Liepnieks JJ, editors. XIVth International symposium on amyloidosis 2014 "Amyloid: Insoluble, but solvable". Indianapolis; 2014.

86. Gómez-Casanovas E, Sanmartí R, Solé M, Cañete JD, Muñoz-Gómez J. The clinical significance of amyloid fat deposits in rheumatoid arthritis: a systematic long-term followup study using abdominal fat aspiration. Arthritis Rheum. 2001;44:66–72.

87. Bardarov S, Michael CW, Pu RT, Pang Y. Computer-assisted image analysis of amyloid deposits in abdominal fat pad aspiration biopsies. Diagn Cytopathol. 2009;37:30–5.

88. van Gameren II, Hazenberg BP, Bijzet J, et al. Amyloid load in fat tissue in patients with amyloidosis reflects disease severity and predicts survival. Arthritis Care Res (Hoboken). 2010;62:296–301.

89. Haagsma EB, van Gameren II, Bijzet J, Posthumus MD, Hazenberg BP. Familial amyloidotic polyneuropathy: long-term follow-up of abdominal fat tissue aspirate in patients with and without liver transplantation. Amyloid. 2007;14:221–6.

90. Tsuchiya A, Yazaki M, Kametani F, Takei Y, Ikeda S. Marked regression of abdominal fat amyloid in patients with familial amyloid polyneuropathy during long-term follow-up after liver transplantation. Liver Transpl. 2008;14:563–70.

91. Tsuchiya-Suzuki A, Yazaki M, Kametani F, Sekijima Y, Ikeda S. Wild-type transthyretin significantly contributes to the formation of amyloid fibrils in familial amyloid polyneuropathy patients with amyloidogenic transthyretin Val30Met. Hum Pathol. 2011; 42:236–43.

92. Ihse E, Suhr OB, Hellman U, Westermark P. Variation in amount of wild-type transthyretin in different fibril and tissue types in ATTR amyloidosis. J Mol Med. 2011;89:171–80.

93. Ihse E, Rapezzi C, Merlini G, et al. Amyloid fibrils containing fragmented ATTR may be the standard fibril composition in ATTR amyloidosis. Amyloid. 2013;20:142–50.

94. van Gameren II, van Rijswijk MH, Bijzet J, Vellenga E, Hazenberg BP. Histological regression of amyloid in AL amyloidosis is exclusively seen after normalization of serum free light chain. Haematologica. 2009;94:1094–100.

95. Nilsson KP, Ikenberg K, Åslund A, et al. Structural typing of systemic amyloidosis by luminescent-conjugated polymer spectroscopy. Am J Pathol. 2010;176:563–74.

96. Sjölander D, Bijzet J, Hazenberg BP, Nilsson KP, Hammarström P. Sensitive and rapid assessment of amyloid by oligothiophene fluorescence in subcutaneous fat tissue. Amyloid. 2015;22(1):19–25.

97. Poitou C, Viguerie N, Cancello R, et al. Serum amyloid A: production by human white adipocyten and regulation by obesity and nutrition. Diabetologia. 2005;48:519–28.

98. Upragarin N, Landman WJ, Gaastra W, Gruys E. Extrahepatic production of acute phase serum amyloid A. Histol Histopathol. 2005;20:1295–307.

99. Kluve-Beckerman B, Liepnieks JJ, Wang L, Benson MD. A cell culture system for the study of amyloid pathogenesis. Amyloid formation by peritoneal macrophages cultured with recombinant serum amyloid A. Am J Pathol. 1999;155:123–33.

100. Elimova E, Kisilevsky R, Szarek WA, Ancsin JB. Amyloidogenesis recapitulated in cell culture: a peptide inhibitor provides direct evidence for the role of heparan sulfate and suggests a new treatment strategy. FASEB J. 2004;18:1749–51.

101. Magy N, Benson MD, Liepnieks JJ, Kluve-Beckerman B. Cellular events associated with the initial phase of AA amyloidogenesis: insights from a human monocyte model. Amyloid. 2007;14:51–63.

102. Ishii W, Liepnieks JJ, Yamada T, Benson MD, Kluve-Beckerman B. Human SAA1-derived amyloid deposition in cell culture: a consistent model utilizing human peripheral blood mononuclear cells and serum-free medium. Amyloid. 2013;20:61–71.

103. Fat aspiration procedure for the detection of amyloid—instruction video. http://www.amyloid.nl/investigations.htm. Accessed 14 July 2014.

104. Kettwich LG, Sibbitt Jr WL, Emil NS, et al. New device technologies for subcutaneous fat biopsy. Amyloid. 2012;19:66–73.

105. Devata S, Hari P, Markelova N, Li R, Komorowski R, Shidham VB. Detection of amyloid in abdominal fat pad aspirates in early amyloidosis: role of electron microscopy and Congo red stained cell block sections. Cytojournal. 2011;8:11.

106. Shidham VB, Hunt B, Jardeh SS, Barboi AC, Devata S, Hari P. Performing and processing FNA of anterior fat pad for amyloid. J Vis Exp. 2010;30(44). pii: 1747.

107. Jager PL, Hazenberg BP, Franssen EJ, Limburg PC, van Rijswijk MH, Piers DA. Kinetic studies with iodine-123-labeled serum amyloid P component in patients with systemic AA and AL amyloidosis and assessment of clinical value. J Nucl Med. 1998; 39:699–706.

108. Commercial kit for SAA ELISA. http://www.hycult-biotech.com/products/innate-immunity/acute-phase-proteins/acute-phase-proteins-saa-human-elisa-kit-p11209-html. Accessed 14 July 2014.

Generic Diagnosis of Amyloid: A Summary of Current Recommendations and the Editor's Comments on Chapters 13–16

17

Maria M. Picken

This chapter provides a brief summary of recommendations on current standards for the diagnosis of amyloidosis. It is based on the results of a consensus session held at the XIIth and XIIIth International Symposium on Amyloidosis, organized by the International Society of Amyloidosis [1, 2] and the recently published updated recommendations on amyloid diagnosis and nomenclature [3] agreed upon at the XIVth Symposium of the International Society of Amyloidosis. The latter includes an acknowledgement that, besides apple-green birefringence, other anomalous colors, such as yellow or orange, are also diagnostic of amyloid. An assessment of current practices in amyloid diagnosis, based on a survey of amyloid centers and practicing renal pathologists, is also included [1, 4]. The editor's comments, in connection with the corresponding prior chapters, are also provided.

Clinical Diagnosis: The "Gold Standard"

Currently, a clinical diagnosis of amyloidosis is made by the histochemical demonstration of amyloid deposits in organs and tissue sections.

M.M. Picken, MD, PhD (✉)
Department of Pathology, Loyola University Medical Center, Loyola University Chicago, Building 110, Room 2242, 2160 South First Avenue, Maywood, IL 60153, USA
e-mail: mpicken@luc.edu; MMPicken@aol.com

Congo red stain continues to be the generally accepted standard in amyloid detection [1–3].

According to the most recent publication of the nomenclature committee of the International Society of Amyloidosis, "an amyloid fibril protein is defined as the protein (which) must occur in body tissue deposits and exhibit affinity for Congo red and green, yellow or orange birefringence when the Congo red stained deposits are viewed with polarized light " [3]. Thus, while the apple-green birefringence of Congo red positive material is typically described in conventional pathology terminology as the most specific finding, it has been recognized that other anomalous colors (yellow or orange) are also diagnostic [3].

This expanded definition of the diagnostic results of Congo red stain birefringence acknowledges that while pure green can be seen under *ideal optical conditions*, more often than not are green and yellow also present, caused by strain birefringence, or green and orange caused by uncrossing of the polarizer and analyzer [3, 5–7]. Figures 17.1 and 17.2 illustrate this point [8, 9].

The concept of "anomalous colors" rather than "pathognomonic apple-green birefringence" was postulated earlier by Howie et al. [5–7] and is explained in more detail by Howie in an earlier chapter in this book. Anomalous colors are those produced by birefringent effects. Thus, as stated by Howie, "strictly speaking, Congo red-stained amyloid should be said to show anomalous colors when examined between a polarizer and a

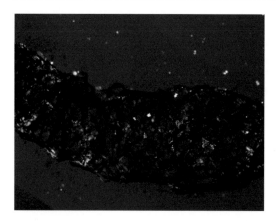

Fig. 17.1 Fat needle biopsy. *Congo red*-stained slide viewed under polarized light showing *apple green* as well as *yellow* anomalous colors. Specimen obtained using a 16-gauge needle (Reprinted with permission from [9])

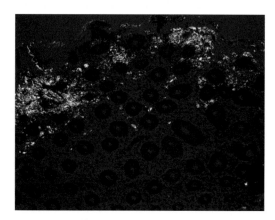

Fig. 17.2 Colon biopsy with deposits of amyloid seen in the superficial lamina propria. *Congo red*-stained slide viewed under polarized light showing *apple green* as well as *yellow* anomalous colors (Reprinted with permission from [8])

crossed polarizer" [7]. This property of the different absorption of polarized light, depending on its orientation, is called dichroism.

In the primary care situation, in particular, there is a need for enhanced clinical suspicion in order to instigate the initial investigation of amyloidosis by histochemical methods. It is important to stress that the use of H&E-stained slides alone is insufficiently sensitive to elicit a suspicion of amyloid. A special stain, preferably Congo red (alkaline Congo red), must be performed in order to not only confirm the presence of amyloid but also to rule it out.

Worldwide, many centers use in-house reagents; however, currently available commercial kits for Congo red stain, which can be used with automated stainers, have also been reported to be satisfactory by those who use them [1, 4]. Standard quality assurance measures need to be routinely applied and a control slide examined with each run. In the author's own experience, occasional runs may result in weaker stains, which need to be repeated and investigated. Preanalytical steps, involving prolonged tissue fixation in formaldehyde, or prolonged storage of the cut sections, should be avoided [10].

For diagnosis of amyloid, apart from correct fixation and a proper staining protocol, a high-quality microscope, a strong light source, pupil accommodation, a rotating table, and *experience in interpretation* are also mandatory.

It is critical to have a high-quality microscope with a powerful light source and a commercial polarizer set with rotatable table capabilities (discussed by Howie, Linke, Bijzet, et al. in this book). There is absolutely no room for "homemade" substitutes. A rotating table, in particular, is critical for exposing the entire area containing amyloid deposits by gradually rotating the table and, thereby, "unmasking" areas of amyloid deposition that were initially obscured by the phenomenon of "polarization shadow" (see Chap. 14 in this book) or exposing other "anomalous colors" as described by Howie in Chap. 13. As the section is rotated on the microscope stage, the bright and dark areas in amyloid deposits will be seen to change positions depending on their relation to the plane of the polarizer: different colors are seen in areas that are roughly perpendicular to each other, they appear to rotate as the section is rotated, and they exchange positions when the stage is rotated by 90°. The role of optics in achieving perfect polarization results, including "strain birefringence," is discussed by Howie in this book (see Chap. 13).

Given the degree of complexity and expertise involved, it is not surprising that difficulties in the interpretation of Congo red stain were commonly reported. Interestingly, variability in Congo red stain was reported by 75 % of responders and was particularly noted in AL [1, 4]. While collagen is notorious for showing anomalous birefringence and may render certain sections difficult to interpret, in the author's own experience, red blood cells that are present in small capillaries, or in a small hemorrhage, may also, at times, produce birefringence similar to that of amyloid. A similar observation has also been noted by Verga et al. (see Chap. 22 on amyloid typing in this book). Thus, Congo red stain birefringence should always be correlated with the bright field appearance of tissue.

There are many reports in the literature of amyloid proteins being detectable by immunohistochemistry in the absence of Congo red positivity. This has been noted, in particular, in experimental amyloidosis and Alzheimer's disease [11–14] but also in extracerebral amyloidoses such as those found in patients with hereditary ATTR [15–17]. It is now widely accepted that such deposits represent a preamyloidotic stage of tissue deposition and that these preamyloidotic, nonfibrillar deposits are cytotoxic, perhaps even more so than fully formed fibrils [18, 19]. This is in contrast to the situation with preclinical amyloid deposits, which are detectable in tissues by standard methods, seemingly in the absence of clinical symptoms.

Thickness of Paraffin Sections for Congo Red Stain

Thicker sections, 4–8 µm, are *helpful* in the detection of small deposits for two reasons: (1) in thicker sections, amyloid deposits are already visible by bright field microscopy as salmon-pink-stained areas, and (2) in thicker sections, sample error is less likely to occur. This is particularly relevant in the early stages of amyloidosis, where small deposits of amyloid may not be present in each section. As discussed earlier in this book, by Linke, the pathognomonic Congo red birefringence seen under polarized light can be demonstrated only in sections that are cut within *standard* thicknesses. In particular, when sections are cut with a thickness of less than 1 µm, the anisotropy changes from apple green to bluish white. While sections that are too thin may fail to exhibit bire-

fringence, in the author's own experience, the sections typically used in renal pathology are quite adequate. The thinnest paraffin sections used in renal pathology are at least 2 µm thick, with 3 µm being cut most frequently. In the editor's own experience, these thicknesses do not interfere with polarization, providing that appropriate equipment is used. Diagnostic birefringence can be seen, even though no salmon-pink color is apparent by bright field illumination (please see also, in this book, Chap. 14, Fig. 1C by Linke). It is also true that small deposits may be easily missed in thinner sections. In order to minimize sampling error, the author routinely stains two slides with Congo red (and more if clinically indicated), preferably obtained from different levels within the block. Again, the importance of proper optics in the evaluation of Congo red-stained slides cannot be overstressed. Please note also that specimens that are too thick may be difficult to interpret; for example, thick fat smears (please see also Chap. 14 by Linke in this book).

Sampling Error

Sampling error is one of the most important and also one of the most common pitfalls encountered in the diagnosis of amyloid. It is defined as the apparent absence of amyloid in a tissue section from a patient with amyloidosis. As noted by Linke, elsewhere in this book, a negative diagnosis of amyloid, based on examination of a single section, can never be conclusive. Therefore, in patients with a higher level of suspicion, on both clinical as well as on pathologic grounds, but where initial slides are negative for amyloid, the editor routinely evaluates multiple Congo red-stained sections. Moreover, repeated biopsies may be needed (e.g., repeated abdominal fat biopsies) in order to conclusively establish the diagnosis. Not uncommonly, amyloid deposits may be detected later in the course of the disease, with earlier biopsies being truly negative. Sampling error may also be responsible for reports of the detection of amyloid-like fibrils by electron microscopy but with negative Congo red stain results.

Other Stains and/or Modifications of the Congo Red Stain that Are Worth Considering and Strongly Recommended

The birefringence with anomalous colors, that is found when Congo red-stained amyloid is examined with polarized light and which is considered to be the most specific finding, is, however, even under optimal circumstances, less sensitive than some other stains. However, these other stains are, in turn, less specific. Despite this lesser specificity of polarization alternatives, the use of fluorochromes is particularly worthwhile due to their markedly increased sensitivity. Interestingly, Congo red itself can be used as a fluorochrome when examined under fluorescent light. This application offers the added benefit of examining the same section using two different techniques: namely, fluorescence and polarization (as shown by Linke elsewhere in this book). Among other fluorochromes, Thioflavin T and S are particularly useful in the diagnosis of amyloid (discussed in this book in Chap. 15, see also Chap. 29) [20].

The use of fluorescence for the detection of amyloid is gaining in popularity. Elimination of the "polarization shadow" phenomenon through the use of fluorescence results in a significant increase in the sensitivity of detection of small deposits. Briefly, using polarization microscopy, at any given time, only a portion of the amyloid deposit shows diagnostic orange–green–yellow birefringence—only by further rotation of the stage, other parts will become visible while, in turn, the formerly visible areas will be obscured by the "polarization shadow." Thus, at any given time, only a portion of the amyloid is visualized (please see also the Chaps. 13 and 14 in this book). Hence, the enhanced sensitivity of Thioflavin and Congo red stains as fluorochromes for the detection of amyloid is, in part, due to visualization of the entire area containing amyloid, at the same time. The absence of "polarization shadow" makes the detection of small deposits much more sensitive (Fig. 17.3a–c).

Note particularly that different filters may be used in the Congo red fluorescence technique, including a filter for detecting fluorescein isothiocyanate (FITC) with an absorption maximum of 495 (blue) and an emission maximum of 525 nm (green), and tetramethylrhodamine isothiocyanate (TRITC) with an absorption maximum of 555 nm (green) and an emission maximum of 580 nm (red). With the former filter, amyloid deposits appear orange while, with the latter filter, deposits are red. In the editor's own experience, the red fluorescence (TRITC) filter gives a cleaner and more-easily discernible visualization of amyloid (Fig. 17.3c, see also Chap. 28, Fig. 28.6d). For detecting amyloid in laser microdissection techniques, a newer generation of filters is being used, i.e., the BGR filter cube; here also, red fluorescence is used preferentially. A practical approach would be to try different filters and see which gives the best results with the microscope/optics available in a given laboratory.

As noted in the chapter devoted to the Thioflavin stain, this is easy to perform, the outcome is predictable and interpretation is much easier than with the Congo red stain (see Chap. 15). The Thioflavin T stain is used extensively in the research setting and, given the advantages listed above, it should be considered as a desirable screening test for use in the clinical setting as well. As can be seen from other chapters in this book, several laboratories have used Thioflavin stains (T or S) successfully in amyloid diagnosis (please see also Chap. 29, Figs. 29.1c, 29.2h, i, and 29.8c, g). For the detection of amyloid with the Thioflavin stain, different filters may also be used as shown in Chap. 29. Other issues, namely the need for a fluorescence microscope, or the fading of sections, are relatively minor. While such equipment may not be readily available in general surgical pathology laboratories, it is standard equipment in renal pathology/dermatopathology laboratories, and renal pathologists, in particular, also have the necessary experience for handling such microscopes. Also, faded sections can be restained. In sum, the thioflavin stain is a desirable option for screening purposes and is worthy of inclusion in most laboratory protocols, in particular, those that also have renal/dermathopathologists on the staff.

Fig. 17.3 *Congo red*-stained slide viewed under bright light (**a**), the same slide viewed under polarized light (**b**) and under fluorescence light (**c**) using TRITC filter showing abundant deposits of amyloid in various compartments of the kidney

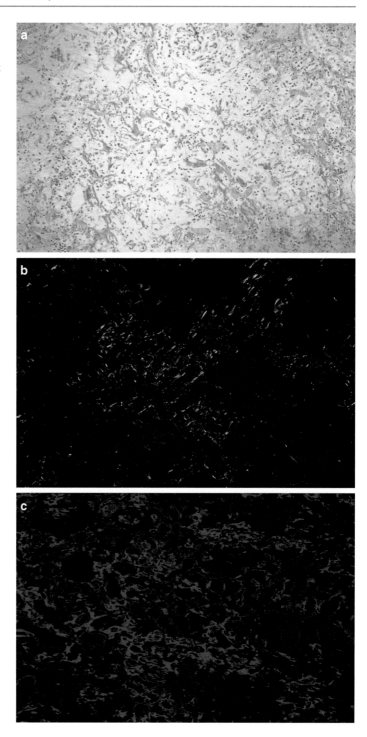

The combination of Congo red and immuno-histochemistry on a single slide (the "overlay technique") is discussed extensively by Linke in Chap. 14 in this book. However, while the combi-nation of Congo red stain with immunohisto-chemistry results in enhanced sensitivity for amyloid detection, prior knowledge of the amy-loid type is necessary. This is possible in certain clinical situations; for example, when patients with rheumatoid arthritis, or periodic fevers, are monitored for the development of AA amyloidosis, or when patients with a known mutation associated with one of the hereditary amyloidoses are monitored for development of the corresponding amyloidosis (see chapter by Linke, Chap. 14, and Refs. [15, 17]). Another approach to consider is the use of immunostain for amyloid P component, which, being invariably associated with deposits of amyloid, may allow its early detection and localization [21, 22] (see also discussion regarding amyloid P component in chapters on amyloid typing).

The concept of "amyloid signature" has been introduced in amyloid proteomics. Since several compounds, most notably amyloid P component and Apolipoprotein E, are invariably associated with all deposits of amyloid, regardless of their amyloid protein precursor type, their presence in abundant amounts, above the "baseline," is considered indicative of the presence of amyloid deposits (please see chapters on mass spectrometry) in this part of the book.

Other Stains that Are Less Useful and/or Obsolete

Other stains: sulfated alcian blue (SAB), crystal violet, methyl violet, various cotton dyes (e.g., pagoda red, Sirius red), other fluorescent dyes (Phorwhite BBU), periodic acid-Schiff (PAS), and even other fabric dyes (RIT Scarlet No. 5, and RIT Cardinal Red No. 9 [yielding a bright orange color]) have been used to detect amyloid, with variable results. The presence of carbohydrate moieties in amyloid fibrils has also encouraged some investigators to use carbohydrate stains, such as alcian blue or even periodic acid-Schiff, to demonstrate amyloid deposits; however, dye uptake is variable and generally poor with these methods. SAB identifies glycosaminoglycans (GAGs) that are present in all types of amyloid, similar to amyloid P component. Likewise, metachromatic stains, such as crystal violet or methyl violet, capitalize on the carbohydrate content of amyloid fibrils, but their staining

is not very specific, and the low sensitivity of these methods has caused them to fall into disfavor; these stains also fade with time. Sirius red F3B (but not Sirius red F4B) stains amyloid rose-red while the background is clear to pale pink. However, the Sirius red stain is not specific for amyloid as it also binds to all types of collagen and, for this reason, has been used as a stain for collagen.

The Diagnosis of Amyloid: Summary of Options for Clinical Diagnosis

While the use of alternatives to the Congo red stain may be helpful (in particular, the use of stains/modifications yielding increased sensitivity), ultimately, the results will have to be confirmed against the generally accepted gold standard, i.e., the Congo red stain. Nonetheless, stains with increased sensitivity are helpful in screening and can be instrumental in assuring that potential true-positive cases are not missed. If needed, help from a specialized laboratory should be obtained with regard to both stain performance and/or interpretation. The editor's own preference is for a combined approach using both Congo red stain polarization as well as Congo red stain + fluorescence and/or Thioflavin stain. The appropriate equipment and environment are important. It is advisable to have a high-quality polarizer (with stage rotation capability) fitted into a fluorescence microscope, which also has bright-field capabilities. Evaluation of the same section-field under various types of illumination is an excellent approach and is extensively discussed by Linke in this book. Installing the polarizer set in a fluorescence microscope will also ensure that specimens are routinely evaluated in the dark, which allows for pupil accommodation and the easier detection of small deposits. The editor's advice follows that of Linke—i.e., to take advantage of the more sensitive methods first and, thereby, to progressively "narrow down" the detection area until it can be viewed by the "gold-standard" of Congo red stain under polarized light. Some minute deposits can be seen by polarized light only under higher magnification; thus, in order to confirm the fluorescence results by polarization, an area of interest may need to be examined at higher magnification than that typically used for fluorescence. As mentioned earlier, the polarization (and fluorescence) results should always be correlated with the bright-field appearance, in order to avoid certain pitfalls (red blood cells, etc.).

Electron Microscopy

Electron microscopy, which demonstrates the fibrillar structure of amyloid, is not practical for screening purposes because of the high levels of magnification involved and, therefore, the relatively small screening area. Electron microscopic examination is not required in routine clinical practice and, in a recent survey [1, 4], it was performed routinely by 45–72 % of all respondents, mostly as part of a routine native kidney biopsy workup, while others performed this study either occasionally, rarely, or when possible. It is felt that the interpretation of small amyloid-like deposits is inherently difficult when based on electron microscopy alone, and is particularly difficult in the kidney, as renal glomeruli not uncommonly show vaguely fibrillary areas, in particular associated with scarring (as discussed by Herrera elsewhere in this book). Thus, for clinical purposes, the diagnosis of renal amyloid based solely on electron microscopy, in the absence of a positive Congo red or Thioflavin stain, is considered insufficient for a definite diagnosis of amyloid and should be discouraged. Congo red negative deposits with amyloid-like fibrils, detectable only by electron microscopy, were reported by 39 % of survey respondents. At present, the clinical significance of these findings is not clear but sampling error and/or low sensitivity of Congo red stain may be responsible for this discrepancy, at least in part. However, electron microscopy is critical for the detection and characterization of various other organized deposits that should be in the differential diagnosis (fibrillary and immunotactoid deposits, powdery deposits in light chain deposition disease, and various crystalline inclusions such as those

seen in light chain proximal tubulopathy or crystal-storing histiocytosis); these are discussed extensively in Part II of this book [23, 24]. While many such deposits are systemic, some are exclusively or predominantly detected in the kidney (Part II). All of these other types of deposits are Congo red stain negative.

The Choice of Tissue Specimen: Fat as an Underutilized Source of Tissue for Amyloid Detection, Typing, Monitoring Therapy and Diagnosis of Related Diseases

In order to confirm a clinical suspicion of amyloidosis, a tissue specimen is needed. While biopsy of the diseased organ itself, in particular, a kidney or myocardial biopsy, is the most sensitive diagnostic method and may detect causes other than amyloid, the invasive nature of the procedure is disadvantageous. Alternatively, rectal or gingival, minor salivary gland biopsies have been utilized successfully for amyloidosis screening for decades with a good sensitivity of about 80 % [17]. In recent years, aspirated subcutaneous abdominal fat tissue has been used to screen for *systemic* amyloidosis. This technique is noninvasive, safe, cheap, elegant, fast, and can be performed as an outpatient procedure. As discussed, the procedure has a good sensitivity if performed and analyzed *properly*. However, in common practice, the amount and quality of tissue available for examination may be too small to allow testing with confidence. Not uncommonly, the procedure is performed by inexperienced trainees and the needles used are too narrow. As discussed by Bijzet et al., elsewhere in this book, 16 gauge needless should be used routinely (Fig. 17.1). Thus, in the editor's own experience, surgical fat biopsy is an excellent alternative to fat aspirates and avoids the pitfalls associated with inadequate tissue collection. The editor routinely receives a surgical biopsy consisting of 1–2 cm^3 of subcutaneous fat (Fig. 17.4). The specimen is received either fresh, in saline, or in fluorescence transport medium (particularly if submitted from an outside institution). Such a specimen is abundant

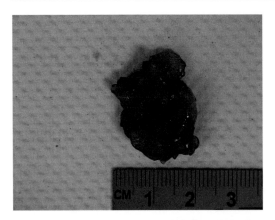

Fig. 17.4 Surgical fat biopsy. Such a sample provides abundant material for amyloid detection as well as amyloid typing. Multiple levels can be examined and false negative results owing to sample error can be easily avoided. In contrast to fine needle aspiration biopsy, blood contamination is minimal (Reprinted with permission from [8])

and 35 these patients may develop amyloid at sites of repeated subcutaneous insulin injection and thus may develop iatrogenic insulin amyloid deposits. In these patients, deposits of amyloid should not be considered as a manifestation of either systemic amyloidosis or localized non-insulin derived amyloid; amyloid typing should be performed if needed. Recently, two patients with skin reactions at the sites of enfuvirtide administration had biopsies that showed Congo red positivity suggestive of amyloidosis [25]. Finally, other deposits, such as those seen in crystal storing histiocytosis (see Chap. 12) and the light chain deposition diseases may be detected in adipose tissue [23, 24] but these deposits are Congo red negative. Hence, stains for kappa and lambda light chains should be considered in all patients with underlying plasma cell dyscrasia who are screened for amyloid.

enough to allow processing of 1/3 for paraffin sections and freezing of the remainder for possible amyloid typing.

If necessary, repeated fat specimens (aspirates or surgical biopsies) can be obtained, in order to monitor for the development of systemic amyloidosis in patients with known risk factors, such as plasma cell dyscrasia, mutations associated with hereditary amyloidosis, or chronic inflammatory states, including periodic fevers; repeated fat biopsies should also be considered in such patients when the initial biopsies are negative.

Other applications, discussed in this book by Bijzet et al., in Chap.16, include amyloid typing, as well as quantitation and monitoring of therapy. It should also be pointed out that the presence of amyloid in subcutaneous fat is usually associated with systemic amyloidosis. Thus, abdominal fat biopsy is also useful in amyloidosis staging where distinction between a systemic versus a localized process is needed for treatment strategies (see Part I and VI in this book). While a negative fat biopsy may not rule out the systemic process, a positive result supports it. However, there is one important consideration in diabetic patients who depend on repeated injections of insulin, typically administered into the abdominal subcutaneous tissue. As discussed in Chaps. 7,

Clinical Diagnosis: Current Challenges and Possible Solutions

As in prior years, the emphasis is on early detection of amyloid deposits and the need for increased awareness of the disease, the available diagnostic and treatment options, and enhanced clinical suspicion of amyloid diseases among pathologists and clinicians. However, it has been universally agreed that the Congo red stain is not easy to interpret and that, besides technical variables, the observer's experience is of paramount importance. It should be emphasized that the identification of amyloid in tissue is not straightforward and considerable experience is required. In general, Renal Pathologists are involved in the diagnosis of amyloid more frequently than other surgical pathologists, are more familiar with polarization and fluorescence microscopy, and are, therefore, more likely to be more experienced in the handling of such specimens. Furthermore, the necessary equipment is usually already in place in Renal Pathology Laboratories or can be easily modified. Thus, not surprisingly, a recent survey demonstrated that many Renal Pathology Laboratories are already handling non-renal specimens that were submitted for amyloid testing [4]. It is also strongly recommended that, given the level of difficulty involved, the expertise required, and the relatively low incidence of positive specimens, within each group of pathologists, a dedicated person should be assigned to the handling of *all* "amyloid" specimens, whether by way of consulting, triaging and/or advising with regard to available options.

Finally, the reporting of amyloid should include the following: (1) anatomic site (if known), (2) histologic structure(s) involved by amyloid (if known, list all), (3) distinction between vascular limited versus stromal; distinctive patterns should also be described (glomerular vs. extraglomerular, sinusoidal vs. portal, interstitial vs. endocardial, etc.), (4) scoring should be provided for fat, according to established criteria (scoring for bone marrow, liver, kidney is currently under discussion/development), and (5) stain/method upon which the diagnosis was based [2]. Please see also Part VI, Chaps. 36–38.

Amyloid Diagnosis in the Future?

It is apparent that, despite the Congo red stain being employed since the 1920s for the detection of amyloid, there are still major problems associated with its use, mainly as a consequence of the difficulties encountered in its interpretation by pathologists. Clearly, more sensitive and easier screening procedures for amyloid detection are needed.

Several years ago, Nilsson et al., reported that luminescent-conjugated thiophene polymers (LCP) were able to sensitively detect and even type amyloid deposits [26, 27]. Thus, a European Union project "LUPAS" (Luminescent Polymers for in vivo imaging of Amyloid Signatures) was initiated, with the goal of developing novel tools for the diagnosis and therapy of Alzheimer and prion diseases. Luminescent-conjugated oligothiophenes (LCOs) have been developed with the goal of targeting preamyloid states on the misfolding pathway and discriminating between different stages of amyloid formation in vitro and in vivo. The LCOs constitute a new set of fluorophores that preferentially bind to amyloid

deposits and, upon doing so, change its spectral signature [28, 29]. Spectral imaging fluorescence microscopy, in combination with atomic force microscopy (AFM), was used to evaluate the formation of different misfolded conformations. Using animal models of prionosis, size exclusion chromatography, Fluorescence lifetime imaging (FLIM), and 2-photon excitation microscopy have also been used to monitor fibrillogenesis.

Only rare reports pertain to amyloid detection in body fluids. Although amyloid can be seen, on occasion, in certain body fluids (urine, synovial fluid), in general there is a difficulty in diagnosing urinary/body fluid amyloid in the absence of clinical suspicion [30–32]. Urinary exosomes have been explored for potential application to the diagnosis of plasma cell dyscrasia-related kidney diseases [33]. However, no advances applicable to daily practice in surgical pathology, examination of body fluids, and/or the possibility of automation have been reported as yet.

Summary and Conclusions

Thus far, all available tests for the diagnosis of amyloid (as well as recently published developments) are based on the examination of tissue sections; this makes the anatomic pathologist/histopathologist indispensable to the process. Currently, no data are available on the prospects for diagnosis based on the examination of body fluids and/or the possibility of automation.

Most importantly, it must be emphasized that the diagnosis of amyloid is not trivial and practical experience is the most significant factor in the successful diagnosis of amyloidosis, in particular, at the early stages when therapy may be most successful. Therefore, development of an advanced level of expertise by a dedicated pathologist within each group is strongly recommended. In case of difficulty, a second opinion, from another expert laboratory, should be obtained. Currently, effective and highly sensitive screening in the primary practice setting is needed, with the possibility of increased specificity being provided via specialized laboratories. In this regard, the wider application of fluorochromes to clinical diagnosis may be helpful. Also, the wider application of fat biopsy to early amyloidosis detection and staging is encouraged.

Conclusions

1. There is an urgent need for increased awareness of the amyloidoses among pathologists and clinicians, as well as available diagnostic and treatment options.
2. There is a need to develop expertise in the diagnosis of amyloidosis
3. There is a need to concentrate on early detection.
4. The detection of amyloid, the initial step, is the most critical and is entirely dependent upon the skill of the pathologist! Higher sensitivity methods should be used in screening protocols and consultation with reference laboratories should be sought to help with and/or confirm the diagnosis.
5. Reporting—the following information should be included in the pathology report: (1) anatomic site(s), (2) histologic structure(s) involved by amyloid, (3) distinctive patterns of involvement, (4) scoring where applicable, and (5) method (stain) by which amyloid was diagnosed [2].

References

1. Picken MM, Westermark P. Amyloid detection and typing: summary of current practice and recommendations of the consensus group. Amyloid. 2011;18 Suppl 1:48–50.
2. Picken MM, Hazenberg BPC, Westermark P. Early detection of amyloid and its reporting: where are we now and where are we heading? In: Hazenberg BPC, Bijzet J, editors. The Proceedings of the XIIIth International Symposium on Amyloidosis; Netherlands: GUARD (Groningen Unit for Amyloidosis Research & Development) UMC Groningen; 2013. p. 459–465.
3. Sipe JD, Benson MD, Buxbaum JN, Ikeda S, Merlini G, Saraiva MJ, Westermark P. Nomenclature 2014: amyloid fibril proteins and clinical classification of
the amyloidosis. Amyloid. 2014;21(4):221–4. Epub 2014 Sep 29.
4. Picken MM. Current practice in amyloid detection and typing among renal pathologists. Amyloid. 2011;18 Suppl 1:73–5.
5. Howie AJ, Brewer DB, Howell D, Jones AP. Physical basis of colors seen in Congo red-stained amyloid in polarized light. Lab Invest. 2008;88:232–42.
6. Howie AJ, Owen-Casey MP. Discrepancies between descriptions and illustrations of colours in Congo red-stained amyloid, and explanation of discrepant colours. Amyloid. 2010;17(3–4):109–17. Epub 2010 Nov 2.
7. Howie AJ, Owen-Casey MP. 'Apple-green birefringence' of amyloid stained by Congo red. Letter to the editor. Kid Int. 2012;82:114.
8. Picken MM. Modern approaches to the treatment of amyloidosis—the critical importance of early detection in surgical pathology. Adv Anat Pathol. 2013;20(6):424–39.
9. Picken MM. Amyloidosis—where are we now and where are we heading? Arch Pathol Lab Med. 2010;134:545–51.
10. Della Speranza V. Histologic preparations: common problems and their solutions College of American Pathologists; 2009. p. 133–137. http://www.cap.org/apps/docs/cap_press/Amyloid.pdf
11. Rostagno A, Lashley T, Ng D, Meyerson J, Braendgaard H, Plant G, Bojsen-Møller M, Holton J, Frangione B, Revesz T, Ghiso J. Preferential association of serum amyloid P component with fibrillar deposits in familial British and Danish dementias: similarities with Alzheimer's disease. J Neurol Sci. 2007;257(1–2):88–96.
12. Rahimi F, Shanmugam A, Bitan G. Structure-function relationships of pre-fibrillar protein assemblies in Alzheimer's disease and related disorders. Curr Alzheimer Res. 2008;5(3):319–41.
13. Guerreiro N, Staufenbiel M, Gomez-Mancilla B. Proteomic 2-D DIGE profiling of APP23 transgenic mice brain from pre-plaque and plaque phenotypes. J Alzheimers Dis. 2008;13(1):17–30.
14. Tomidokoro Y, Rostagno A, Neubert TA, Lu Y, Rebeck GW, Frangione B, Greenberg SM, Ghiso J. Iowa variant of familial Alzheimer's disease: accumulation of posttranslationally modified AβD23N in parenchymal and cerebrovascular amyloid deposits. Am J Pathol. 2010;176(4):1841–54.
15. Sousa MM, Cardoso I, Fernandes R, Guimarães A, Saraiva MJ. Deposition of transthyretin in early stages of familial amyloidotic polyneuropathy: evidence for toxicity of nonfibrillar aggregates. Am J Pathol. 2001;159(6):1993–2000.
16. Santos SD, Fernandes R, Saraiva MJ. The heat shock response modulates transthyretin deposition in the peripheral and autonomic nervous systems. Neurobiol Aging. 2010;31(2):280–9.
17. Ando Y, Coelho T, Berk JL, Cruz MW, Ericzon BG, Ikeda S, Lewis WD, Obici L, Planté-Bordeneuve V,

Rapezzi C, Said G, Salvi F. Guideline of transthyretin-related hereditary amyloidosis for clinicians. Orphanet J Rare Dis. 2013;8:31.

18. Pattison JS, Robbins J. Protein misfolding and cardiac disease: establishing cause and effect. Autophagy. 2008;4(6):821–3.

19. Shi J, Guan J, Jiang B, Brenner DA, Del Monte F, Ward JE, Connors LH, Sawyer DB, Semigran MJ, Macgillivray TE, Seldin DC, Falk R, Liao R. Amyloidogenic light chains induce cardiomyocyte contractile dysfunction and apoptosis via a non-canonical p38alpha MAPK pathway. Proc Natl Acad Sci USA. 2010;107(9):4188–93.

20. Biancalana M, Koide S. Molecular mechanism of Thioflavin-T binding to amyloid fibrils. Biochim Biophys Acta. 2010;1804(7):1405–12.

21. Gallo G, Picken M, Frangione B, Buxbaum J. Nonamyloidotic monoclonal immunoglobulin deposits lack amyloid P component. Mod Pathol. 1988;1(6):453–6.

22. Picken MM. Immunoglobulin Light and Heavy chain amyloid: renal pathology and differential diagnosis. Contrib Nephrol. 2007;153:135.

23. Picken MM, Frangione B, Barlogie B, Luna M, Gallo G. Light chain deposition disease derived from the kappa I light chain subgroup. Biochemical characterization. Am J Pathol. 1989;134(4):749–54.

24. Kapur U, Barton K, Fresco R, Leehey D, Picken MM. Expanding the pathologic spectrum of immunoglobulin Light Chain Proximal Tubulopathy. Arch Pathol Lab Med. 2007;131:1368.

25. D'Souza A, Theis JD, Vrana JA, Dogan A. Pharmaceutical amyloidosis associated with subcutaneous insulin and enfuvirtide administration. Amyloid. 2014;21(2):71–5. Epub 2014 Jan 22.

26. Nilsson KP, et al. Conjugated polyelectrolytes–conformation-sensitive optical probes for staining and characterization of amyloid deposits. Chembiochem. 2006;7(7):1096–104.

27. Nilsson KP, Ikenberg K, Aslund A, Fransson S, Konradsson P, Röcken C, Moch H, Aguzzi A. Structural typing of systemic amyloidoses by luminescent-conjugated polymer spectroscopy. Am J Pathol. 2010;176(2):563–74.

28. Magnusson K, Simon R, Sjölander D, Sigurdson CJ, Hammarström P, Nilsson KP. Multimodal fluorescence microscopy of prion strain specific PrP deposits stained by thiophene-based amyloid ligands. Prion. 2014;8(4):319–29. Epub 2014 Nov 1.

29. Sjöqvist J, Maria J, Simon RA, Linares M, Norman P, Nilsson KP, Lindgren M. Toward a molecular understanding of the detection of amyloid proteins with flexible conjugated oligothiophenes. J Phys Chem A. 2014;118(42):9820–7. Epub 2014 Oct 8.

30. Picken MM. Diagnosis of amyloid in urine cytology specimens. In: Hazenberg BPC, Bijzetthe J, editors. Proceedings of the XIIIth International Symposium on Amyloidosis; 2012 May 6–10; Groningen, Netherlands: GUARD; 2013. p. 161–2.

31. Klooster P, Bijzet J, Hazenberg BPC. Amyloid arthropathy in a patient with ATTR-Val122Ile amyloidosis. In: Hazenberg BPC, Bijzet J, editors. The Proceedings of the XIIIth International Symposium on Amyloidosis; Netherlands: GUARD (Groningen Unit for Amyloidosis Research & Development), UMC Groningen; 2013. p. 344–7.

32. Toll AD, Ali SZ. Urinary cytopathology in primary bladder amyloidosis. Acta Cytol. 2013;57(3):271–5. Epub 2013 Apr 25.

33. Ramirez-Alvarado M, Ward CJ, Huang BQ, Gong X, Hogan MC, Madden BJ, Charlesworth MC, Leung N. Differences in immunoglobulin light chain species found in urinary exosomes in light chain amyloidosis (AL). PLoS ONE. 2012;7(6):e38061. Epub 2012 Jun 18.

Typing of Amyloid for Routine Use on Formalin-Fixed Paraffin Sections of 626 Patients by Applying Amyloid type-Specific Immunohistochemistry: A Review

18

Reinhold P. Linke

Introduction and Overview

All forms of amyloidosis are diagnosed using tissue sections and when amyloid has been diagnosed (see Chaps. 13–17), it needs to be classified by identification of the chemical constituents of their amyloidogenic proteins. The currently known amyloid syndromes have been found to be associated with one of approximately 30 chemically different proteins [1] by which the amyloid diseases differ. The amyloidotic protein therefore needs to be identified routinely in each patient in order to get information concerning the prognosis and the design of a pathogenetically adequate therapy (see other chapters).

The classification of amyloid deposits can be performed *directly* on isolated amyloid fibril proteins by amino acid sequencing [2] or by proteomics on isolated amyloid fibrils [3]. Although these direct methods provide the highest level of precision, they are both laborious and time consuming and, hence, are less practical for routine clinical work. On the other hand, routinely fixed paraffin sections have been used for the typing of amyloid, either by immunohistochemistry (IHC)

or mass spectrometry (MS) ([4–10]; see other chapter). Both IHC and MS are much faster and are therefore applicable to routine practice. The IHC procedure identifies amyloidotic proteins under the microscope by evaluating the antibody binding pattern obtained using amyloid type-specific antibodies in situ. In contrast, MS, the most recently devised method, analyses the likelihood of the presence of peptides generated from tissue extracts taken from tissue slides [6, 7]. Since both IHC and MS examine unseparated amyloid fibrils, the results obtained are, therefore, *indirect* in these two latter methods. They were specifically developed for the classification of amyloid proteins in the formalin-fixed and paraffin-embedded tissue sections that are used in routine pathologic work, and have subsequently been introduced into clinicopathological practice [11, 13].

In this chapter, amyloid classification (or typing) through IHC is presented. The principal aim is not only to explain the special features of IHC typing of amyloid using amyloid antibodies, to show its validity, its ease of use, and its performance as a highly sensitive method applicable to routine practice, but also to show how to recognize pitfalls and avoid drawbacks [8, 10–13].

Finally, a note is added concerning the progress of two projects that compare (in double-blind studies) IHC and MS (Ring study I and II) in order to obtain well-substantiated data on a comparison of the two methods with respect to

R.P. Linke, MD, PhD (✉)
Reference Center of Amyloid Diseases amYmed.
Innovation Center of Biotechnology,
Am Klopferspitz 19, Martinsried D-82152, Germany
e-mail: linke@amymed.de

© Springer International Publishing Switzerland 2015
M.M. Picken et al. (eds.), *Amyloid and Related Disorders*, Current Clinical Pathology,
DOI 10.1007/978-3-319-19294-9_18

their performance and practicability for routine clinical work, at the international level.

Tissues, Amyloid type-specific Antibodies, Immunohistochemistry, and Execution

The basis for the development of a reliable classification of amyloid by IHC was dependent on two key features: *firstly,* the availability of **prototype amyloid tissues** and, *secondly,* the availability **of amyloid type-specific antibodies.** Prototype amyloid tissues are tissues from patients whose amyloid type is known based on analysis of the extracted amyloid fibril protein by chemical or immunochemical means such as partial or complete amino acid sequence analysis or Western blotting [4, 5, 10–13]. We collected more than 153 prototype amyloids of various amyloid classes, mostly through the courtesy of colleagues, but also as a result of chemical identification in our laboratory over many years [4, 13].

The **amyloid type-specific antibodies** used were custom antibodies generated and produced by the author, which were selected based on their reactivity with prototype amyloids in formalin-fixed and paraffin-embedded tissue sections [4, 13]. Briefly, precursor proteins or the ex vivo fragments thereof were used as immunogens while, in some cases, also synthetic peptides coupled to immunogenic carriers were used. Both, polyclonal and monoclonal antibodies were used as reviewed [4, 5, 8, 10, 13].

An initial set of antibodies was tested with the common amyloid types [4]. Later, this antibody panel was extended to include also rare, and even very rare, amyloid types [5, 13]. It was important to test the antibodies against the amyloidotic proteins in situ since antibodies directed against the native precursor proteins may show only limited reactivity with the corresponding amyloidotic proteins in tissue sections. Therefore, antibodies tested against the native protein may not meet the full requirements for a safe IHC amyloid typing procedure (reviewed in [4, 9, 13]).

The requisite criteria for an antibody to be included in the IHC amyloid typing panel were as follows: (a) An antibody against a specific amy-loid type should bind, by IHC, to *all* amyloids of this type in fixed tissue sections. (b) The IHC reaction should be strong, uniform, and consistent (see Figs. 18.1–18.5). (c) The antibody should not bind to any other amyloid type strongly and consistently. (d) Two further considerations also influenced the selection of the antibodies for the standard panel: (d') when one antibody did not meet the above-mentioned criteria in full, more than one antibody was used, and (d") a proper application and evaluation of a panel of antibodies for a definite classification of amyloidotic proteins in tissue sections requires a comparative evaluation (see below); (e) the antibody panel should be available to anyone, now and in the future, and the results obtained should be reproducible in other laboratories. Currently, these antibodies (and the protocols for their application) are available commercially [5, 13].

The antibody set used for routine typing in this chapter, and in prior reports [4, 13], comprises a panel of ten antibodies that are able to simultaneously classify eight different amyloid types. This panel covers more than 97 % of all amyloid-containing tissues submitted consecutively to our center for amyloid typing by physicians and patients. The standard set of antibodies is directed against amyloid of the classes AA, ALλ (lambda), ALκ (kappa), AHγ (gamma), ATTR, Aβ$_2$M (beta), AFib, and ApoAI. Further antibodies against ALys, AGel, ACys, Aß, APrP, AIAPP (see Table 18.1), and other types (to be published), are available when results from the standard panel indicate that they might be necessary [5, 11, 13].

The IHC technique used for amyloid typing by our laboratory (and also by others) is the unlabeled IHC technique of Sternberger (cited in ref. [4]), in which a peroxidase–anti-peroxidase (PAP) complex is applied as the final amplification system, or its more sensitive variant—the ABC technique which uses a biotin–avidin complex for amplification. Before beginning the IHC staining procedure, one section must be examined in order to verify the presence of amyloid in the submitted biopsy. When smaller amounts of amyloid are present, or if it is suspected that a sampling error might occur (see "sampling error" in Chap. 14), approximately 15 sections

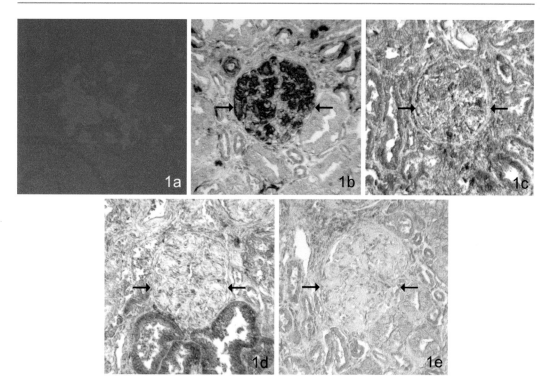

Fig. 18.1 Immunohistochemical classification using amyloid type-specific antibodies. Figures 18.1, 18.2, 18.3, and 18.4 show the classification of four different amyloid types as AA, ALλ, ALκ, and ATTR, respectively. Here, stains using four antibodies are presented [5, 8, 10] to illustrate the principle of comparative amyloid typing. The results of CRF are shown in row (**a**), the reaction with anti-AA antibodies across the different amyloid types in row (**b**), the reactivities against ALλ, ALκ, and ATTR are shown in rows (**c, d**, and **e**), respectively. The diagnostic reaction is always the strongest and most consistent (see text)

are prestained for 10–20 s with Congo red (CR) using a modified Puchtler method [4]. This procedure incorporates the absolute minimum time necessary for staining so that the CR staining will show up only by Congo red fluorescence (CRF), a more sensitive technique than the classical CR method employing bright light [4, 13]. This brief prestaining treatment therefore ensures that the CR staining will not interfere with the IHC procedure. Amyloid that fluoresces by CRF needs to be verified by polarization microscopy, when the pathognomonic green birefringence (GB) should be seen [4]. Sections that show the presence of amyloid are then chosen for IHC staining. Whenever the procedure needs to be changed, consequent to the inclusion of new solutions, other reagents, new personnel, etc., we routinely include seven positive controls (one for each of the five major amyloid classes) in order to make sure that the applied technique will be of a simi-

lar high standard and that the results will be comparable to former IHC stains. Positive controls, after evaluation, can be destained (using 80 % acetic acid dropped onto the section for 2 min) and reused for IHC. In our laboratory, we routinely reuse positive control slides up to approximately six times [4]. The staining procedure utilizes routine methods with AEC (3-aminoethyl carbazol) as the chromogen, followed by a weak counterstain with Mayer's hemalum, and embedding in Kaiser's glycerin jelly [4].

Evaluation of Immunohistochemical Reactivities

The reading of IHC-stained slides is performed without any prior knowledge of either laboratory data or clinical picture. Positive standard slides are first evaluated in order to provide assurance

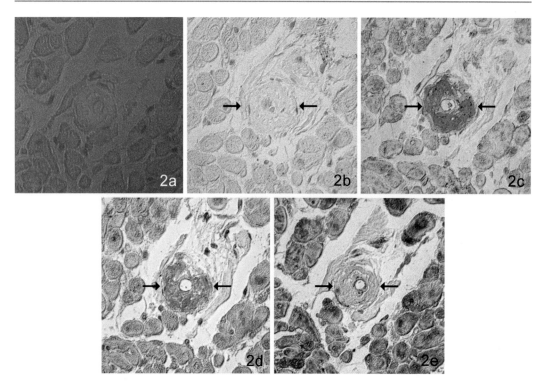

Fig. 18.2 Immunohistochemical classification using amyloid type-specific antibodies. Figures 18.1, 18.2, 18.3, and 18.4 show the classification of four different amyloid types as AA, ALλ, ALκ, and ATTR, respectively. Here, stains using four antibodies are presented [5, 8, 10] to illustrate the principle of comparative amyloid typing. The results of CRF are shown in row (**a**), the reaction with anti-AA antibodies across the different amyloid types in row (**b**), the reactivities against ALλ, ALκ, and ATTR are shown in rows (**c, d**, and **e**), respectively. The diagnostic reaction is always the strongest and most consistent (see text)

that the "unknown" slides of submitted tissue sections have been stained properly with the set of antibodies employed. The second stage of the procedure is then to read the ten stained slides and evaluate their IHC reactivities. This requires some experience since amyloid represents a complex mixture of many proteins and other constituents [8–10, 13] that will show various reactivities. The latter need to be categorized by distinguishing strong uniform and consistent IHC reactions from the more inconsistent ones in order to separate the specific and *diagnostic* from the *nonspecific* reactivities.

This is shown in Figs. 18.1, 18.2, 18.3, and 18.4. The amyloid typing is illustrated here using the four most prevalent amyloid types: AA, ALλ (lambda), ALκ (kappa), and ATTR (more types have been illustrated in [10, 13]). CRF was used to identify the presence of amyloid in each of the four presented cases since it is the most sensitive method for confirming the presence of amyloid (see Chap. 14). Amyloid is shown by CRF in the "a-row" of all cases in Figs. 18.1, 18.2, 18.3, and 18.4. IHC typing of amyloid was performed on adjacent sections, to which the above-described panel of amyloid type-specific antibodies was applied. All three forms of illumination used for identifying amyloid (triple illumination) were applied to all amyloid types, as exemplified in the ATTR case in Fig. 18.4b.

In Fig. 18.1a–e, characteristic reactivities are shown for renal autopsy tissue with glomerular **AA amyloid** (in a case of Muckle-Wells syndrome, see ref. in [4]) as identified by CRF (Fig. 18.1a) and a very consistent and strongly congruent diagnostic reaction with anti-AA only (Fig. 18.1b, between arrows) while anti-ALκ and anti-ATTR (Fig. 18.1d, e) were nonreactive. The

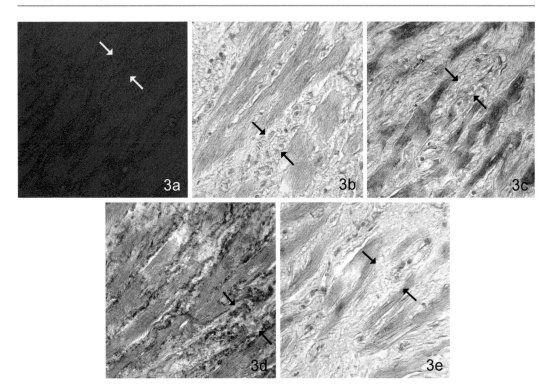

Fig. 18.3 Immunohistochemical classification using amyloid type-specific antibodies. Figures 18.1, 18.2, 18.3, and 18.4 show the classification of four different amyloid types as AA, ALλ, ALκ, and ATTR, respectively. Here, stains using four antibodies are presented [5, 8, 10] to illustrate the principle of comparative amyloid typing. The results of CRF are shown in row (**a**), the reaction with anti-AA antibodies across the different amyloid types in row (**b**), the reactivities against ALλ, ALκ, and ATTR are shown in rows (**c, d,** and **e**) respectively. The diagnostic reaction is always the strongest and most consistent (see text)

anti-ALλ (lambda) antibody (Fig. 18.1c) showed a distinct reactivity; however, this was weak in comparison to the reactivity shown in Fig. 18.1b which, being the strongest, was considered diagnostic of the amyloid type. Please note that light chain amyloid antibodies also react strongly with amyloid-free tissue structures such as tubular cells (Fig. 18.1c, d).

In Fig. 18.2a–e, IHC identified **ALλ (lambda) amyloid** as the type; here, amyloid is seen only in the cardiac vessels in a patient with cardiac decompensation and MGUS (free λ-L 343 mg/l serum). The cardiac functional decompensation resulted from severe narrowing of the vessels by amyloid (Fig. 18.2b–e, between arrows) leading to functional impairment, despite the cardiac muscle being virtually free of amyloid. The amyloid was barely stained with Congo red (not shown) but was visible with CRF illumination (Fig. 18.2a). Diagnosis of the amyloid type was based on identification of a single, consistent, and very strong IHC reaction (corresponding to the location of amyloid deposits by CRF) with anti-ALλ (lambda) only (Fig. 18.2c). In contrast, the anti-ALκ (kappa) (Fig. 18.2d) stain was less strong and less uniform. There was almost no reactivity with anti-AA (Fig. 18.2b) and anti-ATTR (Fig. 18.2e) except for a few reactive and inconsistent spots in the latter. Please note that considerable reactivity is present with anti-ATTR in cardiomyocytes, which does not, however, correspond in location to the areas positive for amyloid by CRF and, therefore, is not specific for amyloid.

Figure 18.3a–e displays severe interstitial cardiac **ALκ (kappa)-amyloid** as identified in a patient with MGUS (free kappa-L 916 mg/l serum). ALκ (kappa) amyloidosis was diagnosed

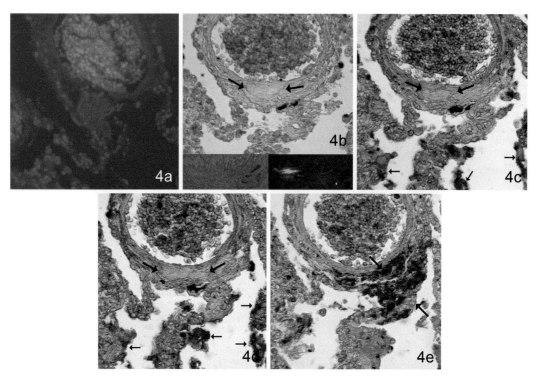

Fig. 18.4 Immunohistochemical classification using amyloid type-specific antibodies. Figures 18.1, 18.2, 18.3, and 18.4 show the classification of four different amyloid types as AA, ALλ, ALκ, and ATTR, respectively. Here, stains using four antibodies are presented [5, 8, 10] to illustrate the principle of comparative amyloid typing. The results of CRF are shown in row (**a**), the reaction with anti-AA antibodies across the different amyloid types in row (**b**), the reactivities against ALλ, ALκ, and ATTR are shown in rows (**c, d**, and **e**) respectively. The diagnostic reaction is always the strongest and most consistent (see text)

based on CRF detection of an interstitial bright orange-red web of somewhat kinked amyloid bundles (Fig. 18.3a, between arrows). This corresponds with a similar kinked web-like reactivity with anti-ALκ (kappa) in Fig. 18.3d (between arrows). Anti-AA (Fig. 18.3b) and anti-ATTR (Fig. 18.3e) were nonreactive, but some ALλ (lambda)-reactivity was seen (Fig. 18.3c, between arrows), which was, however, far weaker and more inconsistent when compared to the diagnostic kappa reaction in Fig. 18.3d.

Figure 18.4a–e shows IHC typing of pulmonary **ATTR amyloid** in a 91-year-old patient who died of pneumonia after a heart infarction. The amyloid seen in CRF illumination (Fig. 18.4a) gave a consistent, and therefore diagnostic, reaction with Anti-ATTR antibody only (Fig. 18.4e, between arrows), while anti-AA (Fig. 18.4b) was nonreactive and anti-ALλ (lambda) (Fig. 18.4c) and anti-ALκ (kappa) (Fig. 18.4d) showed only minor reactivities. The inset in Fig. 18.4b shows the CRF and green birefringence (GB) of adjacent amyloid deposits that were used for evaluating this amyloid (indicated by two larger arrows in Fig. 18.4b–e). The smaller arrows in Fig. 18.4c, d point to intensive collateral reactivities, which do not represent amyloid. They can easily be distinguished from amyloid by CR prestaining followed by an IHC overlay and subsequent examination of the same frame with bright light as compared to fluorescent light illumination (by switching the light source) in order to verify which reactive areas represent amyloid. Using this technique, the amyloid specificity of the IHC stain is ensured [4].

In summary, in Figs. 18.1, 18.2, 18.3, and 18.4, the CRF (**a-row**) shows an intense bright orange-red fluorescence of high sensitivity for all

Antibodies		1	2	3	4	5	6
Patient #	Amyloid Type	AA mcC	ALλ HAR	ALκ SIN	Aβ$_2$M WOE	ATTR TIE	FibAα
1	AA	+++	(++)	(+)	0	(+)	0
2	AA	+++	0	0	0	0	0
3	ALλ	0	+++	(++)	(+)	(+)	(+)
4	ALλ	0	++-+++	0	0	0	0
5	ALλ	0	(++)	+++	0	0	(+)
6	ALκ	0	0	+++	0	0	0
7	Aβ$_2$M	0	(+)	0	+++	0	0
8	Aβ$_2$M	0	0	0	+++	0	0
9	ATTR	(+)	(++)	(+)	0	+++	0
10	ATTR	0	0	0	0	++-+++	0
11	AFibAα	0	(+++)	(+)	0	0	+++
12	AFibAα	0	0	0	0	0	++-+++

Legend: Consistency of reaction: ▨ consistent   ( ) inconsistent

Strength of reaction: +++ very strong reaction   ++ strong reaction   + definite reaction   0 no reaction

Fig. 18.5 Immunohistochemical patterns of comparative immunohistochemistry. The *shaded reactivities* are the diagnostic ones while the unshaded reactivities are the non-specific ones (see text)

amyloid deposits, regardless of type. The **b-row** shows the specificity of the AA antibodies across the different amyloid types. There is only a single, very strong reactivity against AA amyloid and no reactivity with the other amyloid types. AA reactivity with monoclonal antibodies [4, 13] shows the highest level of selectivity. The **c-row** shows representative anti-ALλ reactivities. Although anti-ALλ reacts with most amyloids, the strongest reaction (which is therefore considered to be amyloid-specific) occurs only with ALλ (lambda) amyloid deposits as shown in Fig. 18.2c. The λ (lambda)-reactivities of many amyloids have plagued amyloid IHC studies for many years [4, 9, 13], leading to misdiagnoses, as discussed above, and has intensified a search for remedies. The resolution of this problem, some 15 years ago, led to the adoption of the method of "comparative IHC" (reviewed in [4, 10, 13]; see below). As shown above, this method of comparative IHC is based on selection of the *strongest amyloid-specific reactivity*. The **d-row** presents the performance of the κ (kappa) reactivities and the **e-row** presents the performance of the ATTR antibodies across the four different amyloid types. Only the corresponding ATTR amyloid reacts strongly, as in the case of most ATTR amyloidosis seen in patients.

Comparative Amyloid type-Specific Immunohistochemistry as a Routine Method for Amyloid Typing

The following example is instructive of the use of this technique. Recently, in 2011, we received tissue sections of a reported AA amyloidosis with a request for a second opinion. The amyloid had been classified using a single monoclonal AA antibody, which was reported as reactive. Similar instances of amyloid typing, based on evaluation using a single antibody, have also been reported [8]. Subsequently, they were all found to be incorrect results. In cases where an incomplete antibody panel is used, and the antibody that corresponds to the particular type of amyloid present in the specimen is missing from the panel, collateral nonspecific reactions can occur that have been misinterpreted as positive, diagnostic results. This type of false-positive result has been reported in cases that were subsequently diagnosed as: AFib, AApoAI [8], and as AHγ (gamma)-amyloid (Ring study I and II [13]).

The deficiencies associated with the use of a single antibody in the typing of amyloid deposits can be further illustrated with reference to Fig. 18.1. From Fig. 18.1, it is apparent that the single reactivities seen in Figs. 18.1c and 18.2d would result in the misdiagnosis ALλ (lambda) and ALκ (kappa) amyloidosis, if the homologous, diagnostic antibodies were not available, or if they had reacted inappropriately in Figs. 18.1b and 18.2c. This should be clear from the reasoning of the paragraph above: the only way to arrive at a firm identification of the correct chemical amyloid type is by comparison of the different IHC reactions and, thus, by **separating the diagnostic from the nonspecific reaction.** How this can be done is shown in Figs. 18.1, 18.2, 18.3, and 18.4 using comparative IHC with antibodies that meet the above-mentioned criteria. The results of many such comparative amyloid analyses are listed in Fig. 18.5. The visible reactions are graded based on their intensity as illustrated and described in Fig. 18.1. Thus, the homologous reactions in Figs. 18.1b, 18.2c, 18.3d, and 18.4e are graded as +++ since they are very strong and uniform. By contrast, the negative reactions in the b-row are graded negative 0, as are also the reactions in Figs. 18.1e and 18.3e. However, Fig. 18.2d is graded as (++) in brackets to denote a reaction that is weaker and inconsistent as compared to the diagnostic reaction in Fig. 18.2c. Accordingly, Figs. 18.3c and 18.4c, d are graded as inconsistent (+ - ++), while Figs. 18.1d, 18.2e, and 18.3e are graded as (+), displaying the lowest level of reactivity with a signal that consists of only of a few spots, as in Fig. 18.2e.

Figure 18.5 shows a summary of the above-described grading approach, which was applied over several years to a large number of patients who were diagnosed with six of the most common amyloid types (the typing of additional amyloid classes is described in [10, 11, 13]). As can be seen from Fig. 18.5 (and additional publications), this comparative IHC evaluation scheme, involving the differentiation of truly diagnostic from non-specific reactions, can be applied to many different amyloid types. However, particular attention must be paid to light-chain amyloid antibodies, since they have a tendency to be detectable also in different amyloid types [4, 10, 13], with variable intensities. Thus, to address this issue, light chain derived are typically tested with several antibodies, and a consistently observable reactivity must be seen in order to diagnose the respective ALλ (lambda) or ALκ (kappa) amyloids [13]. Note that while the consistent and strong reactivities are readily apparent, the inconsistent reactivities are more variable.

The **validity of the above IHC typing of amyloid** is based on several key points: (a) All IHC reactions were tested with **seven positive controls**, representing prototype amyloids. (b) The ten different amyloid antibodies that were used intrinsically provided several built-in controls and typically yielded only **one diagnostic reaction, while allowing the exclusion of all other amyloid types** through the recognition of nonspecific reactions, as described above. (c) In all cases where clinical information was available, the **IHC results were consistent with the type of amyloidosis suspected on clinical grounds.** (d) In one patient ([4], not part of this review), **more than one type of amyloid was detected by IHC**, and this correlated with the microscopic morphology seen in the tissues, suggesting different sites for amyloidogenesis of each amyloid type. The recognition of such rare cases clearly shows the advantage of IHC as compared to MS. (e) This panel of antibodies has been **used by numerous other laboratories**, with similar results. Many of these cooperative studies are cited in Ref. [13]. (f) Additional data supporting the validity, high sensitivity, and precision of the comparative IHC typing of amyloid, using the above panel of amyloid antibodies, has been obtained from the **first two international blinded comparisons** of IHC versus MS (Ring study I and II as in part reported [13]).

High-Sensitivity Classification of Single Minute Amyloid Deposits

At one time, it was requested that we perform IHC typing on a single tissue section that contained one small area of amyloid of approximately the size of 2 macrophages. We attempted, for the first time, the sequential application of one amyloid type-specific antibody after another, with destaining (see above) between each application. The resultant diagnosis was ATTR amyloidosis (published in 1984, Feurle, H.E. et al. cited in [4]). This amyloid was later genotyped as a rare ATTR variant. Similarly, the detection of very small, single amyloid deposits in the initiating phase of AA amyloidosis in Juvenile Rheumatoid Arthritis, missed by former evaluators, has been summarized and illustrated in Chap. 14, Fig. 18.4. Over the years, numerous patients have been diagnosed, based on the evaluation of small deposits of amyloid present in biopsies with very early amyloidosis that were too small to be evaluated by other typing methods, including MS [13].

Performance and Prevalence

This section presents the overall results of amyloid typing, using comparative IHC with a diagnostic panel of amyloid type-specific antibodies. Only patients with a single amyloid type have been included. The results of amyloid typing in patients with more than one amyloid type, and the typing of amyloids in animals (which both follow the same principles as discussed above) will be presented elsewhere (manuscript in preparation). In addition, the non-amyloidotic proteinthesauroses, such as λ- and κ-LCDD, have not been included in this list.

In these studies, 153 prototype amyloids were employed in order to ensure the specificity of the

Table 18.1 Prevalence of different amyloid types among 626 samples submitted and typed by comparative immunohistochemistry

Amyloid class	No. of patients	% of total
ALλ	271	43.3
ALκ	118	18.8
(AL, sum)	(389)	(62.1)
ATTR	93	14.9
AA	80	12.8
AFib	14	2.2
Aβ$_2$M	11	1.8
ALys	6	1.0
AApoAI	5	0.8
Aβ	4	0.6
APrP	2	0.3
ACys	2	0.3
AHγ	2	0.3
AGel	2	0.3
AApoAII	1	0.2
SAA$_4$	1	0.2
Unknown	14	2.2
Sum total	626	100

amyloid antibodies [10, 13]. All 153 (100 %) of the prototype amyloids could be typed correctly using comparative IHC. The results of amyloid typing in 626 patients evaluated at the Reference Center of Amyloid Diseases are presented in Table 18.1. Of the 626 samples received, in 612 patients (97.8 %), the amyloid type could be diagnosed and verified by the use of appropriate controls. Light chain derived amyloid was the most prevalent form, being diagnosed in 389 patients (62.1 % of all samples submitted), with 271 patients having ALλ (43.3 %) and 118 having ALκ (18.8 %). The second and the third most numerous classes were: ATTR in 14.9 % and AA in 12.8 %, respectively. All other amyloid classes were rare, or very rare, with AFib (2.2 %) representing the most numerous among the rare amyloid classes encountered.

Among the 14 unknown samples, in two patients, amyloid derived from semenogelin was subsequently diagnosed, and the corresponding specific antibody had already been prepared [11]. Two other amyloids were analyzed by amino acid sequence analysis and identified as ALκ amyloid (one published in [12] and the other identified by courtesy of J.J. Liepnieks and M.D. Benson). Six other unknown amyloids, which could not be typed by IHC, were analyzed by MS but could not be typed either.

In approximately 60 % of patients, the clinical records were available for evaluation and in almost all cases the clinicopathologic correlation was excellent. In many cases, the IHC typing of amyloid was instrumental in guiding the subsequent clinical management of patients with seemingly uncharacteristic, and even obscure, minor symptoms [2]. Results similar to those presented in this chapter were also obtained independently, in other laboratories, using the same sets of antibodies [4, 13].

In summary, amyloid typing on tissue sections using comparative IHC does not require any prior clinical knowledge or laboratory data. It provides a definitive diagnosis of the amyloid type by detection of the chemical identity of the amyloidotic protein of the fibril in situ without antigenic retrieval. This amyloid typing technique is reliable, very fast, easy, and affordable for all institutes competent in performing immunohistochemistry. In addition, it is of the highest sensitivity since one amyloid spot in a single slide is virtually sufficient for a full classification (see Fig. 14. 4).

In the author's experience, based on 626 submitted samples, and using this comparative approach, the sensitivity of IHC is >97 %, and the specificity even higher; there were no major cross-reacting stains. Other laboratories have also achieved similar reliable results, on a routine basis, using amyloid-specific antibodies [13]. Finally, the reliability of the typing results obtained using amyloid-specific antibodies was confirmed by mass spectrometric analysis on paraffin sections with different amyloid-types in two collaborative international comparative studies in blinded fashion [13].

Pitfalls and Remedies

(a) An inherent problem in the classification of amyloid is that amyloid is **not a pure substance but a very heterogeneous complex,** which is comprised of various aggregated and polymerized proteins and their fragmented or point-mutated variants. In addition, this complex is saturated with various, variable, extracellular constituents, including, in particular, serum proteins that can be adsorbed to this amyloid complex to varying extents ([4, 9, 13]; see Fig. 18.1). Both methods, IHC and MS, have to cope with this situation. Since the pathogenetically most important and unique constituents are the amyloid fibril proteins, we have produced antibodies that preferentially recognize these. In this report, it is described how these special antibodies can distinguish amyloid from its contaminants.

(b) The histomorphological evaluation of amyloid that is possible with IHC is very helpful in coping with the plethora of constituents found associated with amyloid deposits. Since the amyloid fibrils remain intact and in place during the typing process, even in tissues with the smallest deposits, a spatial correlation between the site of antibody reactivity and the amyloid deposit can be made (see Figs. 18.1–18.5; Chap. 14).

(c) The rare instances when more than one amyloid type can be diagnosed in a single patient [9] can also be addressed by using this panel of antibodies for comparative amyloid typing as illustrated in [4].

(d) In instances where the antibodies produce a stronger stain with structures other than amyloid deposits (a common occurrence, in particular, in the immunoglobulin-derived amyloids, AIg,[1] since the extracellular space is washed with IgGs, see Fig. 18.1), prestaining of the section with CR, followed by an IHC overlay, allows correlation of the spatial distribution of the CRF and the IHC staining patterns (i.e., whether they occur in the same area of the section) and determination of which region with the strongest reaction is congruent with the amyloid deposit.

(e) When problems arise, consultation with an expert center for **diagnosis of the amyloid type** should be considered [9].

---

[1] AIg is proposed here as a practical acronym for the combination of AL and AH.

Take Home Message

1. The immunohistochemical diagnosis of amyloid type is fast and very precise when performed by an expert laboratory. It can be performed in every institute that is competent in the techniques of immunohistochemistry, after some degree of training.
2. For immunohistochemical typing, an appropriate panel of amyloid type-specific antibodies is needed for comparative evaluation without antigenic retrieval, since "one antibody—one diagnosis" does not lead to a safe assessment of the amyloid type.
3. Evaluation of the IHC patterns generated by these antibodies needs a certain amount of histopathologic training in order to recognize a true diagnostic reaction, which is characterized by its strong and consistent appearance, and to distinguish the latter from the inconsistent and weak reaction typical of a false-positive result (see Fig. 18.1).
4. To distinguish non-amyloidotic structures from amyloidotic ones, prestaining with CR and the use of CRF in combination with IHC is very helpful and even some small amyloid deposits can be correctly typed.
5. When problems arise, an expert reference center needs to be consulted [9].

Report for Clinicians

The **report to the clinician** should be **candid** and present both **the strengths and the limitations of the procedures under which the classification was performed**. This ensures that the clinician has confidence in the findings on which he or she must base the appropriate therapy. The first issue to be addressed should be the **quality of the biopsy**, its size, and the amount of amyloid. In cases where the presence or absence of amyloid is not clear, an **independent expert should be consulted** to clarify the issue. Amyloid typing should always be performed as a double-blind study, preferably without any prior knowledge of the clinical data, since the latter can, at times, also be misleading.

Acknowledgments This work was only possible as a result of contributions by many colleagues over several decades. Full acknowledgement of some of these contributions can be found in an in-depth review [13]. Here, I would like to thank Prof. Dr. R. Huber, director emeritus of the Max-Planck-Institute of Biochemistry in Martinsried, who provided laboratory space, and supported some of the technicians and coworkers involved in the laboratory work. They include Mrs. A. Rail, Mrs. A. Kerling, Mrs. R. Oos, Mrs. A. Meinel, and Dr. N. Wiegel. For secretarial work, I thank Mrs. A. Feix, Martinsried, Germany, and for the artwork Ms. A. K. M. Linke, Essen/Germany.

References

1. Sipe JD, Benson MD, Buxbaum JN, Ikeda S, Merlini G, Saraiva MJ, Westermark P. Nomenclature 2014: amyloid fibril proteins and clinical classification of the amyloidosis. Amyloid. 2014;21(4):221–4. 2014 Sep 29.
2. Merlini G, Westermark P. The systemic amyloidosis: clearer understanding of the molecular mechanisms offer hope for more effective therapies. J Intern Med. 2004;255:159–78.
3. Lavatelli F, Perlman DH, Spencer B, et al. Amyloidogenic and associated proteins in systemic amyloidosis proteome of adipose tissue. Mol Cell Proteomics. 2008;7:1570–83.
4. Linke RP. Congo red staining of amyloid. Improvements and practical guide for a more precise diagnosis of amyloid and the different amyloidosis. Chapter 11.1. In: Uversky VN, Fink AL, editors. Protein misfolding, aggregation and conformational diseases, Protein Reviews, vol. 4. New York: Springer; 2006. p. 239–76.
5. Schroeder R, Deckert M, Linke RP. Novel isolated cerebral ALλ (lambda) amyloid angiopathy with widespread subcortical distribution and leukoencephalopathy due to atypical monoclonal plasma cell proliferation, and terminal systemic gammopathy. J Neuropathol Exp Neurol. 2009;68(3):286–99.
6. Murphy CL, Wang S, Williams T, et al. Characterization of systemic amyloid deposits by mass spectrometry. Methods Enzymol. 2006;412:48–62.
7. Vrana JA, Gamez JD, Madden BJ, Theis JD, Bergen 3rd HR, Dogan A. Classification of amyloidosis by laser micro dissection and mass spectrometry based proteomic analysis in clinical biopsy specimens. Blood. 2009;114(24):4957–9.
8. Linke RP, Oos R, Wiegel NM, Nathrath WBJ. Classification of amyloidosis: misdiagnosing by way of incomplete immunohistochemistry and how to prevent it. Acta Histochem. 2006;108:197–208.
9. Picken MM, Herrera GA. The burden of "sticky" amyloid: typing challenges. Arch Pathol Lab Med. 2007;131(6):850–1.
10. Linke RP. Classifying of amyloid on fixed tissue sections for routine use by validated immunohistochemistry. Amyloid. 2011;18 Suppl 1:67–70.

11. Linke RP, Joswig R, Murphy CL, et al. Seminogelin I is the amyloidogenic protein in senile seminal vesicles. In: Grateau G, Kyle RA, Skinner M, editors. Amyloid and amyloidosis. Boca Raton, FL: CRC Press; 2004. p. 471–3.

12. Wiegel NM, Mentele R, Kellermann J, Meyer L, Riess H, Linke RP. ALkappa(I) (UNK)—primary structure of an AL-amyloid protein presenting an organ-limited subcutaneous nodular amyloid syndrome of long duration. Case report and review. Amyloid. 2010;17(1):10–23.

13. Linke RP. On typing of amyloidosis using immunohistochemstry. Detailed illustrations, review and a note on mass spectrometry. Progr Histochem Cytochem. 2012;47:61–132.

Amyloid Typing: Experience from a Large Referral Centre

19

Janet A. Gilbertson, Julian D. Gillmore, and Philip N. Hawkins

Introduction

Since our last review [1], the NAC continues to grow and more than 14,000 patients have been evaluated at the centre since it opened in 1999. In 2013 alone, 1583 histology samples were reviewed, taken from 1130 patients who were referred to the NAC in that year, requiring interpretation of 20,453 Congo red-stained and immunohistochemically stained slides.

At the NAC, Congo red staining that produces characteristic apple green birefringence under cross polarised light remains the gold standard for confirming the presence of amyloid in tissues [2, 3]. Whilst immunohistochemical staining of amyloid with a panel of monospecific antibodies against known amyloid-forming fibril proteins remains the most accessible means to identify the amyloid fibril protein, it does have many pitfalls [4]. Proteomic analysis of microdissected amyloid material is of late being increasingly utilised at the NAC in conjunction with immunohistochemistry to characterise the amyloid fibril

J.A. Gilbertson, CSci, FIBMS (✉) • J.D. Gillmore, MBBS, MD, PhD, FRCP • P.N. Hawkins, PhD, FRCP, FRCPath, FMedSci
UCL Division of Medicine, National Amyloidosis Centre, Royal Free Hospital, Rowland Hill Street, NW3 2PF, London, UK
e-mail: j.gilbertson@ucl.ac.uk; j.gillmore@ucl.ac.uk; p.hawkins@ucl.ac.uk

protein and, hence, make a definitive diagnosis. This new diagnostic tool involves laser dissection of amyloidotic material from tissue sections, proteolytic digestion, separation of individual peptides and protein identification through mass spectrometry [5]; it can be performed using remarkably small quantities of formalin-fixed amyloidotic tissue.

Biopsies

Biopsies are usually taken to investigate the cause of organ dysfunction and sometimes specifically in the context of a suspicion of amyloidosis. Approximately 10,000 biopsy specimens have been examined at our centre to date from almost every anatomical site. Each year we receive ~50–60 different types of tissues for analysis. The sensitivity of rectal and/or subcutaneous fat biopsies in patients with systemic AA or AL amyloidosis is reportedly >90 % [6, 7]; as a result we receive a large number of rectal biopsies for histological review. The role of fat tissue analysis in management of patients with amyloidosis is now well established [8], and fat biopsies are frequently obtained when patients attend their outpatient appointment at the NAC. Seventeen percent of all biopsies reviewed were fat biopsies taken in the NAC clinic, with only small numbers received from elsewhere. Other tissue specimens include bone marrow trephines (BMT) (21 %), renal

© Springer International Publishing Switzerland 2015
M.M. Picken et al. (eds.), *Amyloid and Related Disorders*, Current Clinical Pathology,
DOI 10.1007/978-3-319-19294-9_19

(17 %) and gastrointestinal (11 %). Biopsy methods have generally become safer and, as a result, a much greater number of endomyocardial biopsies have recently been received at the NAC, although the proportion of the total has remained largely stable (4–8 %). One third of biopsies are from other sites including testis, spine, lung, omentum and incidental brain amyloid. Nearly all biopsies are formalin fixed, paraffin embedded (FFPE); they are only very rarely unfixed. In the UK, in general, paraffin immunohistochemistry is used in renal pathology rather than immunofluorescence in frozen sections.

As previously reported [1] it is vital to appreciate that a negative biopsy does not exclude the possibility of amyloidosis but merely excludes the presence of amyloid in the precise tissue section being examined. Amyloid is a patchy disease, and tissue sections typically cover only a few micrometres such that the deposits may be missed. Furthermore, if, for example, only the mucosa of a rectal biopsy is sectioned and examined, amyloid deposits within the submucosa, which is where they are typically found, may be missed.

Congo Red

All biopsy tissue is routinely stained with Congo red to determine the presence or absence of amyloid. Every year our conclusions in this regard differ from that of the patients' local hospitals in a substantial proportion of cases; we find a 4–8 % false-positive rate (i.e. no amyloid present in our opinion) and an 8–11 % false-negative rate (i.e. amyloid deposits present which were missed locally); the latter figure represents the percentage among patients who have been referred to the NAC due to clinical suspicion of amyloid. Incorrect results can, as mentioned previously, be due to a tissue specimen being orientated inappropriately in the paraffin block or not cut sufficiently deeply for the amyloid to be included in the specimen. Alternatively, false-positive and false-negative results may be associated with the variety of different Congo red methodologies used in different pathology departments or incor-

rect microscope or polarising filter assembly. At the NAC we recommend the Puchtler method, which has no operator intervention and thus less scope for error. However, false positives and false negatives still do occur in our own laboratory, and on occasion, we have been unable to demonstrate amyloid with the Puchtler method in material from patients with proven systemic amyloidosis and compelling clinical evidence of involvement within the relevant tissue. Amyloid in some such cases was demonstrated using the Highman's or Stokes methods [9, 10]. Another factor contributing to false negatives at the centre is receipt of unstained sections that are cut too thinly for optimal Congo red staining; the recommended section thickness is 6–8 μm. False-positive cases usually result from methodologies which include a differentiation step, causing other tissue components to become overstained and exhibit white or extremely pale green birefringence under crossed polarised light. In a recent study [11] several renal biopsies were reported by the referring hospital not to show amyloid and were diagnosed with minimal change disease (MCD). Re-staining of tissue from the original block and review at the NAC however, prompted by a clinical suspicion of amyloid in each case, sometimes as long as 4 years later, resulted in discovery of amyloid deposits within the glomeruli and interstitium (Fig. 19.1).

Another diagnosis that may cause difficulty is that of light chain deposition disease (LCDD).

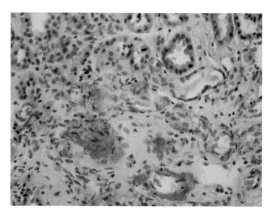

Fig. 19.1 Renal biopsy diagnosed MCD showing amyloid deposition with *Congo red* staining

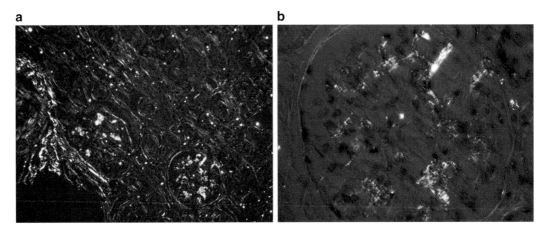

Fig. 19.2 Renal biopsy reported as LCDD containing amyloid deposition within the glomeruli (**a**) and at a higher magnification (**b**), stained with Congo red and viewed under crossed polars

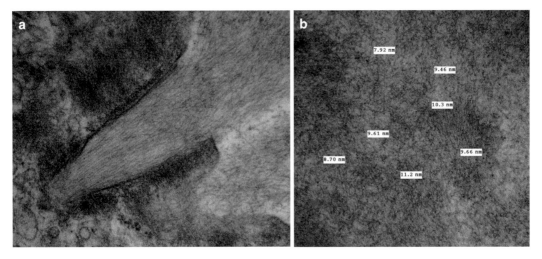

Fig. 19.3 EM micrograph confirming amyloid fibrils (**a**) ×67,000 magnification and (**b**) ×80,000 magnification in the biopsies reported as LCDD

Of late, we were referred a case that had been reported as LCDD but showed amyloid on Congo red staining (Fig. 19.2) and with an antibody against lambda light chains. Subsequently EM was performed at the referring hospital and amyloid fibrils were identified (Fig. 19.3).

Immunohistochemistry for Amyloid at the NAC

Immunohistochemistry is a widely used technique for characterisation of amyloid fibril type and the presence of normal or aberrant proteins/

epitopes and can be used to determine the amyloid fibril protein in a substantial proportion of cases. Antisera to all known amyloidogenic proteins are commercially available, and most are reliable in identifying the fibril type. Once amyloid has been confirmed, we stain the biopsy with a panel of monospecific antibodies against known amyloidogenic proteins (Table 19.1). Morphology of amyloid in certain tissues can give important clues regarding the fibril protein. For example, fibrinogen amyloid is virtually restricted to the glomeruli [12] (Fig. 19.4), and anti-fibrinogen antisera will always be included in the antibody panel when this pattern is identified.

Table 19.1 Antibodies used routinely at the NAC

Antibody	Raised in	Dilution	Cat No.	Source	Absorbed by
P component	Rabbit	1:1200	A0302	DAKO	Human SAP
AA (REU 86.2)	Mouse	1:100	2232MREU	Euro Diagnostica	Human SAA
Kappa	Rabbit	1:20,000	A0191	DAKO	Human serum
Lambda	Rabbit	1:20,000	A0193	DAKO	Human serum
Lysozyme	Rabbit	1:1000	A099	DAKO	Pure antigen
Fibrinogen α chain	Sheep	1:300	CA1023	Cambiochem	Human plasma
TTR	Rabbit	1:4000	A002	DAKO	Pre-albumin
Insulin	Mouse	1:100	NCL-insulin	Novocastra	
apoA1	Goat	1:4000	PBA0313	Genzyme	HD lipoprotein
β 2 Microglobulin	Rabbit	1:500	A0072	DAKO	
Lect2	Goat	1:600	AF722	R&D systems	

All human serum is from a normal pool
Reprinted from Gilbertson, Janet A C.Sci., F.I.B.M.S. Amyloid Typing: Experience from a Large Referral Centre, in Amyloid and Related Disorders, 1st Ed., Jan 2012, with kind permission from Springer Science and Business Media

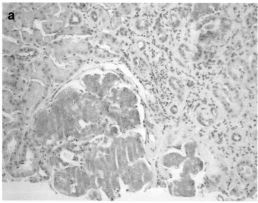 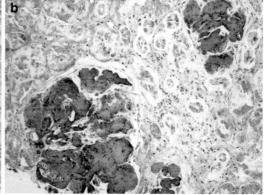

Fig. 19.4 (**a**) *Congo red staining* of a renal biopsy with amyloid deposition within the glomeruli. (**b**) Anti-fibrinogen A immunohistochemistry staining of the glomeruli (Reprinted from Gilbertson, Janet A C.Sci., F.I.B.M.S. Amyloid Typing: Experience from a Large Referral Centre, in Amyloid and Related Disorders, 1st Ed., Jan 2012, with kind permission from Springer Science and Business Media)

AA amyloid deposits are typically extensive in the renal medulla and are always stained in biopsies showing amyloid. In our experience of a small group of Punjabi Indians, ALECT2 amyloid is found throughout renal tissue and can sometimes have a predominance of glomerular deposition. ALECT2 amyloid generally shows bright congophilia with a 'sparkly glistening' apple green birefringence when renal tissue is viewed under crossed polarised light (Fig. 19.5). ATTR amyloid also has a distinct appearance and typically displays a 'honeycomb' pattern within affected cardiac tissue. ATTR amyloid

in the gut is typically identified in submucosal vessels, though it can also present as diffuse amorphous deposition throughout the submucosa (Fig. 19.6). ATTR deposits may be found in other sites such as the bladder, prostate and BMT [13]. Therefore, anti-TTR staining should routinely be carried out on these specimens as part of a panel. In skin biopsies, insulin-induced amyloid is always considered especially in specimens larger than 2 cm^2, as we have seen several cases over the years. Buccal cavity biopsies are always stained for apolipoprotien A-I (apoA1) amyloid. All biopsies are stained with anti-amyloid

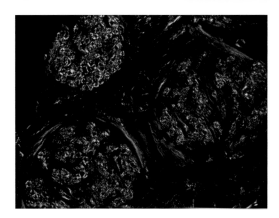

Fig. 19.5 'Sparkly' *apple green* birefringence morphology of LECT2 amyloid

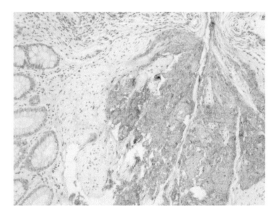

Fig. 19.6 Anti-TTR immunohistochemistry staining of a rectal biopsy showing diffuse amorphous deposition throughout the submucosa of a rectal biopsy (Reprinted from Gilbertson, Janet A C.Sci., F.I.B.M.S. Amyloid Typing: Experience from a Large Referral Centre, in Amyloid and Related Disorders, 1st Ed., Jan 2012, with kind permission from Springer Science and Business Media)

P component (AP) so that a comparison can be made with that of a negative Congo red. AP, identical to and directly derived from the normal plasma protein serum amyloid P component (SAP), is present in all human amyloid deposits, though in variable quantities. AP/SAP staining thus corroborates the presence of amyloid deposits of all kinds, though the same protein is also found naturally in basement membranes and some other connective tissue components.

Whilst completely specific antibodies are available to the various proteins from which amy-

loid is derived, the major conformational transformation from the native soluble proteins to the insoluble β-pleated amyloid fibril forms can result in specific peptide epitopes being lost. Further, protein epitopes can be masked by fixation of the tissue due to the cross-linking of amino acid side groups. In the early days of amyloid immunohistochemistry, it was thought that antigen retrieval was needed to demonstrate the fibril type, and various antigen retrieval methods were used with varying success. However, in our hands, we find that antigen retrieval is of little, if any, use for the detection of amyloid fibril type with the exception of TTR immunohistochemistry where oxidation with 1 % aqueous Na-m-periodate and 0.1 % di-NA borohydride for 10 min each followed by 4 h incubation with high-molarity guanidine treatment [14] is always performed. Without this retrieval, TTR staining is often negative or very weak. This retrieval step is needed due to the β-pleated conformation of amyloid 'hiding' some antigenic sites, of which TTR is one. Nowadays retrieval methods are commonplace in most laboratories, and since each antibody differs in the epitope that it recognises, it is important to try the whole range of available antigen recovery methods for each new antiserum.

As well as testing various retrieval methods, the correct way to evaluate the specificity of immunoreactions is to absorb antiserum with its specific antigen [15]. This is routine practice at the NAC.

Although relatively rare, amyloid is a differential diagnosis that ought to be not infrequently considered. Although antisera for AA and AL amyloid are available in most hospitals, if the clinical phenotype is consistent with hereditary systemic amyloidosis (ATTR, AApoAI, AGel, ALys, AFib, etc.), then discussion with or preferably referral to a specialist centre for a full 'amyloid evaluation' including detailed immunohistochemistry is advised so that available tissue can be best used to identify the amyloid fibril type.

At the NAC we cut 22 serial sections from each biopsy where possible, though the limiting factor is often the amount of tissue left in the block. Sections are cut at 2 μm for immunohisto-chemistry and at 6 μm for a Congo red overlay. Congo red overlay is a very useful technique that was adopted by NAC some years ago [16]. After completing the immunohistochemistry, a Congo red method is performed over the top of the immunostain; this allows the amyloid with the aid of cross polarisation to be visualised as the bire-fringence shows through the brown DAB stain-ing. Immunohistochemistry at the NAC is carried out using the Sequenza™ (Thermo Shandon, UK) system with Impress™ (Vector Laboratories, UK) detection kits. We follow the standard method as outlined in the Vector kit and use a metal-enhanced DAB Substrate kit (Thermo Scientific) for visualising the immuno-compound. Anti-human SAP immunostaining is performed on the Leica Bond Max according to their proto-col using their kits (Leica Microsystems UK).

Interpretation of all stained slides is carried out blindly by two experienced people. In an average year, approximately 34 % of all biopsies examined at the NAC contain no amyloid. On average among amyloidotic biopsies, immuno-histochemistry will positively identify 8 % AA, 14 % ATTR, 1 % of other types (insulin, LECT2, AFib, β 2 microglobulin, AapoA1) and 77 % AL amyloid. In patients with compelling evidence of AL amyloidosis, immunohistochemistry in our experience definitively identifies about 9 % of cases as AL-kappa and 38 % as AL-lambda types. Whilst other fibril types can often be con-fidently excluded, for example, AA, ~30 % of amyloid specimens do not stain immunohisto-chemically. This generally supports a diagnosis of AL amyloid but does not prove it. In our recent study [17], polyclonal antibodies to free light chains rather than conventional antibodies to light chains gave slightly cleaner background and sharper discrimination to amyloid deposits; how-ever, in routine, not all amyloid deposits are eas-ily identified by this panel. This failure to stain AL amyloid is due to the fact that the fibrils are composed from the variable domain of immuno-globulin light chains, in addition to which there may be highly soluble background monoclonal light chain staining throughout the tissue, due to presence of high light chain concentration in

patients' sera [7]. When the immunohistochem-istry is non-diagnostic of amyloid fibril type, we now routinely perform laser microdissection of amyloid and mass spectrometry in tandem.

Laser Capture Microdissection and Mass Spectrometry Dissection Mass Spectrometry

Laser capture microdissection and tandem mass spectrometry has been well documented as a novel method for typing amyloid [18]. Although it has been proposed as the new gold standard for amyloid detection and typing, it remains largely unvalidated as a clinical test and results are not always clear-cut [19]. Since 2012, proteomics has routinely accompanied Congo red histology and immunohistochemistry at the NAC in order to evaluate its role in diagnosis and amyloid fibril typing.

Proteomics in our centre is performed on the Velos platform and analysed using MASCOT software. Like immunohistochemistry, interpre-tation is performed blindly by two independent experienced investigators. To date we have ana-lysed over 1000 samples by this method, taken from over 30 different tissue types. In our hands, the fibril protein is unequivocally determined in approximately 30 % cases and identified with a high degree of certainty in a further 15 % but remains uncertain in ~32 % cases. The remain-ing 23 % cases show the 'amyloid signature' by proteomics [20], but there are insufficient proteins present to determine the amyloid type. Figure 19.7 shows a large vessel in a fat pad biopsy stained with Congo red observed under TRITC filters that gave positive staining with anti-TTR; however, insufficient proteins were present in the microdissected sample to confirm the immunohistochemical findings. A similar case is highlighted in Fig. 19.8 which shows a nerve biopsy from a patient with a rare TTR vari-ant. Congo red histology demonstrated amyloid within the nerve bundles which stained immuno-specifically with anti-TTR antibody. The amy-loid was laser captured, and whilst TTR was present in the sample, the 'amyloid signature' proteins were not detected such that the diagnosis was not clear.

Nevertheless, we have found that proteomic analysis can be a very useful adjunct to immuno-

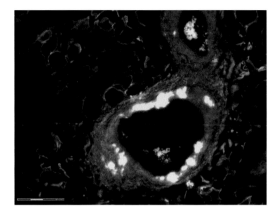

Fig. 19.7 Fat pad under TRITC filters showing amyloid as *bright yellow* against a *red background*

histochemistry, especially when the clinical details are not known. For example, a 69-year-old male from abroad presented to a local hospital during a vacation in the UK with advanced renal impairment. He had no past medical history and no inflammatory condition, and his serum light chain ratio was within normal limits. On review of his renal biopsy at the NAC, there was scanty amyloid within the glomeruli (Fig. 19.9), which did not stain with antibodies against AA protein or light chain proteins. Laser microdissection and capture mass spectrometry unexpectedly identified fibrinogen α chain as the fibril protein, later confirmed by genetic analysis and immunohistochemistry. We have also identified three cases of immunoglobulin heavy chain (AH) amyloidosis by mass spectrometry, though these results have not been confirmed by IHC or any further tests.

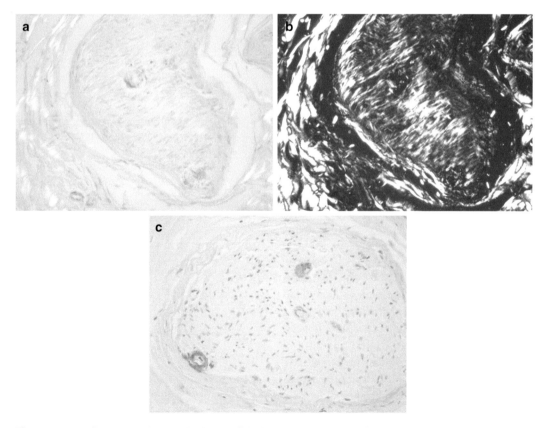

Fig. 19.8 Nerve biopsy showing two distinct amyloid deposits with *Congo red* (**a**) and *apple green* birefringence (**b**) and stained with anti-TTR IHC (**c**) ×200 magnification

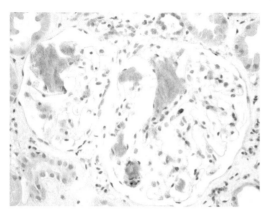

Fig. 19.9 Atypical morphological appearance of a glomerulus with fibrinogen-A-type amyloid

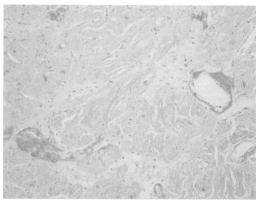

Fig. 19.10 *Congo red*-stained cardiac biopsy showing two distinct intensities of amyloid staining

Anomalies

It is exceptionally rare, although not completely unknown, for a patient to have two coexisting types of amyloid [21]. A routine cardiac biopsy was stained with Congo red and showed amyloid deposits throughout the tissue section, some of which were intensely congophilic (Fig. 19.10) and some of which showed pale diffuse congophilia. On immunohistochemistry, the areas of intense congophilia stained with anti-lambda antibody (Fig. 19.11) and the pale diffusely stained amyloid, stained with anti-TTR (Fig. 19.12). Laser capture microdissection of the two separate areas followed by tandem mass spectrometry confirmed the presence of two distinct types of amyloid within the one heart. We have also found two different types of amyloid in the rectal biopsies of two other patients, although in these cases the different amyloids were present in different tissue compartments: AL (lambda) amyloid in the mucosa and TTR amyloid in the submucosal vessels. The immunohistochemical findings were again confirmed by proteomic analysis. Such cases are rare and careful consideration should be given to clinical relevance of the amyloid in question. Interestingly, we have never knowingly identified two different amyloid fibril types within a single amyloid deposit, despite anti-AA staining in thousands of patients with AL amyloidosis, some of whom have had a chronic inflammatory disorder at the time of the

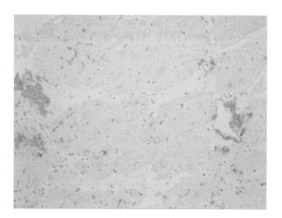

Fig. 19.11 AL-lambda immunohistochemistry staining the areas of *darker Congo red*-stained amyloid

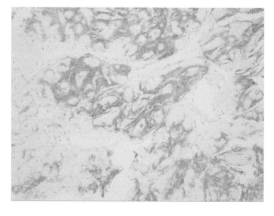

Fig. 19.12 Transthyretin immunohistochemistry staining the areas of paler *Congo red*-stained amyloid

diagnosis of amyloid. Thus, unlike the mouse in which it seems that any type/species of inoculated amyloidotic material can act as a seed for deposition of mouse AA amyloid in the presence of an acute phase response, induction and propagation of amyloid in man seems to be utterly protein/fibril specific.

Summary

The tools available today to determine the amyloid fibril protein from amyloidotic tissue include immunohistochemistry, proteomics and direct fibril sequencing (the latter only possible when sufficient fresh tissue is available). Indirect investigations, which may be very helpful, include searches for monoclonal immunoglobulins using conventional electrophoresis and immunoassays of serum and urine free light chain, assessment of the acute phase response by measuring SAA and CRP and, where indicated, genetic sequencing of known amyloid fibril protein genes. A definitive diagnosis of the presence and type of amyloid at the NAC relies on the results of most of these investigations, undertaken simultaneously in most patients.

At the NAC, the use of SAP scintigraphy allows in vivo diagnosis as well as monitoring of accumulation and regression of amyloid deposits, for example, in response to therapeutic intervention [22, 23]. Unfortunately SAP scintigraphy is of limited use in visualising amyloid deposition within cardiac tissue due to the fact that the heart contains much 'blood pool' and is a moving organ. The bone scanning agent DPD, labelled with technetium (^{99m}Tc-3,3-diphosphono-1,2-propanodicarboxylic acid), was serendipitously discovered to have extraordinarily high affinity for cardiac ATTR amyloid deposits [24, 25], and Tc-DPD scanning is now routinely undertaken at the NAC as an additional diagnostic test in those suspected to have cardiac ATTR amyloidosis.

Positive immunohistochemistry with antisera to amyloid P/SAP may be useful when used in conjunction with Congo red staining, though it must be remembered that elastin and collagen fibres will also stain. It is essential in cases of amyloid to determine the fibril protein in order to guide clinical management. Whilst most laboratories may be able to type AA and certain patients with AL amyloid by immunohistochemistry, it is sufficiently rare that referral of cases of amyloid to the National Centre can be justified.

In our experience, immunohistochemical typing of amyloid and even routine Congo red histology remain challenging. Immunohistochemical identification of the amyloid fibril protein continues to improve, but the precise diagnosis can often be determined only after additional highly specialised, expensive tests such as genetic sequencing and mass spectrometry. Early receipt of biopsy tissue from patients who are referred to the NAC for a clinical evaluation is recommended, since a firm diagnosis by the time the patient attends maximises the potential for a detailed discussion of treatment and prognosis with such patients.

References

1. Gilbertson JA, Hunt T, Hawkins PN. Amyloid typing: experience from a large referral centre. In: Picken MM, Dogan A, Herrera GA, editors. Amyloid and related disorders. New York, NY: Humana; 2012. p. 231–8.
2. Puchtler H, Sweat F, Levine M. On the binding of Congo red by amyloid. J Histochem Cytochem. 1962;10:355–64.
3. Picken MM. Amyloidosis—where are we now and where are we heading? Arch Pathol Lab Med. 2010; 134:545–51.
4. Gilbertson JA, Thesis JD, Hunt T, et al. A comparison of immunohistochemistry and mass spectrometry for determining the amyloid fibril protein from formalin fixed biopsy tissue. XIIIth International Symposium on Amyloidosis; 2012. pp. 183–5.
5. Loo D, Mollee PN, Renaut P, et al. Proteomics in molecular diagnosis: typing of amyloidosis. J Biomed Biotechnol. 2011;2011:1–9.
6. Westermark P, Stenkvist B. A new method for the diagnosis of systemic amyloidosis. Arch Intern Med. 1973;132(4):522–3.
7. Pepys MB. Amyloid P component and the diagnosis of amyloidosis. J Int Med Res. 1992;232(6):519–21.
8. Bijzet J, van Gameren I, Hazenberg BPC. Fat tissue analysis in the management of patients with systemic amyloidosis. In: Picken MM, Dogan A, Herrera GA, editors. Amyloid and related disorders. New York: Humana; 2012. p. 191–207.
9. Highman B. Improved methods for demonstrating amyloid in paraffin sections. Arch Pathol. 1946;41:559.
10. Stokes G. An improved Congo red method for amyloid. Med Lab Sci. 1976;33:79.

11. Sayed RH, Gilbertson JA, Hutt DF, et al. Misdiagnosing renal amyloidosis as minimal change disease. Nephrol Dial Transplant. 2014;29(11):2120–6.

12. Lachmann H, Chir B, Booth D, et al. Misdiagnosis of hereditary amyloidosis as AL (primary) amyloidosis. N Engl J Med. 2002;346(23):1786–91.

13. Sachchithanantham S, Gillmore JD, Gilbertson JA, et al. Painless haematuria is a manifestation of senile systemic amyloidosis. XIV International Symposium on Amyloidosis; 2014. PC-45.

14. Costa PP, Jacobsson B, Collin VP, et al. Unmasking antigen determinants in amyloid. J Histochem Cytochem. 1986;34(12):1683–5.

15. Westermark GT, Johnson KH, Westermark P. Staining methods for identification of amyloid in tissue. Methods Enzymol. 1999;309:3–25.

16. Tennent GA, Cafferty KD, Pepys MB, et al. Congo red overlay immunohistochemistry aids classification of amyloid deposits. In: Kyle RA, Gertz MA, editors. Amyloid and amyloidosis 1998. Pearl River: Parthenon; 1999. p. 160–2.

17. Owen-Casey MP, Sim R, Cook HT, et al. Value of antibodies to free light chains in immunoperoxidase studies of renal biopsies. J Clin Pathol. 2014;67(8):661–6.

18. Vrana JA, Gamez JD, Madden BJ, et al. Classification of amyloidosis by laser microdissection and mass spectrometry-based proteomic analysis in clinical biopsy specimens. Blood. 2009;114:4957–9.

19. Kaul E, Pilichowska M, Vullaganti M, et al. Twists and turns of determining amyloid type and amyloid-related organ damage: discordance and clinical skepticism in the era of proteomic typing. Amyloid. 2014; 21(1):62–5.

20. Vrana JA, Theis JD, Dasari S, et al. Clinical diagnosis and typing of systemic amyloidosis in subcutaneous fat aspirates by mass spectrometry-based proteomics. Haematologica. 2014;99(7):1239–47.

21. Mahmood S, Gilbertson JA, Rendell N, et al. Two types of amyloid in a single heart. Blood. 2014; 124(19):3025–7.

22. Hawkins PN, Richardson S, Vigushin DM, et al. Serum amyloid P component scintigraphy and turn-over studies for diagnosis and quantitative monitoring of AA amyloidosis in juvenile rheumatoid arthritis. Arthritis Rheum. 1993;36(6):842–51.

23. Hawkins PN. Studies with radiolabelled serum amyloid P component provide evidence for turnover and regression of amyloid deposits in vivo. Clin Sci (Colch). 1994;87(3):289–95.

24. Rapezzi C, Quarta CC, Guidalotti PL, et al. Usefulness and limitations of 99mTc-3,3-diphosphono-1,2-propanodicarboxylic acid scintigraphy in the aetiological diagnosis of amyloidotic cardiomyopathy. Eur J Nucl Med Mol Imaging. 2011;38:470–8.

25. Bokhari S, Castano A, Pozniakoff T, et al. 99mTc-pyrophosphate scintigraphy for differentiating light-chain cardiac amyloidosis from the transthyretin-related familial and senile cardiac amyloidoses. Circ Cardiovasc Imaging. 2013;6:195–201.

Options for Amyloid Typing in Renal Pathology: The Advantages of Frozen Section Immunofluorescence and a Summary of General Recommendations Regarding Immunohistochemistry Methods

20

Maria M. Picken

As may be seen from prior chapters and recent surveys, amyloid typing by antibody-based methods continues to play a major role in current clinical practice [1–6]. However, it must be stressed that the immunohistochemistry of amyloid differs markedly from that encountered in other areas of general surgical pathology. In this chapter, another form of immunohistochemistry, namely immunofluorescence performed on frozen sections, will be discussed. This technique is routinely used by renal pathology laboratories in North America and many other parts of the world and contributes significantly to amyloid typing in clinical practice. As a consequence, there is an abundant literature pertaining to the use of immunofluorescence in renal pathology; hence, only a brief summary will be provided here, focusing on issues that are of particular relevance to amyloid typing [1–4, 7, 8].

M.M. Picken, MD, PhD (✉)
Department of Pathology, Loyola University Medical Center, Loyola University Chicago, Building 110, Room 2242, 2160 South First Avenue, Maywood, IL 60153, USA
e-mail: mpicken@luc.edu; MMPicken@aol.com

Frozen Section Immunofluorescence Amyloid Typing

The clinical workup of a native kidney biopsy typically includes paraffin sections, a panel of immunofluorescence stains performed on frozen sections, and, in most instances, also electron microscopy. Thus, frozen section immunofluorescence is a standard component of the workup of native kidney biopsies, which are routinely tested for immunoglobulins G, A, M, immunoglobulin light chains kappa and lambda, complement components (C3, C1q), and fibrinogen; typically, a stain for albumin and control tissues are also included. Figure 20.1 shows a case of amyloid derived from lambda light chain, AL-lambda. Figure 20.1a–c illustrates how stain for a single light chain (i.e., light chain restriction) can be detected as part of a routine biopsy workup, while stains with other antibodies are negative (Fig. 20.1b–c). Note the high signal-to-noise ratio in Fig. 20.1a. In contrast, in Fig. 20.1b, amyloid deposits show only a weak and "dull" appearance, which is, also, not fluorescent and the signal-to-noise ratio is minimal. In contrast to other pathologies associated with light chain restriction (see Part II), amyloid deposits are Congo red positive (Fig. 20.1d). Thus, for a diagnosis of AL, the light chain reactivity pattern must correspond to the

© Springer International Publishing Switzerland 2015
M.M. Picken et al. (eds.), *Amyloid and Related Disorders*, Current Clinical Pathology,
DOI 10.1007/978-3-319-19294-9_20

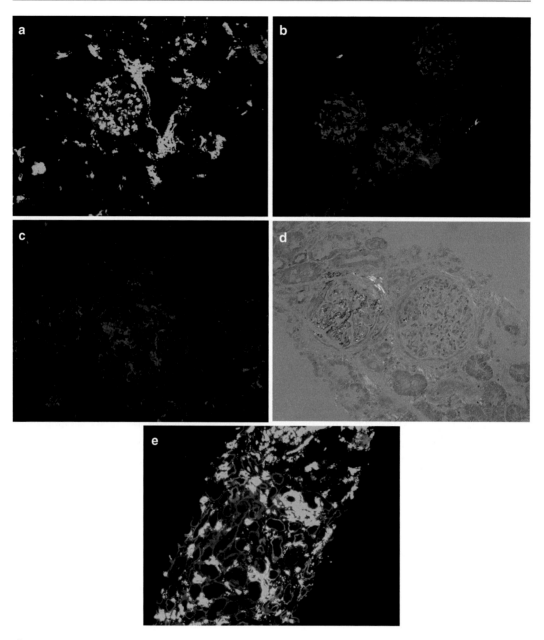

Fig. 20.1 A case of AL-lambda. (**a**) Stain for lambda light chain. Notice the high signal-to noise ratio. (**b**) Stain for kappa light chain. Although the exposure had to be increased for photographic purposes (in order to show the structures clearly), the signal-to-noise ratio is low and the deposits of amyloid are not truly fluorescent but instead show a dull appearance. (**c**) Negative stain for IgG. Please see also comments for (**b**) above regarding the signal-to-noise ratio. (**d**) Congo red stain viewed under polarized light. (**e**) Stain for AP showing bright fluorescence, with a high signal-to-noise ratio, highlighting deposits of amyloid

spatial distribution of Congo red-positive deposits. To this end, stain for amyloid P component (AP) can also be helpful (Fig. 20.1e). Despite the biochemical diversity of amyloid fibril proteins, all types of amyloid have been shown to contain AP component, which can be readily visualized by immunohistochemical methods as shown in Fig. 20.1e [9]. In contrast, the deposits of monoclonal (light or heavy chain) immunoglobulin deposition disease lack AP component [9]. Thus,

regulatory issues, e.g., the validation of such antibodies as analyte-specific reagents (ASR), have not been uniformly addressed. Interestingly, however, the extent of the various antibody reactivities with amyloid fibril proteins is variable and appears also to be technique dependent. Thus, as shown in two subsequent chapters, antibody typing using commercial antibodies by immuno-electron microscopy techniques gives better results than typing in paraffin sections; similarly, amyloid typing by the immunoblotting (Western blot) technique has been shown to be more reliable than by immunohistochemistry in paraffin sections.

The question therefore arises as to how we can explain this variability in apparent sensitivity between the various antibody-based techniques used in amyloid typing, and particularly in the case of AL? While, in some instances, the use of custom anti-amyloid fibril antibodies and greater proficiency in antibody testing techniques may be responsible for such variability, other factors need to be considered as well. One such factor may be that our collective knowledge and perception of the composition of amyloid fibrils in AL is limited and continues to evolve. For example, it has been postulated for decades that the fibrils are composed of light chain fragments. However, as data from more sophisticated antibody-based techniques (such as immuno-electron microscopy, Western blot) and mass spectrometry (MS) accumulate, they increasingly suggest that most ALs contain, at the very least, a significant portion of the constant region and that those composed predominantly of the V region are rare. Even in the case of the MS method of amyloid typing, diagnosis is dependent on finding a match with *known* protein fragments. Thus, the increased sensitivity of antibody binding may depend on the presence of significant segments of the constant region present in the fibrils. While further consideration of these issues lies outside the scope of this chapter, it seems clear that there are significant aspects of amyloid fibril structure/composition (particularly in the case of AL) that are still incompletely understood.

Rare cases of amyloidoses derived from the immunoglobulin heavy chain, AH, have been reported. Cases derived either from γ or μ- heavy chain, typically, have had deletions in the C_H1 and C_H2 regions [7]. Specific antibodies to the intact heavy chains are routinely used, and hence the fibrils, being derived from a truncated protein, may not be reactive; thus, it is not clear how many cases may be missed using current methods. More recently, Sethi et al. [23] described clinicopathologic findings in four cases of renal immunoglobulin heavy chain amyloidosis, which, in two cases, also showed reactivity for heavy chains together with light chains. Subsequent studies reported additional cases of amyloidosis where both light and heavy chains were detected and the authors coined the term "immunoglobulin amyloidosis" to encompass the apparent spectrum of amyloidoses derived from various immunoglobulin components, including also light+heavy chain [24]. Whether these findings indicate that the fibrils are truly composed of both light+heavy chains is an open question at the present time [25]. Thus far, light/heavy chain amyloidosis has not been officially included in the classification and nomenclature of the amyloidoses [26].

Other Factors

Amyloid deposits do not contain pure fibril proteins but represent a rather heterogeneous complex that also includes, besides the amyloid fibril protein itself, other components such as AP component, Apolipoprotein E, glycosaminoglycans, variable extracellular components, and even lipids [7]. All of these may affect antibody binding. AP component and Apolipoprotein E have been recognized as "amyloid signature" elements.

Paraffin Versus Frozen Sections

It has been shown that antigenic sites may be altered during fixation to a variable degree, and, therefore, it is not surprising that many antibodies perform better in frozen than in paraffin sections. This is especially evident in the case of serum protein detection in kidney biopsies, as well as the detection of light chain restriction in general and in AL in particular [27–29]. The use of antigen retrieval in amyloid immunohisto-chemistry is controversial, and experience, expertise, and validation are critical ([30], please see also Chaps. 18 and 19 by Linke and Gilbertson et al. respectively).

Another important factor to consider is the fact that most amyloid fibril proteins also have their native counterparts present in the serum. Thus, in paraffin sections, the plasma proteins may have been fixed in the tissues and, if they are to be removed, they must be removed by a digestion process. Their incomplete elimination creates a background stain that may compete with the signal from the amyloid protein and result in a low signal-to-noise ratio. In contrast, in frozen sections, plasma proteins can be removed simply by washing [8]. However, to some extent, even in vivo, various serum proteins can be adsorbed to amyloid deposits. As can be seen from the above, in renal pathology, the issues of limited antibody reactivity and background staining appear to be less of an impediment to successful amyloid typing, largely due to the application of immuno-fluorescence performed on frozen sections.

General Comments Regarding Antibody Typing by Frozen Section Immunofluorescence

Based on the author's own experience, the majority of renal and extra-renal systemic amyloidoses can be successfully typed using commercial antibodies and immunofluorescence on frozen sections; a similar experience was also published by others [4, 7, 13, 20]. While not all ALs are reactive with commercial antibodies and, in rare instances, may not even react with custom antibodies (please see chapters by Linke, Gilbertson et al. and Verga et al. in this book in Chaps. 18, 19 and 22 respectively), in the author's own experience, based on immuno-fluorescence on frozen sections, up to 85 % of ALs can be confidently typed with commercial antibodies. Similar results were also reported by Collins, using immunofluorescence on frozen sections for the typing of cardiac amyloid [20].

However, this technique is still underutilized in general surgical pathology, since tissues are routinely fixed in formalin. In certain situations, setting aside a portion of tissue for potential immunofluorescence testing on frozen sections is advisable. This is particularly recommended for native myocardial biopsies and fat biopsies performed for amyloid testing. If necessary, an abdominal fat biopsy can be repeated (please see Chap. 16 and 17 in part II). In connection with these procedures, it should be added that commercially available immunofluorescence transport medium now allows the shipment of tissue at ambient temperature, with refrigeration upon arrival. Also, the antibody panel can be expanded, depending on the type of biopsy (renal, cardiac, or liver), the clinical setting, or even the geographic area and/or ethnicity; in particular, in patients on dialysis, testing for β_2-microglobulin should be performed. Ultimately, however, maintaining an extended amyloid antibody testing panel may not be practical in laboratories with a low volume of amyloid specimens. As is the case in general surgical pathology, low volume tests are best outsourced to a reference laboratory. Therefore, in all negative and inconclusive cases, typing is best undertaken by reference laboratories, where a wider selection of antibodies and techniques are available.

A certain amount of experience in the interpretation of *amyloid* immunofluorescence stains is needed, and this is variable. Consequently, the published rates of successful typing by immuno-fluorescence are also variable but still, in general, better than the usual experience with paraffin sections [4, 20, 31–33]. Importantly, however, an inconclusive result derived from immunohisto-chemistry, regardless of the technique employed, should be reported as such and these cases should be tested further by a reference laboratory. Any attempt at "guessing" the amyloid type is wholly unacceptable in clinical practice and is frankly dangerous. For example, Lachman et al. [34] studied 350 patients with systemic amyloidosis, in whom the diagnosis of AL had been suggested by clinical and laboratory findings, and by the absence of a family history. This study showed that 10 % of patients actually had familial amyloi-dosis; interestingly, a low-grade monoclonal gam-mopathy was detected in 24 % of these patients.

Subsequent studies reported similar results [35]. Conversely, patients can have a potentially amyloidogenic mutation and AL [36, 37]. Thus, although the vast majority of patients (in the USA approximately 85 %) are ultimately diagnosed with AL, this diagnosis may never be assumed. Given the implications for clinical management, which in the case of AL is markedly different from that of other amyloidoses, correct diagnosis of the amyloid type is critical [3, 11, 21].

Summary Comments Regarding Amyloid Typing

Amyloid immunohistochemistry is complex and is also not directly comparable to immunohistochemistry testing in other areas of general surgical pathology. Thus, the interpretation of amyloid immunohistochemistry stains is not trivial and a certain amount of experience is necessary.

Immunofluorescence in frozen sections continues to be the most common and convenient method of amyloid typing and should be the first step when feasible. It is most useful in cases of amyloid derived from immunoglobulin components, which are also the most prevalent type [3, 11]. It is a fast, inexpensive, and widely accessible method. The critical issues are strict adherence to the typing criteria and determining when a more sophisticated approach is needed.

Laser microdissection/mass spectrometry (LMD/MS) has emerged as a new and extremely valuable technology (see Chaps. 19, 23, 24 in this book). It takes advantage of the fact that the amyloid fibril protein is the most abundant protein in the tissue under study. However, even with sample enrichment, via laser dissection of amyloidotic areas, it is still a protein extract, rather than pure amyloid fibrils, that is subjected to LMD/MS studies. The proteins in the extract are identified based on their fingerprinting pattern, which is then compared with published databases and the predominant protein is presumed to be the amyloid fibril protein. In the absence of immunoglobulin light chains, other proteins are presumed to be the amyloid fibril proteins. The validation of LMD/MS results has been done, thus far, by conventional immunohistochemistry. The greatest advantage of the LMD/MS technique is its role in the diagnosis of rare amyloid types and the discovery of new amyloid types [3].

It is unlikely that, in the future, we will rely on a single method for amyloid typing. Amyloidosis is a relatively rare diagnosis, and, as a consequence, most pathologists examine only a few specimens. In surgical pathology, many low number and/or higher complexity tests are referred to specialized laboratories. Thus, given the complexity of amyloid typing, it is highly advisable, and more practical, to concentrate on screening for amyloid and to refer specimens for amyloid typing to specialized laboratories.

Finally, a brief comment regarding the use of the term typing versus sub-typing (semantics) is also warranted. Amyloid is a generic term that is applicable to all amyloids, which are divisible into different types. In this context, the use of the term "sub-typing" appears to be redundant.

Recommendations

Listed below are current recommendations and standards for the clinical diagnosis of amyloidosis as formulated at the XIIth International Symposium on Amyloidosis [1]:

1. Emphasis should be placed on the early detection of amyloid through increasing awareness of amyloidoses, and the diagnostic and treatment options available, from pathologists and clinicians.
2. Diagnosis of the amyloid type must be based on identification of the amyloid protein in deposits and should not be based solely on clinical suspicion or genetic testing. While clinicopathologic correlation is mandatory, it is not a substitute for amyloid protein identification.
3. Accurate diagnosis of the amyloid protein type is critical. Immunohistochemical typing must be done with caution and only clear-cut results should be reported in clinical practice. All equivocal (or negative) results should be

studied by other techniques, including mass spectrometric methods, which are available in laboratories specializing in amyloidosis diagnosis. These other techniques are at present considered complementary to immunohistochemistry and their standardization is under development.

4. A second opinion is strongly encouraged before administering aggressive therapy, particularly, in cases where amyloid typing was performed in a non-specialized laboratory.

References

1. Picken MM, Westermark P. Amyloid detection and typing: summary of current practice and recommendations of the consensus group. Amyloid. 2011;18 Suppl 1:48–50.
2. Picken MM. Current practice in amyloid detection and typing among renal pathologists. Amyloid. 2011;18 Suppl 1:73–5.
3. Leung N, Nasr SH, Sethi S. How I treat amyloidosis: the importance of accurate diagnosis and amyloid typing. Blood. 2012;120(16):3206–16.
4. Picken MM. Amyloid typing in surgical pathology—experience of a single institution. In: Skinner M, Berk JL, Connors LH, Seldin DC, editors. XIth International Symposium on Amyloidosis; Boca Raton, FL: CRC Press; 2007. p. 289–91.
5. Schönland SO1, Hegenbart U, Bochtler T, Mangatter A, Hansberg M, Ho AD, Lohse P, Röcken C. Immunohistochemistry in the classification of systemic forms of amyloidosis: a systematic investigation of 117 patients. Blood. 2012;119(2):488–93. doi:10.1182/blood-2011-06-358507. Epub 2011 Nov 21.
6. Linke RP. On typing amyloidosis using immunohistochemistry. Detailed illustrations, review and a note on mass spectrometry. Prog Histochem Cytochem. 2012;47(2):61–132. Epub 2012 Jul 20.
7. Herrera GA, Picken MM. Renal diseases associated with plasma cell dyscrasias, amyloidoses, waldenstrom macroglobulinemia and cryoglobulinemic nephropathies. In: Jennette JC, Olson JL, Silva FG, Agati VD', editors. Heptinstall's pathology of the kidney. 7th ed. Philadelphia, PA: Lippincott Williams & Wilkins; 2006. p. 951–1014.
8. Walker PD, Cavallo T, Bonsib SM. Ad hoc committee on renal biopsy guidelines of the renal pathology society. Practice guidelines for the renal biopsy. Mod Pathol. 2004;17(12):1555–63.
9. Gallo G, Picken MM, Buxbaum J, Frangione B. Nonamyloidotic monoclonal immunoglobulin deposits lack amyloid P component. Mod Pathol. 1988;1:453–6.
10. Fermand JP, Bridoux F, Kyle RA, Kastritis E, Weiss BM, Cook MA, Drayson MT, Dispenzieri A, Leung N. International kidney and monoclonal gammopathy research group. How I treat monoclonal gammopathy of renal significance (MGRS). Blood. 2013;122(22):3583–90. Epub 2013 Oct 9.
11. Picken MM. New insights into systemic amyloidosis: the importance of diagnosis of specific type. Curr Opin Nephrol Hypertens. 2007;16(3):196–203.
12. von Hutten H, Mihatsch M, Lobeck H, Rudolph B, Eriksson M, Röcken C. Prevalence and origin of amyloid in kidney biopsies. Am J Surg Pathol. 2009;33(8):1198–205.
13. Picken MM. Amyloidosis-where are we now and where are we heading? Arch Pathol Lab Med. 2010;134(4):545–51.
14. Said SM, Sethi S, Valeri AM, Leung N, Cornell LD, Fidler ME, Herrera Hernandez L, Vrana JA, Theis JD, Quint PS, Dogan A, Nasr SH. Renal amyloidosis: origin and clinicopathologic correlations of 474 recent cases. Clin J Am Soc Nephrol. 2013;8:1515–23.
15. Larsen CP, Walker PD, Weiss DT, Solomon A. Prevalence and morphology of leukocyte chemotactic factor 2-associated amyloid in renal biopsies. Kidney Int. 2010;77(9):816–9.
16. Said SM, Sethi S, Valeri AM, Chang A, Nast CC, Krahl L, Molloy P, Barry M, Fidler ME, Cornell LD, Leung N, Vrana JA, Theis JD, Dogan A, Nasr SH. Renal leukocyte chemotactic factor 2-associated amyloidosis. Kidney Int. 2014;86:370–7. Published online 22 Jan 2014.
17. Larsen CP, Kossmann RJ, Beggs ML, Solomon A, Walker PD. Renal leukocyte chemotactic factor 2 amyloidosis (ALECT2): a case series detailing clinical, morphologic, and genetic features. Kidney Int. 2014;86:378–82. Published online 12 Feb 2014.
18. Picken MM. Alect2 amyloidosis: primum non nocere (first, do no harm). Kidney Int. 2014;86(2):229–32.
19. Mereuta OM, Theis JD, Vrana JA, Law ME, Grogg KL, Dasari S, Chandan VS, Wu TT, Jimenez-Zepeda VH, Fonseca R, Dispenzieri A, Kurtin PJ, Dogan A. Leukocyte cell-derived chemotaxin 2 (LECT2)–associated amyloidosis is a frequent cause of hepatic amyloidosis in the United States. Blood. 2014;123(10):1479–82.
20. Collins AB, Smith RN, Stone JR. Classification of amyloid deposits in diagnostic cardiac specimens by immunofluorescence. Cardiovasc Pathol. 2009;18(4):205–16.
21. Picken MM. Modern approaches to the treatment of amyloidosis—the critical importance of early detection in surgical pathology. Adv Anat Pathol. 2013;20(6):424–39.
22. Owen-Casey MP, Sim R, Cook HT, Roufosse CA, Gillmore JD, Gilbertson JA, Hutchison CA, Howie AJ. Value of antibodies to free light chains in immunoperoxidase studies of renal biopsies. J Clin Pathol. 2014;67:661–6.
23. Sethi S, Theis JD, Leung N, Dispenzieri A, Nasr SH, Fidler ME, Cornell LD, Gamez JD, Vrana JA, Dogan

A. Mass spectrometry-based proteomic diagnosis of renal immunoglobulin heavy chain amyloidosis. Clin J Am Soc Nephrol. 2010;5(12):2180–7.
24. Nasr SH, Said SM, Valeri AM, Sethi S, Fidler ME, Cornell LD, Gertz MA, Dispenzieri A, Buadi FK, Vrana JA, Theis JD, Dogan A, Leung N. The diagnosis and characteristics of renal heavy-chain and heavy/light-chain amyloidosis and their comparison with renal light-chain amyloidosis. Kidney Int. 2013;83(3):463–70. Epub 2013 Jan 9.
25. Picken MM. Non-light-chain immunoglobulin amyloidosis: time to expand or refine the spectrum to include light+heavy chain amyloidosis? Kidney Int. 2013;83(3):353–6.
26. Sipe JD, Benson MD, Buxbaum JN, Ikeda S, Merlini G, Saraiva MJ, Westermark P. Nomenclature 2014: amyloid fibril proteins and clinical classification of the amyloidosis. Amyloid. 2014;21(4):221–4. 2014 Sep 29.
27. Mölne J, Breimer ME, Svalander CT. Immunoperoxidase versus immunofluorescence in the assessment of human renal biopsies. Am J Kidney Dis. 2005;45(4):674–83.
28. Furness PN. Acp. Best practice no 160. Renal biopsy specimens. J Clin Pathol. 2000;53(6):433–8.
29. Nasr SH, Galgano SJ, Markowitz GS, Stokes MB, D'Agati VD. Immunofluorescence on pronase-digested paraffin sections: a valuable salvage technique for renal biopsies. Kidney Int. 2006;70(12):2148–51.
30. Larsen C. Leukocyte chemotactic factor 2 amyloidosis can be reliably diagnosed by immunohistochemical staining. Hum Pathol. 2014;45(10):2179. Epub 2014 Jul 16.
31. Novak L, Cook WJ, Herrera GA, Sanders PW. AL-amyloidosis is underdiagnosed in renal biopsies. Nephrol Dial Transplant. 2004;19(12):3050–3.
32. Satoskar AA, Burdge K, Cowden DJ, Nadasdy GM, Hebert LA, Nadasdy T. Typing of amyloidosis in renal biopsies: diagnostic pitfalls. Arch Pathol Lab Med. 2007;131(6):917–22.
33. Picken MM, Herrera GA. The burden of "sticky" amyloid: typing challenges. Arch Pathol Lab Med. 2007;131(6):850–1.
34. Lachmann HJ, Booth DR, Booth SE, Bybee A, Gillbertson JA, Gillmore JD, Pepys MB, Hawkins PN. Misdiagnosis of hereditary amyloidosis as AL (primary) amyloidosis. N Engl J Med. 2002;346(23):1786–91.
35. Comenzo RL, Zhou P, Fleisher M, Clark B, Teruya-Feldstein J. Seeking confidence in the diagnosis of systemic AL (Ig light-chain) amyloidosis: patients can have both monoclonal gammopathies and hereditary amyloid proteins. Blood. 2006;107(9):3489–91. Epub 2006 Jan 26.
36. Picken MM, Hazenberg BPC, Obici L. Report from the diagnostic interactive session. In: Skinner M, Berk JL, Connors LH, Seldin DC, editors. XIth International Symposium on Amyloidosis; Boca Raton, FL: CRC Press; 2007. p. 377–82.
37. Rowczenio D, Dogan A, Theis JD, Vrana JA, Lachmann HJ, Wechalekar AD, Gilbertson JA, Hunt T, Gibbs SD, Sattianayagam PT, Pinney JH, Hawkins PN, Gillmore JD. Amyloidogenicity and clinical phenotype associated with five novel mutations in apolipoprotein A-I. Am J Pathol. 2011;179(4):1978–87. Epub 2011 Aug 5.

Amyloid Typing in Plastic-Embedded Tissue by Immune-Gold-Silver Method

21

Anne Räisänen-Sokolowski and Tom Törnroth

Introduction

In this short chapter, we present an immune stain-ing method which was originally developed in our laboratory for the evaluation of kidney biop-sies and which we subsequently adapted for amy-loid typing. This method was originally developed as an alternative method for kidney biopsies where fresh tissue was not available for routine immunofluorescence.

Development of the immune-gold-silver labeling method in plastic-embedded tissue

For many years, we have routinely used plastic embedding for all kidney biopsies that were fixed in paraformaldehyde, since plastic sections produced far superior light microscopic morphology than paraffin sections. Although immunoperoxidase and immunofluorescence on paraformaldehyde-fixed, plastic-embedded tissues were also tested, they never produced satisfactory results. This led us to the development of a gold-labeled, silver-enhanced

method, which is based on a technique originally developed for electron microscopy.

Thus, we have developed an immune-gold-silver method that uses a direct double-layer tech-nique to detect different amyloid types. In this method, the unconjugated antibody binds to the protein and is then visualized by a gold-labeled secondary antibody and silver developer, result-ing in a strong black or dark brown precipitate. The stains are evaluated by routine light micros-copy. A positive stain is one that colocalizes with a positive Congo red stain with birefringent areas.

This method is particularly sensitive and spe-cific for immunoglobulin light chains; however, stains for heavy chains also work well. We rou-tinely stain for kappa and lambda light chain and transthyretin. A stain for AA amyloid protein is performed by immunoperoxidase (Ventana). Gelsolin is added if the prior stains are negative and/or depending on the clinical scenario, since Finland is an endemic area for amyloid derived from gelsolin, AGel [1]. Hence, if clinically indicated, and/or in cases that are negative in the routine antibody panel, we add a stain for gelsolin. We have successfully applied this method to a variety of specimens, including: kidney biopsies, myocardium, fat, peripheral nerve, gastrointesti-nal biopsies, skin, etc.

Over several years, we have used this method to evaluate approximately 12–14 amyloid speci-mens per year and were able to successfully type 88 % of specimens. Among the specimens, which

A. Räisänen-Sokolowski, MD, PhD (✉) • T. Törnroth
Transplantation Laboratory-HUSLAB,
Helsinki University Central Hospital,
P.O. Box 400, Helsinki 00029, HUS, Finland
e-mail: Anne.Raisanen-Sokolowski@hus.fi;
tom.tornroth@gmail.com

M.M. Picken et al. (eds.), *Amyloid and Related Disorders*, Current Clinical Pathology,
DOI 10.1007/978-3-319-19294-9_21

could not be typed by this method were mostly minute biopsies or specimens with very small or sparse amyloid. We did not encounter positive stains for more than one amyloidotic protein.

We are not able to provide a cogent explanation of why immune stains work well on plastic sections. However, other laboratories, using plastic-embedded tissues for amyloid typing, have also reported results that were superior to those obtained with immunohistochemistry performed on paraffin sections ([2–4], see also chapter by Verga et al. elsewhere in this book). Our method, despite being used for several decades, has not thus far been published. The technique is presented below. We have also tried immuno-gold-method on paraffin sections, as suggested by Aurion [5], but never got satisfactory results.

Immune-Gold-Silver Method for Amyloid Typing in Plastic-Embedded Tissue

Paraffin-embedded tissue is deparaffinized and re-embedded in glycolmethacrylate [6]. After polymerization the tissue is cut into 1 μm thick sections and prepared with three sections on each slide. A positive control is included on each slide. After drying the slides on a hot plate, the staining protocol is performed as follows:

1. Lugol's iodine solution (stock: potassium iodide 2 g, iodine 1 g, distilled water ad 100 ml. For use dilute 1:20) for 5 min
2. Rinse with water
3. 2.5 % Sodium thiosulfate 10 min
4. Wash with water for 35 min on magnetic stirrer
5. Washing buffer (PBS and 0.1 % BSA-c [Aurion 900.022]) 3×5 min on magnetic stirrer
6. Circle the sample and control with hydrophobic barrier pen
7. Blocking solution (Aurion 905.002) for 20 min
8. Primary antibody incubation for 30 min in humid chamber:
   (a) Polyclonal rabbit-anti-human kappa light chains (DAKO A0192, dilution 1:1000)

   (b) Polyclonal rabbit-anti-human lambda light chain (DAKO A0193, dilution 1:100)
   (c) Polyclonal rabbit-anti-human prealbumin (transthyretin) (DAKO A0002, dilution 1:100)
9. Washing buffer for 3×5 min on magnetic stirrer
10. Secondary antibody incubation for 60 min in humid chamber (gold-labeled goat-anti-rabbit UltraSmall, Aurion 100.011)
11. Washing buffer PBS and 0.1 % BSA-c (Aurion 900.022) for 3×5 min on magnetic stirrer
12. Wash with water for 3×5 min on magnetic stirrer
13. Silver development with R-GENT developer and R-GENT enhancer (Aurion 500.011) that are mixed (1:2) just prior to use. Incubation for 30 min in humid and dark chamber
14. Wash with water for 3×5 min on magnetic stirrer
15. Dip the slides in increasing concentrations of alcohol until placing them in xylene
16. Coverslip the slides

Interpretation of stains is done in conjunction with Congo red stain results. We routinely stain for kappa and lambda light chain, AA amyloid protein and transthyretin; stain for gelsolin is performed if the prior stains are negative. The positive stain is that which colocalizes with Congo red positive areas (Figs. 21.1, 21.2, and 21.3).

Conclusions

Amyloid detection and correct typing are critical in patient management. In our experience, amyloid typing in plastic-embedded tissue by the above immune-gold-silver method represents a reliable and sensitive method for the identification of amyloid fibril proteins in various tissues and can correctly characterize the amyloid protein in most cases.

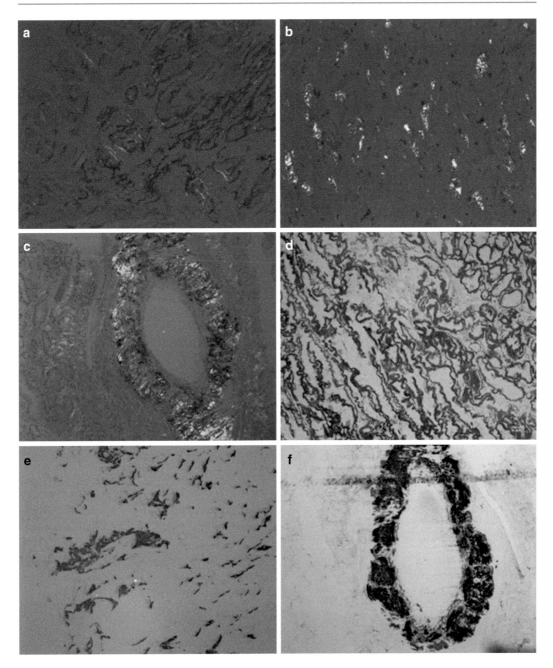

Fig. 21.1 In microphotographs (**a**) heart, (**b**) heart, and (**c**) kidney amyloid deposits are seen by Congo staining. Microphotographs (**d**), (**e**), and (**f**) show: lambda light chain deposits (**d**), transthyretin (**e**) and kappa light chains (**f**)

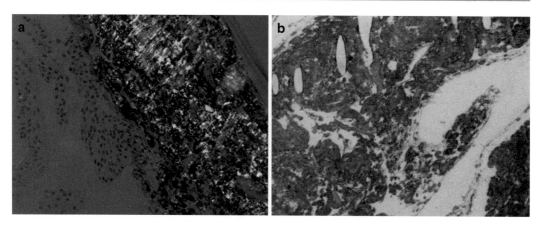

Fig. 21.2 Renal pelvis amyloid. (**a**) *Congo red* stain viewed under polarized light. (**b**) Positive stain for lambda light chain. Stain for kappa light chain was negative (not shown)

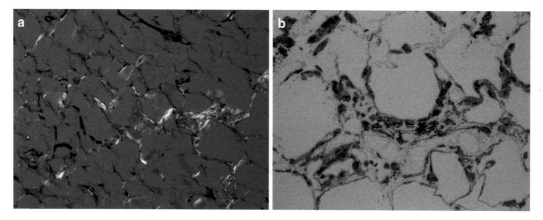

Fig. 21.3 Perirenal adipose tissue. (**a**) *Congo red* stain viewed under polarized light. (**b**) Positive stain for kappa light chain. Stain for lambda light chain was negative (not shown)

References

1. Pihlamaa T, Suominen S, Kiuru-Enari S. Familial amyloidotic polyneuropathy type IV-gelsolin amyloidosis. Amyloid. 2012;19 Suppl 1:30–3.
2. Arbustini E, Morbini P, Verga L, Concardi M, Porcu E, Pilotto A, Zorzoli I, Garini P, Anesi E, Merlini G. Light and electron microscopy immunohistochemical characterization of amyloid deposits. Amyloid Int J Exp Clin Invest. 1997;4:157–70.
3. Arbustini E, Verga L, Concardi M, Palladini G, Obici L, Merlini G. Electron and immuno-electron microscopy of abdominal fat identifies and characterizes amyloid fibrils in suspected cardiac amyloidosis. Amyloid. 2002;9:108–14.
4. Palladini G, Verga L, Corona S, Obici L, Morbini P, Lavatelli F, Donadei S, Sarais G, Roggeri L, Foli A, Russo P, Zenone Bragotti L, Paulli M, Magrini U, Merlini G. Diagnostic performance of immuno-electron microscopy of abdominal fat in systemic amyloidoses. Amyloid. 2010;17:59–60.
5. Datasheet: Aurion Blocking Solution. Aurion R-GENT SE-LM, Aurion, Wageningen, The Netherlands.
6. Datasheet: Leica Historesin Embedding Kit. Leica Biosystems Nussloch GmbH, Heidelberg, Germany.

The Role of Immuno-Electron Microscopy in Amyloid Typing: The Experience of the Pavia Referral Center

Laura Verga, Patrizia Morbini, Giovanni Palladini, Laura Obici, Gian Luca Capello, Marco Paulli, and Giampaolo Merlini

Introduction: The Role of Electron Microscopy in the Diagnosis of Amyloidosis

The diagnosis of amyloidosis requires demonstration of amyloid deposits in a tissue biopsy. The examination, under polarized light, of Congo red-stained abdominal fat smears or tissue biopsies is still the reference method used in the detection of amyloid deposits. Nevertheless, in some instances, interpretation of the Congo red stain birefringence pattern under polarized light may prove difficult, especially if performed by centers with limited experience in these techniques. Notably, in tissues with abundant collagen fibers, such as subcutaneous abdominal fat (Figs. 22.1 and 22.2b), birefringence of the collagen itself may be misinterpreted as amyloid [1]. Collagen typically shows some degree of birefringence under polarized light after Congo red staining, although this is yellowish and not "apple green" (Fig. 22.3a, b). In such instances, expert review of the slides can be of help. However, in selected cases, electron microscopic confirmation of amyloid fibrils is the only means to reach a definitive diagnosis.

In most centers, the routine diagnostic protocol for patients suspected of having amyloidosis, but with a negative abdominal fat aspirate, usually includes either minor salivary gland or rectal biopsy and, when both give negative results, a biopsy is obtained from an involved "target" organ. In the latter case, either fibrosis or other pathologies, i.e., fibrillary glomerulopathy, may sometimes be misdiagnosed as amyloid at the light microscopic level [2]. The ultrastructural examination of biopsy samples is capable of confirming or ruling out the diagnosis of amyloidosis [3] and can identify even very small deposits of amyloid fibrils [1]. By electron microscopy, whatever the amyloidogenic protein may be, amyloid deposits typically appear as randomly oriented, non-branching fibrils measuring 8–10 nm in diameter (Fig. 22.2a), quite differ-

L. Verga, DVM, PhD (✉) • P. Morbini, MD, PhD
Pathology Unit, Department of Molecular Medicine, University of Pavia and Fondazione IRCCS Policlinico San Matteo, Via Forlanini 16, 27100 Pavia, Italy
e-mail: l.verga@smatteo.pv.it; p.morbini@smatteo.pv.it

M. Paulli • G.L. Capello, BS
Foundation IRCCS Policlinico San Matteo, Pavia, Italy

Department of Molecular Medicine, University of Pavia, Pavia, Italy
e-mail: m.paulli@smatteo.pv.it; gcapello2002@libero.it

G. Palladini • L. Obici, MD • G. Merlini, MD
Departments of Molecular Medicine and Amyloidosis Research and Treatment Center, Foundation IRCCS Policlinico San Matteo and University of Pavia, Piazzale Golgi, 2, 27100 Pavia, Italy
e-mail: g.palladini@smatteo.pv.it; l.obici@smatteo.pv.it; gmerlini@unipv.it

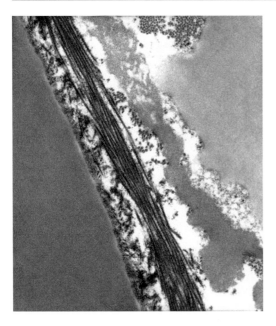

Fig. 22.1 Abdominal fat aspirate. In the middle a bundle of collagen fibers is seen and *on the left*, a lipid *droplet* in the cytoplasm of an adipocyte. Uranyl acetate, lead citrate ×13,000

ent from collagen fibers, which are much thicker and appear darker with routine stains (Fig. 22.2b).

Usually, only one amyloidogenic protein forms amyloid fibrils in each type of amyloidosis [4]. However, rare exceptions with mixed pathology (e.g., AL and $Abeta_2M$) have been reported [5]. Definitive identification of the deposited amyloidogenic protein is crucial for a correct diagnosis, appropriate treatment, assessment of prognosis, and genetic counseling, when applicable [6]. Thus, once amyloid fibrils have been identified in a biopsy sample (Fig. 22.4), it is necessary to characterize the amyloid fibril protein [3, 7]. Light microscopic immunohistochemical differentiation among different types of amyloid fibril proteins, by means either of immunofluorescence or of other methods such as immunoperoxidase, may be sometimes difficult and carries a high rate of false-positive results due to unspecific stain [1, 8–11]. In contrast, immuno-electron microscopy can correctly characterize amyloid deposits in over 99 % of specimens, including tissues that are easy to sample, such as abdominal fat and minor salivary glands [12, 13].

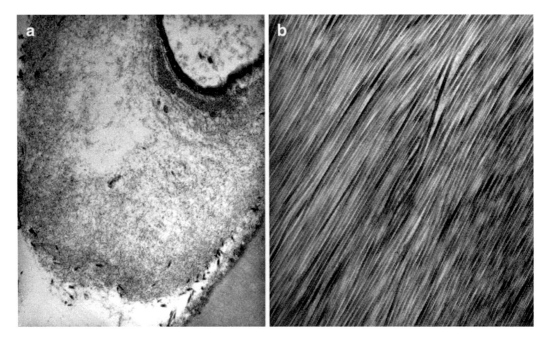

Fig. 22.2 (**a**) Abdominal fat aspirate. Amyloid fibrils surround a blood vessel (*in the upper right corner*). Uranyl acetate, lead citrate ×10,000. (**b**) Abdominal fat, surgical biopsy. Bundles of collagen fibers are seen showing the typical striated pattern. Uranyl acetate, lead citrate ×10,000

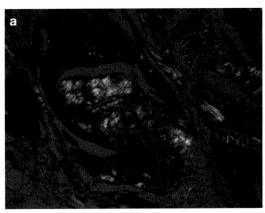 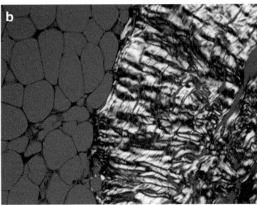

Fig. 22.3 (**a**) Abdominal fat, surgical biopsy. Amyloid deposits show *apple-green* birefringence and an absence of structure under polarized light. *Congo red* staining, ×20.

(**b**) Abdominal fat, surgical biopsy. Bundles of collagen fibers show *yellowish* birefringence and a coarse fascicular structure under polarized light. *Congo red* staining, ×20

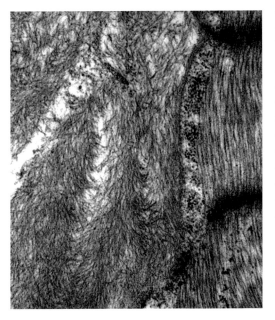

Fig. 22.4 Endomyocardial biopsy. *On the left*, amyloid fibrils are seen and *on the right*, part of the cytoplasm of a myocardial cell with myofibrils. Uranyl acetate, lead citrate ×35,000

Table 22.1 Processing of formalin-fixed paraffin-embedded tissues for conventional ultrastructural examination

Extract selected area (1–2 mm³) from paraffin block with a scalpel blade	
Xylene	2 h
Ethyl alcohol, absolute	20 min (minutes)
Ethyl alcohol 95 %	20 min
Ethyl alcohol 80 %	10 min
Ethyl alcohol 70 %	10 min
Ethyl alcohol 50 %	15 min
Ethyl alcohol 30 %	15 min
Cacodylate buffer 0.2 M, pH 7.3	10 min
OsO₄ 1 % in cacodylate buffer	1 h

Dehydration and resin embedding as usual

Electron and Immuno-Electron Microscopy

Techniques of Electron Microscopy

Samples for electron microscopy do not usually undergo routine formalin fixation and paraffin embedding, but formalin-fixed paraffin-embedded (FFPE) samples can be processed for ultrastructural examination and immuno-electron microscopy (Table 22.1), allowing the use of stored material for the characterization of amyloid proteins. Comparison of the paraffin block with a Congo red-stained slide can help to select the most relevant areas for ultrastructural study. Small portions of tissue are then extracted from the paraffin block, deparaffinized in xylene, rehydrated in a graded series of ethyl alcohols, washed in cacodylate buffer, post-fixed in osmium tetroxide, dehydrated, and embedded in epoxy resin as usual (see below).

The processing of fresh biopsy samples for electron microscopy is summarized in Table 22.2. A small sample size is important in order to obtain good fixation of the tissue. Thus, specimens greater

Table 22.2 Processing of fresh tissues for a conventional ultrastructural examination

Karnovsky solution 0.5 %[a]	4 h or longer at 4 °C
Cacodylate buffer 0.2 M pH 7.2–7.3	1 h or longer at 4 °C
Post-fixation in OsO_4 1 %	1 h at room temperature
Cacodylate buffer 0.2 M pH 7.2–7.3	10 min (minutes) or longer at room temperature
Ethyl alcohol 30 %	10 min at 4 °C
Ethyl alcohol 50 %	10 min at 4 °C
Ethyl alcohol 70 %	10 min at 4 °C
Ethyl alcohol 80 %	10 min at room temperature
Ethyl alcohol 95 %	20 min × 2 at room temperature
Ethyl alcohol, absolute	15 min × 3 at room temperature
Propylene oxide	30 min at room temperature
Propylene oxide-epoxy resin 1:1	1 h at room temperature
Propylene oxide-epoxy resin 1:3	Overnight at room temperature
Epoxy resin	48 h at 60 °C

[a]Modified Karnovsky solution: 0.5 % glutaraldehyde, 2 % paraformaldehyde in 0.2 M cacodylate buffer, pH 7.3

than 2–3 mm³ show poor morphology due to poor penetration of the fixing solution. The specimens are fixed by immersion in a modified Karnovsky solution [14] (see below), then washed in caco-dylate buffer, dehydrated through a graded series of ethyl alcohols, and embedded in epoxy resin (Table 22.2). After polymerization at 60 °C, ultrathin sections 600–800 Å (Angstrom) thick are cut with an ultramicrotome, stained with ura-nyl acetate and lead citrate (Reynolds' solution [15]), and observed with an electron microscope.

Principles of Immuno-Electron Microscopy

Immuno-electron microscopy can be applied to virtually every tissue, either specifically fixed for ultrastructural examination or previously formalin fixed and paraffin embedded. The only limitations include good tissue fixation and the availability of antibodies to the amyloid protein under test. Many protocols have been developed since the introduction of colloidal gold to ultrastructural immunohisto-chemistry. Immuno-electron microscopy, using antibody probes conjugated with gold particles, permits high-resolution detection and local-ization of antigens either within the cells, on their surface, or in the interstitium. The two techniques most widely used in transmission electron microscopy consist of either immu-nolabeling before the specimens are embedded in resin (preembedding immunogold label-ing) or immunolabeling after embedding in resin (postembedding immunogold labeling). Nonetheless, immunogold histochemistry has some general limitations, such as antigen pres-ervation and antibody specificity. Successful detection and localization depends on the antigen-recognition specificity of the primary antibodies for the investigated antigen, on the preservation of the antigenicity of the target proteins, and on the ability of the antibodies to bind to the antigens. Antigenicity is frequently lost during the dehydration and embedding procedures. Suppression of immunoreaction in resin-embedded tissues may be due to intra- and inter-cross-links within aldehyde-treated proteins and the destruction of secondary and tertiary protein structures during dehydration [16]. Specimens embedded in acrylic resins without osmium tetroxide fixation show poor preservation of membranes and low contrast of tissue components, thus making it difficult to correlate the immunostains with tissue details.

For all the above reasons, fixation is one of the most important aspects of sample preparation [17] for immuno-electron microscopy because it affects the strength of the immunoreaction and the preservation of fine cellular structures. In general, fixatives that provide good morphology cross-link macromolecules rapidly and tightly, forming a gel-like structure in the tissues, and, thus, directly modify epitopes and severely inhibit immunore-actions. Due to these undesirable effects, many kinds of fixatives, fixation conditions, and proce-dures have been employed to label each antigen. Although glutaraldehyde is an excellent fixative for the preservation of morphology, it severely inactivates the immunoreactivity of many antigens and, hence, a better fixative for immuno-electron microscopy is a mixture of paraformaldehyde and a low concentration of glutaraldehyde (modified Karnovsky's solution [7]).

Techniques of Immuno-Electron Microscopy

In our Pathology Unit of IRCCS Policlinico San Matteo/University of Pavia, electron microscopy is routinely used to confirm the diagnosis of amyloidosis. When ultrastructural examination demonstrates amyloid fibrils, immuno-electron microscopy is subsequently performed to identify the amyloidogenic protein. We use a postembedding method, i.e., immunostaining is performed on ultrathin sections on nickel grids, as summarized in Table 22.3.

Table 22.3 Postembedding immunogold on epoxy resin-embedded ultrathin sections

MWO[a] 350 W	3 min (minutes)[b]
or	
Trypsin 0.05 % in PBS[c]	15 min 37 °C[b]
PBS	10 min
NGS[d] 1:20 or egg albumin 1 % in PBS	15 min
Primary antibody	Overnight 4 °C
PBS-BSA[e] 1 %	5 min×2
Gold-conjugated secondary antibody	1 h
PBS-BSA 1 %	8 min
PBS	5 min×2
DW[e]	5 min×2

[a]Microwave oven
[b]Only for weak antigens/antibodies
[c]Phosphate buffer saline
[d]Normal goat serum
[e]Distilled water

Usually, for diagnostic purposes, a panel of four primary antibodies is sufficient. This panel covers the commonest forms of amyloidosis: AL (kappa and lambda), AA, and ATTR; in selected cases we also perform immunogold labeling with antibodies directed against apolipoprotein AI and beta-2-microglobulin. Fibrinogen and lysozyme have also been investigated in rare instances with negative results. We have never so far encountered rarer forms of kidney amyloidosis such as ALect2. Enzymatic predigestion with trypsin can be used in some cases to unmask antigenic epitopes modified by fixation-induced protein cross-links, as is commonly performed in light immunohistochemistry. The optimal conditions (antibody source and dilutions, type and duration of pretreatment) must be determined in each laboratory. Table 22.4 gives an example of the conditions used in our laboratory.

When immunogold reactions are examined with the electron microscope, colloidal gold particles decorate amyloid fibrils and allow the recognition of the amyloidogenic protein (Fig. 22.5).

Abdominal Fat

Tissues and organs containing amyloid deposits are fragile and at increased risk of bleeding. This, and the ready accessibility of alternative sites, discourages organ biopsy in patients in whom amyloidosis is suspected. In our experience at the Amyloidosis Research and Treatment Center of Pavia, fine-needle aspiration of abdominal fat and, secondarily, minor salivary gland biopsy represent the first and second preferred options, respectively,

Table 22.4 Antibodies and working conditions for characterization of amyloid

Primary antibody	Source	Dilution	Pretreatment	Secondary antibody
Polyclonal anti-kappa light chains	DAKO	1:100	0.05 % trypsin	GAR 15
Polyclonal anti-lambda light chains	DAKO	1:50	None	PA-GOLD 15
Monoclonal anti-amyloid A	DAKO	1:1	None	GAM 15
Polyclonal anti-transthyretin	DAKO	1:50	0.05 % trypsin	GAR 15
Polyclonal anti-apoA1	DAKO	1:100	None	PA-GOLD 15
Polyclonal anti-beta-2-microglobulin	DAKO	1:100	0.05 % trypsin	GAR 15

GAR goat anti-rabbit, *PA* protein A, *GAM* goat anti-mouse, *apoA1* apolipoprotein A1
The number 15 indicates the size of gold particles, i.e., 15 nm

in the diagnostic workup and serve as valid alternatives to a biopsy of the involved organ.

Table 22.5 shows results of the diagnostic performance of light and electron microscopy in abdominal fat aspirates from 745 consecutive patients suspected for systemic amyloidosis who were referred to the Amyloidosis Research and Treatment Center of Pavia between May 2003 and December 2010.

The apparent lower sensitivity of electron microscopy as compared to light microscopy examination of abdominal fat smears can be explained by the focal distribution of amyloid

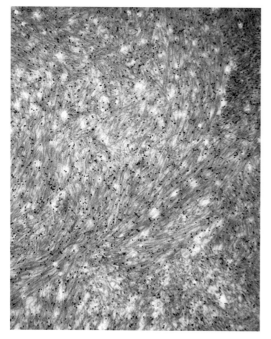

Fig. 22.5 Amyloid fibrils immunostained with a rabbit polyclonal antibody directed against kappa light chains are shown; the reporter system consists of goat anti-rabbit immunoglobulins conjugated with *gold particles* 15 nm in diameter. Uranyl acetate, lead citrate ×35,000

deposits in abdominal fat, which may not be present in the limited samples processed for electron microscopy. The lower specificity of light microscopy, on the other hand, with a relatively high rate of false-positive results, can be due to the technical limitations of Congo red staining (collagen fibers or blood showing nonspecific birefringence) as discussed earlier.

Out of 745 abdominal fat aspirates, amyloid was detected in 458 specimens. In 90 patients in whom abdominal fat did not show amyloid deposits, the diagnosis was subsequently established based on examination of a minor salivary gland or biopsy of the affected organ and amyloid protein was subsequently characterized by IEM and/or proteomics; in hereditary forms of amyloidosis, DNA analysis was performed to support the diagnosis of the amyloid type at the molecular level.

Immuno-electron microscopy was performed on all samples in which amyloid fibrils were observed. Characterization of the amyloid protein was achieved in all of the 458 samples, out of 745, in which amyloid deposits were identified ("positive samples"). Proteomics was also used to confirm the characterization in selected cases [18] (see next chapter on proteomics).

Figures 22.6, 22.7, 22.8, 22.9, 22.10, 22.11, and 22.12 show examples of abdominal fat aspirates that were positive for amyloid deposits, processed with the postembedding immunogold technique. Immunostaining is very specific and intense with the primary antibody directed against the amyloid fibril protein. Immunostained amyloid fibrils were located in the interstitium (Figs. 22.6, 22.8, 22.11, and 22.12), around blood vessels (Figs. 22.6 and 22.10), and along the basement membrane (Figs. 22.7, 22.9, and 22.10). Some amyloid deposits were very focal and small (Fig. 22.9). The focality of amyloid deposits con-

Table 22.5 Diagnostic performance of light and electron microscopy of abdominal fat aspirate in systemic amyloidosis

	Light microscopy % (CI 95 %)	Immuno-electron microscopy % (CI 95 %)	p-significance
Sensitivity	79 (74.7–82.7)	76.1 (71.7–80.1)	Not significant
Specificity	79.7 (74.4–84.2)	100 (98.4–100)	$p < 0.001$
Negative predictive value	71.6 (66.2–76.4)	74 (69.2–78.2)	Not significant
Positive predictive value	85.4 (81.4–88.7)	100 (98.4–100)	$p < 0.001$

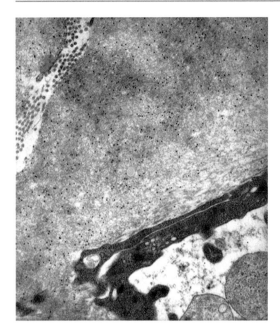

Fig. 22.6 Abdominal fat aspirate. Postembedding immu-nostaining with polyclonal anti-lambda light chain anti-body. In the *upper left corner*, *small circles* represent collagen fibers in cross section. On the *lower right*, a blood vessel is seen. Uranyl acetate, lead citrate ×17,000

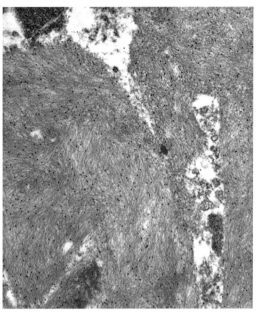

Fig. 22.8 Abdominal fat aspirate. Postembedding immu-nostaining with polyclonal anti-lambda light chain anti-body. Uranyl acetate, lead citrate ×17,000

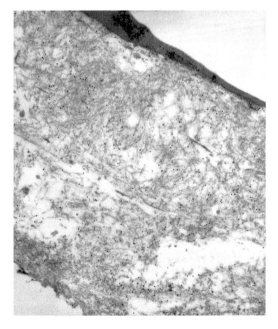

Fig. 22.7 Abdominal fat aspirate. Postembedding immu-nostaining with polyclonal anti-lambda light chain anti-body. Uranyl acetate, lead citrate ×17,000

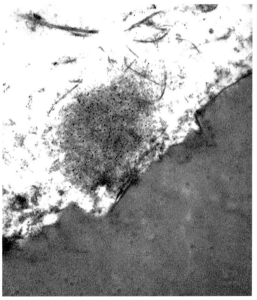

Fig. 22.9 Abdominal fat aspirate. A small, focal deposit of amyloid is seen near the adipocyte. The amyloid fibrils are reactive with polyclonal antibody directed against lambda light chains. Uranyl acetate, lead citrate ×13,000

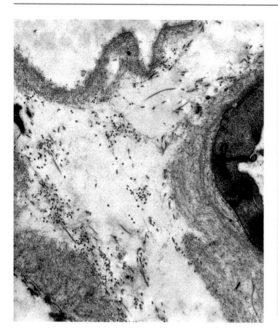

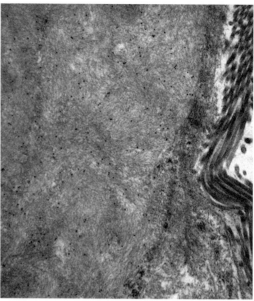

Fig. 22.10 Abdominal fat aspirate. Bundles of amyloid fibrils are seen along the cell membrane of adipocytes (*lower and upper left*) and the blood vessel (*on the right*). The fibrils are immunostained with a polyclonal anti-lambda light chain antibody. Uranyl acetate, lead citrate ×13,000

Fig. 22.12 Abdominal fat biopsy. Postembedding immunostaining with monoclonal anti-SAA antibody. *On the right*, bundles of collagen fibers. Uranyl acetate, lead citrate ×17,000

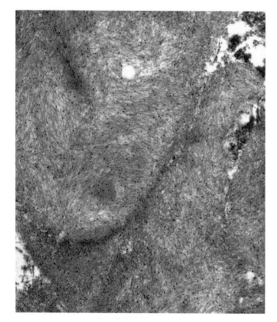

Fig. 22.11 Abdominal fat biopsy. Postembedding immunostaining with polyclonal anti-lambda light chain antibody. Uranyl acetate, lead citrate ×13,000

tributes to the limitations of the electron microscopy technique, since specimens are small in size and scarce deposits may, therefore, be missed. On the other hand, however, minute deposits of amyloid fibrils reacting with antibodies were readily identified by immuno-electron microscopy, allowing early diagnosis of the disease. However, in cases where more tissue is needed, a surgical abdominal fat biopsy that is more generous in size (Figs. 22.11 and 22.12) may be indicated.

Salivary Gland Biopsy

In patients with suspected systemic amyloidosis in whom abdominal fat aspirate is negative for amyloid deposits, a salivary gland biopsy may be subsequently performed; this approach may allow biopsy of the affected organ, such as the kidney or myocardium, to be avoided.

In our experience, the diagnostic sensitivity of light and electron microscopic examination of salivary gland biopsy in patients with negative fat aspirate was 58 %, the specificity of immuno-electron microscopy was 100 %, and the negative predictive value was 91 % [13].

Figures 22.13 and 22.14 show two minor salivary gland biopsies with amyloid fibrils immunostained with anti-lambda light chain and anti-SAA antibodies, respectively.

Clinically Affected Organ Biopsy

When both the abdominal fat and salivary gland biopsies do not show amyloid deposits but systemic amyloidosis is suspected, and in patients with localized amyloidosis, a biopsy of the affected organ or site is needed for diagnosis. In these cases too, electron microscopy and immuno-electron microscopy are of help in identifying amyloid deposits and typing amyloid proteins. Figures 22.15 and 22.16 show two kidney biopsies. Figure 22.15 shows amyloid fibrils

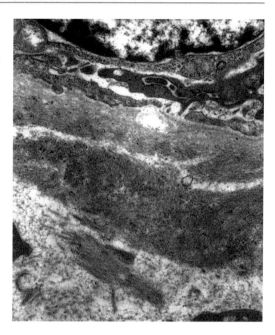

Fig. 22.14 Minor salivary gland biopsy. Amyloid fibrils immunostained with a monoclonal anti-SAA antibody. *At the top* a salivary gland cell is seen. Uranyl acetate, lead citrate ×17,000

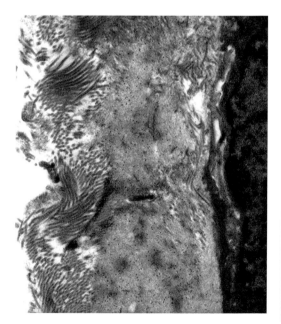

Fig. 22.13 Minor salivary gland biopsy. *On the left*, bundles of collagen fibers are seen. In the middle, amyloid fibrils are immunostained with an anti-lambda light chain polyclonal antibody. *On the right*, a salivary gland epithelial cell is seen. Uranyl acetate, lead citrate ×13,000

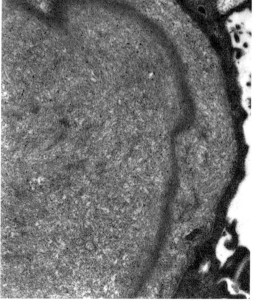

Fig. 22.15 Kidney biopsy. Postembedding immunostaining with a monoclonal antibody directed against SAA. Uranyl acetate, lead citrate ×17,000

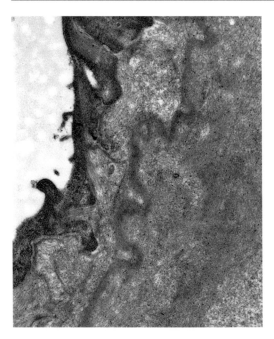

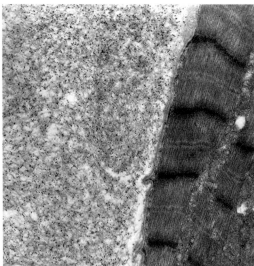

Fig. 22.17 Endomyocardial biopsy, postembedding immunostaining with a polyclonal antibody directed against transthyretin. Uranyl acetate, lead citrate ×12,000

Fig. 22.16 Kidney biopsy. Postembedding immunostaining with a monoclonal antibody directed against SAA. Notice bundles of amyloid fibrils "pushing" the inner surface of a glomerular epithelial cell. Uranyl acetate, lead citrate ×13,000

diffusely infiltrating the subepithelial aspect of the glomerulus in a patient with AA amyloidosis. The basement membrane itself is traversed by the amyloid fibrils, which form bundles "pushing" toward the epithelial cells; there is also effacement of the epithelial cell foot processes.

Cardiac amyloidosis sometimes represents a diagnostic challenge, especially in elderly patients with isolated heart involvement and a monoclonal gammopathy. In these cases, it is very important to differentiate senile cardiac amyloidosis due to the deposition of wild-type transthyretin, hereditary TTR, or AL cardiac amyloidosis. Figure 22.17 shows an endomyocardial biopsy from a patient with TTR heart amyloidosis. In some clinically ambiguous cases, it is possible to address the diagnosis by means of noninvasive imaging techniques such as scintigraphy [19, 20]. Nevertheless, an endomyocardial biopsy is needed for a definite diagnosis [21]. In our experience, we have never observed with immunogold staining the coexistence of two

amyloid types, as recently reported by Blood (Nov. 2014) in heart tissue.

Localized forms of amyloidosis can also be diagnosed and typed with immuno-electron microscopy. Figure 22.18 shows an example of cutaneous amyloidosis with heavy deposition of fibrils immunoreactive with a polyclonal antibody directed against kappa light chains.

Immuno-electron microscopy can also help to distinguish between amyloidosis and light chain deposition disease (LCDD). The non-fibrillary deposits of light chains are immunodecorated by antibodies (Fig. 22.19) and are easily distinguished from fibrillar depositions of amyloid (Fig. 22.20) which are immunostained with isotypic antibodies.

Conclusions

Amyloid detection and typing is vital for correct patient management, and the specific challenges of this task often require specialized resources. In our experience, electron microscopy represents a sensitive tool for the identification of amyloid fibrils in various tissues, and immuno-electron microscopy can correctly characterize the amyloid

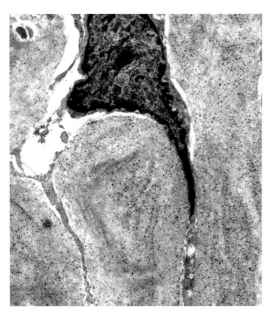

Fig. 22.18 Skin biopsy. Postembedding immunostaining with a polyclonal antibody directed against kappa light chains. Uranyl acetate, lead citrate ×10,000

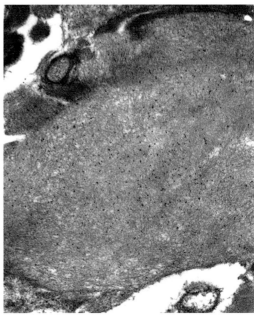

Fig. 22.20 Lung biopsy, amyloidosis. Amyloid fibrils immunostained with a polyclonal antibody directed against lambda light chains. Uranyl acetate, lead citrate ×17,000

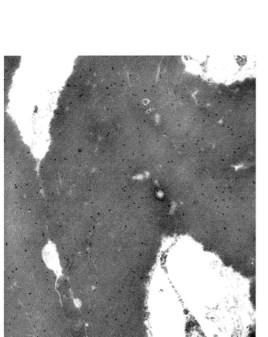

Fig. 22.19 Lung biopsy, LCDD. Amorphous material immunostained with a polyclonal antibody directed against lambda light chains. Uranyl acetate, lead citrate ×17,000

protein in most cases. Immuno-electron microscopy is sparsely employed worldwide for the diagnosis and typing of amyloidosis, despite the fact that almost every Pathology Unit, at least in major institutions, is equipped with an electron microscopy laboratory. The processing of specimens is not particularly complex, neither is it too time-consuming. Moreover, commercially available antibodies can be used for immuno-electron microscopy staining of the most common forms of amyloid proteins, and the limited amount needed for each reaction (a few microliters) contributes to cost containment. In our Pathology Unit, unsatisfactory experiences with light microscopic immunohistochemistry, mostly because of the ambiguous results obtained in paraffin-embedded samples, led us to discontinue this diagnostic test. Currently, when we receive paraffin blocks for consultation from other institutions, we review Congo red-stained slides in order to select tissue areas for amyloid typing by immuno-electron microscopy. In our experience, false-positive referral cases are mostly due to the misinterpretation of collagen fibers in Congo red stains performed by less experienced centers, especially with regard to abdominal fat samples. Major pitfalls in amyloid typing, as evidenced by immuno-electron microscopy, consist of ATTR misdiagnosed as AL by light immunohistochemistry, as reported also by Cowan et al. [18], or suspected AA cases that turn out to be AL or AApoAI.

References

1. Picken MM. Amyloidosis—where are we now and where are we heading? Arch Pathol Lab Med. 2010;134:545–51.
2. Casanova S, Donini U, Zucchelli P, Mazzucco G, Monga G, Linke RP. Immunohistochemical distinction between amyloidosis and fibrillar glomerulopathy. Am J Clin Pathol. 1992;97:787–95.
3. Arbustini E, Morbini P, Verga L, Concardi M, Porcu E, Pilotto A, Zorzoli I, Garini P, Anesi E, Merlini G. Light and electron microscopy immunohistochemical characterization of amyloid deposits. Amyloid: Int J Exp Clin Invest. 1997;4:157–70.
4. Sipe JD, Benson MD, Buxbaum JN, Ikeda S, Merlini G, Saraiva M, Westermark P. Amyloid fibril protein nomenclature committee of the International Society of Amyloidosis. Amyloid. 2010;17:101–4.
5. Bandini S, Bergesio F, Conti P, Mancini G, Cerretini C, Cirami C, Rosati A, Caselli GM, Arbustini E, Merlini G, Ficarra G, Salvadori M. Nodular macroglossia with combined light chain and beta-2 microglobulin deposition in a long-term dialysis patient. J Nephrol. 2001;14:128–31.
6. Merlini G, Bellotti V. Molecular mechanisms of amyloidosis. N Engl J Med. 2002;349:583–96.
7. Arbustini E, Verga L, Concardi M, Palladini G, Obici L, Merlini G. Electron and immuno-electron microscopy of abdominal fat identifies and characterizes amyloid fibrils in suspected cardiac amyloidosis. Amyloid. 2002;9:108–14.
8. Lachmann HJ, Booth DR, Booth SE, Bybee A, Gilbertson JA, Gillmore JD, Pepys MB, Hawkins PN. Misdiagnosis of hereditary amyloidosis as AL (primary) amyloidosis. N Engl J Med. 2002;346:1786–91.
9. Palladini G, Obici L, Merlini G. Hereditary amyloidosis. N Engl J Med. 2002;347:1206.
10. Satoskar AA, Burdge K, Cowden DJ, Nadasdy GM, Hebert LA, Nadasdy T. Typing of amyloidosis in renal biopsies: diagnostic pitfalls. Arch Pathol Lab Med. 2007;131:917–22.
11. Solomon A, Murphy CL, Westermark P. Unreliability of immunohistochemistry for typing amyloid deposits. Arch Pathol Lab Med. 2008;132:14.
12. Palladini G, Verga L, Corona S, Obici L, Morbini P, Lavatelli F, Donadei S, Sarais G, Roggeri L, Foli A, Russo P, Zenone Bragotti L, Paulli M, Magrini U, Merlini G. Diagnostic performance of immuno-electron microscopy of abdominal fat in systemic amyloidoses. Amyloid. 2010;17:59–60.
13. Foli A, Palladini G, Caporali R, Verga L, Morbini P, Obici L, Russo P, Sarais G, Donadei S, Montecucco C, Merlini G. Role of minor salivary gland biopsy in the diagnosis of systemic amyloidosis: results of a prospective study in 62 patients. Amyloid. 2011;18(S1):80–2.
14. Karnovsky MJ. A formaldehyde-glutaraldehyde fixative of high osmolarity for use in electron microscopy. J Cell Biol. 1965;27:137A.
15. Reynolds ES. The use of lead citrate at high pH as an electron-opaque stain in electron microscopy. J Cell Biol. 1963;17:208–12.
16. Roth J, Bendayan M, Orci L. Ultrastructural localization of intracellular antigens by the use of protein A-gold complex. J Histochem Cytochem. 1978;26:1074–81.
17. Perkins EM, McCaffery JM. Conventional and immunoelectron microscopy of mitochondria. Methods Mol Biol. 2007;372:467–83.
18. Cowan AJ, Skinner M, Berk JL, Sloan JM, O'hara C, Seldin DC, Sanchorawala V. Macroglossia—not always AL amyloidosis. Amyloid. 2011;18:83–6.
19. Rapezzi C, Quarta CC, Guidalotti PL, Pettinato C, Fanti S, Leone O, Ferlini A, Longhi S, Lorenzini M, Reggiani LB, Gagliardi C, Gallo P, Villani C, Salvi F. Role of (99m)Tc-DPD scintigraphy in diagnosis and prognosis of hereditary transthyretin-related cardiac amyloidosis. JACC Cardiovasc Imaging. 2011;4(6):659–70.
20. Quarta CC, Obici L, Guidalotti PL, Pieroni M, Longhi S, Perlini S, Verga L, Merlini G, Rapezzi C. High 99mTc-DPD myocardial uptake in a patient with apolipoprotein AI-related amyloidotic cardiomyopathy. Amyloid. 2013;20(1):48–51.
21. Briani C, Cavallaro T, Ferrari S, Taioli F, Calamelli S, Verga L, Adami F, Fabrizi GM. Sporadic transthyretin amyloidosis with a novel TTR gene mutation misdiagnosed as primary amyloidosis. J Neurol. 2012;259(10):2226–8.

Classification of Amyloidosis by Mass Spectrometry-Based Proteomics

23

Ahmet Dogan

Over 30 different proteins have been shown to cause amyloidosis [1]. Most important amyloid types that cause morbidity and mortality are systemic in nature and include SAA (so-called secondary or AA-type), TTR (so-called ATTR, senile, or hereditary) and immunoglobulin kappa (IGK) or lambda light chains (IGL) (so-called primary or AL-type) [2]. These four proteins account for over 85 % of systemic amyloidosis. The current management of amyloidosis relies on treatment of the underlying etiology often by high risk-aggressive treatment modalities such as high dose chemotherapy and peripheral blood autologous stem cell transplantation (for AL-type amyloidosis) [3] or liver transplantation (for hereditary TTR-type amyloidosis) [4, 5]. Given the critical nature of these management decisions, accurate subtyping of amyloid deposits in routine clinical biopsy specimens is of paramount importance.

In routine practice, the diagnosis of amyloidosis is made at the tissue level by histological examination and special histochemical stains such as Congo red which, due to physical structure of the amyloid, gives anomalous colors under polarized light [6]. Further subtyping is often challenging as immunohistochemistry, the most common method used, is problematic because of high background staining due to serum contamination, epitope loss due to the protein cross-linking after formalin fixation, and lack of specific antibody reagents that can detect all different amyloid types [7–9]. Although more sophisticated analytical tools such as high performance liquid chromatography (LC) and/or mass spectrometry (MS) has been used to type amyloid deposits, these often require quantities of tissue not readily available in routine clinical setting and suffer from lack of specificity as they contain nonamyloid tissues and serum, which is a rich source of amyloidogenic proteins [10–12]. To address these difficulties, methods combining specific sampling by laser microdissection (LMD) and analytical power of nano-flow liquid chromatography (LC tandem MS (MS/MS)-based proteomics have been developed [13, 14]. LMD- and LC–MS/MS-based proteomic assays are not dependent on antibodies or a predetermined knowledge of the patient's amyloid subtype, and could analyze small amounts of amyloid that could be obtained from routine paraffin embedded clinical biopsy specimens.

Laser Microdissection

LMD technology offers the ability to analyze selected microanatomical compartments of tissue for molecular or proteomic analysis. There are a

A. Dogan, MD, PhD (✉)
Departments of Pathology and Laboratory Medicine, Memorial Sloan Kettering Cancer Center, 1275 York Avenue, New York, NY 10065, USA
e-mail: dogana@mskcc.org

© Springer International Publishing Switzerland 2015
M.M. Picken et al. (eds.), *Amyloid and Related Disorders*, Current Clinical Pathology,
DOI 10.1007/978-3-319-19294-9_23

number of different technologies available. All current LMD technologies rely on examination of a frozen or paraffin section of the representative tissue under a specially modified microscope, selection of microscopic area of interest, removal of this area by laser dissection from the section into a tube or a tube cap for further analysis. The process requires specialized slides that could be manipulated by the energy provided by the laser beam. Often, the sections are deparaffinized and stained by conventional histochemical or immunohistochemical methods. Some LMD technologies place the sections on slides covered by a membrane, and the laser is used to cut the membrane with the tissue. Others use slides coated with heat/energy-sensitive film that is released from the glass surface with the tissue when hit by the laser beam. Once the tissue is microdissected, the fragments are collected into a tube by a variety of approaches including simple gravitational fall or sticky membranes. In the context of amyloidosis, LMD offers the possibility of acquiring pure amyloid plaques with minimal background tissue for downstream analysis by proteomic methods.

High-Performance Liquid Chromatography (LC) Tandem Mass Spectrometry (MS/MS)-Based Proteomics

In the last 10 years, LC–MS/MS-based proteomic analysis has revolutionized the way proteins could be analyzed and detected. LC–MS/MS has become the preferred methodology for identifying the proteome in cell and tissue samples, gels, and immunoprecipitates. There are two basic approaches to LC–MS/MS-based proteomics: (1) shotgun proteomics, which aims to identify all proteins in a complex mixture; (2) targeted proteomics, which tries to identify specific proteins in a complex mixture. Merits and disadvantages of these two approaches are summarized in Table 23.1. Both approaches require processing of the tissue samples to extract the protein content, and digestion of the proteins to peptide fragments that could be detected by LC–

MS/MS. In fresh or frozen samples, this requires the use of conventional methods of protein extraction. In formalin-fixed paraffin-embedded (FFPE) tissues, special methods to release the proteins are necessary as the proteins are chemically cross-linked by formalin and are not readily soluble by detergents. To overcome this difficulty, a number of methods to break the cross-linkages have been developed. The most widely available methodology uses an approach similar to heat-mediated antigen retrieval as applied in immunohistochemistry [15, 16]. Using such approaches, investigators have shown that protein yields obtained from FFPE are comparable to the yields obtained from fresh/frozen cells or tissues [17, 18].

Once the protein is extracted, it is necessary to cut the protein into peptides as most LC–MS/MS technologies are best suited for measuring peptide fragments 5–25 amino acids long. There are a numerous proteases that can digest proteins into peptides. In proteomic studies, the most commonly used protease is trypsin which cleaves the proteins at lysine and arginine residues. When a protein sample is treated with trypsin, a peptide complex composed of peptides flanked by either a lysine or an arginine residue is generated (Table 23.2). The peptide complex generated by trypsin digestion is then separated by LC. The most commonly used LC approaches use solvent gradients to separate and resolve the peptides based on hydrophobic characteristics. In this way, peptides with similar chemical characteristics move together and are sprayed into the MS for mass detection. MS could only

Table 23.1 Comparison of shotgun and targeted proteomics methodologies

Shotgun proteomics	Targeted proteomics
Tries to identify every protein in a mixture	Tries to identify specific protein targets
Analogous to gene expression profiling	Analogous to RTPCR or immunoassays
Semiquantitative	Quantitative
Discovery tool	Clinical tool
Complex, slow, and expensive	Simple, fast, and cheap

Table 23.2 Predicted tryptic peptides of transthyretin at positions 21–147

Mass	Position	Peptide sequence
833.3999	21–29	GPTGTGESK
690.3677	30–35	CPLMVK
672.4039	36–41	VLDAVR
1366.7589	42–54	GSPAINVAVHVFR
1394.6222	56–68	AADDTWEPFASGK
2455.1510	69–90	TSESGELHGLTTEEEFVEGI YK
704.3825	91–96	VEIDTK
583.2875	97–100	SYWK
2451.2051	101–123	ALGISPFHEHAEVVFTANDSGPR
2360.2384	125–146	YTIAALLSPYSYSTTAVVTN PK

measure the mass of a peptide, if the peptide carries an ionic charge. As most native peptides are charge neutral, ionization of the peptides is required before they are loaded to MS. For peptides in solution as described here, this is achieved by electrospray ionization (ESI). After separation by LC, the solution containing the peptides is forced through a very fine needle exposed to high voltage which leads to the removal of the solvent carrying the peptides and ionization of the peptides. The ionized peptides are sprayed into the MS. In tandem MS/MS analysis, the first MS measures the mass to charge (m/z) ratio of the parent peptide. Then, peptides selected based on predetermined criteria are directed to a collusion cell where the peptides are fragmented upon collusion with an inert gas such as helium. This process is called collusion-induced dissociation (CID). The fragments formed by the CID are measured in the second MS. Each peptide present in the human proteome has a unique CID pattern which makes it possible to predict the amino acid sequence of the peptide being analyzed by MS/MS. A number of complex computational algorithms have been developed to predict the amino acid sequences. The algorithms compare the observed fragmentation pattern of each peptide to the theoretical fragmentation pattern of all human tryptic peptides predicted by the reference human genome, and assign a probability score for individual peptide as well as a protein probability score for identification of a given protein often based on multiple peptides derived from that

protein [19]. Although this is essentially a computational process, and not true sequencing of a protein, the MS instruments have such a high precision and computational methods have become so sophisticated that the results are extremely accurate and reproducible. The work flow for LC–MS/MS-based proteomic analysis is summarized in Fig. 23.1.

The MS-based proteomic analysis has a number of limitations. A given protein can only be identified if peptide fragments with appropriate size for MS can be generated after enzymatic digestion. For example, a number of human proteins contain large areas lacking trypsin cutting residues lysine or arginine; therefore, no peptides suitable for LC–MS/MS detection can be generated. In shotgun proteomic approaches, it may be difficult to detect low abundance proteins/peptides as signals from these peptides may be buried among massive amount of information obtained from more abundant proteins, and MS simply may not be able to scan them. The other important limitation of MS-based proteomics is the reliance of computational predictive algorithms to a reference human genome obtained from publicly available databases such as Swissprot. The algorithms could only match the observed peptide fragmentation data to the protein sequences available in the public databases. Therefore, germline polymorphisms or somatic mutations that are not represented in public databases cannot be identified despite MS data from these peptides would have been captured.

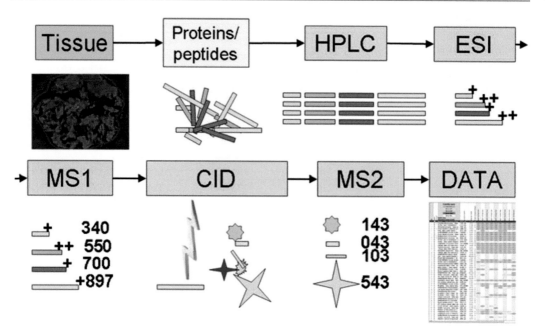

Fig. 23.1 Work flow for LC–MS/MS-based proteomic classification of amyloidosis in FFPE clinical biopsy specimens. Amyloid plaques are laser microdissected (LMD) from *Congo red*-stained section visualized under fluorescent light. The proteins are extracted and digested into peptides with trypsin. The peptides are separated by high-performance liquid chromatography (HPLC), ionized by electron spray ionization, and sprayed into first MS. MS1 measures the parent mass of the peptide and selects the peptides for collusion-induced dissociation (CID). Upon collusion with a neutral gas, the peptides are fragmented and the size of each fragment derived from the parent peptide mass is measured by MS2. These measurements are used to predict the peptide amino acid sequence, and the data are presented as a list ranked according to the relative abundance of each protein identified

Classification of Amyloidosis by LC–MS/MS-Based Proteomics

Biochemical composition of amyloid plaques are complex and contain, in addition to causative protein, other proteins such as serum amyloid P component that stabilizes the amyloid plaques, other abundant serum proteins such as albumin, and complex carbohydrate groups. Despite the complexity, the amyloid plaque's most abundant component is the causative protein. This makes amyloid an ideal matrix for LC–MS/MS-based proteomic diagnostics as the most abundant proteins would dominate the analysis. When combined with specific microdissection of amyloid plaques to reduce the background signal from the tissue of interest, LC–MS/MS provides very powerful tool for identification causative proteins of amyloidosis. Such LC–MS/MS-based

approaches have been initially used in research studies in amyloidosis [13] but more recently, the technology has been validated for clinical use on FFPE clinical biopsy specimens [14] and fresh fat aspirate specimens [20, 21]. The first clinical validation study on FFPE has shown 100 % specificity and sensitivity in a retrospective analysis of 50 cases diagnosed according to previous clinicopathological gold standards. In prospective validation studies, LC–MS/MS method was able to detect amyloid type in 98 % of the cases [14].

When applied to FFPE specimens, LC–MS/MS method requires microdissection of the amyloid plaque (Figs. 23.2a, 23.3a, and 23.4a). The FFPE tissue sections are stained with Congo red and the amyloid deposits are identified under fluorescent light with their characteristic reflective qualities and microdissected by laser. The sensitivity of current LC–MS/MS means

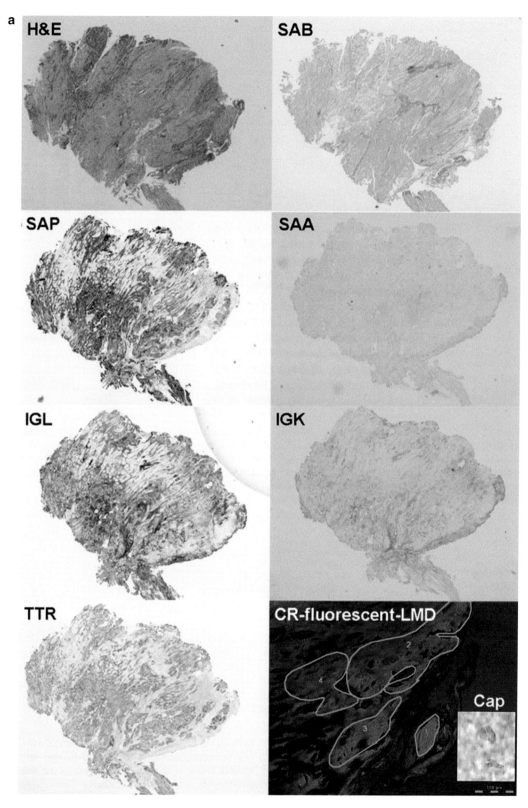

Fig. 23.2 FFPE cardiac biopsy specimen involved by ATTR (transthyretin) amyloidosis classified by LC–MS/MS-based proteomic analysis. (**a**) Hematoxylin and eosin (H&E) and sulfated alcian blue (SAB)-stained sections show interstitial amyloid deposition in the myocardium. By immunohistochemistry, the amyloid deposits are positive for serum amyloid P—component (SAP) but negative for serum amyloid A protein (SAA) and immunoglobulin

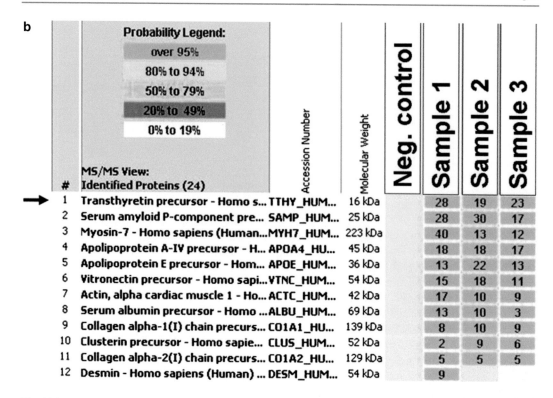

Fig. 23.2 (continued) kappa light chain (ALK). However, amyloid is positive for both immunoglobulin lambda light chain (ALL) and transthyretin (TTR). Congo red (CR)-stained section show bright fluorescence under fluorescent light source. Areas selected for laser microdissection (LMD) are highlighted by *yellow lines*. The inset shows the LMD fragment collected into the cap for proteomic analysis. (**b**) LC–MS/MS-based proteomic analysis shows that the main component of the amyloid plaque is TTR (*arrow*). No evidence IGL deposition is identified, suggesting that immunohistochemistry reactivity for IGL was nonspecific

Fig. 23.3 An FFPE renal biopsy specimen involved by AL (lambda) amyloidosis classified by LC–MS/MS-based proteomic analysis. (**a**) Congo red (CR)-stained section under bright field, polarized, and fluorescent light source is shown. A single glomerulus selected for microdissection is labeled by *blue line*. The glomerulus could be identified in the cap after LMD. The inset shows higher magnification of the glomerulus captured for proteomic analysis. (**b**) LC–MS/MS-based proteomic analysis identifies immunoglobulin lambda light chain constant and variable region as the main components of the amyloid plaque consistent (*arrows*). Other proteins represent serum proteins such as Apolipoprotein E (APOE) that are frequently incorporated into the amyloid plaques and stromal components of the glomerulus

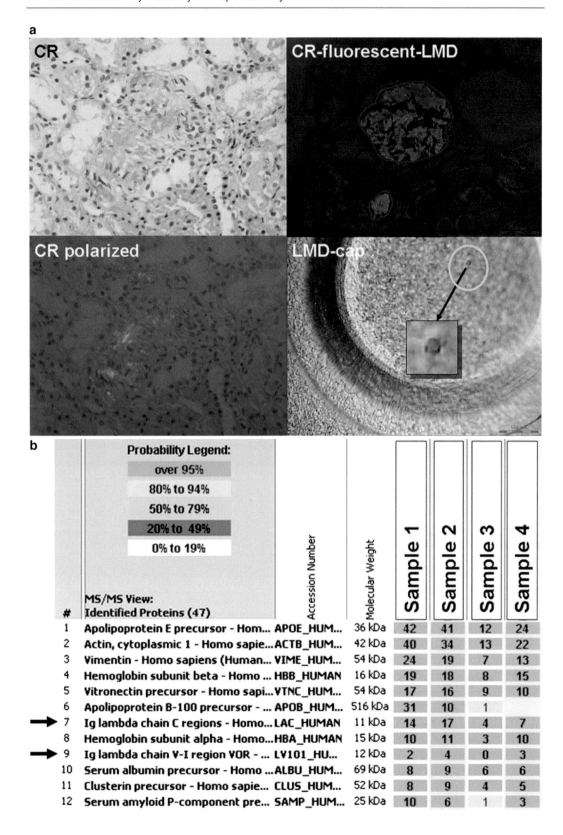

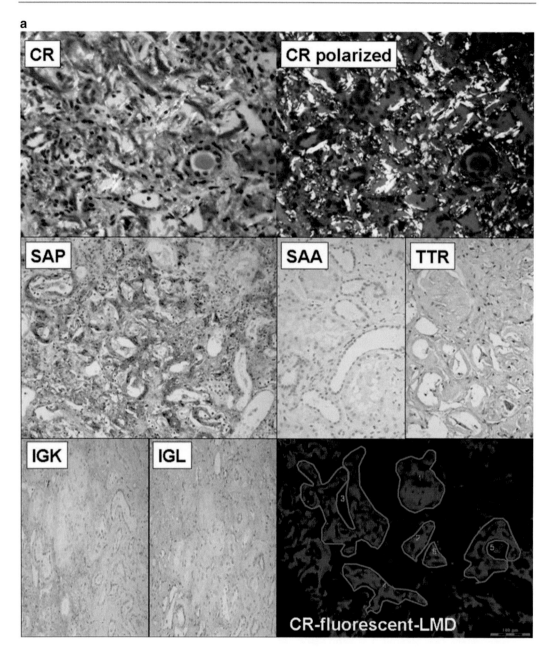

Fig. 23.4 An FFPE renal biopsy specimen involved by ALECT2 (leukocyte cell-derived chemotaxin-2) amyloidosis classified by LC–MS/MS-based proteomic analysis. (**a**) Congo red (CR)-stained section shows striking amyloid deposition in the renal medulla under bright field and polarized light source. By immunohistochemistry, the amyloid deposits are positive for serum amyloid P—component (SAP) but negative for serum amyloid A protein (SAA), transthyretin (TTR), immunoglobulin kappa light chain (ALK), and immunoglobulin lambda light chain (ALL). Amyloid deposits show bright fluorescence under fluorescent light source. Areas selected for laser microdissection (LMD) are highlighted by *blue lines*. (**b**) LC–MS/MS-based proteomic analysis identifies leukocyte cell-derived chemotaxin-2 (LECT2) as the main component of the amyloid plaque (*arrow*). Other proteins represent serum proteins such as Apolipoprotein E (APOE) and SAP that are frequently incorporated into the amyloid plaques and stromal components of the renal medulla

b

Probability Legend:

over 95%

80% to 94%

50% to 79%

20% to 49%

0% to 19%

MS/MS View:

# Identified Proteins (24)	Accession Number	Molecular Weight	Neg. control	Sample 1	Sample 2	Sample 3
1 Vitronectin precursor - Homo sapi...VTNC_HUM...		54 kDa		33	19	32
2 Hemoglobin subunit beta - Homo ... HBB_HUMAN		16 kDa		27	15	13
3 Actin, cytoplasmic 1 - Homo sapie...ACTB_HUM...		42 kDa		17	8	22
4 Apolipoprotein E precursor - Hom... APOE_HUM...		36 kDa		10	7	13
➡ 5 Leukocyte cell-derived chemotax...LECT2_HUM...		16 kDa		10	6	11
6 Hemoglobin subunit alpha - Homo...HBA_HUMAN		15 kDa		11	7	10
7 Serum amyloid P-component pre... SAMP_HUM...		25 kDa		18	7	7
8 Serum albumin precursor - Homo ...ALBU_HUM...		69 kDa		8	1	15
9 Collagen alpha-2(I) chain precurs... CO1A2_HU...		129 kDa		10	5	8
10 Collagen alpha-1(I) chain precurs... CO1A1_HU...		139 kDa		8	4	7
11 Clusterin precursor - Homo sapie... CLUS_HUM...		52 kDa		7	3	3
12 Complement factor H-related pro... FHR1_HUM...		38 kDa		4	2	2
13 Actin, alpha cardiac muscle 1 - Ho... ACTC_HUM...		42 kDa		4	1	4
14 Vimentin - Homo sapiens (Human... VIME_HUM...		54 kDa		4		7
15 Complement C3 precursor [Contai...CO3_HUMAN		187 kDa		1		0

Fig. 23.4 (continued)

that an amyloid plaque area equivalent to single glomeruli is sufficient to obtain diagnostic information in a single LC–MS/MS run (Figs. 23.2a, 23.3a, and 23.4a). The tissue fragments are processed and digested to peptides as previously described. The peptide solution is separated by LC, ionized by ESI, and sprayed into the MS instrument for analysis. The raw MS data are searched using three different algorithms (Mascot, Sequest, and X!Tandem) and the results are assigned peptide and protein probability scores. The results were then combined and displayed using a display program called Scaffold (Proteome Software, Portland, OR, USA). The display program provides a list of protein identified from the amyloid plaque using relative abundance determined by spectral counts for each protein identified. For clinical precision, three to four different microdissections are run per

case. The most abundant amyloidogenic protein identified in all samples is considered to be the causative protein (Figs. 23.2b, 23.3b, and 23.4b). The method has been successfully used to diagnose amyloidosis in a variety of tissues including heart, kidney, skin, gastrointestinal tract, liver, brain, peripheral nerve, bone marrow, upper respiratory tract, urinary tract, prostate, soft tissues, and decalcified bone marrow specimens [13, 14, 22]. It has been possible to identify virtually all known causes for amyloidosis including amyloidosis caused by immunoglobulin heavy (AH) [22] and light chains (AL) [14] (Fig. 23.3), serum amyloid-associated protein (SAA) [14], transthyretin (both hereditary and senile ATTR) [14, 23, 24] (Fig. 23.2), leukocyte derived chemotaxin-2 (LECT2) [23] (Fig. 23.4), fibrinogen alpha [25], lysozyme [26], gelsolin [24], apolipoprotein A1 [27], Apolipoprotein A2, insulin [28], beta-2-microglobulin [29], prolactin, calcitonin, semenogelin, and atrial natriuretic peptide. In addition, it has been possible to identify variant proteins causing hereditary amyloidosis in amyloid by developing specially curated protein databases containing all pathogenic mutations [24, 27].

Abdominal subcutaneous fat aspiration is one of the most practical, sensitive, and specific methods for the diagnosis of systemic amyloidosis. One limitation of this method has remained the technical difficulties in further subtyping in a clinical setting. To overcome this difficulty, LC–MS/MS-based proteomic approaches similar to those described for FFPE biopsy specimens have been developed [20, 21] (Fig. 23.5). Such methods have similar specificity (98 % specificity) but marginal lower sensitivity (87 % sensitivity). The lower sensitivity observed compared to FFPE biopsy specimens most likely reflect sampling differences between two approaches. In FFPE biopsy specimen, every sample studied contains the microdissected amyloid plaque. In contrast, in fat aspirate specimens, one half of the specimen is stained with Congo red for diagnosis and other half is analyzed by LC–MS/MS without prior microdissection. It is likely that in a subset of the cases, the half used for microdissection may not contain sufficient amyloid for identification. Nevertheless, the method is rapid and readily applicable in a clinical setting and has greatly improved screening and management of amyloidosis patients (Fig. 23.6).

Conclusions

The developments in LMD- and LC–MS/MS-based proteomic technologies have created unprecedented opportunities for identification of proteins in routine clinical biopsy specimens. The application of the technology to classification of amyloidosis has resulted in the first clinical

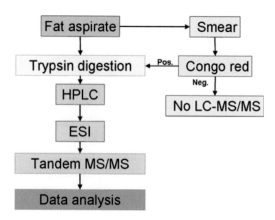

Fig. 23.5 Work flow for LC–MS/MS-based proteomic classification of amyloidosis in fresh fat aspirate specimens. The fat aspirate is obtained and separated into two halves. One half is stained with Congo red. If amyloid is detected, the second half will be processed for LC–MS/MS-based proteomic analysis as described in Fig. 23.1

application of shotgun proteomics. In the context of amyloid classification, LMD- and LC–MS/MS-based proteomics offer many advantages over immunoassay-based methods and clinical surrogates. The method is readily applicable to FFPE or fresh/frozen routine clinical biopsy specimens and requires very little tissue (often, a single section and an area equivalent to a single glomerulus are sufficient). Unlike immunoassays, which require good reagents for each target, LC–MS/MS can detect all amyloidogenic proteins in a single analysis. Although the initial layout for LC–MS/MS-based technology is considerably higher, the reagent costs per case is minimal compared to immunoassay-based technologies, and in the long run, LC–MS/MS is cheaper to perform on a case to case basis. Given these analytical and operational advantages, and the far superior specificity and sensitivity offered by LMD- and LC–MS/MS-based methods, LMD- and LC–MS/MS-based analysis is now considered the gold standard for classification of amyloidosis.

Probability Legend:
- over 95%
- 80% to 94%
- 50% to 79%
- 20% to 49%
- 0% to 19%

Bio View:

#	Identified Proteins (252)	Accession Number	Molecular Weight	AL-K Patient S1	AL-K Patient S2	AL-L Patient S1	AL-L Patient S2	AA Patient S1	AA Patient S2	ATTR Patient S1	ATTR Patient S2	ALys Patient S1	ALys Patient S2
1	Apolipoprotein E OS=Homo sapi...	APOE_HU...	36 kDa	47	48	72	65	9	6	36	28	29	24
2	Apolipoprotein A-IV OS=Homo s...	APOA4_H...	45 kDa			85	50			47	39	32	20
3	Ig lambda chain C regions OS=H...	LAC_HUMAN	11 kDa			99	80						
4	Ig kappa chain C region OS=Ho...	IGKC_HUM...	12 kDa	66	65								
5	Transthyretin OS=Homo sapiens...	TTHY_HU...	16 kDa							65	50		
6	Lysozyme C OS=Homo sapiens ...	LYSC_HUM...	17 kDa									57	46
7	Apolipoprotein A-I OS=Homo sa...	APOA1_H...	31 kDa			36	30	3	10	12	11	3	
8	Serum amyloid P-component OS...	SAMP_HU...	25 kDa	18	21	9	5					2	
9	Serum amyloid A protein OS=Ho...	SAA_HUMAN	14 kDa					20	20				
10	Ig kappa chain V-III region NG9...	KV303_HU...	11 kDa	10	10								
11	Collagen alpha-3(VI) chain OS=...	CO6A3_H...	344 kDa	83	178	61	58	53	33	163	207	158	165
12	Vimentin OS=Homo sapiens GN=...	VIME_HUM...	54 kDa	66	94	73	73	116	61	99	85	128	141
13	Annexin A2 OS=Homo sapiens G...	ANXA2_H...	39 kDa	34	34	54	46	112	44	114	133	61	60
14	Perilipin-1 OS=Homo sapiens GN...	PLIN1_HU...	56 kDa	41	60	28	39	78	58	101	86	94	88
15	Basement membrane-specific he...	PGBM_HU...	469 kDa	30	157	27	41			37	37	139	128
16	Protein KIAA1881 OS=Homo sap...	K1881_HU...	134 kDa	29	52	14	14	45	47	91	90	89	95
17	Actin, cytoplasmic 1 OS=Homo s...	ACTB_HU...	42 kDa	36	44	55	45	89	49	51	53	69	55
18	Membrane primary amine oxidas...	AOC3_HU...	85 kDa	29	38	33	34	57	46	66	79	62	62
19	Collagen alpha-1(VI) chain OS=...	CO6A1_H...	109 kDa	40	69	23	32	18	15	70	74	54	47
20	Hemoglobin subunit beta OS=Ho...	HBB_HUMAN	16 kDa	43	46	93	80	14	11	36	30	33	28
21	Hemoglobin subunit alpha OS=H...	HBA_HUMAN	15 kDa	36	36	88	58	9	8	17	21	27	22
22	Platelet glycoprotein 4 OS=Hom...	CD36_HU...	53 kDa	7	16	20	23	42	38	47	46	29	22
23	Collagen alpha-2(VI) chain OS=...	CO6A2_H...	109 kDa	13	45	21	19	8	4	56	53	45	43
24	Collagen alpha-1(I) chain OS=H...	CO1A1_H...	139 kDa	17	27	39	45	13	42	30	29	19	21
25	Collagen alpha-2(I) chain OS=H...	CO1A2_H...	129 kDa	12	26	37	33	19	41	34	22	20	15

Fig. 23.6 LC–MS/MS proteomic analysis of Congo red positive fat aspirate specimens form five different patients affected by five different types of amyloidosis. The identified proteins are listed according to the relative abundance that was represented in five patients. Top 25 proteins are shown from a total of 252 proteins. At least two different samples (S1 and S2) were run for each patient (left to right, AL-K(kappa), AL-L(lambda), AA, ATTR, ALys). Each patient's fat aspirate proteome contains only one type causative amyloidogenic protein. The columns show the protein name, UniProt protein accession code (UniProt database, http://www.uniprot.org/), the molecular weight of the protein, and two samples from each of the five patients. The numbers indicate number of total peptide spectra identified for each protein in each sample. Each patient's fat aspirate proteome contains only one type causative amyloidogenic protein (row 3, AL-L; rows 4 and 10, AL-K; row 5, ATTR; row 6, ALys, row 9 AA). Rows 1 (APOE), 2 (APOA4), 7 (APOA1), and 8 (SAP) are proteins incorporated most amyloid plaques irrespective of etiology

References

1. Sipe JD, Benson MD, Buxbaum JN, Ikeda S, Merlini G, Saraiva MJ, Westermark P. Nomenclature 2014: amyloid fibril proteins and clinical classification of the amyloidosis. Amyloid. 2014;21:221–4.
2. Merlini G, Bellotti V. Molecular mechanisms of amyloidosis. N Engl J Med. 2003;349:583–96.
3. Merlini G, Seldin DC, Gertz MA. Amyloidosis: pathogenesis and new therapeutic options. J Clin Oncol. 2011;29:1924–33.
4. Holmgren G, Ericzon BG, Groth CG, et al. Clinical improvement and amyloid regression after liver transplantation in hereditary transthyretin amyloidosis. Lancet. 1993;341:1113–6.
5. Stangou AJ, Hawkins PN. Liver transplantation in transthyretin-related familial amyloid polyneuropathy. Curr Opin Neurol. 2004;17:615–20.
6. Howie AJ, Brewer DB, Howell D, Jones AP. Physical basis of colors seen in Congo red-stained amyloid in polarized light. Lab Invest. 2008;88:232–42.
7. Picken MM, Herrera GA. The burden of "sticky" amyloid: typing challenges. Arch Pathol Lab Med. 2007;131:850–1.
8. Solomon A, Murphy CL, Westermark P. Unreliability of immunohistochemistry for typing amyloid deposits. Arch Pathol Lab Med. 2008;132:14–5.
9. Picken MM. New insights into systemic amyloidosis: the importance of diagnosis of specific type. Curr Opin Nephrol Hypertens. 2007;16:196–203.
10. Murphy CL, Eulitz M, Hrncic R, et al. Chemical typing of amyloid protein contained in formalin-fixed paraffin-embedded biopsy specimens. Am J Clin Pathol. 2001;116:135–42.
11. Murphy CL, Wang S, Williams T, Weiss DT, Solomon A. Characterization of systemic amyloid deposits by mass spectrometry. Methods Enzymol. 2006;412:48–62.

12. Kaplan B, Martin BM, Livneh A, Pras M, Gallo GR. Biochemical subtyping of amyloid in formalin-fixed tissue samples confirms and supplements immuno-histologic data. Am J Clin Pathol. 2004;121: 794–800.

13. Rodriguez FJ, Gamez JD, Vrana JA, et al. Immunoglobulin derived depositions in the nervous system: novel mass spectrometry application for protein characterization in formalin-fixed tissues. Lab Invest. 2008;88:1024–37.

14. Vrana JA, Gamez JD, Madden BJ, Theis JD, Bergen 3rd HR, Dogan A. Classification of amyloidosis by laser microdissection and mass spectrometry-based proteomic analysis in clinical biopsy specimens. Blood. 2009;114:4957–9.

15. Hood BL, Darfler MM, Guiel TG, et al. Proteomic analysis of formalin-fixed prostate cancer tissue. Mol Cell Proteomics. 2005;4:1741–53.

16. Prieto DA, Hood BL, Darfler MM, et al. Liquid tissue: proteomic profiling of formalin-fixed tissues. Biotechniques. 2005;38(Suppl):32–5.

17. Palmer-Toy DE, Krastins B, Sarracino DA, Nadol Jr JB, Merchant SN. Efficient method for the proteomic analysis of fixed and embedded tissues. J Proteome Res. 2005;4:2404–11.

18. Guo T, Wang W, Rudnick PA, et al. Proteome analysis of microdissected formalin-fixed and paraffin-embedded tissue specimens. J Histochem Cytochem. 2007;55:763–72.

19. Dasari S, Theis JD, Vrana JA, et al. Clinical proteome informatics workbench detects pathogenic mutations in hereditary amyloidosis. J Proteome Res. 2014;13: 2352–8.

20. Brambilla F, Lavatelli F, Di Silvestre D, et al. Reliable typing of systemic amyloidosis through proteomic analysis of subcutaneous adipose tissue. Blood. 2012;119:1844–7.

21. Vrana JA, Theis JD, Dasari S, et al. Clinical diagnosis and typing of systemic amyloidosis in subcutaneous fat aspirates by mass spectrometry-based proteomics. Haematologica. 2014;99:1239–47.

22. Sethi S, Theis JD, Leung N, et al. Mass spectrometry-based proteomic diagnosis of renal immunoglobulin heavy chain amyloidosis. Clin J Am Soc Nephrol. 2010;5:2180–7.

23. Dogan A, Theis JD, Vrana JA, et al. Clinical and pathological phenotype of leukocyte cell-derived chemotaxin-2 (LECT2) amyloidosis (ALECT2). Amyloid. 2010;17:69–70.

24. Klein CJ, Vrana JA, Theis JD, et al. Mass spectrometric-based proteomic analysis of amyloid neuropathy type in nerve tissue. Arch Neurol-Chicago. 2011;68:195–9.

25. Miller DV, Dogan A, Sethi S. New-onset proteinuria with massive amorphous glomerular deposits. Am J Kidney Dis. 2010;55:749–54.

26. Lacy MQ, Theis JD, Vrana JA, et al. Lysozyme amyloidosis (ALys) affecting a family with a new variant of lysozyme gene (LYZ) and hereditary haemorrhagic telangiectasia. Amyloid. 2010;17:125.

27. Rowczenio D, Dogan A, Theis JD, et al. Amyloidogenicity and clinical phenotype associated with five novel mutations in Apolipoprotein A-I. Am J Pathol. 2011;179:1978–87.

28. D'Souza A, Theis JD, Vrana JA, Dogan A. Pharmaceutical amyloidosis associated with subcutaneous insulin and enfuvirtide administration. Amyloid. 2014;21:71–5.

29. Valleix S, Gillmore JD, Bridoux F, et al. Hereditary systemic amyloidosis due to Asp76Asn variant beta2-microglobulin. N Engl J Med. 2012;366:2276–83.

The Role of Differential Proteomics in Amyloid Typing: The Experience of the Pavia Referral Center

24

Francesca Lavatelli, Francesca Brambilla,
Andrea Di Fonzo, Giovanni Ferraro,
Giovanni Palladini, Pierluigi Mauri,
and Giampaolo Merlini

Introduction: Proteomics in the Diagnosis of Amyloidosis

The diagnosis of amyloidosis requires demonstration of amyloid deposits in a tissue biopsy, followed by amyloid typing, i.e., definition of the protein originating the fibrils [1].

Extensive description of the methods available for amyloid detection, based on specific Congo red staining and microscopic examination, and/or by ultrastructural visualization of the 8–10 nm-wide fibrils, is provided in the pertinent chapters of this book. The traditional and still most widely used approaches for amyloid typing are based on probing the tissue with an array of antibodies against the common known amyloid types and evaluating the staining of the amyloid deposits by optical or electron microscopy. Although the performances of antibody-based techniques are critically dependent on the experience of the pathologist and are generally better in referral centers, it is recognized that immunological methods, especially immunohistochemistry, can suffer from a lack of specificity and sensitivity in this pathological context [2–4]. High success rates are achieved with immuno-electron microscopy typing [5, 6], in centers where this technique is routinely performed.

However, all antibody-based techniques for amyloid typing may present specific and often unpredictable issues, related principally to the altered conformation and extensive posttranslational processing of the deposited amyloid proteins, which may not be recognized by the available antibodies (raised against the native proteins), and to the presence of serum contamination in fixed biopsies, which may lead to high background staining and false identifications. Moreover, antibody-based techniques can only be informative if the panel of antibodies includes those directed against the specific amyloid protein present in the sample, and are blind towards novel or unexpected amyloid types.

The word "proteome" indicates the ensemble of proteins present in a sample at a given state and time point; proteomics, accordingly, is the term used for indicating the comprehensive study of the protein constituents of a biological

F. Lavatelli, MD, PhD • A. Di Fonzo, PhD
G. Ferraro, MSc • G. Palladini, MD, PhD
G. Merlini, MD (✉)
Department of Molecular Medicine and Amyloidosis
Research and Treatment Center, Foundation IRCCS
Policlinico San Matteo and University of Pavia,
Viale Golgi, 19, 27100 Pavia, Italy
e-mail: francesca.lavatelli@unipv.it;
a.difonzo@smatteo.pv.it; fg1983@tin.it;
giovanni.palladini@unipv.it; gmerlini@unipv.it

F. Brambilla, PhD • P. Mauri, PhD
Department of Proteomics and Metabolomics,
Institute for Biomedical Technologies (ITB-CNR),
Via Fratelli Cervi, 93, 20090 Segrate, Italy
e-mail: francesca.brambilla@itb.cnr.it;
pierluigi.mauri@itb.cnr.it

© Springer International Publishing Switzerland 2015
M.M. Picken et al. (eds.), *Amyloid and Related Disorders*, Current Clinical Pathology,
DOI 10.1007/978-3-319-19294-9_24

sample, centered on analysis by mass spectrometry (MS). Proteomics does not provide morphological information but allows molecular identification of the various protein species in the sample, based on amino acid sequencing by means of the mass spectrometer. MS-based amyloid identification [7–11] is especially useful when immunohistochemistry or immuno-electron microscopy does not provide conclusive typing. Indeed, proteomics requires specialized equipment and ad hoc trained personnel, and both of these features are not yet available to most clinical pathology laboratories. In the experience of the Pavia Amyloid Center, in collaboration with investigators at ITB-CNR, the results of proteomics and immuno-electron microscopy, the two typing techniques used as first-line approaches, were shown to be in agreement in all cases [7]. In the cases in which immuno-EM is not conclusive in typing the amyloid fibrils, proteomics provides confident identification [8]. Choice of either approach as first-line typing technique is largely dictated by practical considerations, among which are experience of each center, availability of instruments and trained personnel, suspicion of a novel or rare amyloid type for which antibodies may not be available, and biopsy site (some sites are unpractical in terms of availability of adequate negative controls for proteomics).

The principles of proteomic techniques in use by the Pavia/ITB-CNR team, analyzed tissues, and diagnostic applications are described in this section.

Differential Proteomics for Amyloid Characterization

Principles of Differential Proteomics

In a typical proteomics workflow, tissue proteins are extracted from the tissue and enzymatically digested; the resulting peptides are separated by liquid chromatography (LC) and analyzed in the mass spectrometer, in so-called LC-MS. Within this instrument, the peptides can be further fragmented (tandem mass spectrometry, MS/MS), allowing to deduce their sequence from the progressive loss of amino acid residues. The identified peptide sequences permit the identification of related proteins.

The output of a proteomic analysis is a list of identified proteins, associated with the probability of correct identification and confidence parameters of identification, such as the number of identified peptides (spectral count) and percentage of sequence coverage. In addition, using specific softwares, it is possible to plot each protein list on a virtual 2D map (according to isoelectric point and molecular weight). As an example, Fig. 24.1 shows the virtual 2D map obtained from LC-MS analysis of adipose tissue proteome.

In differential proteomics, samples are compared in order to detect qualitative and quantitative differences. Various experimental approaches are available for this purpose. In particular, starting from the lists of identified proteins in unlabeled specimens (i.e., in specimens that have not been differently tagged by chemical modifications) analyzed by LC-MS, bioinformatics tools exist to calculate semiquantitative differences in protein abundance (label-free differential proteomics) [12, 13].

The diagnostic proteomics approaches in use at the Pavia Amyloid Research and Treatment Center are based on the LC-MS analysis of proteins extracted from unfractionated tissue samples, combined with label-free quantitation. These approaches rely on the comparison of the tissue proteome profile in each patient with the profile of the same tissue from unaffected controls. The proteins deposited as amyloid are assumed to be specifically present or overrepresented in patients, and typing is achieved by comparing the relative abundance of the different amyloidogenic species. This approach implies that an adequate reference map is available for the tissue under analysis. Besides giving information on amyloid composition, whole tissue analysis also provides knowledge on changes in tissue-resident proteins. This information is precious for understanding the bases of amyloid tissue toxicity and for identifying tissue dysfunction biomarkers [9, 10].

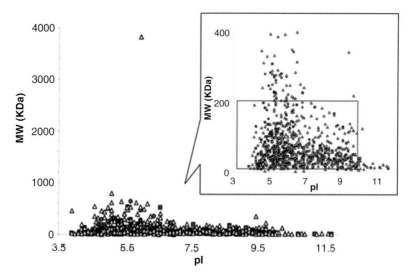

Fig. 24.1 Virtual 2D map, showing the distribution of proteins identified by LC-MS in a representative subcutaneous fat tissue aspirate, according to isoelectric point and molecular weight. The *inset* and *red box* show the range typically covered by gel-based proteomics (Reprinted with permission from Brambilla et al. JPR 2013; 12: 5642–55. Copyright 2013 American Chemical Society)

Differential Proteomic Techniques Used in Amyloid Typing

The analysis of the whole tissue proteome requires powerful separation methods to allow sensitive and specific detection and quantification of the different proteins in each sample. This can be achieved by gel-based (two-dimensional polyacrylamide gel electrophoresis, 2D-PAGE, coupled to MS) or gel-free approaches (LC-MS-based methods). The first method is very powerful in providing immediate visualization of the abnormal species [8, 10, 11]. The digital images of the 2D-PAGE gels from patients and controls samples are overlaid, to detect and identify the abnormal protein spots, which are then cut from the gel, digested, and identified by MS. However, this approach is more labor intensive and less automatable than gel-free approaches and, for the clinical purposes, has generally been abandoned in favor of the latter.

The gel-free (so-called "shotgun") methodologies employ enzymatic digestion of the protein sample (usually with trypsin) prior to analysis, and separation of the peptides by one-dimensional (reverse phase on C18 resin columns) or two-dimensional (reverse phase coupled to strong cation exchange) chromatography. The second approach is employed in the MudPIT technology (Multidimensional Protein Identification Technology), in use by the Pavia/ITB-CNR center (Fig. 24.2). 2D chromatography separates the peptides, which can directly enter the mass spectrometer, where their mass, and the mass of their fragments, is measured. A list of identified proteins is provided after searching the MS data against protein sequence databases (such as NCBInr). The diseased vs. control proteome comparison is performed through dedicated softwares (such as MaProMa [7, 9], developed in-house at ITB-CNR, or commercial ones).

An important step in sample preparation, especially when working with unfixed specimens, is blood removal through washing. In fact, the systemic amyloidosis precursors are blood-borne, and traces of their normal counterparts may be detected in case of blood carryover. Since minor amounts of blood contaminants are often detected in samples, we have developed an algorithm that provides a quantitative parameter (designated α-value [7]) to evaluate the overrepresentation of a specific amyloidogenic protein

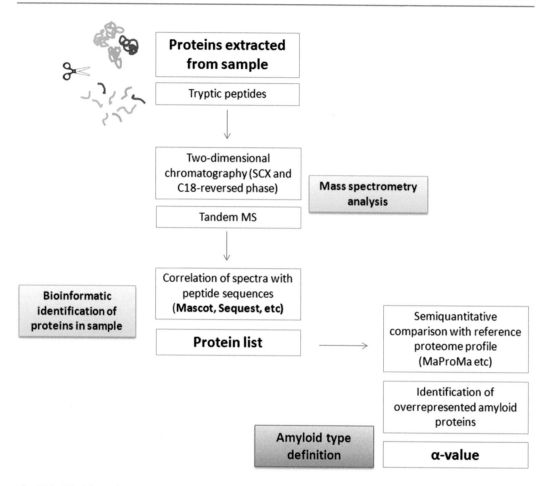

Fig. 24.2 Workflow of MudPIT approach for amyloid typing. *SCX* strong cation exchange

compared to the other ones. This simplifies the interpretation of proteomic results: amyloid type attribution is achieved not only from the presence of an amyloidogenic protein in the list of identified species but also from its greater abundance (Fig. 24.3).

Subcutaneous Abdominal Fat

Abdominal subcutaneous fat, acquired by fine-needle aspiration or by surgical biopsy, can be effectively analyzed by diagnostic proteomics. The tissue preparation workflow is shown in Fig. 24.4 [7–11]. Adipose tissue must be collected in clean microcentrifuge tubes and stored frozen (−80 °C) without fixatives. Care must be paid in freezing the sample as soon as possible

(not later than 30 min, during which time it must be kept on ice), in order to prevent protein degradation. Protein extraction is achieved by manually crushing the sample (10–20 mg) in a lysis buffer. Our preferred lysis buffer contains chaotropes (8 M urea, or 7 M urea plus 2 M thiourea), detergents (4 % CHAPS), and a reducing agent (0.1 M DTT). This buffer has been demonstrated to effectively solubilize the proteins species present in amyloid deposits, including those forming amyloid fibrils. Short pulses of sonication help disaggregate the tissue and extract proteins. Delipidation must be performed after protein extraction and prior to further processing, and is obtained through centrifugation (12,000–16,000 rpm). The clear solution below the floating lipids must be carefully recovered using a gel-loader tip. This protein extract would now be

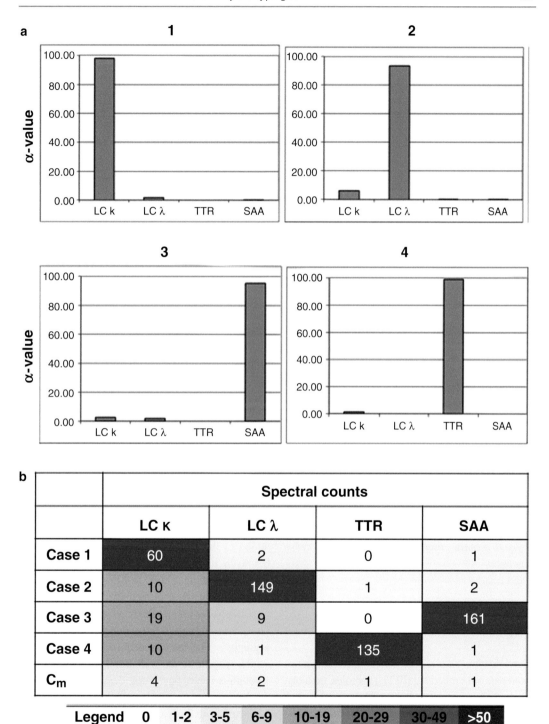

Fig. 24.3 Calculated α-value (**a**) and corresponding spectral counts (**b**) for the major amyloidogenic proteins in four representative patients (proteomic analysis of sub- cutaneous fat). Spectral counts in controls (Cm, averaged count [7]) are provided for comparison

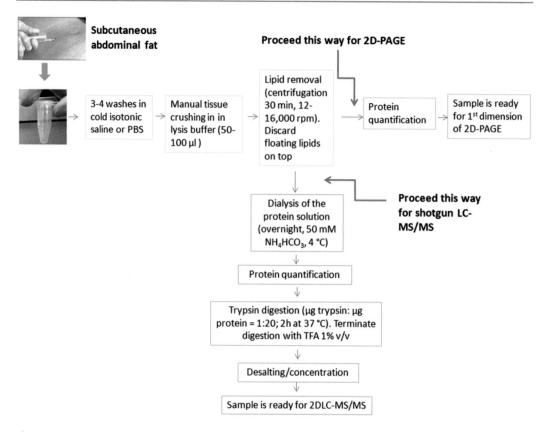

Fig. 24.4 Processing of fresh subcutaneous fat tissue aspirates for LC-MS/MS proteomic analysis or 2D-PAGE

ready for protein quantification and 2D-PAGE analysis [10, 11]. In order to proceed to gel-free proteomic analysis, instead, detergents and other interfering buffer components must be removed [7] and proteins must be subjected to protease digestion.

Formalin-Fixed Paraffin-Embedded Biopsies

Amyloid typing can also be performed on formalin-fixed paraffin-embedded (FFPE) samples. Notably, aldehyde fixation cross-links proteins and makes these samples unsuited for 2D-PAGE separation. The tissue (1–2 slices, 10-μm thick) is subjected to paraffin removal by incubation in 100 % xylene (3 times, 5 min each), followed by rehydration through consecutive incubations in absolute ethanol, 70 % ethanol, and water. The deparaffinized

samples are incubated in a buffer containing 100 mM NH_4HCO_3 at 100 °C for 20 min and then at 100 °C for 2 h. Prior to trypsin digestion, the MS-compatible surfactant Rapigest (Waters) is added to the sample, to a final concentration of 0.5 % in 10 % acetonitrile. Proteins are digested with sequencing grade trypsin in a ratio 1:50 enzyme–substrate and incubated at 37 °C overnight. Peptides are desalted and loaded for LC-MS analysis (using mono- or two-dimensional chromatography). The mass spectrometry and bioinformatic workflow, as well as data interpretation through α-value, have been described above, and are analogous to what performed for proteins extracted from fresh adipose tissue. For each tissue type, a reference proteome map derived from unaffected individuals is used as comparison. Our center currently performs amyloid typing on heart, liver, kidney, lymph nodes, intestine, and salivary glands, using LC-MS.

The "Amyloid Signature" Proteome in Diagnosis; Novel Proteomic Biomarkers of Tissue Dysfunction

Proteomics allows identifying, in a single analysis, the various proteins present in the sample. These include, along with the deposited amyloidogenic species, also tissue-resident proteins and proteins known to be common constituent of the amyloid deposits, such as apolipoproteins A-IV and E, serum amyloid P, vitronectin, heparan-sulfate proteoglycans, and clusterin [7, 9, 14, 15]. In affected adipose tissue analyzed by differential proteomics, these proteins are often overrepresented [7, 9]. Especially in AL amyloidosis, this proteomic "amyloid signature" is detected in the vast majority of patients (Table 24.1), and, when present, is strongly indicative of the presence of amyloid deposits.

In addition, analysis of unfractionated subcutaneous fat by differential proteomics has revealed a set of tissue-resident proteins, belonging to different compartments and networks, which are differentially represented in amyloid patients compared to controls [9, 10]. These proteins include, among others, extracellular matrix components (heparan sulfate proteoglycan core protein and other proteoglycans, collagen VI, components of the basal lamina), species involved in protein folding (including αB-crystallin, HSP47, HSP70), and proteins implicated in adipose tissue-specific and energetic metabolism

(including perilipins, adipocyte fatty acid binding protein FABP4, ATP synthase components).

Describing this proteome remodeling in affected tissues is extremely important to gain insight into the molecular pathogenesis of amyloid diseases. Moreover, these differential proteins could be used as histological or circulating indicators of amyloid tissue dysfunction; if validated, as single analytes or in combination, they could represent novel, sensitive markers of amyloid deposition and indicators of amyloid-associated damage.

Conclusions

Proteomics is the most recent entry among the array of instruments for amyloid typing but has gained immediate popularity. This relays on the maturity and robustness reached by MS-based protein analysis and on the fact that proteomics identification employs completely distinct mechanisms from those used in antibody-based typing techniques. However, proteomics as well presents caveats in the field of amyloid typing. Possible pitfalls are especially related to the fact that variant amyloidogenic protein sequences, as well as specific immunoglobulin light chain sequences, may not be present in protein databases. Thus, peptide mass spectra containing amino acid substitutions, or derived from a light chain's variable region, may not be assigned, impairing protein identification and quantification.

We indeed believe that proteomics is an extremely powerful tool, which has opened novel perspectives in terms of amyloid typing. It undoubtedly outperforms antibody-based methods in typing rare or novel amyloidoses, and was proven to be useful in typing samples for which immuno-EM had not been informative. The existence of a specific amyloid proteome signature could also be exploited as a novel instrument, in parallel to specific staining and electron microscopy, to demonstrate the presence of amyloid in a sample [7, 9]. Moreover, the tissue-resident proteins that were shown to change in affected tissues could be studied as possible future biomarkers [9, 10].

Table 24.1 Amyloid signature proteins, overrepresented in adipose tissue of patients with systemic AL amyloidosis

Accession	Protein	ALλ	ALκ
93163358	Apolipoprotein AIV	+	+
4557325	Apolipoprotein E	+	+
42740907	Clusterin	+	+
24212664	Basement-membrane heparan-sulfate proteoglycan core protein	+	−
88853069	Vitronectin	+	+
576259	Serum Amyloid P	+	−

Adapted from Brambilla et al. (2012); 119: 1844–7 [7]
"+" overrepresented proteins in more than 50 % of patients

The Pavia Amyloid Center is exploiting the information offered by proteomics, using this approach in complement with immuno-electron microscopy. As mentioned in the dedicated chapter, the latter technique is more widely diffuse and could be effectively implemented in most institutions. We devise two situations, however, in which proteomic typing, performed by specialized centers, is mandatory:

1. When antibody-based techniques provide dubious results (for lack or weakness of staining, or multiple positivity) or results not in accordance with the clinical picture
2. When a novel or a rare amyloidosis type is suspected (the correct antibody may not be available or not be included in the diagnostic panel)

Indeed, the automation of the proteomics approach, and its positive performances for amyloid typing, may launch its future routine use in the clinical practice in equipped laboratories.

Today, correctly exploiting the advantages of the available techniques can allow amyloid typing in virtually all patients.

References

1. Sipe JD, Benson MD, Buxbaum JN, Ikeda SI, Merlini G, Saraiva MJ, Westermark P. Nomenclature 2014: amyloid fibril proteins and clinical classification of the amyloidosis. Amyloid. 2014;29:1–4.
2. Lachmann HJ, Booth DR, Booth SE, Bybee A, Gilbertson JA, Gillmore JD, Pepys MB, Hawkins PN. Misdiagnosis of hereditary amyloidosis as AL (primary) amyloidosis. N Engl J Med. 2002;346:1786–91.
3. Satoskar AA, Burdge K, Cowden DJ, Nadasdy GM, Hebert LA, Nadasdy T. Typing of amyloidosis in renal biopsies: diagnostic pitfalls. Arch Pathol Lab Med. 2007;131:917–22.
4. Solomon A, Murphy CL, Westermark P. Unreliability of immunohistochemistry for typing amyloid deposits. Arch Pathol Lab Med. 2008;132:14.
5. Palladini G, Verga L, Corona S, Obici L, Morbini P, Lavatelli F, Donadei S, Sarais G, Roggeri L, Foli A, Russo P, Zenone Bragotti L, Paulli M, Magrini U, Merlini G. Diagnostic performance of immuno-electron microscopy of abdominal fat in systemic amyloidoses. Amyloid. 2010;17:59–60.
6. Foli A, Palladini G, Caporali R, Verga L, Morbini P, Obici L, Russo P, Sarais G, Donadei S, Montecucco C, Merlini G. Role of minor salivary gland biopsy in the diagnosis of systemic amyloidosis: results of a prospective study in 62 patients. Amyloid. 2011;18(S1):80–2.
7. Brambilla F, Lavatelli F, Di Silvestre D, Valentini V, Rossi R, Palladini G, Obici L, Verga L, Mauri P, Merlini G. Reliable typing of systemic amyloidoses through proteomic analysis of subcutaneous adipose tissue. Blood. 2012;119(8):1844–7.
8. Lavatelli F, Valentini V, Palladini G, Verga L, Russo P, Foli A, Obici L, Sarais G, Perfetti V, Casarini S, Merlini G. Mass spectrometry-based proteomics as a diagnostic tool when immunoelectron microscopy fails in typing amyloid deposits. Amyloid. 2011;18(S1):64–6.
9. Brambilla F, Lavatelli F, Di Silvestre D, Valentini V, Palladini G, Merlini G, Mauri P. Shotgun protein profile of human adipose tissue and its changes in relation to systemic amyloidoses. J Proteome Res. 2013;12(12):5642–55.
10. Lavatelli F, Perlman DH, Spencer B, Prokaeva T, McComb ME, Théberge R, Connors LH, Bellotti V, Seldin DC, Merlini G, Skinner M, Costello CE. Amyloidogenic and associated proteins in systemic amyloidosis proteome of adipose tissue. Mol Cell Proteomics. 2008;7(8):1570–83.
11. Valentini V, Lavatelli F, Obici L, Donadei S, Perlini S, Palladini G, Merlini G. Proteomic characterization of amyloid deposits in transthyretin amyloidosis associated with various mutations. Amyloid. 2011;18(S1):61–3.
12. Park SK, Venable JD, Xu T, Yates 3rd JR. A quantitative analysis software tool for mass spectrometry-based proteomics. Nat Methods. 2008;5(4):319–22.
13. Mauri PL, Dehò G. A proteomic MudPIT approach to the analysis of RNA degradosome composition in Escherichia coli. Methods Enzymol. 2008;447:99–117.
14. Sethi S, Vrana JA, Theis JD, Leung N, Sethi A, Nasr SH, Fervenza FC, Cornell LD, Fidler ME, Dogan A. Laser microdissection and mass spectrometry-based proteomics aids the diagnosis and typing of renal amyloidosis. Kidney Int. 2012;82(2):226–34.
15. Vrana JA, Theis JD, Dasari S, Mereuta OM, Dispenzieri A, Zeldenrust SR, Gertz MA, Kurtin PJ, Grogg KL, Dogan A. Clinical diagnosis and typing of systemic amyloidosis in subcutaneous fat aspirates by mass spectrometry-based proteomics. Haematologica. 2014;99(7):1239–47.

Part IV

Ancillary Studies of Amyloidosis

Laboratory Support for Diagnosis of Amyloidosis

David L. Murray and Jerry A. Katzmann

Introduction

The definitive diagnosis of amyloidosis requires identification and characterization of amyloid plaques. Serum- and urine-based laboratory testing are important initial observations in helping to guide both the differential diagnosis of primary amyloidosis (AL) and the testing for identifying and characterizing tissue amyloid. The purpose of this chapter is to describe the methods used to detect plasma cell proliferation disorders and to identify excess monoclonal free light chain (FLC) synthesis. Specifically, the value of protein electrophoresis (PEL), immunofixation electrophoresis (IFE), quantitative serum FLC and serum-based mass spectrometry analysis will be presented. These tests are not only useful in the differential diagnosis of amyloidosis but also have a role in early disease detection, prognosis, and monitoring of AL.

Primary amyloidosis is a plasma cell proliferative disorder. The plasma cell proliferative disorders are characterized by a clonal expansion of plasma cells and can be subgrouped into malignant diseases (multiple myeloma, plasma cell leukemia, plasmacytoma, Waldenström's macroglobulinemia), premalignant syndromes (monoclonal gammopathy of undetermined significance, smoldering multiple myeloma), and protein conformation disorders (AL, light chain deposition disease, cryoglobulinemia). Due to the clonal plasma cell proliferation, most of these diseases are also characterized by the presence of a monoclonal immunoglobulin, and are therefore often described as monoclonal gammopathies. The monoclonal protein serves as a surrogate marker for the clonal plasma cell expansion and was one of the first (and remains one of the best) clonal cell markers. Monoclonal immunoglobulins are recognized, characterized, and quantitated by PEL and IFE. These two assays are illustrated in Fig. 25.1. A normal serum is analyzed in Fig. 25.1a, and the smooth distribution of proteins in the gamma fraction is indicative of polyclonal (or normal) immunoglobulins. An abnormal serum is presented in Fig. 25.1b, and the discrete protein band in the gamma fraction of the PEL is consistent with a monoclonal immunoglobulin. The IFE identifies the discrete band as an IgG lambda monoclonal gammopathy. The identification of this monoclonal IgG lambda is not diagnostic for any of the specific diseases listed above, but it is diagnostic for a plasma cell proliferative disorder. In addition, the demarcation and integration of the PEL band allows quantitation of the monoclonal protein (M-spike) separate from any polyclonal immunoglobulin in the gamma fraction. Changes in the quantitation

D.L. Murray, MD, PhD (✉) • J.A. Katzmann, PhD
Department of Laboratory Medicine and Pathology,
Mayo Clinic, Rochester, MN 55905, USA
e-mail: murray.david@mayo.edu

© Springer International Publishing Switzerland 2015
M.M. Picken et al. (eds.), *Amyloid and Related Disorders*, Current Clinical Pathology,
DOI 10.1007/978-3-319-19294-9_25

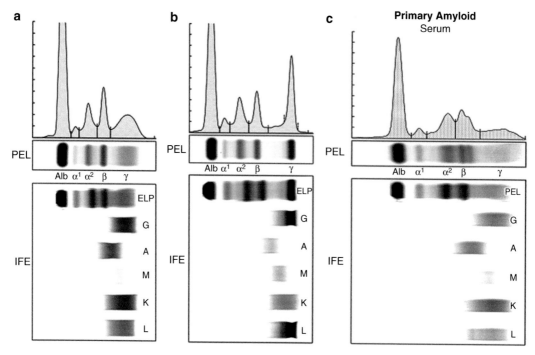

Fig. 25.1 (**a**) Protein Electrophoresis (PEL) and Immunofixation electrophoresis (IFE) of normal serum: the proteins in the gamma fraction on the PEL gel and the precipitated immunoglobulins on the IFE gel exhibit a smooth Gaussian distribution indicating a polyclonal distribution. (**b**) Protein Electrophoresis (PEL) and Immunoelectrophoresis (IFE) of a serum containing a monoclonal IgG Lambda: the proteins in the gamma fraction on the PEL gel and the precipitated immunoglobulins on the IFE gel exhibit a discrete band indicating a mono-clonal protein. The *upper most graph* is a scan of the PEL gel, and the area under the monoclonal protein spike is used in conjunction with the serum total protein concentration to quantitate the amount of monoclonal immunoglobulin. (**c**) Protein Electrophoresis (PEL) and Immunoelectrophoresis (IFE) of patient with Primary Amyloidosis (AL): the proteins in the gamma fraction on the PEL gel and the precipitated immunoglobulins on the IFE gel exhibit only a small abnormality in the beta region reflecting the low plasma cell burden in this patient

of the M-spike reflect changes in the size of the plasma cell clone and can be used to monitor disease or response to therapy.

Not all plasma cell proliferative disorders, however, produce a quantifiable or even detectable monoclonal protein. Nonsecretory multiple myeloma, for example, does not secrete an easily detectable monoclonal protein even though the bone marrow may be packed with malignant plasma cells containing cytoplasmic monoclonal immunoglobulin light chain. In AL patients with significant disease, it may also be difficult to detect a monoclonal protein and often impossible to quantitate. An AL patient with very small amounts of monoclonal free lambda light chain is illustrated in Fig. 25.1c. There is an almost imperceptible asymmetry in the lambda lane of the IFE, and there is clearly no way to monitor and quantitate the hematologic response of this patient.

The distribution of monoclonal gammopathies in our clinical practice is listed in Table 25.1. By far, the most common plasma cell proliferative disorder is monoclonal gammopathy of undetermined significance (MGUS). In the normal population older than 50 years, MGUS has a prevalence of 3 % [1]. The prevalence increases with age: between ages, 50 and 60 the prevalence is 1.7 % and in ages greater than 80 years, the prevalence is 6.6 %. This very common premalignant disorder has no clinical symptoms, but these patients have a 1 % per year progression

Table 25.1 Distribution of plasma cell proliferative disorders in clinical practice

Monoclonal gammopathy of undetermined significance	61 %
Multiple myeloma	17 %
Amyloidosis AL	9 %
Lymphoproliferative disease	3 %
Smoldering myeloma	4 %
Solitary or extramedullary plasmacytoma	2 %
Macroglobulinemia	2 %
Other	2 %

From the Mayo Clinic Dysproteinemia data base, 1960–2003; $n = 31,479$.

to diseases such as multiple myeloma or AL [2]. The diagnosis of MGUS requires the absence of related organ or tissue impairment (e.g., no end organ damage or bone lesions), less than 10 % clonal bone marrow plasma cells, and less than 3 g/dL of serum monoclonal protein. The diagnosis of multiple myeloma requires greater than 10 % clonal bone marrow plasma cells as well as clinical symptoms such as hypercalcemia, renal disease, anemia, and/or bone lesions due to the clonal plasma cell proliferation. Multiple myeloma has an incidence of approximately 40 per million per year in Caucasians, and the incidence is 2–3-fold higher in African American populations [3]. There are approximately 13,000 new cases each year in the USA.

By contrast, AL is a relatively rare plasma cell proliferative disorder. It is one-fifth as common as multiple myeloma with approximately 2500 new patients diagnosed in the USA every year. Multiple myeloma and AL can occur together, with the myeloma commonly being diagnosed before or at the time AL is discovered [4, 5]. Like all forms of amyloid, diagnosis requires histologic identification of amyloid fibrils in tissue [6]. Because AL is a monoclonal gammopathy, the identification of a monoclonal protein is a useful initial screen for patients with AL. The 3 % prevalence of MGUS in the population over 50 years and the increased prevalence in African Americans, however, mean that some of these coincident findings will be unrelated. Over a 6-year period at Memorial Sloan-Kettering Cancer Center, 369 consecutive patients with systemic amyloidosis were evalu-

ated for clonal plasma cell disease and 30 % of them were screened for hereditary transthyretin mutations (ATTRm). ATTRm was identified in 5.4 % (20/369) of the patients. Of the 20 patients with ATTRm, 50 % (10 of 20) had an associated monoclonal gammopathy. Ultimately, four of the six with a gammopathy and mutant TTR were diagnosed with ATTRm, while the other two had AL [7]. This study highlights a potential pitfall of relying on monoclonal protein screening alone. Immunohistochemical staining or some other direct characterization of the amyloid fibrils may be necessary to confirm the type of amyloidosis [8].

The fibrils in AL are derived from intact or fragmented monoclonal immunoglobulin light chains. These patients often have free monoclonal immunoglobulin light chains detected in the serum and/or urine. The FLCs are secreted from the plasma cells without being bound to heavy chain in intact immunoglobulin molecules and the monoclonal light chains or fragments are precursor components for the amyloid fibrils. Unlike patients with multiple myeloma, AL patients may have a very small population of clonal plasma cells in the bone marrow. The long-term continuous secretion of the amyloidogenic monoclonal FLC results in amyloid fibril deposition and eventual organ failure. The presence of small clonal plasma cell populations and the small amount of secreted monoclonal FLC may make it difficult to document the monoclonal gammopathy by serum and/or urine IFE [9].

Free Light Chain Quantitation

Bence Jones proteins are monoclonal FLC that are detected in concentrated urine using PEL and IFE. These urinary FLCs are low molecular weight peptides that are removed from serum by the kidneys and are either metabolized or excreted in the urine. An alternative strategy to detect and quantitate the Bence Jones proteins would be to directly quantitate the FLC in serum. Early approaches used the size difference between intact immunoglobulins and FLC to separate the molecules, and then quantitated the FLC with

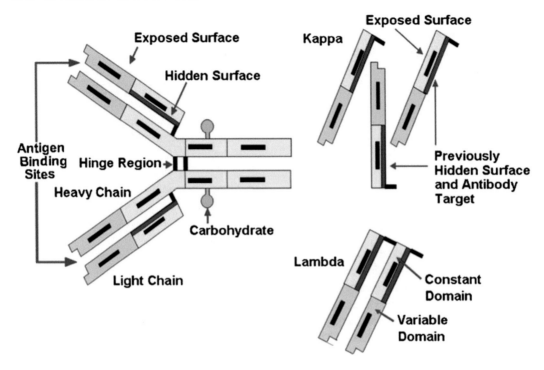

Fig. 25.2 Cartoon of immunoglobulin G showing the intact tetrapeptide as well as FLC. The hidden surfaces of the light chains are tightly bound to the heavy chains by noncovalent interactions. When no longer bound to heavy chain, these surfaces provide the specific targets for the FLC antisera (Courtesy of The Binding Site, Inc., reprinted with permission)

light chain immunoassays. These multistep procedures never migrated into clinical laboratories. Subsequent approaches were based on using antisera that were specific for immunoglobulin light chain epitopes that were obscured when the light chain peptides were bound to the heavy chain peptides (Fig. 25.2). The specificity for these "cryptic" light chain epitopes meant that FLC could be accurately quantitated even in the presence of the large concentrations of intact immunoglobulin found in serum. The introduction of automated assays for the quantitation of immunoglobulin FLC has given clinical laboratories a new tool for evaluating AL. The FLC assays have increased the diagnostic sensitivity for identification of light chain diseases such as AL, and in addition they have improved disease monitoring and prognosis. The FLC assay was described by Bradwell and colleagues in 2001 [10]. The method is an automated nephelometric assay that uses a commercially available reagent set of polyclonal antibodies to quantitate both κ FLC and λ FLC by immunonephelometry (FREELITE™: The Binding Site, San Diego, Calif.). The antibodies show no reactivity by IFE or by Western blots to light chains contained in intact immunoglobulin. Sensitive hemagglutination assays showed reactivity to the appropriate FLC at dilutions above 1:16,000 and no reactivity to light chains contained within intact Ig at antisera dilutions >1:2. The assay reagents therefore appear to have a minimum of a 10,000-fold difference in reactivity to FLC compared to light chain contained within intact Ig. This high specificity allows κ and λ FLC to be quantitated in the presence of a large excess of serum IgG, IgA, and IgM. Similar to the quantitation of elevated immunoglobulins, elevations in FLC concentrations do not indicate monoclonality. The relationship between κ and λ light chain secretion, however, is predictable in normal plasma cell populations. The ratio of κ to λ light chain synthesis is approximately 2:1. Significant deviations from this ratio suggest clonal light chain synthesis. If the ratio of κ to λ FLC (rFLC) is significantly greater than normal, it suggests clonal proliferation of a κ-producing plasma cell. If the ratio is below normal, it suggests clonal excess of λ FLC.

A reference range study was performed with sera from healthy donors aged 21–90 years [11] whose sera were screened by PEL and IFE to exclude samples with a monoclonal protein [e.g., unknown MGUS patients]. The κ FLC and λ FLC concentrations were assessed, and the rFLC was calculated. This reference range study revealed an apparent effect of age on the 2 FLC concentrations, but the rFLC showed no age dependence. Cystatin C (a marker of renal clearance) showed the same apparent age dependence as the 2 FLC concentrations. The increase in serum FLC concentrations with age is most likely due to reduced renal clearance, and the use of the rFLC ratio normalizes the effects of reduced clearance.

Concentrations of κ and λ FLC may be abnormal due to immune suppression, immune stimulation, reduced renal clearance, or monoclonal plasma cell proliferative diseases. Serum from patients with either polyclonal hypergammaglobulinemia or renal impairment for example, often have elevated κ FLC and λ FLC due to increased synthesis or reduced renal clearance, respectively. The rFLC, however, usually remains normal in these conditions [11]. A significantly abnormal rFLC should only be due to a plasma cell proliferative disorder that secretes excess clonal FLC and disturbs the normal balance between κ and λ secretion. An abnormally high ratio suggests expansion of a kappa-producing plasma cell clone, whereas an abnormally low ratio suggests expansion of a lambda-producing plasma cell clone. The κ and λ FLC reference ranges were defined as 95 % reference ranges, but a "diagnostic range" for the rFLC was defined by 100 % of the normal sample study (Table 25.2).

Recently, Barnidge et al. [12] described the application of a mass spectrometry (MS)-based platform routinely used by pharma for monoclonal therapeutic quality control, microLC-ESI-Q-TOF MS, for the rapid detection, quantification,

Table 25.2 FLC quantitation: serum FLC reference intervals and diagnostic range

	95 % reference interval (normal range)	Diagnostic range
Kappa FLC	0.33–1.94 mg/dL	
Lambda FLC	0.57–2.63 mg/dL	
FLC K/L ratio	0.3–1.2	0.26–1.65

and isotyping of monoclonal immunoglobulin in patient sera. Using reduced Ig-enriched serum, these authors utilized the mass distribution measurements to identify isotype and quantify the distribution of light chains. Figure 25.3 demonstrates the mass spectrum distribution in the presence and absence of a monoclonal protein. Limits of detection were significantly lower than existing serum measurements and the technique was able to detect residual M-protein in samples negative by PEL, IFE, and FLC. This methodology represents a major shift in the characterization of monoclonal immunoglobulins. Rather than using gel electrophoresis and anti-isotypic antibody reagents, the authors combine molecular mass and constant region fragment ions to create a more sensitive technique for detecting and monitoring monoclonal immunoglobulins.

Diagnostic Sensitivity for Identification of Monoclonal FLC

The concept of using the alteration of the rFLC as a sensitive marker of monoclonal FLC synthesis was not obvious. There had been many previous attempts to use the total κ to λ ratio as a tool to screen for monoclonal gammopathies. The ratio of the total light chains, however, is a very insensitive marker of clonal expansion. One of the first clinical studies with rFLC assays evaluated 28 patients with nonsecretory multiple myeloma. Drayson and colleagues found that although some patients had no detectable serum or urine monoclonal protein by PEL or IFE, 19 (68 %) had abnormal rFLC ratios [13]. In another study of 262 AL patients, Lachmann and colleagues detected abnormal serum rFLC in 98 % of the AL patients, whereas the serum or urine IFE was positive in only 79 % [14]. This increase in

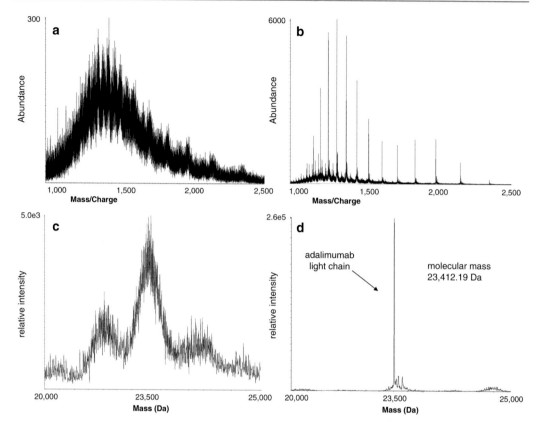

Fig. 25.3 Mass spectra from (**a**) a normal serum sample and (**b**) normal serum spiked with 0.5 g/dL of the IgG kappa recombinant mAb adalimumab. The normal serum mass spectrum displays a broad range of unresolved peaks, whereas the normal serum spiked with 0.5 g/dL of adalimumab shows a clearly defined multiply charged protein ions. (**c**) Converted spectrum for the normal serum sample displaying a broad range of unresolved peaks. (**d**) Converted mass spectrum for the normal serum spiked with 0.5 g/dL of adalimumab showing a single peak at an average molecular mass of 23 412.19 Da. This mass is in excellent agreement with the calculated average molecular mass of 23 412.13 Da for the kappa light chain of adalimumab (reprinted with permission from Ref. [12])

diagnostic sensitivity of the serum FLC assay for monoclonal light chain diseases such as AL was an unexpected diagnostic advance and has been confirmed by other authors [15, 16]. In a prospective study to further evaluate the diagnostic performance in clinical practice, we confirmed the increased sensitivity for monoclonal light chain diseases in a series of all newly diagnosed patients that were seen in our practice in 1 calendar year [17]. In 110 untreated AL patients, the FLC assay was more sensitive (91 %) than the serum or urine IFE assay (69 and 83 % sensitivity, respectively). In addition, the IFE and FLC assays were complementary for the detection of monoclonal FLC in AL patients. If both the

Table 25.3 Diagnostic sensitivity in AL ($n = 110$)

Assay	Sensitivity (%)
FLC κ/λ ratio	91
Serum IFE	69
Urine IFE	83
Serum IFE ± Urine IFE	95
FLC κ/λ ratio + Urine IFE	91
FLC κ/λ ratio + Serum IFE	99
All 3 assays	99

serum IFE and FLC assay were performed, 109 of the 110 AL patients (99 %) had an abnormal result in at least one of the two tests (Table 25.3). The inclusion of urine testing did not increase the diagnostic sensitivity. This enhanced ability to detect monoclonal FLCs does not address whether the light chains are amyloidogenic, but supports the need to search for amyloid deposits as well as the classification of the amyloid.

The high diagnostic sensitivity for AL when using both serum IFE and FLC assays suggests that the recommended diagnostic screening algorithm for monoclonal gammopathies may not be the simplest or best approach. The recommended laboratory testing for patients suspected of having MM, AL, or related disorders has previously been PEL and IFE of both serum and urine. In initial laboratory evaluations, however, urine is only submitted in approximately 30 % of the cases. The lack of submitted urine samples reduces the diagnostic sensitivity in AL, light chain deposition disease, and light chain MM (LCMM). The FLC assays can be performed on serum, and because of the sensitivity of the serum FLC assays for the light chain diseases, it is not apparent that urine studies are still necessary as part of the diagnostic screening algorithm. In a study of 224 patients with LCMM, it was reported that serum IFE and FLC identified 100 % of the patients and that urine IFE added no additional information [18]. Similarly, in the study described above, it was found that 109 of 110 patients with AL had abnormal results in either serum IFE or rFLC and that urine studies did not add to the sensitivity for identifying monoclonal FLC [17]. Because of these reports suggesting that urine studies may not add sensitivity to a screening panel of serum IFE and FLC, the inconvenience in routinely obtaining a 24-h urine sample, and the additional patients detected by serum FLC assays, it is reasonable to replace urine IFE studies with serum FLC assays. The danger of using these studies to dismiss the 24-h urine IFE as part of the screen for monoclonal gammopathies is that none of these

disease-specific studies addressed the broader use of urine testing as part of the detection of monoclonal gammopathies. We therefore used a large cohort of patients with an assortment of plasma cell proliferative diagnoses and a monoclonal urine protein who had urine PEL and IFE as well as serum PEL, IFE, and FLC testing [19]. The study was designed to assess the spectrum of plasma cell proliferative diseases and to determine which patients would have been undiagnosed in the absence of urine studies. There were 428 patients who had positive urine studies and also had serum PEL, IFE, and FLC performed. These patients had diagnoses of MM ($n=148$), AL ($n=123$), monoclonal gammopathy of undetermined significance ($n=69$), smoldering multiple myeloma ($n=59$), solitary plasmacytomas ($n=5$), and other less frequently detected monoclonal gammopathies. All 428 had a monoclonal urine protein (by definition of the cohort), and 86 % had an abnormal serum rFLC, 91 % had an abnormal serum PEL, and 93 % had an abnormal serum immunofixation. Using all three serum assays, only two cases had no serum abnormality. Both of these cases had monoclonal gammopathy (idiopathic Bence Jones proteinuria). Discontinuation of urine studies and reliance on a diagnostic algorithm using solely serum studies (IFE, IFE, and FLC) missed 0.5 % of the 428 monoclonal gammopathies with urinary monoclonal proteins, and these two cases required no medical intervention. Two large subsequent studies confirmed the high sensitivity of using serum IFE and FLC to screen for monoclonal gammopathies. Both studies showed good sensitivity with serum IFE and FLC but that omission of urine studies resulted in missing the monoclonal abnormality in 1 % of patients with AL [20, 21]. A summary of the results from one of these studies is presented in Table 25.4.

Table 25.4 Diagnostic sensitivity of screening panels

Diagnosis (n)	Serum PEL/IFE/FLC urine IFE (all assays) (%)	Serum PEL/IFE/FLC (3 serum assays) (%)
Multiple Myeloma (467)	100	100
Waldenström's Macroglobulinemia (26)	100	100
Primary amyloid (581)	98.1	97.1

As stated earlier, it is important to remember that an abnormal rFLC is not specific for AL. A clinical entity representing the FLC equivalent of conventional MGUS has been identified. Prevalence of light-chain MGUS is 0.8 % (95 % CI 0.7–0.9). Risk of progression to multiple myeloma in patients with light-chain MGUS is 0.3 % (0.1–0.8) per year [22]. An abnormal rFLC ratio warrants further clinical correlation and may not require intervention. The enhanced sensitivity for detecting monoclonal FLC does not of course address whether the light chains are amyloidogenic, but supports the need to search for amyloid deposits. Clinicians ordering the FLC assay should be sensitized to this important point. An abnormal rFLC should place AL on their differential diagnosis and the clinical findings were reviewed in this light. This is true even when serum PEL and IFE show no or small monoclonal proteins.

Monitoring Disease Activity

Once the diagnosis of AL is confirmed, the FLC serum assay provides a quantitation of the involved monoclonal FLC (iFLC) and therefore a way to monitor the plasma cell clone analogous to the electrophoretic M-spike [23]. This allows an assessment of the hematologic response to therapy in the absence of a serum or urine M-spike and provides a faster assessment than organ-based response criteria. Lachmann and colleagues detected abnormal serum rFLC in 98 % of AL patients tested, and only 79 % of the same patients showed an abnormal IFE [14]. Equally interesting, however, was the observation that 46 % of the 262 AL patients had no serum or urine M-spike which could be used to monitor treatment. For AL, therefore, the serum rFLC provided a more sensitive diagnostic tool and the quantitative assessment of iFLC provided a tool to monitor disease activity. Just as a 50 % reduction in M-spike values is used as a response criterion when monitoring MM, a 50 % reduction in the iFLC indicated a therapeutic response and was predictive of a significant survival advantage in AL. Dispenzieri et al. [16] have reported that

rather than assessing the percent reduction of serum iFLC, normalization of rFLC after stem cell transplant predicted organ response in AL patients. Kumar et al. [24] recommended using the difference between the involved FLC (monoclonal FLC) and "uninvolved" FLC as a way to account for reduced renal clearance, and that a 90 % decrease in this FLC difference (dFLC) predicted better survival. In a detailed study of the relationship between dFLC and clinical features in 730 patients with newly diagnosed AL, it was found that the overall survival was shorter among those with a higher dFLC, and in multivariate analysis, dFLC was independent of other prognostic factors. In addition to dFLC correlating with survival, the type of light chain impacted the spectrum of organ involvement [25].

In summary, the quantitation of serum FLC has proved to be a useful biomarker in the monoclonal gammopathies in general and in AL in particular. The rFLC in conjunction with serum IFE defines a sensitive diagnostic screen for AL and reduces the need for urine in the screening algorithm, the differences of serum FLC (dFLC) concentrations independently predicts survival, and the iFLC or dFLC provides a simple way to monitor the disease process and hematologic response.

Future Directions

The greatest potential for future gains in laboratory testing for AL will come from methods that increase specificity for AL. The combination of IFE and rFLC has nearly 99 % sensitivity for detecting cases of AL, but the specificity of these findings is relatively poor. This lack of specificity comes from our current inability to assess the amylogenic nature of the monoclonal protein. Investigations into this subject are numerous, yet a single unifying feature of the proteins responsible for AL plaque formation has been elusive. Although the LC amyloid-forming propensity has been traditionally attributed to the LC variable region, fibrils also contain full-length LC comprising both variable-joining V(L) and constant C(L) regions. Recent studies are demonstrating the importance of the constant regions in amyloid formation [26, 27]. In addition, the role of Amyloid P component (AP) and apolipoprotein E (Apo E), which are known to be highly associated with almost all amyloid deposits, is still unfolding. Recent advances in mass spectroscopy proteomics are giving us deeper chemical insight to the nature of the light chains and associated amylogenic proteins. Perhaps when the chemical nature of these entities become known, it may be possible to risk-stratify patients with monoclonal immunoglobulins in regard to amyloid formation.

References

1. Kyle RA, et al. Prevalence of monoclonal gammopathy of undetermined significance. N Engl J Med. 2006;354(13):1362–9.
2. Kyle RA, et al. A long-term study of prognosis in monoclonal gammopathy of undetermined significance. N Engl J Med. 2002;346(8):564–9.
3. Landgren O, et al. Risk of monoclonal gammopathy of undetermined significance (MGUS) and subsequent multiple myeloma among African American and white veterans in the United States. Blood. 2006;107(3):904–6.
4. Rajkumar SV, Gertz MA, Kyle RA. Primary systemic amyloidosis with delayed progression to multiple myeloma. Cancer. 1998;82(8):1501–5.
5. Madan S, et al. Clinical features and treatment response of light chain (AL) amyloidosis diagnosed in patients with previous diagnosis of multiple myeloma. Mayo Clin Proc. 2010;85(3):232–8.
6. Steensma DP. "Congo" red: out of Africa? Arch Pathol Lab Med. 2001;125(2):250–2.
7. Hoffman JE, Hassoun H, Landau H, Comenzo RL. Coincindal gammopathies in patients with systemic amyloidosis and transthyretin gene mutations. Proceedings of the 52nd ASH annual meeting, Orlando, FL; 2010.
8. Strege RJ, Saeger W, Linke RP. Diagnosis and immunohistochemical classification of systemic amyloidosis. Report of 43 cases in an unselected autopsy series. Virchows Arch. 1998;433(1):19–27.
9. Gertz MA, Lacy MQ, Dispenzieri A. Amyloidosis: recognition, confirmation, prognosis, and therapy. Mayo Clin Proc. 1999;74(5):490–4.
10. Bradwell AR, et al. Highly sensitive, automated immunoassay for immunoglobulin free light chains in serum and urine. Clin Chem. 2001;47(4):673–80.
11. Katzmann JA, et al. Serum reference intervals and diagnostic ranges for free kappa and free lambda immunoglobulin light chains: relative sensitivity for detection of monoclonal light chains. Clin Chem. 2002;48(9):1437–44.
12. Barnidge DR, et al. Using mass spectrometry to monitor monoclonal immunoglobulins in patients with a monoclonal gammopathy. J Proteome Res. 2014;13(3):1419–27.
13. Drayson M, et al. Serum free light-chain measurements for identifying and monitoring patients with nonsecretory multiple myeloma. Blood. 2001;97(9):2900–2.
14. Lachmann HJ, et al. Outcome in systemic AL amyloidosis in relation to changes in concentration of circulating free immunoglobulin light chains following chemotherapy. Br J Haematol. 2003;122(1):78–84.
15. Abraham RS, et al. Quantitative analysis of serum free light chains. A new marker for the diagnostic evaluation of primary systemic amyloidosis. Am J Clin Pathol. 2003;119(2):274–8.
16. Dispenzieri A, et al. Absolute values of immunoglobulin free light chains are prognostic in patients with primary systemic amyloidosis undergoing peripheral blood stem cell transplantation. Blood. 2006;107(8):3378–83.
17. Katzmann JA, et al. Diagnostic performance of quantitative kappa and lambda free light chain assays in clinical practice. Clin Chem. 2005;51(5):878–81.
18. Bradwell AR, et al. Serum test for assessment of patients with Bence Jones myeloma. Lancet. 2003;361(9356):489–91.
19. Katzmann JA, et al. Elimination of the need for urine studies in the screening algorithm for monoclonal gammopathies by using serum immunofixation and free light chain assays. Mayo Clin Proc. 2006;81(12):1575–8.
20. Palladini G, et al. Identification of amyloidogenic light chains requires the combination of serum-free light chain assay with immunofixation of serum and urine. Clin Chem. 2009;55(3):499–504.
21. Katzmann JA. Screening panels for monoclonal gammopathies: time to change. Clin Biochem Rev. 2009;30(3):105–11.
22. Dispenzieri A, et al. Prevalence and risk of progression of light-chain monoclonal gammopathy of undetermined significance: a retrospective population-based cohort study. Lancet. 2010;375(9727):1721–8.
23. Gertz MA, et al. Definition of organ involvement and treatment response in immunoglobulin light chain amyloidosis (AL): a consensus opinion from the 10th international symposium on amyloid and amyloidosis, Tours, France, 18–22 April 2004. Am J Hematol. 2005;79(4):319–28.
24. Kumar SK, et al. Changes in serum-free light chain rather than intact monoclonal immunoglobulin levels predicts outcome following therapy in primary amyloidosis. Am J Hematol. 2011;86(3):251–5.
25. Kumar S, et al. Serum immunoglobulin free light-chain measurement in primary amyloidosis: prognostic value and correlations with clinical features. Blood. 2010;116(24):5126–9.
26. Yamamoto K, et al. The amyloid fibrils of the constant domain of immunoglobulin light chain. FEBS Lett. 2010;584(15):3348–53.
27. Klimtchuk ES, et al. The critical role of the constant region in thermal stability and aggregation of amyloidogenic immunoglobulin light chain. Biochemistry. 2010;49(45):9848–57.

Bone Marrow Biopsy and Its Utility in the Diagnosis of AL Amyloidosis

John C. Lee, Lawreen H. Connors, and Carl J. O'Hara

Bone Marrow Biopsy Procedure and General Findings

A bone marrow core biopsy should be at least 1.0–1.5 cm in length and contain adequate cellularity for optimal evaluation. Of note, subcortical bone marrow may be disproportionately hypocellular and may not be representative. At our institution, bone marrow biopsies are fixed in a formalin-based fixative B-Plus Fix (Gorilla Scientific) for at least 4 h, decalcified with RapidCal-Immuno (BBC Biochemical) for 30 min, and then washed under running water for 10 min before loading onto the tissue processor. Bone marrow aspirates are not typically indicated for AL amyloidosis. Histomorphology is more

Supported by National Institutes of Health, RO1AG031804 (L.H.C), the Young Family Amyloid Research Fund, and the Amyloid Research Fund at Boston University School of Medicine.

J.C. Lee, MD (✉)
Departments of Pathology and Laboratory Medicine,
Boston University School of Medicine,
Boston, MA 02118, USA
e-mail: JohnCho.Lee@bmc.org

L.H. Connors, PhD • C.J. O'Hara, MD
Departments of Pathology and Laboratory Medicine,
Boston University School of Medicine,
Boston, MA 02118, USA

Amyloidosis Center, Boston University School of Medicine, Boston, MA 02118, USA
e-mail: lconnors@bu.edu; Carl.Ohara@bmc.org

accurate than cytomorphology in the assessment for amyloid and enumeration of plasma cells. Amyloid identification is more obvious on a hematoxylin and eosin (H&E) stained core biopsy compared to a Wright-Giemsa stained aspirate smear. In addition, accurate enumeration of plasma cells on aspirate smears is often limited by the cell count differential and the fact that plasma cells often cluster around vessels, which are obscured in the thick part of spicules. We do not routinely perform bone marrow aspiration unless there is some other reason to do so, that is, suspected myelodysplasia or concerns for a B-cell lymphoma with plasmacytic differentiation.

The general appearance of the bone marrow on H&E stain is essentially unremarkable in AL amyloidosis (Fig. 26.1). In a review of 100 bone marrow biopsies, we observed relatively normal trilineage hematopoiesis [1]. While the overall cellularity tends to be within normal limits on initial diagnosis, hypocellularity is not uncommon especially among older patients and those who have received prior chemotherapy. The myeloid and erythroid elements are usually present in normal numbers with a normal myeloid to erythroid ratio of 1–3:1 [1]. The myeloid and erythroid elements also exhibit normal maturation [1]. Megakaryocytes are typically present in normal numbers and exhibit normal morphology [1]. Occasionally isolated aggregates of small lymphocytes are seen, especially in elderly patients, which on further workup usually prove

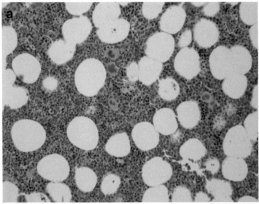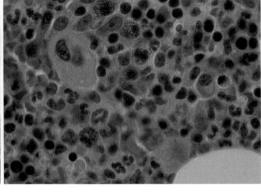

Fig. 26.1 H&E-stained (**a**) normocellular bone marrow (60 % cellularity) from a 41-year-old woman with AL amyloidosis and (**b**) normal hematopoietic bone marrow exhibiting normal maturation of myeloid and erythroid elements, normal megakaryocytes, and rare mature plasma cells

to be nonspecific and reactive [1]. Plasma cells are often minimally to mildly increased in AL amyloidosis [1]. However, identifying a mild plasmacytosis is often difficult on the H&E stain. The plasma cells are often singly scattered, but occasionally occur as small clusters both around and away from blood vessels [1]. In addition, they show mature morphology with clumped chromatin and absent to inconspicuous nucleoli [1]. Enumerating plasma cells is best done using CD138 immunohistochemistry (IHC) [1].

Detecting Amyloid Deposits

Amyloid can be suspected on H&E stain as a lightly eosinophilic, amorphous, "smudgy" deposit seen particularly within arterioles. The deposits often obscure the nuclei of arteriole smooth muscle cells. Occasionally, the degree of amyloid deposition is more advanced with involvement beyond the arteriole and infiltration into the bone marrow interstitium. In a few cases, the extent of amyloid deposition is so severe with geographic deposits replacing entire intertrabecular spaces. Interstitial amyloid deposits, especially when they are not associated with a vessel, should be differentiated from "bone dust" (an artifact seen as the result of the bone marrow biopsy procedure), fibrin, and serous fat atrophy.

Congo red is the most specific stain for amyloid and yields the characteristic orange/pink or "salmon" color [2]. We have devised a scale to convey the presence and degree of amyloid deposition that ranges from no amyloid deposition (0), amyloid localized to blood vessels (1+), and involvement of the interstitium less than two high power fields in size (2+) or greater than two high power fields in size (3+) (Fig. 26.2) [3]. For gold standard confirmation, the Congo red stain demonstrates the characteristic "apple green" birefringence when viewed under polarized light (Fig. 26.3) [2]. Congo red can be particularly helpful in detecting amyloid deposition in the periosteum, where clearance likely takes longer compared to the bone marrow and other organs. Mimics such as "bone dust" can appear Congophilic; however, it will not demonstrate "apple green" birefringence with polarized light. Also of note, not all birefringence is the same, for example collagen fibers in lamellar bone will emit a "silvery" birefringence in contrast to the "apple green" birefringence seen in amyloid.

In our case series of 462 bone marrow biopsies from AL amyloidosis patients, 268 had amyloid deposition in the bone marrow whereas 194 did not (Table 26.1). Of the 268 bone marrows showing demonstrable amyloid involvement, 74 % had 1+, 15 % had 2+, and 11 % had 3+ involvement. We have come to find that this grading scale has no predictive ability for hemato-

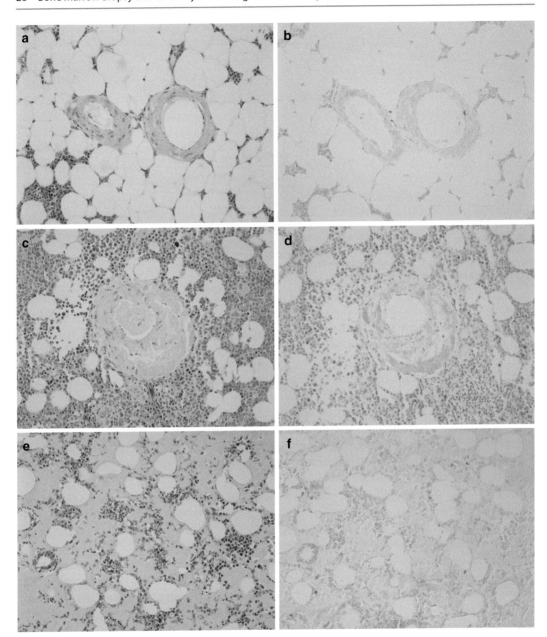

Fig. 26.2 (**a**) H&E and (**b**) *Congo red* appearance of amyloid deposit present in blood vessel (1+). (**c**) H&E and (**d**) *Congo red* appearance of amyloid deposit present in blood vessels with focal infiltration into the bone marrow interstitium (2+). (**e**) H&E and (**f**) *Congo red* appearance of diffuse amyloid deposit present in the bone marrow interstitium (3+)

logic status, bone marrow stem cell mobilization after administering colony stimulating factor, bone marrow engraftment after ablative chemotherapy, or degree of involvement or function in other organs. Lastly, bone marrow amyloid deposition can be seen in non-AL amyloidosis such as AA type amyloidosis [3]. Hence, finding amyloid deposition in the bone marrow is usually, but not always, attributable to an amyloidogenic plasma cell clone (AL amyloidosis).

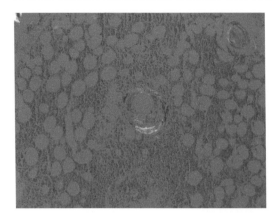

Fig. 26.3 *Congo red* stain of a blood vessel showing amyloid deposition emitting *apple green* birefringence using polarizing light microscopy. Note the contrasting silvery birefringence seen with the bone trabeculae

Table 26.1 Bone marrow core biopsy analysis in 462 newly diagnosed and untreated cases of AL amyloidosis

Congo red	
Positive, *n* (%)	268 (58)
1+	198 (43)
2+	40 (9)
3+	30 (6)
Negative, *n* (%)	194 (42)
% Plasma cells, median (range)	10 (<5–25)
Clonality testing	
Positive, *n* (%)	407 (88)
Kappa	102 (22)
Lambda	305 (66)
Negative, *n* (%)	55 (12)

Establishing a Diagnosis of a Plasma Cell Neoplasm

In AL amyloidosis, demonstrating the clonality [1, 4–6] and measuring the volume [5, 6] of plasma cells are the most important parameters from the bone marrow biopsy in facilitating the diagnosis [1, 4–6] and predicting prognosis [5, 6], respectively. Plasma cells can be identified on H&E stain, but precise enumeration is difficult especially when dealing with small volumes. Unlike multiple myeloma, the plasma cell volume in AL amyloidosis is often low and is on average around 10 % of all nucleated cells (Table 26.1). Our ability to enumerate plasma cells in the face of such low volumes has been greatly enhanced with the use of IHC directed at the CD138 antigen, a marker specific for plasma cells in the bone marrow (Fig. 26.4). IHC with CD138 highlights all plasma cells including the amyloidogenic clone and normal plasma cells. Rarely, amyloid may show nonspecific "sticky" staining with CD138 IHC, which may make plasma cell enumeration difficult especially when amyloid deposits are geographic. As an alternative, MUM1 IHC can be used in these situations in enumerating plasma cells. Of the few cases in which we have used MUM1, the amyloid deposits have not shown nonspecific staining.

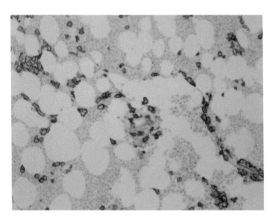

Fig. 26.4 IHC stain for CD138 highlighting plasma cells estimated to comprise 5–10 % of the bone marrow nucleated cell cellularity

Identification of a plasma cell clone requires the demonstration of either kappa or lambda light chain predominance. Plasma cells can only express a single light chain and there are up to three times as many kappa expressing plasma cells as lambda (which is applicable to both bone marrow and extramedullary sites). The normal kappa:lambda ratio is 1–3:1 based on the fact that a B-cell will try to rearrange both kappa light chain genes before attempting to rearrange either of the lambda light chain genes. A mixture of plasma cells with a kappa:lambda ratio of 1–3:1 is presumably polyclonal. Light chain predominance is seen when either the kappa:lambda ratio exceeds 3:1 or a kappa:lambda ratio is less than

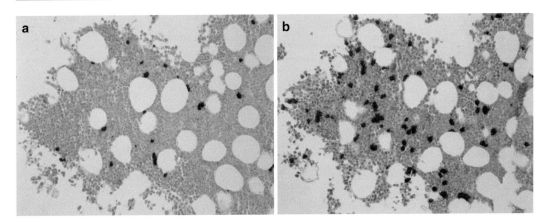

Fig. 26.5 (a) CISH stain for kappa light chain showing distinct *blue-black* staining of plasma cells. (b) CISH staining for lambda light chain on the same case. A tan- dem comparison shows that there is a lambda light chain predominance, which is consistent with the presence of a lambda-restricted plasma cell neoplasm

1:1, denoting either kappa or lambda light chain predominance, respectively [1]. Once light chain predominance is established, it can then be presumed that there is a light chain-restricted clone of the same type upsetting the normal kappa:lambda ratio.

Kappa and lambda light chains can either be stained by targeting the protein (IHC) or the messenger RNA (colorimetric in situ hybridization or CISH). The favored modality of light chain staining is CISH rather than IHC (Fig. 26.5) [7]. In CISH, oligonucleotide probes are directed against the conserved regions of the kappa and lambda light chain messenger RNA [7]. These probes are coupled to a chromogen, which is visualized as blue-black pigment [7]. IHC against the kappa and lambda light chain protein is fraught with nonspecific staining, especially for formalin-based fixatives [1, 7]. Determination of either kappa or lambda light chain predominance requires a tandem comparison of the cellular staining volume seen with kappa versus lambda. In rare cases, amyloid may show dual nonspecific "sticky" staining for both kappa and lambda CISH. If there are geographic amyloid deposits showing nonspecific staining for both kappa and lambda CISH, demonstrating light chain predominance can be difficult or even impossible.

Of the 462 bone marrow biopsies from newly diagnosed and untreated patients with AL amyloidosis who have had clonality studies done in our clinic, 88 % showed a demonstrable plasma cell neoplasm compared to 12 % in which a plasma cell neoplasm was not demonstrable by bone marrow biopsy (Table 26.1). Of the 88 % with a demonstrable plasma cell neoplasm, 66 % were lambda-restricted and 22 % were kappa-restricted, a finding that was consistent with other published reports [4]. An example of a pre- and posttreatment bone marrow evaluation from a patient is shown in Fig. 26.6. The pretreatment bone marrow clearly shows a lambda-restricted plasma cell clone, whereas the posttreatment bone marrow shows polyclonal staining.

Demonstrating the presence of a plasma cell clone can be challenging at times especially for cases with limited total plasma cell volume (5 % or less) and for kappa-restricted cases. However, it is fortuitous in AL amyloidosis that 75 % of cases are of lambda type. Demonstrating lambda light chain predominance is easier than kappa because any excess of lambda over kappa is consistent with a lambda-restricted plasma cell clone. The kappa-restricted cases (25 % of cases) are often more difficult to establish, especially when the kappa:lambda ratio is between 3 and 5:1. Currently at our institution, the presence of light chain predominance is determined by "eye-balling." However, in the future, more objective methods can be instituted such as computerized

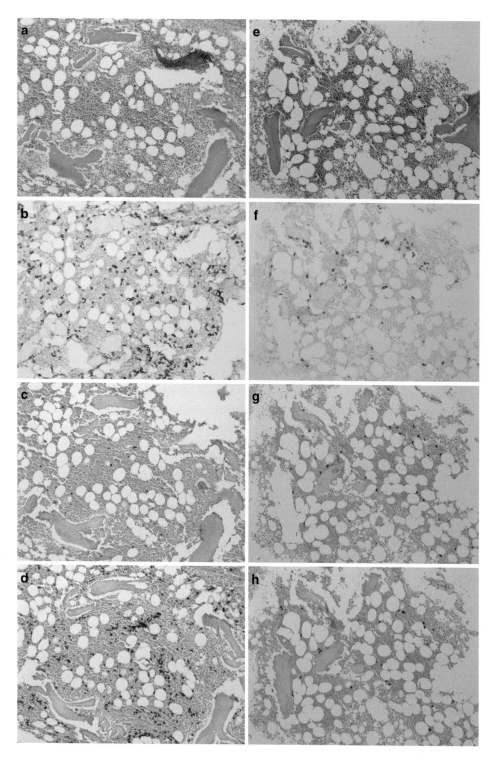

Fig. 26.6 Bone marrow biopsy samples from a 50-year-old woman with AL amyloidosis from pretreatment (*left*) and posttreatment (*right*). The pretreatment bone marrow (**a**) H&E is normal to mildly hypercellular, (**b**) CD138 IHC highlights plasma cells accounting for 5–10 % of cellularity, (**c**) CISH staining of plasma cells for kappa light chain, and (**d**) lambda light chain shows a kappa:lambda ratio of 1:10 consistent with a plasma cell neoplasm. The posttreatment bone marrow (**e**) is normal in cellularity, (**f**) CD138 IHC highlights plasma cells accounting for <5 % cellularity, (**g**) CISH staining of plasma cells for kappa light chain, and (**h**) lambda light chain shows a kappa:lambda ratio of 1–2:1 consistent with no evidence of a plasma cell neoplasm

image staining quantification, which is widely being used for receptor expression analysis in breast cancer for targeted drug therapy.

Comparison of Bone Marrow Biopsy with Serum/Urine Immunofixation Electrophoresis and Serum-Free Light Chain Assay

In a patient with amyloidosis, demonstration of a monoclonal gammopathy and/or plasma cell neoplasm is instrumental in typing the amyloidosis as AL-type [2]. We retrospectively compared diagnostic modalities used to detect a monoclonal gammopathy or plasma cell neoplasm by analyzing results from serum and urine immunofixation electrophoresis (IFE) and bone marrow biopsy IHC from the initial evaluation of confirmed AL amyloidosis patients [8]. A monoclonal gammopathy was found in 76 % of patients on serum IFE and 88 % on urine IFE [8]. When combining the serum and urine IFE, a monoclonal gammopathy was present in 96 % of patients [8]. The bone marrow biopsy CISH showed a plasma cell neoplasm in 89 % of patients [8]. Bone marrow CISH is less sensitive than serum and urine IFE in that the plasma cell neoplasm has to be large enough to create a shift in the overall kappa:lambda ratio [8].

Serum-free light chains were also compared with serum/urine IFE and bone marrow CISH results [8]. When combining those who had an elevated free lambda light chain with known lambda disease (as determined by IFE or IHC) and those who had an elevated free kappa light chain with known kappa disease, 94 % of patients had a respective elevated free light chain [8]. However, 33 % of patients had elevated free light chain of the opposite isotype, which is commonly seen in the setting of renal insufficiency [8]. Rather than looking at free light chain levels, greater specificity (but lower sensitivity) is afforded by using the free light chain ratio [8]. This is evident by an abnormal kappa:lambda free light chain ratio (low in known lambda disease and high in known kappa disease) being seen in 75 % of patients [8].

Flow Cytometry

Flow cytometry can be useful in the evaluation for plasma cell neoplasms. Flow cytometry is most helpful when results show light chain restriction in the plasma cells. Unlike B-cells, which express light chains as part of the surface immunoglobulin, plasma cells contain intracellular light chains. As a result, light chain analysis in plasma cells requires cytoplasmic permeabilization. Flow cytometry can also be helpful in demonstrating an abnormal plasma cell phenotype. Normal plasma cells are CD45−, CD19+, CD20−, and CD56−. However, if there is a deviation from this phenotype (particularly CD56+), this can be used to support a diagnosis of a plasma cell neoplasm.

Despite the potential usefulness of flow cytometry in plasma cell neoplasms, there are also many limitations, particularly in AL amyloidosis. Flow cytometry always underestimates plasma cell volume, due to the fact that plasma cells are fragile and susceptible to rupture. If plasma cell volume is low to begin with, as is often the case in AL amyloidosis, there may be an insufficient number of plasma cells remaining for analysis. In addition, our experience with light chain analysis on cytoplasmic immunoglobulin has shown that these studies can be technically challenging, difficult to interpret, and may not always yield successful results. Lastly, we have found that interpreting and demonstrating an aberrant plasma cell phenotype is not always straightforward, even when attempting to assess aberrant CD56 expression.

There are only a few published reports evaluating the utility of flow cytometry in AL amyloidosis. One group used an aberrant plasma cell phenotype: CD19− and CD56+, as a definition for monotypic plasma cells [9]. Their series included ten untreated AL amyloidosis patients, four positive controls or monoclonal gammopathy of undetermined significance (MGUS) patients, and eight negative control patients with no paraprotein [9]. In their series, the presence of an aberrant plasma cell population was statistically significantly higher in the AL amyloidosis compared to the negative control and even the

MGUS groups [9]. However, all patients, even the negative control patients, had some degree of an "aberrant" plasma cell population albeit very low [9]. In another study, both aberrant plasma cell phenotype and light chain analysis were analyzed in a series of 35 AL amyloidosis patients, most of whom were previously treated [10]. Based on aberrant plasma cell phenotype (CD56+, CD19−, and/or CD45+) or light chain restriction, they were able to detect a plasma cell clone in 34 of 35 patients [10]. However, in their study, they do not exactly specify how many or which of the abnormal phenotypic parameters were used in determining the presence of a plasma cell clone [10]. In addition, they did not specify how many of the cases with a plasma cell clone were determined from light chain analysis [10].

We generally do not perform bone marrow aspirates for flow cytometry on our AL amyloidosis patients, unless there is concern for a B-cell lymphoma with plasmacytic differentiation, that is, an IgM paraprotein. Rarely, B-cell lymphomas with plasmacytic differentiation may secrete an amyloidogenic paraprotein. Albeit rare, the most common B-cell lymphoma with plasmacytic differentiation secreting an amyloidogenic protein in the bone marrow is a lymphoplasmacytic lymphoma; in extranodal sites, it is a marginal zone lymphoma. The presence of monotypic B-cells with the same light chain restriction seen in B-cells (determined by flow cytometry) and plasma cells (determined by either flow cytometry or CISH) is a very helpful finding in the diagnosis of a B-cell lymphoma with plasmacytic differentiation. In addition to light chain analysis, the plasma cell component of a B-cell lymphoma essentially shows the same phenotypic maturation pattern seen in normal plasma cells described previously.

Genetic Pathogenesis of AL Amyloidosis

Recent advances in basic science research in multiple myeloma and MGUS have contributed much to our understanding of AL amyloidosis. One important recent finding is the identification of cyclin D dysregulation as an early unifying patho-

genic event in multiple myeloma [11]. There are numerous translocations seen in multiple myeloma, many of which either directly involve a cyclin D gene or genes involved in regulating cyclin D. These same translocations are also seen in AL amyloidosis. For instance, t(11;14) (q13q32), which involves the *CCND1* (encodes the cyclin D1 protein) and immunoglobulin heavy chain *IGH* genes, was first described in mantle cell lymphoma, later seen in multiple myeloma, and has been more recently described in AL amyloidosis [12–15]. Translocations t(4;14) (p16.3q32) [14, 16] and t(14;16)(q32q23) [14, 15] have also been described in AL amyloidosis, after previous discovery in multiple myeloma. The former is involved in a translocation between either the *FGFR3* and *MMSET* (both found on 4p16.3) and the *IGH* gene, and the latter is involved in a translocation between the *c-MAF* and *IGH* gene. Both of these translocations modulate cyclin D2 expression.

Interestingly, findings from cytogenetic studies can give rise to questions which can be addressed by IHC studies. We evaluated the expression of the cyclin D proteins in AL amyloidosis using IHC [17]. We evaluated cyclin D1, D2, and D3 protein expression in light chain-restricted plasma cells using a double stain that involved light chain CISH followed by cyclin D IHC [17]. The double stains were performed in tandem with both kappa and lambda CISH being performed for each cyclin D: D1, D2, and D3; for every patient in our series [17]. The cyclin D profiles in our patient series (newly diagnosed as well as treated patients) are summarized in Table 26.2 [17]. A figure showing our double stain is shown in Fig. 26.7 [17].

Table 26.2 Cyclin D1, D2, and D3 positivity in 34 cases of both newly diagnosed/untreated cases as well as previously diagnosed/treated cases of AL amyloidosis

	Cyclin D1	Cyclin D2	Cyclin D3
Positive cases (%)	18 (53 %)	5 (15 %)	1 (3 %)
Kappa-restricted (%)	3 (9 %)	1 (3 %)	0 (0 %)
Lambda-restricted (%)	15 (44 %)	2 (6 %)	0 (0 %)
Biclonal (%)	0 (0 %)	2 (6 %)	1 (3 %)

Total cases = 34

Fig. 26.7 Kappa/lambda
CISH and cyclin D IHC
double staining. (**a**) One
the left, cyclin D1 IHC
shows both nuclear and
cytoplasmic positivity; in
the middle, kappa CISH
and cyclin D1 IHC double
staining; on the right,
lambda CISH and cyclin
D1 IHC double staining;
overall cyclin D1 positivity
is restricted to the lambda
plasma cells. (**b**) On the
left, cyclin D2 IHC shows
nuclear positivity; in the
middle, kappa CISH and
cyclin D2 IHC double
staining; on the right,
lambda CISH and cyclin
D2 IHC double staining;
overall cyclin D2 positivity
is restricted to the kappa
plasma cells. (**c**) On the
left, cyclin D3 IHC shows
nuclear positivity; in the
middle, kappa CISH and
cyclin D3 IHC double
staining; on the right,
lambda CISH and cyclin
D3 IHC double staining;
overall cyclin D3 positivity
is seen in both kappa (rare)
and lambda (more
frequent) plasma cells

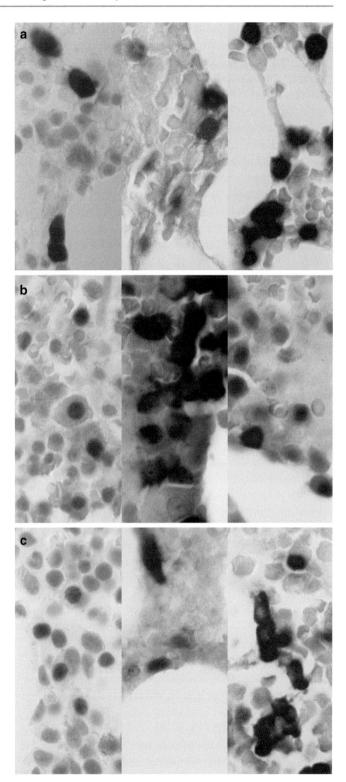

As for numerical chromosome abnormalities, the same abnormalities or aneuploidies seen in multiple myeloma are also seen in AL amyloidosis using multiple myeloma fluorescent *in situ* hybridization (FISH) panels [18]. For instance, monosomy 13 or 13q deletion is commonly seen in multiple myeloma and also frequently seen in AL amyloidosis [13]. Of note, karyotypes derived from both unstimulated and plasma cell mitogen-stimulated cultures are not sensitive in detecting cytogenetic changes in AL amyloidosis due to low plasma cell volume and proliferation. All of these previously described cytogenetic changes have been seen as a result of interphase FISH, which is much more sensitive than karyotype. However, other yet-to-be-discovered aneuploidies and abnormalities may exist that are not currently known due to the absence of a FISH probe. FISH is limited by the number and types of probes found within a panel.

Some cytogenetic abnormalities have been tied to prognosis in AL amyloidosis, much in the same way for multiple myeloma with cytogenetics being a major source for prognostication. For instance, t(11;14)(q13q32) has been associated with a worse prognosis in AL amyloidosis [15], which contrasts with the good prognosis seen in multiple myeloma [19, 20].

Despite the many similarities in AL amyloidosis and multiple myeloma with respect to both structural and numerical cytogenetic abnormalities, these diseases are distinctly different. AL amyloidosis is characterized by very low plasma cell proliferation and a low but steady production of an amyloidogenic paraprotein which forms fibrils that accumulate as deposits in various organs causing dysfunction. In contrast, multiple myeloma is characterized by higher plasma cell proliferation and high paraprotein production which gives rise to complications such as anemia, renal failure, lytic bone lesions, hypercalcemia, and suppression of nonclonal plasma cells. There are also intermediate cases of AL amyloidosis with higher plasma cell volume and multiple myeloma-type (CRAB) symptoms. Additional pathogenic events awaiting discovery may someday account for the duality between AL amyloidosis and multiple myeloma as well as the spectrum of presentation between these two related but different diseases.

Summary

The bone marrow is the site of the amyloidogenic plasma cell clone and light chain production in AL amyloidosis. A bone marrow core biopsy carries great importance in definitively establishing a diagnosis and defining the extent of a plasma cell neoplasm. Bone marrow core biopsies should be obtained at the initial visit for confirming a diagnosis of AL amyloidosis and establishing baseline features. A bone marrow aspirate for flow cytometry or cytogenetic studies can also be supportive in the diagnosis of a plasma cell neoplasm or play a role in predicting prognosis, respectively. For those patients undergoing treatment, bone marrow biopsies should be obtained at intervals of 6–12 months following treatment. Assessing hematologic response to treatment is based on laboratory parameters including the bone marrow biopsy, serum and urine IFEs, serum-free light chain assay, and any markers of organ dysfunction for the respective effected organs.

References

1. Swan N, Skinner M, O'Hara CJ. Bone marrow core biopsy specimens in AL (primary) amyloidosis. A morphologic and immunohistochemical study of 100 cases. Am J Clin Pathol. 2003;120:610–6.
2. Falk RH, Comenzo RL, Skinner M. The systemic amyloidosis. N Engl J Med. 1997;337:898–909.
3. Sungur C, Sungur A, Ruacan S, et al. Diagnostic value of bone marrow biopsy in patients with renal disease secondary to familiar Mediterranean fever. Kidney Int. 1993;44:834–6.
4. Hasserjian RP, Goodman HJ, Lachmann HJ, Muzikansky A, Hawkins PN. Bone marrow findings correlate with clinical outcome in systemic AL amyloidosis patients. Histopathology. 2007;50:567–73.
5. Perfetti V, Colli Vignarelli M, Anesi E, et al. The degrees of plasma cell clonality and marrow infiltration adversely influence the prognosis of AL amyloidosis patients. Haematologica. 1999;84:218–21.

6. Pardanani A, Witzig TE, Schroeder G, et al. Circulating peripheral blood plasma cells as a prognostic indicator in patients with primary systemic amyloidosis. Blood. 2003;101:827–30.

7. Beck RC, Tubbs RR, Hussein M, Pettay J, Hsi ED. Automated colorimetric in situ hybridization (CISH) detection of immunoglobulin (Ig) light chain mRNA expression in plasma cell (PC) dyscrasias and non-Hodgkin lymphoma. Diagn Mol Pathol. 2003;12:14–20.

8. Akar H, Seldin DC, Magnani B, et al. Quantitative serum free light chain assay in the diagnostic evaluation of AL amyloidosis. Amyloid. 2005;12:210–5.

9. Matsuda M, Gono T, Shimojima Y, Hoshii Y, Ikeda S. Phenotypic analysis of plasma cells in bone marrow using flow cytometry in AL amyloidosis. Amyloid. 2003;10:110–6.

10. Paiva B, Vidriales MB, Perez JJ, et al. The clinical utility and prognostic value of multiparameter flow cytometry immunophenotyping in light-chain amyloidosis. Blood. 2011;117:1–6.

11. Bergsagel PL, Kuehl WM, Zhan F, Sawyer J, Barlogie B, Shaugnessy J. Cyclin D dysregulation: an early and unifying pathogenic event in multiple myeloma. Blood. 2005;106:296–303.

12. Hayman SR, Bailey RJ, Jalal SM, et al. Translocations involving the immunoglobulin heavy-chain locus are possibly early genetic events in patients with primary systemic amyloidosis. Blood. 2001;98:2266–8.

13. Harrison CJ, Mazzullo H, Ross FM, et al. Translocations of 14q32 and deletions of 13q14 are common chromosomal abnormalities in systemic amyloidosis. Br J Haematol. 2002;117:427–35.

14. Bochtler T, Hegenbart U, Cremer FW, et al. Evaluation of the cytogenetic aberration pattern in light chain amyloidosis as compared with monoclonal gammopathy of undetermined significance reveals common pathways of karyotypic instability. Blood. 2008;111:4700–5.

15. Bryce AH, Ketterling RP, Gertz MA, et al. Translocation t(11;14) and survival of patients with light chain (AL) amyloidosis. Haematologica. 2009;94:380–6.

16. Perfetti V, Coluccia AM, Intini D, et al. Translocation t(4;14)(p16.3;q32) is a recurrent genetic lesion in primary amyloidosis. Am J Clin Pathol. 2001;158:1599–603.

17. Lee JC, Wu H, Prokaeva T, et al. Expression of D-type cyclins in AL amyloidosis plasma cells. J Clin Pathol. 2012;65:1052–5.

18. Fonseca R, Ahmann GJ, Jalal SM, et al. Chromosomal abnormalities in systemic amyloidosis. Br J Haematol. 1998;103:704–10.

19. Fonseca R, Harrington D, Oken M, et al. Myeloma and the t(11;14)(q13;q32) represents a uniquely defined biological subset of patients. Blood. 2002;99:3735–41.

20. Moreau P, Facon T, Leleu X, et al. Recurrent 14q32 translocations determine the prognosis of multiple myeloma, especially in patients receiving intensive chemotherapy. Blood. 2002;100:1579–83.

Laboratory Methods for the Diagnosis of Hereditary Amyloidoses

27

S. Michelle Shiller, Ahmet Dogan, Kimiyo M. Raymond, and W. Edward Highsmith Jr.

Introduction

As described elsewhere in this volume, amyloid consists of fibrils composed of stacked proteins which have adopted a beta-pleated sheet conformation. The mechanism by which a protein which has substantial alpha helical character refolds into a configuration with a primarily beta-pleated sheet structure is unclear and is the subject of much ongoing research. It is clear, however, that specific amino acid substitutions in

S.M. Shiller, DO (✉)
Department of Laboratory Medicine and Pathology,
Mayo Clinic College of Medicine, 200 First
Street SW, Rochester, MN 55905, USA

Department of Surgical Pathology, Baylor University
Medical Center, 3500 Gaston Avenue, 5Y Wing,
Dallas, TX 75246, USA
e-mail: shirley.shiller@baylorhealth.edu

A. Dogan, MD, PhD
Departments of Pathology and Laboratory Medicine,
Memorial Sloan Kettering Cancer Center, 1275 York
Avenue, New York, NY 10065, USA
e-mail: dogana@mskcc.org

K.M. Raymond, MD • W.E. Highsmith Jr., PhD
Department of Laboratory Medicine and Pathology,
Mayo Clinic College of Medicine, 200 First
Street SW, Rochester, MN 55905, USA
e-mail: raymond.kimiyo@mayo.edu;
Highsmith.w@mayo.edu

a small number of circulating proteins can accelerate or facilitate this process.

All of the hereditary amyloidoses (also known as familial or systemic amyloidoses) are inherited in an autosomal dominant manner, as is the case for other "gain-of-function" mutations in disorders such as Huntington disease, myotonic dystrophy, or the spinocerebellar ataxias. The dominant inheritance of the familial amyloidoses has implications for family members of an affected individual. It is important to understand that siblings and children of an affected individual have a one in two chance of being affected themselves and may benefit from presymptomatic monitoring. Moreover, careful attention to the family history may reveal subclinical symptoms in one parent, which may or may not have received subsequent medical attention. However, even in the setting of a thorough family history, hereditary amyloidosis can be missed and attributed to more common diseases. Thus, after the identification of an amyloidogenic mutation in an individual, it is important to offer testing for at-risk family members so that appropriate monitoring can be carried out for mutation positive family members.

Clinically, it may be difficult to distinguish amyloidosis that is secondary to overproduction of immunoglobulin light chains (AL amyloid), age-related ATTR amyloidosis, or serum amyloid A (AA amyloid) from an amyloidosis that is hereditary in nature. As the treatment for the underlying cause of amyloidosis differs markedly for the different etiologies, it is critical that the amyloid be properly classified. Therapy for plasma cell disease can include chemotherapy and/or bone marrow transplant, and the therapy for AA amyloid involves addressing the underlying cause of inflammation, while the curative treatment for two varieties of familial amyloidosis, including the most common form due to mutant transthyretin (ATTR amyloid), is liver transplant.

To make a diagnosis, including identification of the protein being deposited as amyloid fibrils, it is typically necessary to obtain biopsy material from an affected organ or site. Most often, biopsies are obtained from either the bone marrow, subcutaneous fat (often of the abdomen), or the rectum. Following tissue acquisition, a variety of methods are used in identifying and characterizing amyloid protein, including Congo Red staining, immunoperoxidase staining of histological tissue, mass spectrometry, and genetic evaluation in cases of familial disease. Further, when clinical suspicion of amyloid is high, serum tests for TTR are available [1, 2]. A frequently described method of serum detection of hereditary TTR amyloid is a two-step process using nondenaturing gel electrophoresis in polyacrylamide gel (PAGE) followed by isoelectric focusing (IEF). The varying protein conformations resulting from genetic mutations in the *TTR* gene result in differing patterns of migration seen on IEF. Moreover, the banding patterns are unique to the specific mutation, which has been supported in follow-up genetic analysis [1, 2]. Though this has high specificity, it does not delineate all variants of *TTR* mutation, which do have varying phenotypic presentations and thus may be important clinically. Further, this method cannot be used for hereditary amyloid due to other genes.

While the majority of systemic amyloidosis is due to transthyretin (TTR) mutations, other genes involved in conferring aberrant protein folding with subsequent amyloid deposition have been identified. These additional genes have been documented in a substantially smaller number of individuals than TTR mutations and include ApoA1, ApoA2, gelsolin, lysozyme, and

fibrinogen alpha (FGA). While the most common symptom of amyloidogenic mutations in these genes is nephropathy, mutations in one, gelsolin, demonstrates a predisposition for cranial nerve tissue, lattice corneal dystrophy, and cutis laxia of the facial skin. As gelsolin amyloidosis was originally identified in a large Finnish family [3], and is more common, but not limited to individuals of Finnish descent, it is often referred to as Finnish amyloidosis.

The differential diagnosis of systemic amyloidosis includes light chain disease, Sjögren's syndrome, rheumatoid arthritis, other inflammatory conditions, β2-microglobulinemia, and Familial Mediterranean Fever, as well as other similar conditions. A discussion of a thorough diagnostic evaluation for these conditions is beyond the scope of this chapter. However, a few key laboratory tests can expedite the process: serum protein electrophoresis (assists in the diagnosis of light chain disease or β2-microglobulinemia), and the presence of antinuclear antibody and SSBLa > SSBRo by immunofluorescence for Sjögren's syndrome. The presence of rheumatoid factor raises suspicion for Rheumatoid Arthritis. Detection of serum amyloid A in amyloid deposits by immunohistochemistry elicits a definitive diagnosis of AA amyloid, or amyloid deposition of an inflammatory origin [4].

With respect to AL amyloidosis, serum protein electrophoresis (SPEP) is the classical method of working up this diagnosis, but ruling out coexisting hereditary amyloidosis through DNA interrogation is pivotal. One study showed that 24 % of individuals with hereditary amyloidosis may also demonstrate monoclonal immunoglobulins on SPEP [4]. In the study by Lachmann et al., all of the patients had less than 0.2 g/dL of immunoglobulins in the serum, and no kappa or lambda free light chains by urine protein electrophoresis. Comenzo et al.'s had similar findings, with 6 % of patients with a hereditary amyloidosis presenting with definitive monoclonal gammopathies in a subject population of similar size [5]. In the Lachmann et al.'s study, in addition to the monoclonal gammopathy by SPEP, the patients also demonstrated mutations in a variety of genes for hereditary amyloidosis, whereas in the Comenzo et al.'s study, all patients had *TTR* mutations with concomitant SPEP monoclonal gammopathy. In the absence of DNA analysis, these patients with hereditary amyloidosis masquerading with a monoclonal gammopathy would be misdiagnosed, and the improper clinical management could be implemented.

Mass Spectrometry in TTR

The recent advances in the identification of amyloid proteins in tissue, particularly formalin-fixed, paraffin-embedded material, are covered elsewhere in this volume. Here, we discuss screening for mutant TTR in serum samples. One technique to accomplish this analysis is through affinity chromatography protein isolation, followed by electron-spray mass spectrometry. The process begins by reducing plasma with 12.5 mM dithiothreitol, which removes the cysteine adducts to simplify the mass spectra. Next the plasma/dithiothreitol solution is injected to a column to sequester TTR, followed by elution with pH 2.5, 100 mM glycine/2 % acetic acid, and concentrated on a C4 column. Next the TTR is eluted from the column and introduced to the mass spectrometer (MS). This is a method of qualitative and quantitative investigation for the presence of TTR which includes relative proportions of wild type and mutant. Though this has high sensitivity and specificity, it does not delineate all variants of *TTR* mutation, particularly changes with relatively minimal mass shifts (less than 10 Da). Mass shifts that are this small may be indicated with a slightly wider peak, and can likely be detected with follow-up molecular genetic testing [6]. One of the larger mass shifts is a Gly to Trp or Trp to Gly change, which differs by 129 Da. If a shift is present of 256 Da or more, double mutation is suggested [6–9]. Follow-up confirmation of MS findings with gene sequencing is helpful. Further, this serum-based test for amyloidogenic protein deposition is limited to TTR amyloidosis and does not cover amyloidosis due to the other genes.

Genetic Testing in Amyloidosis

Genetic Evaluation

Gene sequencing is the gold standard to detect aberrations such as substitutions, and small deletions and insertions at the nucleotide level. In genetically heterogeneous diseases, sequencing is particularly useful. The familial amyloidoses display both genetic heterogeneity (multiple genes being involved in a disease) and allelic heterogeneity (multiple mutations in the sample gene being able to cause the disease).

The first step in any DNA sequencing is the extraction, or purification, of DNA, typically from a peripheral blood sample. Many platforms are available for DNA extraction. Following DNA extraction, the samples are prepared for PCR with primers specific to the gene of interest, and the standard PCR constituents (Taq polymerase, buffer, magnesium chloride, and PCR-grade water). Next, the PCR product is treated to remove unincorporated primers and nucleotides. The cleaned PCR product is next combined with a mixture of fluorescently labeled di-deoxynucleotide triphosphates and dNTPs (e.g., BigDye® terminators [Applied Biosystems]), sequencing buffer, PCR-grade water, and a thermostable DNA polymerase. After carrying out the sequencing reaction by thermal cycling and another purification step, this time removing unincorporated fluorescent material, the sample is analyzed by capillary electrophoresis. There are multiple software programs commercially available for base calling, alignments, and mutation detection. One widely used program is Mutation Surveyor® (Soft Genetics) (Fig. 27.1).

Genes Involved in Hereditary Amyloidosis

Notes on Nomenclature

The Human Genome Variation Society (HGVS) has proposed standard nomenclature for variation at both the nucleotide and the protein level (www.hgvs.org/mutnomen/). In this chapter, all

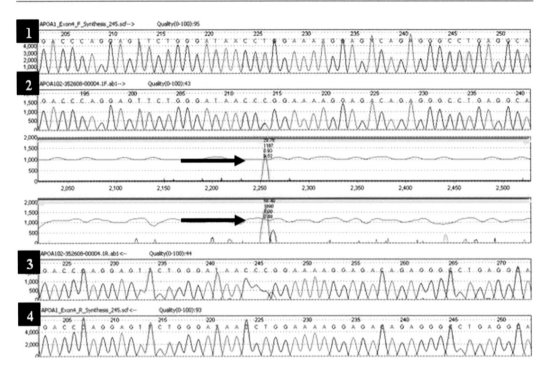

Fig. 27.1 Gene sequencing for ApoA1 showing c. 296T>C, p. Leu99Pro pathogenic mutation in exon 4. The *top* and *bottom* sequences (1 and 4) are the reference sequences against which the sample is compared. Sequences 2 and 3 are the patient sample. The *top* traces (1, 2) are sequenced in the forward direction, and the *bot-* *tom* trace (3, 4) in the reverse. The two *middle* traces are the subtraction plots between the reference sequence and the patient sample. The *pink peak* is the location of the mutation (*arrows*), indicating substitution of a cytosine for a thymine. This substitution can also be seen in the sequences of the patient sample

mutations and variants will be discussed referring to protein sequence, or amino acid changes. Previously, the standard nomenclature was to number the first amino acid of the mature, processed protein as amino acid number one. For secreted proteins (such as those involved in familial amyloidoses), this numbering system neglected the signal peptides and propeptides that are cleaved from the amino terminus after translation as the protein is being processed by the cell for secretion. The HGVS standard nomenclature now recommends that proteins be numbered starting with the initiator methionine as amino acid number one. All of the amino acid changes discussed here will use the HGVS standard nomenclature.

For example, the signal peptide of the TTR protein is 20 amino acids in length. One mutation seen in TTR amyloid is Cys30Arg (new nomenclature). Using historical nomenclature, the mutation is termed Cys10Arg (subtract 20 amino acids that account for the signal peptide in the new nomenclature to derive this). Apolipoprotein A1 (ApoA1) is an example of a protein with a signal peptide and a propeptide. The signal peptide is 18 amino acids in length, and the propeptide is 6. Hence, to extrapolate the historical nomenclature from the new nomenclature for a mutation in ApoA1, Gly50Arg would be Gly26Arg. Please refer to Table 27.1 for a listing of all genes and the conversions.

Transthyretin

The first protein identified in hereditary amyloidosis with amyloid deposition due to coding

Table 27.1 Table depicting nomenclature conversion from historical to new

Protein	Signal peptide/ propeptide	Example (historical → new)
TTR	20	Cys10Arg → Cys30Arg
ApoA1	18/6	Gly26Arg → Gly50Arg
ApoA2	18/5	Stop78S → Stop101S
Gelsolin A	27	Asp187Tyr → Asp214Tyr
Fibrinogen alpha	19	Arg554Leu → Arg573Leu
Lysozyme	18	W112R → W130R

The primary difference is that the new nomenclature includes all codons beginning with the initiating methionine, and the historical nomenclature utilizes only the mature protein. Hence, to convert to the new nomenclature requires adding the appropriate number of codons acting as signal peptides and propeptides, as indicated

sequence missense mutations was transthyretin (TTR). Notably, TTR is by far the most common protein and gene involved in familial amyloidosis, accounting for between 95 and 98 % of reported familial amyloid cases, and often presenting after the age of 50. TTR is a transport protein that has four exons, 127 amino acids, weighs 55 kDa, and is synthesized predominantly in the liver. The function of TTR is to carry thyroxine (T4) and to participate in the thyroxine–retinol binding protein complex. This function is important to bear in mind when testing for mutations in TTR since familial euthyroid hyperthyroxinemia can demonstrate a substitution in position 129 (Ala129Thr, Ala 129 Thr, Ala129Val) of the protein. These patients are clinically euthyroid, with normal free thyroid and triiodothyronine levels, but increased thyroxine due to the thyroxine-binding capacity of TTR [10]. Alternatively, when *TTR* is mutated, aberrant protein folding often results with deposition as described above and the clinical sequelae including most predominantly peripheral polyneuropathy, and/or cardiomyopathy (with or without eye and brain involvement).

Liver transplantation is the treatment of choice for patients with TTR amyloidosis, due to its predominant hepatic synthesis. Since this treatment is vastly different than the cytotoxic chemotherapeutic regimens and/or bone marrow transplant

indicated for AL amyloidosis, the correct diagnosis of these two disorders with supporting laboratory data is paramount. Also, senile amyloid deposition is often composed of wild-type TTR protein. In this case, the conversion of TTR into amyloid fibrils is not driven by pathogenic mutations, and gene sequencing is necessary to distinguish TTR type senile amyloid from a hereditary disorder.

More than 100 mutations have been reported in *TTR*, almost all of them being single base substitutions in the gene, located on chromosome 18 [11] (Fig. 27.2). Common single base substitutions include V50M, L75P, L78H, T80A, and Y134H [12]. A common three-nucleotide/single codon deletion is ΔVal142. Ethnic propensities exist for a number of TTR mutations [2, 13]. For example, M33I is seen in the German population; A45T, Y89I, and Q112K segregate amongst the Japanese. Variants common in the United States are D38N, A45S, F53C, W61L, T69P, L75Q, A101T, and R123S [2]. Phenotypic clustering is seen in some codon changes (Table 27.2), and Tyr89Ile is the only double nucleotide substitution documented to date. Specifically, Tyr89Ile is seen in the Japanese population, with cardiac and connective tissue involvement, and autonomic neuropathy [6].

V122I is another example of a variant with a strong ethnic predisposition, in this case with African American ancestry. Heterozygosity for this mutation is associated with cardiac amyloidosis, congestive heart failure, and mortality in African Americans, typically after the age of 70 [2, 13]. The frequency of the V122I variant is high in the African American population, approximately 4 %. It is interesting to note that this mutation has the same frequency as the most common cystic fibrosis mutation, deltaF508, in the Caucasian population. However, in contrast to the case of CF, where homozygosity for the common mutation is well appreciated, and indeed, is the most common disease-associated genotype, homozygosity for V122I has only infrequently been reported. A recent publication describes 13 homozygous cases—the largest case series reported to date.

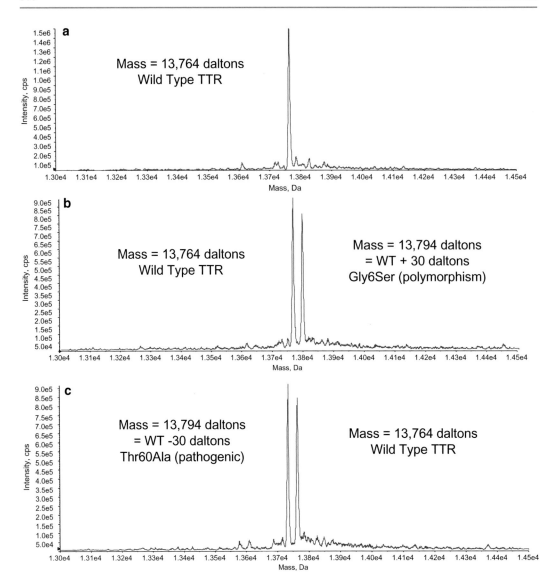

Fig. 27.2 Mass spectra of transthyretin (TTR) immunopu- rified from blood serum. Panel **a** is a normal TTR. Panel **b** shows TTR from an individual heterozygous for the normal TTR and the common Gly6Ser polymorphism. Panel **c** shows the spectra from an individual with hereditary TTR amyloidosis due to the pathogenic Phe44Leu mutation

These investigators found that homozygosity for the V122I mutation was associated with an earlier onset of disease, by approximately 10 years [14]. Whether the small number of reported cases of V122I homozygosity repre- sents a lack of ascertainment of cardiac disease in the elderly African American population, or whether it represents a penetrance that is sub- stantially less than 100 %, is an important ques- tion for future research.

Apolipoprotein A1

Apolipoprotein A1 (ApoA1), another protein involved with hereditary amyloidosis, contains four exons, 243 amino acids, weighs 28 kDa, and is located on chromosome 11q23–q24. ApoA1 is synthesized in the liver and small intestine, con- ferring a plasma protein that is the main protein of high-density lipoprotein particles and has a key role in lipoprotein metabolism. ApoA1 is

Table 27.2 Phenotypic correlations of TTR mutations along with segregation among particular geographic kindreds

Mutation	Clinical features	Geographic kindreds
Phe53Ile	Peripheral neuropathy, eye	Israel
Phe53Leu	Peripheral neuropathy, heart	USA
Phe53Val	Peripheral neuropathy	UK, Japan, China
Ala65Thr	Heart	USA
Ala65Asp	Heart, peripheral neuropathy	USA
Ala65Ser	Heart	Sweden
Ile104Asn	Heart, eye	USA
Ile104Thr	Heart, peripheral neuropathy	Germany, UK
Glu109Gln	Peripheral neuropathy, heart	Italy
Glu109Lys	Peripheral neuropathy, heart	USA
Val142Ile	Heart	USA
ΔVal142	Heart, peripheral neuropathy	USA
Val142Ala	Heart, eye, peripheral neuropathy	USA

Adapted from [17]

Table 27.3 Common ApoA1 mutations

Mutation	Clinical features
Gly50Arg	Peripheral neuropathy, nephropathy
Glu58Lys	Nephropathy
Leu84Arg	Nephropathy
Glu94_Trp96del	HTN, nephropathy
Trp74Arg	Nephropathy
Del84-85insVal/Thr	Hepatic
Leu88Pro	Nephropathy
Del94-96	Nephropathy
Phe95Tyr	Palate
Asn98fs	Nephropathy, gastrointestinal
Leu99Pro	Hepatic
Leu114Pro	Cardiomyopathy, cutaneous
Lys131del	Aortic intima
Ala178fs	Nephropathy
Leu194Pro	Laryngeal
Arg197Pro	Cardiomyopathy, cutaneous, laryngeal
Leu198Ser	Cardiomyopathy
Ala199Pro	Laryngeal
Leu202His	Cardiomyopathy, laryngeal

Adapted from [15–17]

important for the formation of high-density lipoprotein cholesterol esters, promoting efflux of cholesterol from cells [15, 16]. Consequently, mutations in ApoA1 can lead to one of two rare diseases of lipoprotein metabolism: primary hypoalphalipoproteinemia (Tangier's disease) or ApoA1 amyloidosis, which has no pathophysiology linked directly to lipoprotein metabolism, depending on the mutation. The predominant genetic changes seen in ApoA1 amyloidosis are nucleotide substitutions; however, two deletion mutations and deletion/insertion have been described. Most of the mutations are in-frame, with the exception of Asn122fs and Ala202fs. Hence, the mechanism of amyloid production for all of the ApoA1 mutations involves aberrant folding, and the unstable species produced with the Asn122fs and Ala202fs mutations is a truncated protein rather than a full length one.

The clinical presentation of amyloidosis consistent with ApoA1 involves the liver, kidney, larynx, skin, and myocardium most commonly and rarely the testes and adrenal glands [15]. The most common mutations to date include G50R, L99P, A197P, A199P, and L198S [15–17]. Most of these mutations are present in Northern Europeans. Specifically, G50R is common among British, Scandinavians, and North Americans, L99P in Italians, Germans, and North Americans, A197P in Americans and British, and L198S in Italian and Dutch individuals [16] (Table 27.3).

Apolipoprotein A2

Apolipoprotein A2 (ApoA2), similar to ApoA1, is an amyloidogenic protein involved in lipid metabolism. Unlike ApoA1, ApoA2 can be found in senile amyloidosis [18]. As is the case with TTR, gene sequencing is required to determine if ApoA2 deposition in a given case is due to deposition of a wild-type protein (senile amyloid) or a mutant one (familial amyloidosis). Structurally, it is a 77-amino acid, 17.4 kDa protein located on chromosome 1p21-1qter [19]. While comprised of four exons, three exons in ApoA2 are coding: exons 2, 3, and the 5′ end of exon 4. The Apo A2 gene is one of the more recently described forms of hereditary amyloid, with a clinical picture of early adult-onset, rapidly progressive renal failure [17]. There is no neuropathy

Table 27.4 Listing of common mutation for other amyloidogenic proteins

Protein	Mutation	Clinical features
ApoA2	Stop78Gly	Nephropathy
	Stop78Ser	Nephropathy
	Stop78Arg	Nephropathy
Gelsolin A	Asp214Asn	PN, LCD
	Asp214Tyr	PN
Fibrinogen alpha	Arg573Leu	Nephropathy
	Glu545Val	Nephropathy
	1629delG	Nephropathy
	1622delT	Nephropathy
Lysozyme	Ile74Thr	Nephropathy, petechiae
	Asp85His	Nephropathy
	Trp82Arg	Nephropathy
	Phe75Ile	Nephropathy

PN peripheral neuropathy, *LCD* lattice corneal dystrophy

associated with the abrupt renal failure, which occurs in the absence of proteinuria. Mutations in the stop codon are the common genetic change resulting in a 21-amino acid extension at the carboxy terminus of the mature protein [17]. All of these changes occur at codon 101 in exon 4 as follows: Stop101G, Stop101S, and Stop101R (Table 27.4). Geographically, these mutations are seen in North Americans, with the exception of Stop101R, which is also seen in Russians [17].

Gelsolin A

Gelsolin (GSN) protein is associated with actin metabolism. Also known as brevin, or, actin-depolymerizing factor, it acts to prevent toxicity due to the release of actin into the extracellular space in the presence of cell necrosis [20]. The gene is comprised of 17 exons and is located on chromosome 9q34 (centromeric to *ABL*); the protein weighs 82 kDa. In the setting of familial/hereditary amyloidosis, gelsolin variant disease presents with unique features of neuropathy, particularly of the cranial nerves. There are additional clinical features of gelsolin amyloidosis that merit clinical subclassification of the disease. The "Meretoja" subtype is associated with corneal dystrophy, and cutis laxia of facial skin is another clinically distin-

guishing feature [21, 22]. Known pathogenic mutations include D214N in individuals from Finland, North America, Denmark, and Japan, and D214Y (c. 654G>C) in individuals from Finland, Denmark, and the Czech Republic [21]. The D214N and D214Y mutations permit exposure of an otherwise masked cleavage site, which is the initial step of amyloid formation. Both of these mutations result in the production of an aberrant, 68-kDa fragment, likely a carboxy-terminal part of the protein which is suggested to be amyloidogenic [23].

The Meretoja subtype is associated with a single base mutation c. 654G>A (GAC>GAA), p. D214N (Asp214Asn). The pathogenic protein is comprised of 71 amino acids [21, 24]. Regardless of the genotype, the gelsolin variant of amyloid is classically associated with cranial neuropathy, possibly even bilateral, with additional phenotypic features rendering subclassification as described herein [22] (Table 27.4).

To date, only two pathogenic mutations in the gelsolin gene have been described, both at the same codon (above). A novel mutation was recently described in a case of renal amyloid [25]. Interestingly, although this novel missense change was at codon 194, 18 amino acids distant from the codon 214 mutations, when mapped onto the three-dimensional gelsolin crystal structure, it was noted to be adjacent to codon 214. Whether the mechanism of amyloidogenesis is similar to that seen in the codon 214 mutations will be an interesting avenue for future research.

Fibrinogen Alpha

Synthesized in the liver, fibrinogen is a plasma glycoprotein with three structural subunits: alpha (FGA), beta (FGB), and gamma (FGG). Most research regarding fibrinogen in general has been in the setting of hemostasis, where it has a primary functional role. There are two other rare diseases due to mutations in fibrinogen alpha that confer bleeding disorders: afibrinogenemia and dysfibrinogenemia. Afibrinogenemia has an absence of fibrinogen due to a truncating mutation, and dysfibrinogenemia has decreased fibrin production due to a mutation at the cleavage site for thrombin to convert inactive fibrinogen to fibrin. The mutations seen with bleeding are different than those seen in FGA amyloid. Fibrinogen alpha is located on chromosome 4q28, with 6 exons, and varying amino acid lengths as determined by alternative splicing.

Phenotypically, FGA amyloidosis is associated with visceral involvement, specifically renal, with the manifestations including hypertension, proteinuria, and subsequent azotemia [17]. Importantly, renal involvement in amyloid of this genetic origin is associated with rapidly progressive renal failure. Hence, early detection of amyloid with an FGA mutation permits consideration of liver transplant for curative treatment, perhaps avoiding the negative consequences of renal disease [26]. Historically, renal transplantation, which has also been performed, has not had long-term success; thus, this paradigm shift to hepatic transplantation, especially in light of the ability to detect the mutation, is a promising treatment alternative for patients. Thus far, neuropathy has not been seen with FGA amyloidosis, and cardiomyopathy is reported in one case. Hence, neurologic and cardiac involvement would be the exception rather than the rule at this point in time in diagnosing FGA amyloid [27].

To date, there are four common mutations associated with FGA amyloidosis: two point mutations with pathogenic single amino acid substitutions, and two single nucleotide deletions yielding a frameshift in DNA transcription, with subsequent premature termination of protein synthesis [17, 26, 28]. One point mutation, c. 4993 G>T, p. R573L has been identified in a Peruvian family, and another, c. 1674 A>T, p. E545V has been detected in individuals of American and Irish descent [11, 29]. Specifically, the E545V mutation is the one example of cardiac manifestations of FGA amyloid [27]. One deletion, 1629delG, the third base in codon 543, was detected in an American family with hereditary renal amyloidosis. Due to this mutation, a premature stop codon is created at codon 567. Individuals with the 1629delG mutation had a later onset of disease (later thirties and early forties) when compared to those with the R573L mutation [28]. Finally, early renal disease with terminal renal failure has been documented in

French kindred with a single nucleotide deletion c. 1622T, with subsequent frameshift mutation at codon 541 and, similar to 1629delG, premature termination of protein synthesis at codon 567 [26] (Table 27.4). This particular subtype, with its inherently aggressive sequelae, is particularly relevant to consideration of liver transplantation early in the course of disease.

Lysozyme

Lysozyme (LYZ) is an enzyme that catalyzes the hydrolysis of certain mucopolysaccharides of bacterial cell walls. Specifically, lysozyme catalyzes the hydrolysis of the beta [1–4] glycosidic linkages between N-acetylmuramic acid and N-acetylglucosamine. Lysozyme is found in the spleen, lung, kidney, white blood cells, plasma, saliva, milk, and tears. The gene is located on chromosome 12q15 with four exons. Transcription permits a 14.6 kDa protein containing 130 amino acids.

Similarly, with regard to management, early detection of this amyloid variant alters the course of treatment in that individuals with this mutation experience a very early onset of renal disease, and rapid decline (this is similar, in some regards, to some variants of FGA). Unlike FGA, lysozyme amyloidosis patients benefit from renal transplantation [17]. Other manifestations include gastrointestinal involvement (peptic ulcer), cardiac disease, Sicca syndrome, and propensity towards petechiae, hemorrhage, and hematoma, including hepatic hemorrhage. Neuropathy is not a component of this type of amyloid, similar to FGA. In fact, the presence of neuropathy might suggest a different variant, such as gelsolin, depending on the location and type of neuropathy [30, 31].

The mutations documented thus far with lysozyme amyloid have their ancestral roots associated with the United Kingdom, France, America, and Italy (specifically, Piedmont, Italy). The D85H (Asp85His) mutation, which regionalizes to the United Kingdom, has renal disease as the predominant symptom. A tryptophan-to-arginine substitution at codon 82 (W82R) has been documented with a French family, with Sicca syndrome contributing to the phenotype in addition to renal manifestations. Two other mutations,

Phe75Ile (F75I) and Trp82Arg (W82R), are described in an Italian-Canadian family, and an Italian family (Piedmont, Italy), respectively [31, 32]. The W82R variant had predominant gastrointestinal involvement; however, the same mutation in an English man presented with dramatic bleeding and rupture of abdominal lymph nodes [30] Table 27.4.

LECT2: A New Hereditary Amyloidosis Gene?

The most recently described gene in systemic amyloidosis is *LECT2*. LECT2 is a *le*ukocyte *ch*emo*t*actic factor whose synthetic origin is uncertain at this time [33]. Some studies indicate a hepatic origin for LECT2 is expressed in the adult and fetal liver, but follow-up immunohistochemical studies have detected LECT2 in many tissues of the body. LECT2 weighs 16.4 kDa, is comprised of 133 residues (after cleavage of the 18-amino acid signal peptide), and is located on chromosome 5q31.1–q32 [33–36].

Functionally, LECT2 can serve as a cartilage growth factor (chondromodulin II), as well as in neutrophil chemotaxis [33, 36]. With its role in neutrophilic chemotaxis, LECT2 has a presumable role in cell growth and repair after damage. Further, LECT2 has also been detected in hepatocellular carcinoma cell lines, suggesting a role in neoplasia, and also supporting its potential origin within hepatic tissue [33, 36].

To date, LECT2 amyloidosis has been seen primarily in individuals of Mexican American ancestry. A study by Murphy et al. [35] reported a series of 21,985 consecutive renal biopsies, of which 285 had positive Congo Red staining. Seven of ten cases with LECT2 renal amyloidosis were of Mexican descent. In some cases (typically reported in smaller studies), the amyloid was detected after long-standing, slowly progressive renal disease [33, 35].

A case reported by Benson [33] is a patient with a long history of slowly progressive renal failure, without a diagnosis of amyloidosis including its specific subtype until nephrectomy due to renal cell carcinoma. Moreover, since its recent discovery, there is suggestion by Larsen et al. [37] that the incidence of LECT2 amyloid might actually exceed TTR. While a polymorphism has been detected in all of the cases affected with LECT2 amyloid (Ile58Val), no pathogenic mutations are present to date. Thus, whether or not LECT2 will emerge under the category of systemic or hereditary amyloidosis is yet to be determined.

Beta-2 Microglobulin: A New Hereditary Amyloid Gene!

Beta-2 microglobulin (B2M) has long been known to be associated with dialysis-related amyloidosis. B2M is expressed in all nucleated calls and serves to bind to and stabilize major histocompatibility (MHC) class I and CD1 molecules at the cell surface for antigen presentation and T-cell interaction. A small amount of free monomer is found as a plasma protein. There are several circumstances under which the plasma level of B2M is elevated. With normal renal function, B2M levels can be elevated in chronic inflammatory conditions and hematologic malignancies, such as chronic lymphocytic leukemia. Levels can also be elevated in renal disease with impaired glomerular filtration rate. Interestingly, plasma B2M level elevation in inflammation or leukemia is not associated with amyloidosis, while the elevation in kidney disease is. Even though the mature B2M protein is relatively small, 11.7 kDa, it is not typically removed by most dialysis membranes. These conditions, elevated plasma B2M levels under uremic conditions, are associated with dialysis-related amyloidosis (DRA). The physical chemistry and physiology of B2M folding and unfolding has been extensively studies, and was reviewed in 2009 by Heegaard [38]. Even though the effect of multiple amino acid substitutions on the amyloidogenic behavior of the protein has been carried out with in vitro mutated sequences, no naturally occurring B2M mutations associated with familial B2M amyloidosis were reported until 2012.

Valleix and colleagues reported a three-generation French family that presented with progressive bowel dysfunction, visceral B2M amyloid deposition, normal renal function, and normal plasma B2M levels. Gene sequencing revealed a single variant, c. 286G>A, which results in the substitution of an uncharged asparagine residue for the positively charged aspartate at position 76 of the mature protein, Asp76Asn (D76N). The authors carried out extensive genetic and physical studies, which included producing the recombinant mutant protein and obtaining the X-ray crystal structure, conclusively proving that this mutation was responsible for the hereditary amyloidosis in this family [39].

However, understanding the origin of the proteins involved in the subtypes has achieved better control of this process in some types (TTR, FGA).

Acknowledgments The authors would like to thank Steven R. Zeldenrust, MD, PhD Consultant, Division of Hematology, Mayo Clinic, Rochester, Minnesota, for his editorial help and clinical support; Jason Theis and Karen Schowalter for their assistance in the mass spectrometry and molecular genetics laboratories, respectively, at Mayo Clinic, Rochester, Minnesota; Tad Holtegaard and Cindy McFarlin for their technical support; and Debbie Johnson and Pam Carter for their administrative support.

Summary

In summary, many laboratory techniques to detect and characterize the presence of amyloid are available. With these tools, the ability to detect the presence of amyloid has improved, as well as our ability to better understand the varying presentations and pathologic processes associated with the presence of amyloid.

While the understanding of amyloid continues to evolve, so does our ability to detect, diagnose, and treat the varying etiologies. Two techniques pivotal in perpetuating this progress are tissue mass spectrometry and gene sequencing. The refined finesse accomplished by utilizing mass spectrometry and gene sequencing continues to unravel the amyloid puzzle, and reveal more patients, with more unique phenotypic expression of disease. As our ability to identify and characterize systemic amyloidosis improves, and genotype–phenotype correlations become more clear, it will likely be possible in the future to explain seemingly unique manifestations of the disease, such as the cardiac specific presentation seen with the V142I TTR mutation.

The ultimate beneficiary of the utility of the refined laboratory diagnosis of amyloidosis is, of course, the patient. However, the information gathered due to test results is best handled in a multidisciplinary practice with well-established genetic counseling to educate the patient and family regarding the disease process, screening, and treatment considerations. At present, no direct pharmacologic therapy "cures" amyloid.

References

1. Altland K, Benson MD, Costello CE, Ferlini A, Hazenberg BP, Hund E, et al. Genetic microheterogeneity of human transthyretin detected by IEF. Electrophoresis. 2007;28(12):2053–64.
2. Connors LH, Lim A, Prokaeva T, Roskens VA, Costello CE. Tabulation of human transthyretin (TTR) variants, 2003. Amyloid. 2003;10(3):160–84.
3. Maury CP, Baumann M. Isolation and characterization of cardiac amyloid in familial amyloid polyneuropathy type IV (Finnish): relation of the amyloid protein to variant gelsolin. Biochim Biophys Acta. 1990;1096(1):84–6.
4. Lachmann HJ, Booth DR, Booth SE, Bybee A, Gilbertson JA, Gillmore JD, et al. Misdiagnosis of hereditary amyloidosis as AL (primary) amyloidosis. N Engl J Med. 2002;346(23):1786–91.
5. Comenzo RL, Zhou P, Fleisher M, Clark B, Teruya-Feldstein J. Seeking confidence in the diagnosis of systemic AL (Ig light-chain) amyloidosis: patients can have both monoclonal gammopathies and hereditary amyloid proteins. Blood. 2006;107(9):3489–91.
6. Bergen HR, Zeldenrust SR, Butz ML, Snow DS, Dyck PJ, Dyck PJ, et al. Identification of transthyretin variants by sequential proteomic and genomic analysis. Clin Chem. 2004;50(9):1544–52.
7. Bergethon PR, Sabin TD, Lewis D, Simms RW, Cohen AS, Skinner M. Improvement in the polyneuropathy associated with familial amyloid polyneuropathy after liver transplantation. Neurology. 1996;47(4):944–51.
8. Kishikawa M, Nakanishi T, Miyazaki A, Shimizu A, Nakazato M, Kangawa K, et al. Simple detection of abnormal serum transthyretin from patients with familial amyloidotic polyneuropathy by high-performance liquid chromatography/electrospray ionization mass spectrometry using material precipitated with specific antiserum. J Mass Spectrom. 1996;31(1):112–4.
9. Theberge R, Connors L, Skare J, Skinner M, Falk RH, Costello CE. A new amyloidogenic transthyretin variant (Val122Ala) found in a compound heterozygous patient. Amyloid. 1999;6(1):54–8.

10. Saraiva M. Transthyretin mutations in hyperthyroxinemia and amyloid diseases. Hum Mutat. 2001;17: 493–503.

11. Benson MD, Liepnieks J, Uemichi T, Wheeler G, Correa R. Hereditary renal amyloidosis associated with a mutant fibrinogen alpha-chain. Nat Genet. 1993;3(3):252–5.

12. Cendron L, Trovato A, Seno F, Folli C, Alfieri B, Zanotti G, et al. Amyloidogenic potential of transthyretin variants: insights from structural and computational analyses. J Biol Chem. 2009;284(38): 25832–41.

13. Jacob E, Edwards W, Zucker M, D'Cruz C, Seshan S, Crow F, et al. Homozygous transthyretin mutation in an African American Male. J Mol Diagn. 2007;9(1): 127–31.

14. Reddi HV, Jenkins S, Theis J, Thomas BC, Connors LH, Van Rhee F, et al. Homozygosity for the V122I mutation in transthyretin is associated with earlier onset of cardiac amyloidosis in the African American population in the seventh decade of life. J Mol Diagn. 2014;16(1):68–74.

15. Eriksson M, Schonland S, Yumlu S, Hegenbart U, von Hutten H, Gioeva Z, et al. Hereditary apolipoprotein AI-associated amyloidosis in surgical pathology specimens: identification of three novel mutations in the APOA1 gene. J Mol Diagn. 2009;11(3):257–62.

16. Rowczenio D, Dogan A, Theis JD, Vrana JA, Lachmann HJ, Wechalekar AD, et al. Amyloidogenicity and clinical phenotype associated with five novel mutations in apolipoprotein A-I. Am J Pathol. 2011;179(4):1978–87. doi:10.1016/j. ajpath.2011.06.024. Epub 2011 Aug 5.

17. Benson MD. The hereditary amyloidoses. Best Pract Res Clin Rheumatol. 2003;17(6):909–27.

18. Kitagawa K, Wang J, Mastushita T, Kogishi K, Hosokawa M, Fu X, et al. Polymorphisms of mouse apolipoprotein A-II: seven alleles found among 41 inbred strains of mice. Amyloid. 2003;10(4):207–14.

19. Lackner KJ, Law SW, Brewer Jr HB. The human apolipoprotein A-II gene: complete nucleic acid sequence and genomic organization. Nucleic Acids Res. 1985;13(12):4597–608.

20. Lee WM, Galbraith RM. The extracellular actin-scavenger system and actin toxicity. N Engl J Med. 1992;326(20):1335–41.

21. de la Chapelle A, Tolvanen R, Boysen G, Santavy J, Bleeker-Wagemakers L, Maury CP, et al. Gelsolin-derived familial amyloidosis caused by asparagine or tyrosine substitution for aspartic acid at residue 187. Nat Genet. 1992;2(2):157–60.

22. Meretoja J. Genetic aspects of familial amyloidosis with corneal lattice dystrophy and cranial neuropathy. Clin Genet. 1973;4(3):173–85.

23. Paunio T, Kangas H, Kalkkinen N, Haltia M, Palo J, Peltonen L. Toward understanding the pathogenic mechanisms in gelsolin-related amyloidosis: in vitro expression reveals an abnormal gelsolin fragment. Hum Mol Genet. 1994;3(12):2223–9.

24. Maury CP. Gelsolin-related amyloidosis. Identification of the amyloid protein in Finnish hereditary amyloidosis as a fragment of variant gelsolin. J Clin Investig. 1991;87(4):1195–9.

25. Sethi S, Theis JD, Quint P, Maierhofer W, Kurtin PJ, Dogan A, et al. Renal amyloidosis associated with a novel sequence variant of gelsolin. Am J Kidney Dis. 2013;61(1):161–6.

26. Hamidi Asl L, Liepnieks JJ, Uemichi T, Rebibou JM, Justrabo E, Droz D, et al. Renal amyloidosis with a frame shift mutation in fibrinogen aalpha-chain gene producing a novel amyloid protein. Blood. 1997; 90(12):4799–805.

27. Mourad G, Delabre JP, Garrigue V. Cardiac amyloidosis with the E526V mutation of the fibrinogen A alpha-chain. N Engl J Med. 2008;359(26):2847–8.

28. Uemichi T, Liepnieks JJ, Yamada T, Gertz MA, Bang N, Benson MD. A frame shift mutation in the fibrinogen A alpha chain gene in a kindred with renal amyloidosis. Blood. 1996;87(10):4197–203.

29. Uemichi T, Liepnieks JJ, Benson MD. Hereditary renal amyloidosis with a novel variant fibrinogen. J Clin Invest. 1994;93(2):731–6.

30. Granel B, Serratrice J, Disdier P, Weiller PJ, Valleix S, Grateau G, et al. Underdiagnosed amyloidosis: amyloidosis of lysozyme variant. Am J Med. 2005; 118(3):321–2.

31. Granel B, Serratrice J, Valleix S, Grateau G, Droz D, Lafon J, et al. A family with gastrointestinal amyloidosis associated with variant lysozyme. Gastroenterology. 2002;123(4):1346–9.

32. Yazaki M, Liepnieks JJ, Barats MS, Cohen AH, Benson MD. Hereditary systemic amyloidosis associated with a new apolipoprotein AII stop codon mutation Stop78Arg. Kidney Int. 2003;64(1):11–6.

33. Benson MD. LECT2 amyloidosis. Kidney Int. 2010; 77(9):757–9.

34. Benson MD, James S, Scott K, Liepnieks JJ, Kluve-Beckerman B. Leukocyte chemotactic factor 2: a novel renal amyloid protein. Kidney Int. 2008;74(2): 218–22.

35. Murphy CL, Wang S, Kestler D, Larsen C, Benson D, Weiss DT, et al. Leukocyte chemotactic factor 2 (LECT2)-associated renal amyloidosis: a case series. Am J Kidney Dis. 2010;56(6):1100–7.

36. Yamagoe S, Kameoka Y, Hashimoto K, Mizuno S, Suzuki K. Molecular cloning, structural characterization, and chromosomal mapping of the human LECT2 gene. Genomics. 1998;48(3):324–9.

37. Larsen CP, Walker PD, Weiss DT, Solomon A. Prevalence and morphology of leukocyte chemotactic factor 2-associated amyloid in renal biopsies. Kidney Int. 2010;77(9):816–9.

38. Heegaard NH. beta(2)-microglobulin: from physiology to amyloidosis. Amyloid. 2009;16(3):151–73.

39. Valleix S, Gillmore JD, Bridoux F, Mangione PP, Dogan A, Nedelec B, et al. Hereditary systemic amyloidosis due to Asp76Asn variant beta2-microglobulin. N Engl J Med. 2012;366(24):2276–83.

Amyloidoses of the Kidney, the Lower Urinary and Genital Tracts (Male and Female), and the Breast

28

Maria M. Picken and Ahmet Dogan

Abbreviations

AA	AA amyloidosis
AL	Amyloidosis derived from immunoglobulin light chain
ALECT2	Amyloidosis derived from leukocyte chemotactic factor 2
ATTR	Amyloidosis derived from transthyretin

Genitourinary surgical pathology covers the urinary system (kidneys, ureters, urinary bladder, urethra), the male reproductive system, the adrenal glands, and the retroperitoneum. In this chapter, the female genital organs and breast have also been included. Among these different organs of the male and female genitourinary system, the kidney and adrenal glands are the most frequent genitourinary localization of amyloidosis [1, 2].

M.M. Picken, MD, PhD (✉)
Department of Pathology, Loyola University
Medical Center, Loyola University Chicago,
Building 110, Room 2242, 2160 South First Avenue,
Maywood, IL 60153, USA
e-mail: mpicken@luc.edu; MMPicken@aol.com

A. Dogan, MD, PhD
Departments of Pathology and Laboratory Medicine,
Memorial Sloan Kettering Cancer Center,
1275 York Avenue, New York, NY 10065, USA
e-mail: dogana@mskcc.org

While most systemic amyloidoses can affect the genitourinary system, apart from renal and adrenal amyloid deposits, other sites are usually silent or clinically less prominent; however, the clinical relevance of gonadal involvement in young patients is increasingly recognized [3–6]. On the other hand, the involvement of peripheral nerves and autonomic nerves, as seen in amyloidoses derived from immunoglobulin light chain (AL) and transthyretin (ATTR), may cause urinary bladder and erectile dysfunction [7]. Among the localized amyloidoses, the genitourinary tract is one of the more frequently involved sites, where amyloidosis may mimic malignancy [8–12]. While renal parenchymal amyloidosis has been extensively studied and there is an abundance of pertinent literature, the involvement of other parts of the genitourinary system is less well known [1, 13–24]. Moreover, renal amyloidosis is usually handled by renal pathologists. Since this book is primarily directed toward general surgical pathologists, in this chapter, only a brief review will be provided summarizing the key features as they pertain to general surgical pathology.

The Kidney

The kidney parenchyma is one of the most frequent sites of amyloid deposition in AL, AA, ALECT2, and several of the hereditary amyloidoses ([1, 13–24], please see also Chaps. 2–5). Among the

© Springer International Publishing Switzerland 2015
M.M. Picken et al. (eds.), *Amyloid and Related Disorders*, Current Clinical Pathology,
DOI 10.1007/978-3-319-19294-9_28

various systemic amyloidoses, essentially, all can involve the kidney and, conversely, the kidney is the organ most commonly involved by clinically significant amyloid deposits. In general, systemic amyloidoses are considered to be clinically significant (with type-specific treatments being currently available for the most common forms) and renal amyloid is virtually always systemic (please see also Chaps. 2–5 and Chaps. 36–38 in Part VI). In general, experience with amyloid diagnosis is better among renal pathologists than among general surgical pathologists, for at least two reasons:

- Renal amyloidosis is more likely to be associated with clinically detectable symptoms and/or laboratory abnormalities, which are likely to prompt a kidney biopsy;
- Kidney biopsies are, as a routine matter, more extensively investigated than other biopsies in surgical pathology, and, hence, the likelihood of amyloid detection is increased.

Clinical Presentation

The most common clinical presentation is proteinuria with or without renal insufficiency [1, 13–16, 25]. The amount of proteinuria is very variable and depends on the extent of glomerular involvement. In contrast, patients with extraglomerular amyloid deposits typically present with renal failure that is not associated with significant proteinuria. Renal involvement may be the first manifestation of systemic disease, with subsequent studies confirming its systemic nature. Thus, amyloidosis is often diagnosed by renal biopsy and only a minority of patients have an established diagnosis of amyloidosis prior to renal biopsy. The differential diagnosis of amyloidosis in renal pathology is shorter than in other areas of surgical pathology (please see also Chap. 20). Thus, among patients diagnosed with nephrotic syndrome, the differential diagnosis involves minimal change disease, focal and segmental glomerular sclerosis, membranous nephropathy, secondary renal involvement in systemic diseases such as diabetes and

systemic lupus erythematosus, and amyloidosis. Hence, amyloidosis should often be considered in differential diagnoses in renal pathology [1]. Moreover, in the kidney, in particular, there are other pathologies that may mimic amyloid, that are associated with underlying plasma cell dyscrasia (please see Part II), and that, although individually rare, collectively account for a significant number of biopsies [1, 26].

Pathology

Amyloid deposits can be found in any of the renal compartments (Fig. 28.1a–d). Typically, in H&E stained sections, amyloid has an amorphous "hyaline" appearance, is weakly PAS positive, and shows loss of argyrophilia [1]. However, early deposits of amyloid may be inconspicuous in H&E and other stains. Therefore, Congo red stain should be performed, either to confirm the suspicion of amyloid or to rule it out. In the glomerulus, typically, the first deposits are detectable in the mesangium (Fig. 28.1b); subsequently, deposits extend to the capillaries and, ultimately, may replace the entire glomerulus (Fig. 28.2, please see also Fig. 19.4). While bulky deposits may mimic segmental sclerosis or diabetic nephropathy, early deposits may be inconspicuous and may be misdiagnosed by the unwary as minimal change disease. Near complete glomerular obliteration by amyloid is typically seen in amyloidosis derived from fibrinogen (AFib), Fig. 28.2 [27, 28]. While glomerular deposits are reported most frequently, other compartments may be involved (interstitium, extraglomerular vessels), usually accompanying glomerular deposits (Fig. 28.1a). In a study by Hopfer et al. [15], involving >200 native kidney biopsies with amyloidosis, glomerular deposits were seen in 84.6 %, a vascular distribution pattern was seen in 9.4 %, and deposits limited to the tubulointerstitial compartment were seen in 6 % of biopsies (Fig. 28.1d). Rarely, crescents can be seen, in particular, in AA [29]. Crescentic glomerulonephritis, with rapidly progressive glomerulonephritis, was also reported [30]. Crosthwaite et al. [31] recently reported the first clinical case of rapidly

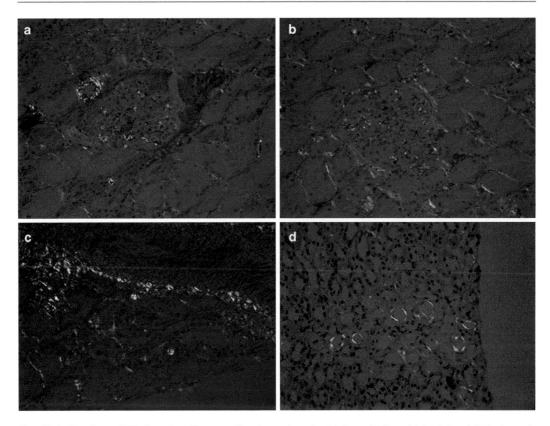

Fig. 28.1 Renal amyloid deposits—*Congo red* stains viewed under polarized light. (**a**) Glomerular and extra-glomerular vessels and interstitial amyloid. (**b**) Glomerular deposits. (**c**) Interstitial amyloid. (**d**) Amyloid in the medullary tubular basement membrane

progressive glomerulonephritis complicating AL renal amyloidosis and multiple myeloma.

Interstitial and peritubular deposits of amyloid are seen in approximately 50 % of cases, in addition to glomerular deposits (Fig. 28.1a). However, in certain amyloidoses, exclusively extraglomerular deposits may be formed (Fig. 28.1c). In many cases of ALECT2, cortical interstitium is typically involved, while glomeruli may be only minimally involved, or not at all [19, 20]. Occasional patients with AA and AApoA-I amyloidosis may show amyloid deposition limited to the medullary interstitium (please see also Fig. 5.6); recently, AApoA-IV deposits were also reported in the medulla [32]. In cases of ATTR that are associated with certain mutations, amyloid may be seen in deep medulla, sparing glomeruli [7]. Scattered aggregates of lymphoplasmacytic cells may be present in AL

at times, accompanied by a multinucleated giant cell reaction.

Renal extraglomerular vessels are often involved, most commonly together with glomerular involvement (Fig. 28.1a). However, in certain patients, there may be an almost exclusive involvement of the extraglomerular vessels in the absence of detectable glomerular amyloid [1, 33–35]. This may be seen in some patients with AA and AApoA-I; however, rare patients with AL, who had vascular amyloid in the absence of detectable glomerular deposits, have also been observed [33–35]. While early deposits may be inconspicuous, more advanced deposits may mimic hyalinosis and even fibrinoid necrosis. There is no correlation between the biochemical type of amyloid and the distribution pattern [15]. Hatakeyama [30] reported a rare case of coexistent focal extracapillary glomerulonephritis with

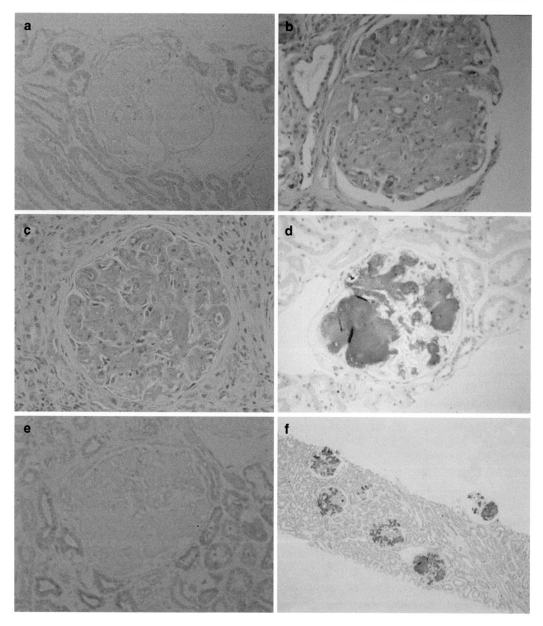

Fig. 28.2 Kidney with AFib. (**a**) Negative stain for amyloid A protein (paraffin section, immunoperoxidase stain, no counterstain). (**b**) Deposits of amyloid are negative for lambda light chain; positivity for this antibody is focally seen in the lumen of glomerular vessels (paraffin section, immunoperoxidase stain, hematoxylin counterstain). (**c**) Stain for kappa light chain showing weak (1+) positivity (paraffin section, immunoperoxidase stain, hematoxylin counterstain). (**d**) Stain for amyloid P component showing strong positivity (3+; paraffin section, immunoperoxidase stain, hematoxylin counterstain). (**e**) Negative stain for TTR (paraffin section, immunoperoxidase stain, no counterstain). (**f**) Paraffin sections of kidney showing abundant deposits that are strongly immunoreactive for fibrinogen (3+) and are limited to glomeruli (paraffin section, immunoperoxidase stain, hematoxylin counterstain). Magnifications: ×280 in **a** through **e**; ×60 in **f**. Reprinted with permission from the publisher ([28]. Picken MM, Linke RP. Nephrotic syndrome due to an amyloidogenic mutation in Fibrinogen A alpha chain. J Am Soc Nephrol. 2009;20:1681–5)

vasculitis and AA renal amyloidosis 3 months after the initiation of infliximab therapy. In rare patients, coexistence of AL amyloidosis and light chain deposition disease (LCDD) in the kidney has been reported [36]. Amyloid is also typically present in the perirenal fat.

Differential Diagnosis of the Renal Amyloidosis Type

In the USA and Europe, AL amyloidosis is currently the most prevalent type of systemic amyloidosis, but ALECT2 and hereditary amyloidoses are being diagnosed with increasing frequency [1, 13–16, 37, 38]. The incidence of AA, however, appears to be declining. In North America, AL contributes 85 % of cases, and worldwide >90 % of renal amyloids are of the AL/AA type with marked regional differences concerning the incidence of AA ([13, 14, 37, 38], please see also Chap. 20). Thus, while, in North America, AA is diagnosed in 3.5–7 % of kidney biopsies, in one large European series the incidence was reported to be 40 % [13, 14, 16, 38], although more recent studies report a declining rate of AA in European patients [39]. Thus, in the kidney, with a declining rate of AA in North America in particular, the non-AL/AA amyloidoses are collectively becoming the second most prominent group of amyloidoses. Discovered in 2008, ALECT2 has emerged as the third most common type of renal amyloidosis in the USA ([14, 19–21, 40], please see also Chaps. 4 and 5). ALECT2 is also systemic and the second most common type of amyloidosis in the liver [41]. Although individual types are rather rare, collectively, the hereditary amyloidoses constitute a significant proportion of patients with systemic amyloidosis, currently estimated at approximately 10 % in the USA (and they may still be underdiagnosed) [37]. While several of the familial disorders are distinctly neuropathic or cardiopathic, virtually all of them can affect the kidneys, although, in some of these amyloidoses, renal deposits may be clinically silent [1]. In the USA, among patients with hereditary amyloidoses, 85 % are diagnosed with ATTR and 5 % with AFib [1, 14, 17, 37, 42, 43] (Fig. 28.2). In contrast, in the United Kingdom, AFib is the most frequent hereditary amyloidosis [42]. Although rare, these forms need to be properly recognized because of the implications for patient management (please see also Chap. 5 and Part VI—Chaps. 36, 37). Amyloid derived from apolipoprotein AIV (AApolipo AIV), apparently not associated with a mutation, was also recently reported in the kidney [32]. Rare patients with mixed renal amyloid deposits have also been reported (AL+AA, AA+ATTR, AL+ATTR) [13].

AL/AH Amyloidosis

AL amyloidosis has been extensively discussed in Chaps. 2, 20, and Part VI—Chap. 36. Significant progress has been achieved in the treatment of AL with chemotherapy and stem cell rescue [25]. Thus, the main issue now centers on early and correct diagnosis of AL and distinguishing it from other types of amyloidosis, which require different treatments. Immunoglobulin heavy chain amyloidosis, AH, is a rare, poorly recognized disease with very few cases thus far reported. It often poses a diagnostic dilemma [22, 43, 44] since immunohistochemistry may be negative and more sophisticated studies are needed for diagnosis. In some patients, the heavy chain may be associated with the light chain [22–24]. The treatment regimen of these immunoglobulin component-derived amyloidoses is similar [25, 26].

AA Amyloidosis

AA amyloidosis is discussed extensively in Chap. 3. It usually arises in the context of an acute phase response such as that seen in the inflammatory arthritides, periodic fevers, chronic infections, and malignancies, including renal cell carcinoma [1]. Significant proteinuria and nephrotic syndrome are the most common presenting symptoms, diagnosed in 97 % of patients in one recent large series [45]. Occasional patients may present with renal failure without significant proteinuria.

These patients have deposits that are limited to the interstitium and affect predominantly the medulla or tubules. Less commonly, crescentic glomerulonephritis may be seen [29, 30]. Rare instances, where AA co-deposits with AL in the kidney, have been reported [1]. Interestingly, while patients with Waldenstrom's macroglobulinemia typically develop AL, instances of AA amyloidosis were also reported in these patients [1]. Familial AA amyloidoses develop in the context of mutations in genes for non-amyloid fibril proteins that play a permissive role in the development of amyloid (please see Chap. 3 and Figs. 3.2 and 3.3). Amyloid deposits in familial Mediterranean fever (FMF) are distributed throughout the body in small vessels with primarily glomerular involvement. While proteinuria is presumptive evidence of amyloidosis, other renal pathologies should also be considered, in particular, in patients treated with colchicine [1]. Also, an increased incidence of vasculitides and Henoch–Schoenlein disease has been reported in patients suffering from FMF. Since albuminuria is an early finding in FMF amyloidosis, patients should undergo periodic urinalyses, especially those who are at high risk.

Non-AL/AA Amyloidoses

ALECT2 amyloidosis (amyloid derived from leukocyte chemotactic factor 2) is the latest type of systemic amyloidosis to be described [14, 19–21, 40]. It was first reported in patients with renal failure; subsequently, some patients with proteinuria/nephrotic syndrome were also reported. Typically, there is amyloid deposition in the cortical interstitium with sparing of the medullary interstitium. However, in at least some patients, glomeruli and extraglomerular renal vessels are also involved (please see also Chaps. 4 and 5 and Fig. 5.18). It is postulated that ALECT2 represents a unique and perhaps not uncommon disease entity, which shows a predilection for certain ethnic groups, most notably Mexican Americans. Based on two large recently published series, it represents 3–10 % of renal amyloidoses in the USA [14, 19, 20]. However,

there are big regional differences. Thus, in the US South-West, where there is a high concentration of Mexican Americans, ALECT2 amyloidosis accounts for 54 % of renal amyloidosis cases [20]. Other ethnic groups affected by ALECT2 include First Nation people in Canada and Punjabi people in a UK series ([19, 20, 46], see also Chaps. 4 and 5). There is no clear evidence, as yet, whether ALECT2 represents a hereditary amyloidosis, since no mutation has been documented. Interestingly, however, two brothers affected by ALECT2 were recently reported [20].

At present, there is no specific treatment available. Hence, it is important not to misdiagnose ALECT2 as AL, or other type, where a specific treatment may be available ([21], please see also Chap. 20, Fig. 20.3).

The hereditary amyloidoses are described in Chap. 5. Here, they are discussed in connection with their pertinence to the kidney.

AFib (amyloid derived from a mutant fibrinogen A-α chain) primarily causes renal amyloidosis, but, increasingly, evidence is emerging that the disease is systemic [27, 28, 47–49]. There is variable penetrance, and de novo mutation has been documented [32]. Clinically, there is a rapid deterioration in kidney function from initial presentation (proteinuria, hypertension, mild renal impairment) to end-stage renal failure, leading to dialysis dependence within 1–5 years [27, 28, 47, 48]. AFib shows a remarkable tropism for the kidney, with a very characteristic histology (Fig. 28.2, please see also Chap. 5 and Fig. 5.12 and Chap. 20 and Fig. 20.2). There is near replacement of the glomeruli by amyloid, without any interstitial or vascular involvement. Deposits stain specifically with antibodies to fibrinogen [27, 28, 47–49].

ATTR (amyloid derived from various mutants of transthyretin) is typically associated with polyneuropathy (with progressive peripheral and autonomic neuropathy) and cardiomyopathy. However, nephropathic and lower genitourinary system deposits have also been found associated with certain mutations [1, 7, 17]. In the kidney, typically, medullary deposits of amyloid are present, but, in some mutations, significant glomerular deposits can also be seen (please see Chap. 5

and Fig. 5.3). Despite being inherited, the disease is not clinically apparent until middle or later life. In general, there is a low penetrance in carriers of the mutation, and, hence, a family history may be absent. In elderly patients, even wild-type transthyretin may form amyloid, which typically shows a cardiac tropism but may also be associated with clinically silent renal interstitial and lower genitourinary tract deposits (please see also Chaps. 5 and 7).

AApoAI (amyloid derived from various mutants of apolipoprotein AI) amyloidosis is due to germline mutations in the APOA1 gene ([4, 50, 51], please see also Chap. 5). Replacement of the leucine residue at position 75 by proline (Leu75Pro) leads to a new hereditary systemic amyloidosis, involving mostly the liver, kidney, and testis [4, 51]. Interestingly, an incidental mutation in the APOA1 gene, in a patient with systemic AL amyloidosis, was also recently documented [51]. Renal amyloid deposition differs, depending on the mutation. In many patients, amyloid deposits are small and limited to large arteries while the glomeruli are generally spared (please see also Chap. 5 and Fig. 5.6). However, other patients also showed glomerular deposits [50]. AApo AII (amyloid derived from various mutants of apolipoprotein AII) amyloidosis is characterized by slowly progressing renal disease with glomerular, interstitial, and vascular deposits (please see also Chap. 5 and Figs. 5.15–5.17).

AGel (amyloid derived from a mutant gelsolin gene) is associated with severe nephrotic syndrome in homozygotic patients and it may be the presenting feature of this disease in young, homozygotic patients when other manifestations are minimal [52]. ALys (amyloid derived from lysozyme) is relatively rare and characterized by nephropathy (with glomerular and vascular deposits), dermal petechiae, gastrointestinal involvement with bleeding, hepatic involvement, and ocular or oral sicca syndrome ([53], please see Chap. 5 and Fig. 5.14). ACys (amyloid derived from cystatin C) is associated with familial cerebral congophilic angiopathy. However, systemic deposits of amyloid were also reported in the kidneys and lower genitourinary tract, where the deposits are clinically silent [54].

Aβ2M

This systemic amyloidosis develops in patients with chronic renal failure undergoing long-term dialysis (please see Chap. 6). For this reason, it is frequently referred to as dialysis-related amyloidosis. Aβ2M (amyloid derived from β2-microglobulin) is deposited in end-stage kidneys, but this has no clinical significance. At autopsy, Mazanec et al. [55] detected amyloid within the stroma of the kidney in one patient with a 15-year history of dialysis, together with foci of calcification. Recently, an autosomal dominant hereditary Aβ2M was reported in individuals with normal kidney function and normal levels of circulating β2M. These individuals were shown to have an inherited mutation together with extrarenal and extra-osteoarticular deposits of amyloid (please see Chap. 6).

Extrarenal Genitourinary Tract

Amyloidosis of the genitourinary tract, outside the kidney parenchyma, is uncommonly reported [1, 8–12, 55–76]. This involvement may be part of a systemic amyloidosis or represent a localized process and this subject will be presented here accordingly.

Extrarenal Genitourinary Tract in Systemic Amyloidoses

Clinical Presentation

Systemic amyloidosis presenting with lower urinary symptoms is exceedingly rare, but it has been reported [57]. Clinically, however, small fiber neuropathy and endocrine involvement with sub/infertility are increasingly being recognized [2–5, 7]. The former, which typically occurs in ATTR, but also in AL, may be responsible for lower urinary dysfunction, including dysuria and incontinence, sensitivity and contractility disturbances of the detrusor muscle, non-relaxing urethral sphincter, dyssynergia, impaired bladder sensation, and erectile dysfunction [7]. Systemic amyloidoses frequently involve the endocrine system and endocrine dysfunction is increasingly recognized [2–7, 50, 77–79]. While, most commonly, thyroid gland dysfunction is clinically apparent, adrenal dysfunction has also been reported [2, 77]. Gonadal involvement, typically seen in males and females in AA and AL, and in males in AApoAI, leads to sub/infertility. Moreover, treatment-related sub/infertility is also recognized in patients with AL and AA [5, 6]. Hence, in young patients of both sexes, semen/oocyte preservation may be considered [3, 6]. Cases of amyloidosis affecting the female genital tract have been associated with menorrhagia. Hemorrhagic complications associated with amyloidosis are most probably due to amyloid angiopathy leading to fragility and impaired contractility of blood vessels due to deposition of amyloid in the vascular wall. Moreover, bleeding may also be secondary to the coagulation abnormalities that are associated with AL amyloidosis.

Pathology

Although autopsy and in vivo amyloid P component scintigraphy studies show that all main types of systemic amyloidoses (AL, AA, ATTR, AApoAI, dialysis-associated amyloidosis) can involve the lower genitourinary tract, such involvement is uncommonly encountered in surgical pathology [12, 45, 47, 55, 57]. In particular, autopsy studies of patients with ATTR and familial amyloid polyneuropathy showed, in addition to deposits in the heart and peripheral nerves, also heavy amyloid deposition in the prostate and testis and moderate deposition in the adrenal gland, urinary bladder, kidney, and sympathetic nerve trunk and pelvic plexus [7].

Urinary Bladder and Prostate

In AL and ATTR, urinary bladder wall thickening may be seen [7, 12, 58, 59] with deposition of amyloid in the detrusor muscle. This is in contrast to localized bladder amyloidosis, which forms a mass within the lamina propria. A rare case of clinically significant prostate amyloid tumor, which led to a diagnosis of systemic AL amyloidosis with successful treatment, has also been reported [80]. Heavy amyloid deposition in the prostate has also been seen at autopsy in patients with ATTR and familial amyloid polyneuropathy [7].

Testis

Testicular involvement is not uncommon in the systemic amyloidoses, in particular in AA, AL, AApolipo A-I amyloidosis, ATTR, and dialysis-associated amyloidosis [3, 4]. Testicular involvement in systemic AA and AApolipo A-I amyloidosis may affect young adults, and, hence, its clinical relevance is increasing [3, 4]. It may be associated with testicular enlargement and lead to abnormal spermatogenesis and secondary infertility [3, 4]. In patients with known amyloidosis or identifiable risk factors (e.g., Familial Mediterranean fever), sperm cryopreservation and early sperm retrieval may be considered [77]. Treatment-related infertility has also been reported in AL and AA [5, 81].

Primary infertility and hypergonadotropic hypogonadism in young patients may be caused by testicular amyloidosis associated with a mutation in the APOA1 gene, resulting in the replacement of proline by leucine at residue 75 of the protein [4]. This hereditary systemic amyloidosis involves mostly the liver, kidney, and testis. In some patients, testicular amyloidosis was the first manifestation of this systemic disease and was associated with macro-orchidism. Testicular biopsies showed abundant deposits of amyloid in the basement membrane of the seminiferous tubules with narrowing of the lumen and varying degrees of replacement of the germinal epithelium and the Sertoli cells by amyloid (Fig. 28.3). Amyloid deposits were also found in the interstitium, and in the walls of arteries, capillaries, and veins. Leydig cells were preserved in normogonadic but not hypogonadic patients. Amyloid deposits were immunoreactive with anti-apoA-I antibody (Fig. 28.3c) [4].

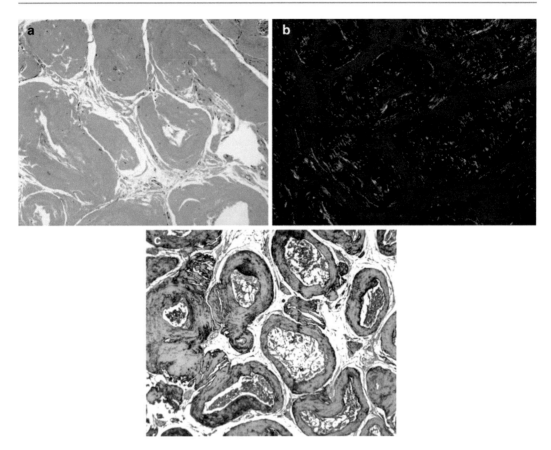

Fig. 28.3 Testicular biopsy. (**a**) Massive deposits of amorphous material along the basement membrane of the seminiferous tubules with complete loss of germinal epithelium; interstitial deposits of amyloid are also focally visible. H & E stain. (**b**) Testicular biopsy, *Congo red* stain viewed under polarized light. (**c**) Immunohistochemical stain with anti-Apo A-I antibody shows diffuse and intense immunostaining of peritubular and interstitial amyloid deposits. Immunohistochemical stain courtesy of C. Rocken. Figures **a** and **c** reprinted with permission from the publisher ([4]. Scalvini T, Martini PR, Obici L, Tardanico R, Biasi L, Gregorini G, Scolari F, Merlini G. Infertility and hypergonadotropic hypogonadism as first evidence of hereditary apolipoprotein A-I amyloidosis. J Urol. 2007;178(1):344–8). Figure **b** courtesy of L. Obici

Interestingly, systemic deposits of amyloid, including testicular deposits, were also reported in patients with hereditary cystatin C amyloid angiopathy, which affects primarily cerebral vasculature, leading to catastrophic strokes at a young age [54].

Female Genital Tract

The female genital tract may be affected by systemic amyloidoses, including hereditary apolipoprotein A-I-associated amyloidosis [50].

Ovary

Sub/infertility, seen in female amyloidosis patients, is most likely multifactorial and consequent to either the actual gonad and/or endocrine gland involvement by amyloidosis, or a side effect of the disease and/or of the treatment [5, 6].

In patients with AL, infertility is likely to be a treatment side effect. Thus, in child-bearing female patients, oocyte preservation may be considered. However, hormonal follicle stimulation therapy, which is needed in such an instance, has been reported to be associated with the development of a severe hypercoagulable state [6].

Familial Mediterranean Fever (FMF) is typically associated with subfertility [5]. Untreated FMF, by itself, can lead to amyloid deposition in the ovary, resulting in infertility; oligomenorrhea is also frequent, but its cause(s) remain(s) unclear. Interestingly, SAA is produced locally in developing ovarian follicles and is also a constituent of follicular fluids, suggestive of its role within the follicular environment. Elevated follicular SAA levels are associated with a decreased pregnancy rate and may signify lower reproductive performance [82].

One patient, on long-term dialysis, with systemic β_2 microglobulin amyloidosis, initially presented with bilateral ovarian masses [76]. Also, massive vascular and interstitial deposits of amyloid in the ovaries were seen in one patient with hereditary apolipoprotein A-I-associated amyloidosis [50].

Adrenal Gland

While amyloid deposits in the adrenal gland are detectable in AL, AA, and ATTR amyloidosis, symptomatic primary adrenal insufficiency rarely occurs, since extensive amyloid deposition is required to produce clinical symptoms [2, 45]. Recently, using whole-body serum amyloid P component scintigraphy, 41 % of patients with AA systemic amyloidosis were found to have adrenal deposits of amyloid [45], but only a few (<1.5 %) required long-term glucocorticoid therapy. Nevertheless, although clinically significant adrenal failure is rare, almost half of patients have a reduced response to adrenal stimulation tests [2].

At autopsy, amyloid deposits in the adrenal gland have also been reported in patients with hereditary ATTR, dialysis-associated amyloidosis, and hereditary cystatin C cerebral amyloid angiopathy [7, 54, 55]. However, except at autopsy, adrenal gland amyloid is rarely evaluated in surgical pathology.

Breast

Mass-forming deposition of amyloid may be seen in the breast in rare patients with systemic AL. In a recent series of mammary gland amyloidosis by Said et al, close to half of patients with breast amyloidosis had systemic AL [83]. In most of these patients, systemic amyloidosis was diagnosed before breast amyloidosis, suggesting that breast involvement is a relatively late event [83]. Nevertheless, the authors recommended a work up to rule out systemic amyloidosis in patients diagnosed with mammary amyloidosis.

In systemic ATTR, mammary gland involvement may be seen even at preclinical stages of the disease, while, in patients with clinically apparent disease, amyloid deposits are more abundant [84]. Interestingly, there is no mass-forming deposition, but amyloid deposits form a network surrounding the lactiferous alveoli and ducts (Fig. 28.4). Please see also below, under localized amyloidosis.

Localized Amyloidosis

Clinical Presentation

In general, most patients who present with urinary tract symptoms (painless hematuria, flank pain, hydronephrosis, mass, irritative bladder symptoms), and who are found to have amyloid deposits, are affected by localized amyloid deposits that involve the urinary tract in the absence of visceral amyloid deposits [8–12, 56–60]. Overall, however, primary localized amyloidosis of the genitourinary tract is a rare entity characterized by small pseudotumors that are localized, most commonly, in the urinary bladder but are also seen in the renal pelvis, ureters, urethra, and glans penis [12, 60–64]; localized retroperitoneal amyloidosis mimicking retroperitoneal fibrosis, and causing obstructive uropathy, has also been reported [65]. Senile seminal vesicle amyloid, associated with the aging process, is one of the most common forms of localized amyloidosis [66, 67]. Female genital organs are involved even less frequently than male genital

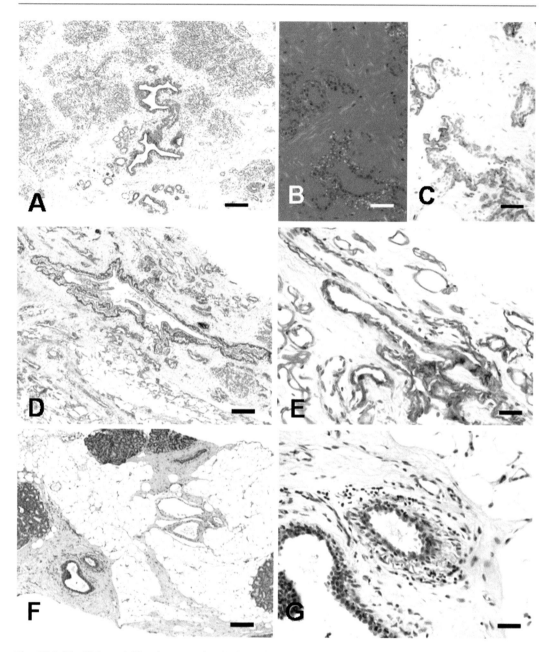

Fig. 28.4 Familial amyloid polyneuropathy (FAP) and systemic amyloidosis derived from transthyretin variant (ATTRVal30Met). Breast biopsy. Case 1 (**a–c**) *Congo red* stain, bright field (**a**), under polarized light (**b**), and immunostain with anti-TTR antibody (**c**). Case 2 (**d, e**) Extensive and heavy deposits of amyloid are shown at both lower and higher magnifications. Case 3 (**f, g**) Minimal deposits of amyloid in adipose tissues (**f**) and periductal areas (**g**). (**a, d, f**) *Bars* = 200 μm; (**b, c, e, g**) *bars* = 50 μm. Reprinted with permission from Tokuda et al. [84]

organs; rare cases of a localized mammary gland amyloidosis have been reported.

Typically, localized amyloid deposits mimic malignancy, both clinically and radiologically. However, with surgical or local therapies, the prognosis for these lesions is excellent [68–70]. Multifocal and bilateral involvement of the genitourinary tract and recurrences, with subsequent obstructions, has also been reported [71, 72]. Hence, surveillance for obstruction is advocated. Renal and ipsilateral urothelial carcinoma with concomitant amyloidosis has also been reported; hence, pathologic examination is warranted. Other complications include the formation of vesico-peritoneal fistula [73]. While localized genitourinary amyloid is most often of the AL type, other types of amyloid have also been detected, including ATTR and AA [74, 75].

Pathogenesis

The reason for localized deposition of amyloid is unknown, but it is hypothesized that deposits result from local synthesis of the amyloid protein. Thus, it is postulated that chronic antigenic stimulation leads to chronic inflammation [9]. To this end, in localized AL deposits, there is frequently an infiltration of plasma cells in the vicinity of the deposits [85]. The plasma cell populations associated with local amyloid deposits have been shown to be clonal (by immunohistochemistry and/or analysis of immunoglobulin heavy chain gene rearrangements) which supports the hypothesis of local production of the amyloid precursor protein ([85], please see also Chap. 7 and Fig. 7.1). Evolution into systemic amyloidosis has not been reported, further supporting the hypothesis of local production of amyloid protein in these cases.

In recent years, localized amyloidosis has been reported with increasing frequency in association with plasma/B-cell proliferative lesions (Fig. 28.5). In particular, extranodal marginal zone lymphoma of mucosa-associated lymphoid tissue (MALT lymphoma) is increasingly reported in this context. MALT lymphoma is also the most prevalent histological subtype of primary malignant lymphoma of the urinary bladder and, although rare, has been reported in the kidney and ureter [86–88]. The reported anatomic sites affected by both entities (amyloid deposits and MALT lymphoma) include the skin/soft tissue, ocular adnexa, lung, upper aerodigestive tract, salivary gland, gastrointestinal tract (small bowel and stomach), and breast [83, 89]. In the urinary bladder, localized AL amyloidosis is also associated with subtle clonal B-cell/plasma cell proliferative lesions, which most likely represent MALT lymphoma (Fig. 28.5).

It is postulated that, in other types of localized deposits, local tissue factors may create a milieu favorable for fibrillogenesis. Secondary deposition of dialysis-associated amyloid deposits in transplanted ureters, presumably facilitated by preexisting ischemic ureteral damage, was also reported [90] in two renal transplant recipients with ureteral amyloid deposits and ureteral stenosis, each of whom received one kidney from the same donor.

Urinary Bladder

There are approximately 120 reported cases of localized amyloid deposits in the urinary bladder [12]. Biopsy demonstrates irregular, mass-forming deposits of amyloid in the bladder mucosa, including the local blood vessels, in the absence of systemic deposits (Fig. 28.6). In contrast to bladder involvement in systemic amyloidosis, deep (detrusor) muscle is not involved. Amyloid may also be detected in cytology specimens [91, 92]. On occasion, amyloid deposits may involve multiple sites (trigone, lower ureters, and prostatic stroma) in the lower urinary tract [62]. The lesions can be confused with bladder neoplasm and can cause obstruction. Recurrences of localized amyloid deposits have also been reported. Thus, Chan et al. [93] reported a case of primary bladder amyloidosis presenting with gross hydronephrosis 3 years after the first diagnosis. Laparoscopic ileal replacement of bilateral ureters was performed with no recurrent ureteric obstruction 2 years after surgery. Thus, localized amyloid may be progressive and a diagnosis of primary bladder amyloidosis warrants long-term surveillance of the upper urinary tract. Rare cases of primary localized non-AL amyloid of the bladder have also been reported

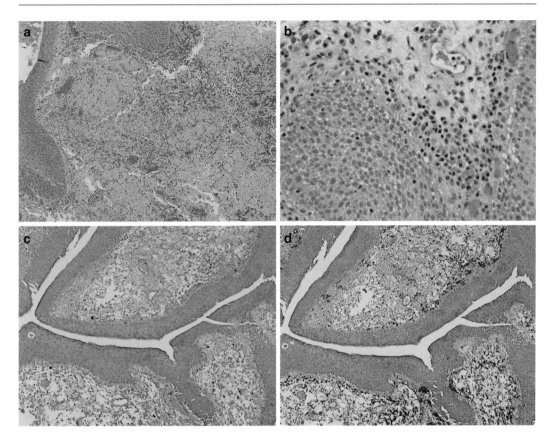

Fig. 28.5 Urinary bladder. Localized bladder amyloidosis in association with plasma cell disorder. (**a**) Amyloid deposits in the lamina propria, (**b**) plasma cells are seen in the vicinity of amyloid deposits, H&E stain. (**c**) Stain for kappa light chain, chromogenic in situ hybridization (CISH) stain, (**d**) stain for lambda light chain, CISH stain. In this case of a localized AL bladder amyloid, lambda light chain positive plasma cells predominate, while only rare cells are positive for kappa light chain. In the majority of cases of localized AL amyloid, the reverse is true

[74, 75]. Amyloidosis of the pelvis and/or ureter was also reported ([94, 95], see also Chap. 21 by Räisänen-Sokolowski, Fig. 21.2).

Prostate

Senile seminal vesicle amyloid clinically mimics mass and presents with hematospermia. The deposits of amyloid tend to be nodular and to affect the subepithelial layer of seminal vesicles (Fig. 28.7, please see also Chap. 7 and Fig. 7.14). Other parts of the ejaculatory system can also be involved, but there are no amyloid deposits in the blood vessels or in the prostatic parenchyma [66, 67]. Kee et al. [67] evaluated the incidence of amyloidosis in seminal vesicles, in a large series, and established it to be 4.7 %. Mass spectrometric analysis of the seminal vesicle amyloid revealed that, in all cases, the fibrils were composed mainly of polypeptide fragments identical in sequence to the N-terminal portion of the major secretory product of seminal vesicles, namely semenogelin. This form of amyloidosis is designated ASemI [66]. Interestingly, seminal vesicle amyloid does not seem to provide absolute or relative protection from seminal vesicle involvement by prostate cancer [96]. Corpora amylacea (extracellular spheroids with amyloid properties) may be found in the prostate in association with aging (please see also Chap. 7 and Fig. 7.17c, d).

Testis, Ovaries, and Adrenal Gland

Amyloid deposits in the testis, ovaries, and adrenal glands are usually associated with systemic

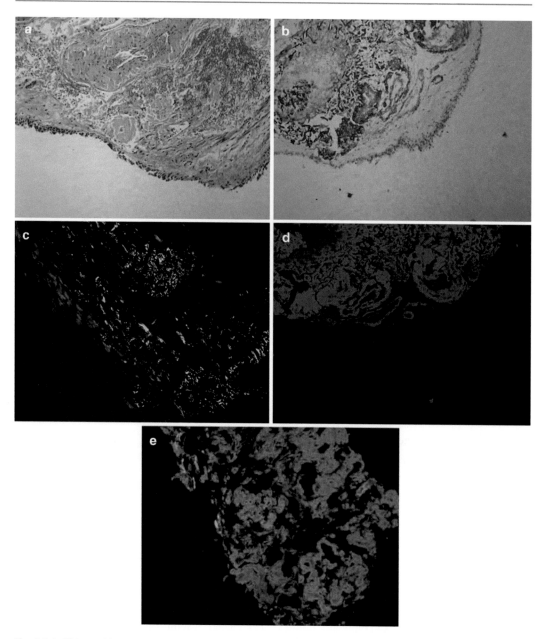

Fig. 28.6 Urinary bladder with abundant deposits of amyloid in the lamina propria. (**a**) H&E stain, (**b**) *Congo red* stain viewed under bright light, (**c**) *Congo red* stain viewed under polarized light, (**d**) *Congo red* stain viewed under fluorescence light (filter *Texas red*), (**e**) stain for lambda light chain, immunofluorescence, FITC stain. Please see also comment to Fig. 28.5 above

amyloidosis (please see above). A case of primary testicular amyloidosis, of undetermined amyloid type, mimicking tumor, in a cryptorchid testis, was also reported [79]. Fibrillar intracellular aggregates with amyloid staining properties have been described in the adrenal cortex (please

see Chap. 7 and Fig. 7.17a). The biochemical characteristics of the proteins are not known.

Penis

Urethral amyloidosis is a rare, probably inflammatory condition, usually presenting with hematuria

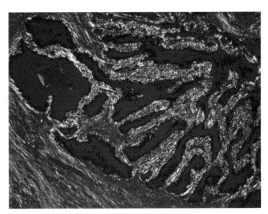

Fig. 28.7 Seminal vesicle amyloid—*Congo red* stain viewed under polarized light

and obstructive urinary symptoms, thus mimicking urethral malignancy [97–101]. Please see also Chap. 9 and Fig. 9.11. It may affect young males and cause urethral stricture [99] or urethrorrhagia occurring only during erection. A single case of amyloid in the urethral corpus spongiosum, with isolated urethrorrhagia during erection, has also been reported [101, 102]. Localized amyloidosis affecting only the glans is a very rare entity, with only seven cases reported [102–104]. Clinically, it may be associated with penile rash [103]. Biopsy of the lesion revealed dermal deposits of amyloid [104].

Female Genital Tract: Uterus, Cervix, Ovaries, Fallopian Tubes, Vulva

While the female genital tract may be affected by systemic amyloidosis, localized amyloid deposits have also been reported, albeit very rarely [105–109]. Localized AL amyloidosis, with a subtle MALT lymphoma involving the fallopian tube, was recently observed by Dr. April Chiu (personal communication), Fig. 28.8. Liu et al. reported six cases of amyloid in uterine leiomyoma [105]. Postmenopausal bleeding has also been associated with rare cases of isolated amyloid deposition in the uterine cervix [108, 109]. All cases reported to date were associated with a primary cervical squamous cell carcinoma; immunohistochemical studies demonstrated cytokeratin, presumably derived from tumor cells, similar to the pathogenesis of primary cutaneous amyloidosis [109].

Breast

Breast amyloidosis is rare. It can be part of a systemic disease or it may be localized to the breast [83, 110–116]. It is typically unilateral, but bilateral involvement has also been described [113]. Some of the reported cases were associated with carcinoma, including in situ, invasive ductal or lobular carcinoma [113, 114]. In addition to single case reports, three series of breast amyloidosis were published [83, 110, 111]. In 2002, Rocken et al. reported three cases of breast amyloidosis and reviewed the 42 previously reported cases; in 2011, Charlot et al. reported seven patients with localized amyloidosis and, in 2013, Said et al. reported 40 cases of breast amyloidosis.

The typical clinical presentation is that of a painless, solitary breast mass, which may or may not be associated with calcifications. Diagnosis is based on characteristic staining with Congo red; multinucleated giant cells are common. Breast amyloidosis has also been diagnosed by cytology, where amyloid was reported to appear as darkblue to purple clumps of acellular material on Diff-Quik stain, accompanied by chronic inflammatory cell infiltrates and multinucleated giant cells, simulating granulomatous inflammation. Papanicolaou stain demonstrated cyanophilic to orangophilic acellular material. However, confirmation with Congo red stain is required for diagnosis of amyloid [117].

While data on the amyloid type are limited, AL is the predominant type associated with mammary amyloidosis. Thus, in Rocken's review: among 18 cases where amyloid type was available, AL was diagnosed in 83 % (15/18 cases) and AH was diagnosed in another case [110]; in remaining two cases mammary AA amyloidosis was diagnosed. However, in the series from the Mayo Clinic, among specimens in which amyloid typing yielded diagnostic results, virtually all were typed as AL and one additional case was diagnosed as IgA/lambda [83]. Noticeably, none of the cases in the Mayo series were of the AA or other types. Prior to 2002 [110], in two cases, mammary amyloid was reported as AA. More recently, Chiang et al. [116] reported one case of breast amyloid associated with Castleman's

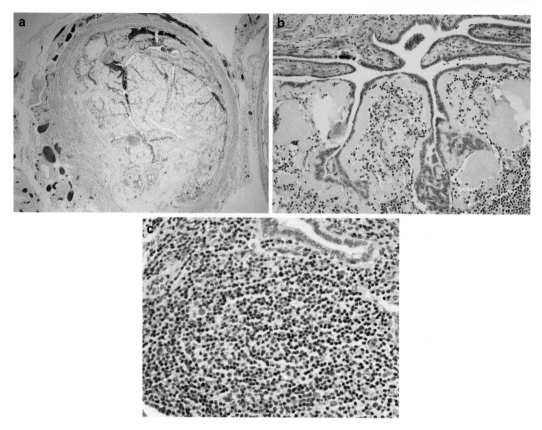

Fig. 28.8 Fallopian tube localized amyloidosis. (**a**) Low magnification demonstrating heavy deposits of amyloid with thickening of the fimbriated ends. (**b**) Plasma cells are seen in the vicinity of amyloid. (**c**) Lymphoid aggregate associated with amyloid deposits. Slides courtesy of Dr. April Chiu, Memorial Sloan Kettering Cancer Center, New York

disease. Since Castleman's disease is known to be associated with systemic AA amyloidosis, the authors presumed (but did not conclusively prove) that their case also represented a case of a mammary AA amyloidosis. Non-tumor forming amyloid deposition in the mammary gland can also be commonly seen in familial amyloid polyneuropathy (FAP), which is associated with systemic deposits derived from a mutant transthyretin [84]. In the series by Said et al., close to half of patients with breast amyloidosis had systemic AL amyloidosis. Since systemic disease was diagnosed before breast amyloidosis in most patients, the authors suggested that breast involvement is a relatively late event [83]. Nevertheless, the authors recommended a work up to rule out systemic amyloidosis in patients with localized mammary amyloidosis.

In localized mammary AL, deposits were derived more commonly from kappa light chain, which is similar to other, non-mammary, cases of localized AL amyloidosis. This is in contrast to systemic AL amyloidosis, where deposits of amyloid are derived more frequently from the lambda light chain. As discussed by Westermark (see Chap. 7), the reason for this is unknown but may be associated with differences in pathogenesis.

Briefly, similar to systemic AL amyloidosis, the amyloid is composed of a monoclonal immunoglobulin light chain, usually C-terminally truncated. However, in localized AL, the precursor light chain is synthesized at the site of deposition by a local clone of plasma cells, possibly initiated by antigenic stimulation causing chronic inflammation (Fig. 28.8). In a series by Said et al., mammary AL amyloidosis was noted to be frequently associated with a concomitant hematologic disorder, most commonly MALT lymphoma. Therefore, MALT lymphoma should be excluded in any patient with mammary amyloidosis. Conversely, breast tissue with MALT lymphoma should be stained for concurrent amyloidosis.

Patients with systemic amyloidosis and/or associated hematologic disorders are treated with chemotherapy, with or without radiation. The prognosis in such patients is guarded and largely dependent on the hematologic disease. In contrast, in patients with truly localized breast amyloidosis, without a systemic hematologic disorder, local treatment with surgery, with or without radiation, is sufficient [83, 110, 111].

In conclusion, breast amyloidosis is predominantly of the AL type. Almost half of the patients have systemic amyloidosis, and concurrent hematologic disorders in the breast are frequently seen. Hence, in patients with breast amyloidosis, further work up to rule out hematologic malignancy and/or systemic amyloidosis is warranted.

References

1. Herrera GA, Picken MM. Renal diseases associated with plasma cell dyscrasias, amyloidoses, Waldenstrom macroglobulinemia and cryoglobulinemic nephropathies. In: Jennette JC, Olson JL, Silva FG, D'Agati V, editors. Heptinstall's pathology of the kidney. 7th ed. Philadelphia, PA: Lippincott Williams & Wilkins; 2014. p. 951–114.
2. Ozdemir D, Dagdelen S, Erbas T. Endocrine involvement in systemic amyloidosis. Endocr Pract. 2010;16(6):1056–63.
3. Ozdemir BH, Ozdemir OG, Ozdemir FN, Ozdemir AI. Value of testis biopsy in the diagnosis of systemic amyloidosis. Urology. 2002;59(2):201–5.
4. Scalvini T, Martini PR, Obici L, Tardanico R, Biasi L, Gregorini G, Scolari F, Merlini G. Infertility and hypergonadotropic hypogonadism as first evidence of hereditary apolipoprotein A-I amyloidosis. J Urol. 2007;178(1):344–8.
5. Mijatovic V, Hompes PG, Wouters MG. Familial Mediterranean fever and its implications for fertility and pregnancy. Eur J Obstet Gynecol Reprod Biol. 2003;108(2):171–6.
6. Piccin A, Vezzali N, Pescosta N, Steurer M, Palladini G, Billio A. Ovarian hyperstimulation syndrome in systemic amyloidosis. Amyloid. 2014;21(1):69–70.
7. Nagasaka T, Togashi S, Watanabe H, Iida H, Nagasaka K, Nakamura Y, Miwa M, Kobayashi F, Shindo K, Shiozawa Z. Clinical and histopathological features of progressive-type familial amyloidotic polyneuropathy with TTR Lys54. J Neurol Sci. 2009;276(1–2):88–94.
8. Biewend ML, Menke DM, Calamia KT. The spectrum of localized amyloidosis: a case series of 20 patients and review of the literature. Amyloid. 2006;13(3):135–42.
9. Merrimen JL, Alkhudair WK, Gupta R. Localized amyloidosis of the urinary tract: case series of nine patients. Urology. 2006;67(5):904–9.
10. Paccalin M, Hachulla E, Cazalet C, Tricot L, Carreiro M, Rubi M, Grateau G, Roblot P. Localized amyloidosis: a survey of 35 French cases. Amyloid. 2005;12(4):239–45.
11. Tirzaman O, Wahner-Roedler DL, Malek RS, Sebo TJ, Li CY, Kyle RA. Primary localized amyloidosis of the urinary bladder: a case series of 31 patients. Mayo Clin Proc. 2000;75(12):1264–8.
12. Zhou F, Lee P, Zhou M, Melamed J, Deng FM. Primary localized amyloidosis of the urinary tract frequently mimics neoplasia: a clinicopathologic analysis of 11 cases. Am J Clin Exp Urol. 2014;2(1):71–5. eCollection 2014.
13. von Hutten H, Mihatsch M, Lobeck H, Rudolph B, Eriksson M, Röcken C. Prevalence and origin of amyloid in kidney biopsies. Am J Surg Pathol. 2009;33(8):1198–205.
14. Larsen CP, Walker PD, Weiss DT, Solomon A. Prevalence and morphology of leukocyte chemotactic factor 2-associated amyloid in renal biopsies. Kidney Int. 2010;77(9):816–9.
15. Hopfer H, Wiech T, Mihatsch MJ. Renal amyloidosis revisited: amyloid distribution, dynamics and biochemical type. Nephrol Dial Transplant. 2011;26(9):2877–84. doi:10.1093/ndt/gfq831. Epub 2011 Mar 21.
16. Said SM, Sethi S, Valeri AM, Leung N, Cornell LD, Fidler ME, Herrera Hernandez L, Vrana JA, Theis JD, Quint PS, Dogan A, Nasr SH. Renal amyloidosis: origin and clinicopathologic correlations of 474 recent cases. Clin J Am Soc Nephrol. 2013;8: 1515–23.
17. Lobato L, Rocha A. Transthyretin amyloidosis and the kidney. Clin J Am Soc Nephrol. 2012;7(8):1337–46. doi:10.2215/CJN.08720811. Epub 2012 Apr 26.
18. Schönland SO, Hegenbart U, Bochtler T, Mangatter A, Hansberg M, Ho AD, Lohse P, Röcken C. Immunohistochemistry in the classification of systemic forms of amyloidosis: a systematic investigation of 117 patients. Blood. 2012;119(2):488–93. doi:10.1182/blood-2011-06-358507. Epub 2011 Nov 21.
19. Said SM, Sethi S, Valeri AM, Chang A, Nast CC, Krahl L, Molloy P, Barry M, Fidler ME, Cornell LD, Leung N, Vrana JA, Theis JD, Dogan A, Nasr SH. Renal leukocyte chemotactic factor 2-associated

amyloidosis. Kidney Int. 2014;86:370–7. Published online 22 January 2014.

20. Larsen CP, Kossmann RJ, Beggs ML, Solomon A, Walker PD. Renal leukocyte chemotactic factor 2 amyloidosis (ALECT2): a case series detailing clinical, morphologic, and genetic features. Kidney Int. 2014;86:378–82. Published online 12 February 2014.

21. Picken MM. Alect2 amyloidosis: primum non nocere (first, do no harm). Kidney Int. 2014;86(2): 229–32.

22. Sethi S, Theis JD, Leung N, Dispenzieri A, Nasr SH, Fidler ME, Cornell LD, Gamez JD, Vrana JA, Dogan A. Mass spectrometry-based proteomic diagnosis of renal immunoglobulin heavy chain amyloidosis. Clin J Am Soc Nephrol. 2010;5(12):2180–7.

23. Nasr SH, Said SM, Valeri AM, Sethi S, Fidler ME, Cornell LD, Gertz MA, Dispenzieri A, Buadi FK, Vrana JA, Theis JD, Dogan A, Leung N. The diagnosis and characteristics of renal heavy-chain and heavy/light-chain amyloidosis and their comparison with renal light-chain amyloidosis. Kidney Int. 2013;83(3):463–70. Epub 2013 Jan 9.

24. Picken MM. Non-light-chain immunoglobulin amyloidosis: time to expand or refine the spectrum to include light+heavy chain amyloidosis? Kidney Int. 2013;83(3):353–6.

25. Leung N, Nasr SH, Sethi S. How I treat amyloidosis: the importance of accurate diagnosis and amyloid typing. Blood. 2012;120(16):3206–16.

26. Bridoux F, Nelson L, Hutchison CA, Touchard G, Sethi S, Fermand JP, Picken MM, Herrera GA, Kastritis E, Merlini G, Roussel M, Fervenza FC, Dispenzieri A, Kyle RA, Nasr SH, on behalf of the International Kidney and Monoclonal Gammopathy Research Group. Diagnosis of monoclonal gammopathy of renal significance. Kid Int. 2015;87(4):698–711. doi:10.1038/ki.2014.408. Epub ahead of print (21 January 2015), http://www.nature.com/doifinder/10.1038/ki.2014.408. Advance Online Publication (AOP) service.

27. Uemichi T, Liepnieks JJ, Benson MD. Hereditary renal amyloidosis with a novel variant fibrinogen. J Clin Invest. 1994;93(2):731–6.

28. Picken MM, Linke RP. Nephrotic syndrome due to an amyloidogenic mutation in Fibrinogen A alpha chain. J Am Soc Nephrol. 2009;20:1681–5.

29. Masutani K, Nagata M, Ikeda H, Takeda K, Katafuchi R, Hirakata H, Tsuruya K, Iida M. Glomerular crescent formation in renal amyloidosis. A clinicopathological study and demonstration of upregulated cell-mediated immunity. Clin Nephrol. 2008;70(6):464–74.

30. Hatakeyama T, Komatsuda A, Matsuda A, Togashi M, Maki N, Masai R, Sawada K, Wakui H. Renal amyloidosis associated with extracapillary glomerulonephritis and vasculitis in a patient with inflammatory bowel disease treated with infliximab. Clin Nephrol. 2008;70(3):240–4.

31. Crosthwaite A, Skene A, Mount P. Rapidly progressive glomerulonephritis complicating primary AL amyloidosis and multiple myeloma. Nephrol Dial Transplant. 2010;25(8):2786–9. Epub 2009 Dec 29.

32. Sethi S, Theis JD, Shiller SM, Nast CC, Harrison D, Rennke HG, Vrana JA, Dogan A. Medullary amyloidosis associated with apolipoprotein A-IV deposition. Kidney Int. 2012;81(2):201–6. doi:10.1038/ki.2011.316. Epub 2011 Sep 7.

33. Itabashi M, Takei T, Tsukada M, Sugiura H, Uchida K, Tsuchiya K, Honda K, Nitta K. Association between clinical characteristics and AL amyloid deposition in the kidney. Heart Vessels. 2010;25(6): 543–8. Epub 2010 Oct 5.

34. Eirin A, Irazabal MV, Gertz MA, Dispenzieri A, Lacy MQ, Shaji Kumar S, Sethi S, Nasr SH, Cornell LD, Fidler ME, Fervenza FC, Leung N. Clinical features of patients with immunoglobulin light chain amyloidosis (AL) with vascular-limited deposition in the kidney. Nephrol Dial Transplant. 2012;27: 1097–101. doi:10.1093/ndt/gfr381. Advance Access publication 7 November 2011.

35. Steffl D, Göbel H, Groth C, Fischer KG, Kühn W, Walz G, Gerke P. Quiz page. Renal AA amyloidosis with vascular predominance, secondary to rheumatoid arthritis. Am J Kidney Dis. 2007;49(2): A49–50.

36. Nakayama N, Fujigaki Y, Tsuji T, Sakakima M, Yasuda H, Togawa A, Suzuki H, Fujikura T, Kato A, Baba S, Takahashi S, Hishida A. Rapid deterioration of renal function in a patient with multiple myeloma associated with amyloid and light chain depositions. Clin Exp Nephrol. 2009;13(6):671–6.

37. Picken MM. Amyloidosis—where are we now and where are we heading? Arch Path Lab Med. 2010;2010(134):545–51.

38. Picken MM. Current practice in amyloid detection and typing among renal pathologists. Amyloid. 2011;18 Suppl 1:73–5.

39. Vasala M, Immonen K, Kautiainen H, Hakala M. More evidence of declining incidence of amyloidosis associated with inflammatory rheumatic diseases. Scand J Rheumatol. 2010;39(6):461–5. Epub 2010 Jun 21.

40. Benson MD, James S, Scott K, Liepnieks JJ, Kluve-Beckerman B. Leukocyte chemotactic factor 2: a novel renal protein. Kidney Int. 2008;74(2):218–22.

41. Mereuta OM, Theis JD, Vrana JA, Law ME, Grogg KI, Dasari S, Chandan VS, Wu TT, Jimenez-Zepeda VH, Fonseca R, Dispenzieri A, Kurtin PJ, Dogan A. Leukocyte cell-derived chemotaxin 2 (LECT2)-associated amyloidosis is a frequent cause of hepatic amyloidosis in the United States. Blood. 2014; 123(10):1479–82.

42. Lachmann HJ, Booth DR, Booth SE, Bybee A, Gillbertson JA, Gillmore JD, Pepys MB, Hawkins PN. Misdiagnosis of hereditary amyloidosis as AL (primary) amyloidosis. N Engl J Med. 2002;346(23): 1786–91.

43. Picken MM. New insights into systemic amyloidosis: the importance of type diagnosis. Curr Opin Nephrol Hypertens. 2007;16:196–203.
44. Miyazaki D, Yazaki M, Gono T, Kametani F, Tsuchiya A, Matsuda M, Takenaka Y, Hosh 2nd Y, Ikeda S. AH amyloidosis associated with an immunoglobulin heavy chain variable region (VH1) fragment: a case report. Amyloid. 2008;15(2):125–8.
45. Lachmann HJ, Goodman HJ, Gilbertson JA, Gallimore JR, Sabin CA, Gillmore JD, Hawkins PN. Natural history and outcome in systemic AA amyloidosis. N Engl J Med. 2007;356(23):2361–71.
46. Hutton HL, DeMarco ML, Magil AB, Taylor P. Renal leukocyte chemotactic factor 2 (LECT2) amyloidosis in First Nations people in Northern British Columbia, Canada: a report of 4 cases. Am J Kidney Dis. 2014;64(5):790–2. Published Online: July 24, 2014.
47. Gillmore JD, Lachmann HJ, Rowczenio D, Gilbertson JA, Zeng CH, Liu ZH, Li LS, Wechalekar A, Hawkins PN. Diagnosis, pathogenesis, treatment, and prognosis of hereditary fibrinogen A alpha-chain amyloidosis. J Am Soc Nephrol. 2009;20(2): 444–51.
48. Stangou AJ, Banner NR, Hendry BM, Rela M, Portmann B, Wendon J, Monaghan M, Maccarthy P, Buxton-Thomas M, Mathias CJ, Liepnieks JJ, O'Grady J, Heaton ND, Benson MD. Hereditary fibrinogen A alpha-chain amyloidosis: phenotypic characterization of a systemic disease and the role of liver transplantation. Blood. 2010;115(15): 2998–3007.
49. Picken MM. Fibrinogen amyloidosis: the clot thickens! Blood. 2010;115(15):2985–6.
50. Eriksson M, Schönland S, Yumlu S, Hegenbart U, von Hutten H, Gioeva Z, Lohse P, Büttner J, Schmidt H, Röcken C. Hereditary apolipoprotein AI-associated amyloidosis in surgical pathology specimens: identification of three novel mutations in the APOA1 gene. J Mol Diagn. 2009;11(3):257–62.
51. Rowczenio D, Dogan A, Theis JD, Vrana JA, Lachmann HJ, Wechalekar AD, Gilbertson JA, Hunt T, Gibbs SD, Sattianayagam PT, Pinney JH, Hawkins PN, Gillmore JD. Amyloidogenicity and clinical phenotype associated with five novel mutations in apolipoprotein A-I. Am J Pathol. 2011;179(4):1978–87. doi:10.1016/j.ajpath.2011.06.024. Epub 2011 Aug 5.
52. Maury CPJ, Kere J, Tolvanen R, de la Chapelle A. Homozygosity for the Asn187 gelsolin mutation in Finnish-type familial amyloidosis is associated with severe renal disease. Genomics. 1992;13(3): 902–3.
53. Yazaki M, Farrell SA, Benson MD. A novel lysozyme mutation Phe57Ile associated with hereditary renal amyloidosis. Kidney Int. 2003;63(5):1652–7.
54. Palsdottir A, Snorradottir AO, Thorsteinsson L. Hereditary cystatin C amyloid angiopathy: genetic, clinical, and pathological aspects. Brain Pathol. 2006;16(1):55–9.
55. Mazanec K, McClure J, Bartley CJ, Newbould MJ, Ackrill PJ. Systemic amyloidosis of beta 2 microglobulin type. Clin Pathol. 1992;45(9):832–3.
56. Esslimani M, Serre I, Granier M, Robert M, Baldet P, Costes V. [Urogenital amyloidosis: clinicopathological study of 8 cases]. Ann Pathol. 1999; 19(6):487–91.
57. Davis P, Corcoran N, Hanegbi U, Bultitude M. Systemic amyloidosis presenting with lower urinary tract symptoms. ANZ J Surg. 2010;80(10): 759–60.
58. Javed A, Canales BK, Maclennan GT. Bladder amyloidosis. J Urol. 2010;183(6):2388–9.
59. DeSouza MA, Rekhi B, Thyavihally YB, Tongaonkar HB, Desai SB. Localized amyloidosis of the urinary bladder, clinically masquerading as bladder cancer. J Clin Rheumatol. 2008;14(3):161–5.
60. Monge M, Chauveau D, Cordonnier C, Noël LH, Presne C, Makdassi R, Jauréguy M, Lecaque C, Renou M, Grünfeld JP, Choukroun G. Localized amyloidosis of the genitourinary tract: report of 5 new cases and review of the literature. Medicine (Baltimore). 2011;90(3):212–22.
61. Borza T, Shah RB, Faerber GJ, Wolf Jr JS. Localized amyloidosis of the upper urinary tract: a case series of three patients managed with reconstructive surgery or surveillance. J Endourol. 2010;24(4):641–4.
62. Singh SK, Wadhwa P, Nada R, Mohan VC, Singh P, Jha V. Localized primary amyloidosis of the prostate, bladder and ureters. Int Urol Nephrol. 2005;37(3):495–7.
63. Duffau P, Imbert Y, De Faucal P, Fleury D, Arlet P, Camou F, Etienne G, Paccalin M. [Primary localized amyloidosis of the urinary tract. A case series of five patients]. Rev Med Interne. 2005;26(4):288–93.
64. Domiciano DS, de Carvalho JF. Primary localized amyloidosis of the ureter. Isr Med Assoc J. 2008; 10(3):237–8.
65. Banerji JS, Gopalakrishnan G, Sriram K, Manipadam MT. Localised retroperitoneal amyloidosis mimicking retroperitoneal fibrosis: a rare cause of obstructive uropathy. Singapore Med J. 2009;50(9):e332–5.
66. Linke RP, Joswig R, Murphy CL, Wang S, Zhou H, Gross U, Rocken C, Westermark P, Weiss DT, Solomon A. Senile seminal vesicle amyloid is derived from semenogelin I. J Lab Clin Med. 2005;145(4):187–96.
67. Kee KH, Lee MJ, Shen SS, Suh JH, Lee OJ, Cho HY, Ayala AG, Ro JY. Amyloidosis of seminal vesicles and ejaculatory ducts: a histologic analysis of 21 cases among 447 prostatectomy specimens. Ann Diagn Pathol. 2008;12(4):235–8.
68. Zaman W, Singh V, Kumar B, Mandhani A, Srivastava A, Kumar A, Kapoor R. Localized primary amyloidosis of the genitourinary tract: does conservatism help? Urol Int. 2004;73(3):280–2.
69. Alsikafi NF, O'Connor RC, Yang XJ, Steinberg GD. Primary amyloidosis of the bladder treated with partial cystectomy. Can J Urol. 2003;10(4):1950–1.

70. Hafron JM, Flanigan RC. Primary localized amyloidosis of the ureter and bladder managed by ileal interposition. Tech Urol. 2000;6(1):50–2.
71. Fushimi T, Takei Y, Touma T, Kudoh S, Yamamoto K, Hoshii Y, Ishihara T, Ikeda S. Bilateral localized amyloidosis of the ureters: clinicopathology and therapeutic approaches in two cases. Amyloid. 2004;11(4):260–4.
72. Patel S, Trivedi A, Dholaria P, Dholakia M, Devra A, Gupta B, Shah SA. Recurrent multifocal primary amyloidosis of urinary bladder. Saudi J Kidney Dis Transpl. 2008;19(2):247–9.
73. Hajji K, Martin L, Devevey JM, Tanter Y, Justrabo E, Rifle G, Mousson C. Rheumatoid arthritis-induced pseudotumoral AA amyloidosis of the bladder with vesico-peritoneal fistula. Clin Nephrol. 2007;67(1):38–43.
74. Akram CM, Al-Marhoon MS, Mathew J, Grant CS, Rao TV. Primary localized AA type amyloidosis of urinary bladder: case report of rare cause of episodic painless hematuria. Urology. 2006;68(6):1343.e15–7.
75. Boorjian S, Choi BB, Loo MH, Kim P, Sandhu J. A rare case of painless gross hematuria: primary localized AA-type amyloidosis of the urinary bladder. Urology. 2002;59(1):137.
76. Mount SL, Eltabbakh GH, Hardin NJ. Beta-2 microglobulin amyloidosis presenting as bilateral ovarian masses: a case report and review of the literature. Am J Surg Pathol. 2002;26(1):130–3.
77. Haimov-Kochman R, Prus D, Ben-Chetrit E. Azoospermia due to testicular amyloidosis in a patient with familial Mediterranean fever. Hum Reprod. 2001;16(6):1218–20.
78. Corvino C, Balloni F, Meliani E, Giannini A, Serni S, Carini M. Testicular amyloidosis. Urol Int. 2002;69(2):162–3.
79. Casella R, Nudell D, Cozzolino D, Wang H, Lipshultz LI. Primary testicular amyloidosis mimicking tumor in a cryptorchid testis. Urology. 2002;59(3):445.
80. Ogawa Y, Nakagawa M, Ikeda S. Prostate amyloid tumor is a clue leading to the diagnosis of systemic AL amyloidosis. Amyloid. 2013;20(3):193–4.
81. Meinzer U, Marie I, Koné-Paut I, Tran TA. Hypofertility in Muckle Wells syndrome and treatment with IL-1 targeting drugs. Pediatr Rheumatol Online J. 2011;9 Suppl 1:P14.
82. Urieli-Shoval S, Finci-Yeheskel Z, Eldar I, Linke RP, Levin M, Prus D, Haimov-Kochman R. Serum amyloid A: expression throughout human ovarian folliculogenesis and levels in follicular fluid of women undergoing controlled ovarian stimulation. J Clin Endocrinol Metab. 2013;98(12):4970–8. Epub 2013 Sep 12.
83. Said SM, Reynolds C, Jimenez RE, Chen B, Vrana JA, Theis JD, Dogan A, Shah SS. Amyloidosis of the breast: predominantly AL type and over half have concurrent breast hematologic disorders. Mod Pathol. 2013;26:232–8. Published online 28 September 2012.
84. Tokuda T, Takei Y, Takayama B, Hoshii Y, Ikeda S. Severe amyloid deposition in mammary glands of familial amyloid polyneuropathy patients. Amyloid. 2007;14(3):249–53.
85. Setoguchi M, Hoshii Y, Kawano H, Ishihara T. Analysis of plasma cell clonality in localized AL amyloidosis. Amyloid. 2000;7:41–5.
86. Al-Maghrabi J, Kamel-Reid S, Jewett M, Gospodarowicz M, Wells W, Banerjee D. Primary low-grade B-cell lymphoma of mucosa-associated lymphoid tissue type arising in the urinary bladder. Report of 4 cases with molecular analysis. Arch Pathol Lab Med. 2001;125:332–6.
87. Garcia M, Konoplev S, Morosan C, Abruzzo LV, Bueso-Ramos CE, Medeiros JL. Malt lymphoma involving the kidney. A report of 10 cases and review of the literature. Am J Clin Pathol. 2007;128:464–73.
88. Otsuki H, Ito K, Sato K, Kosaka T, Shimazaki H, Kaji T, Asano T. Malignant lymphoma of mucosa-associated lymphoid tissue involving the renal pelvis and the entire ureter: a case report. Oncol Lett. 2013;5:1625–8.
89. Ryan RJH, Sloan JM, Collins AB, Mansouri J, Raje NS, Zukerberg LR, Ferry JA. Extranodal marginal zone lymphoma of mucosa-associated lymphoid tissue with amyloid deposition: a clinicopathologic case series. Am J Clin Pathol. 2012;137:51–64.
90. Buchholz NP, Moch H, Gasser TC, Linke RP, Thiel GT, Mihatsch MJ. Ureteral amyloid deposits of beta 2-icroglobuin origin in both kidney recipients of 1 donor. J Urol. 1995;153(2):399–401.
91. Takahashi T, Miura H, Matsu-ura Y, Iwana S, Maruyama R, Harada T. Urine cytology of localized primary amyloidosis of the ureter: a case report. Acta Cytol. 2005;49(3):319–22.
92. Picken MM. Diagnosis of amyloid in urine cytology specimens. In: Hazenberg BPC, Bijzet J, editors. XIIIth International Symposium on Amyloidosis. The Netherlands: GUARD (Groningen Unit for Amyloidosis Research & Development) UMC Groningen; 2013. p. 161–2.
93. Chan ES, Ng CF, Chui KL, Hou SM, Yip SK. Primary bladder amyloidosis—case report of a patient with delayed upper urinary tract obstruction 3 years after the diagnosis. Amyloid. 2010;17(1):36–8.
94. Sparwasser C, Gilbert P, Mohr W, Linke RP. Unilateral extended amyloidosis of the renal pelvis and ureter: a case report. Urol Int. 1991;46(2):208–10.
95. Fugita OE, DeLatorre CG, Kavoussi LR. Primary localized amyloidosis of the ureter. Urology. 2001;58(2):281.
96. Erbersdobler A, Kollermann J, Graefen M, Röcken C, Schlomm T. Seminal vesicle amyloidosis does not provide any protection from invasion by prostate cancer. BJU Int. 2009;103(3):324–6.
97. Ichioka K, Utsunomiya N, Ueda N, Matsui Y, Yoshimura K, Terai A. Primary localized amyloidosis of urethra: magnetic resonance imaging findings. Urology. 2004;64(2):376–8.

98. Biyani CS, Fitzmaurice RJ, Upsdell SM. Localized amyloidosis of the urethra with transitional cell carcinoma of the bladder. BJU Int. 1999;83(6):722–3.
99. Crook TJ, Koslowski M, Dyer JP, Bass P, Birch BR. A case of amyloid of the urethra and review of this rare diagnosis, its natural history and management, with reference to the literature. Scand J Urol Nephrol. 2002;36(6):481–6.
100. Lim JH, Kim H. Localized amyloidosis presenting with a penile mass: a case report. Cases J. 2009;2:160.
101. Cormio L, Sanguedeolce F, Pentimone S, Perrone A, Annese A, Turri FP, Bufo P, Carrieri G. Urethral corpus spongiosum amyloidosis presenting with urethrorrhagia during erection. J Sex Med. 2009; 6(10):2915–7.
102. Ritter M, Nawab RA, Tannenbaum M, Hakky SI, Morgan MB. Localized amyloidosis of the glans penis: a case report and literature review. J Cutan Pathol. 2003;30(1):37–40.
103. Kawsar M, Long S. Localized amyloidosis of glans penis. Int J STD AIDS. 2007;18(10):720–1.
104. Dominguez Dominguez M, Valero Puerta JA, Jimenez Leiro JF, Martinez Ruiz R, Medina Perez M. Primary localized amyloidosis of glans penis. A new case and review of the literature. Actas Urol Esp. 2007;31(2):168–71.
105. Liu J, Zhai F, Ge P, Lu J, Qin Y, Sun X. Investigation of amyloid deposition in uterine leiomyoma patients. Health. 2012;4(8):522–5. http://dx.doi.org/10.4236/health.2012.48083.
106. Kotru M, Chandra H, Singh N, Bhatia A. Localized amyloidosis in endometrioid carcinoma of the uterus: a rare association. Arch Gynecol Obstet. 2007;276(4):383–4. Epub 2007 Apr 4.
107. Gibbons D, Lindberg GM, Ashfaq R, Saboorian MH. Localized amyloidosis of the uterine cervix. Int J Gynecol Pathol. 1998;17(4):368–71.
108. Yamada M, Hatakeyama S, Yamamoto E, Kimura Y, Tsukagoshi H, Yokota T, Uchino F. Localized amyloidosis of the uterine cervix. Virchows Arch A Pathol Anat Histopathol. 1988;413(3):265–8.
109. Tsang WY, Chan JK. Amyloid-producing squamous cell carcinoma of the uterine cervix. Arch Pathol Lab Med. 1993;117(2):199–201.
110. Roecken C, Kronsbein H, Sletten K, et al. Amyloidosis of the breast. Virchows Arch. 2002;440: 527–35.
111. Charlot M, Seldin DC, O'Hara C, Skinner M, Sanchorawala V. Localized amyloidosis of the breast: a case series. Amyloid. 2011;18:72–5.
112. Morris GJ, Schmidt PH, Jagannath S. Two cases of plasma cell dyscrasias with systemic involvement of breast. Semin Oncol. 2014;41(4):e33–7. doi:10.1053/j.seminoncol.2014.06.007. Epub 2014 Jun 26.
113. Gupta D, Shidham V, Zemba-Palko V, et al. Primary bilateral mucosa-associated lymphoid tissue lymphoma of the breast with atypical ductal hyperplasia and localized amyloidosis. A case report and review of the literature. Arch Pathol Lab Med. 2000; 124:1233–6.
114. Sabate JM, Clotet M, Torrubia S, Guerrero R, Pineda R, Lerma E, Capdevila E. Localized amyloidosis of the breast associated with invasive lobular carcinoma. Br J Radiol. 2008;81:e252–4.
115. Toohey JM, Ismail K, Lonergan D, et al. Amyloidosis of the breast mimicking recurrence in a previously treated early breast cancer. Australas Radiol. 2007;51:594–6.
116. Chiang D, Lee M, Gaermaine P, Liao L. Amyloidosis of the breast with multicentric DCIS and pleomorphic invasive lobular carcinoma in a patient with underlying extranodal Castleman's disease. Case Rep Radiol. 2013;2013:190856. 3 pages http://dx.doi.org/10.1155/2013/190856.
117. Sahoo S, Reeves W, DeMay RM. Amyloid tumor: a clinical and cytomorphologic study. Diagn Cytopathol. 2003;28(6):325–8.

Cardiac Amyloidosis

Carmela D. Tan and E. Rene Rodriguez

When the heart is involved by amyloidosis, the amyloid can be deposited in the atrial and ventricular myocardium, the sinoatrial and atrioventricular conduction system, the valves, and the intramural coronary arteries. Amyloid deposition in the cardiovascular system can be age-related or pathologic. It can also occur as a localized phenomenon to the heart or be part of a systemic involvement. Age-related amyloidosis is generally asymptomatic and is seen in three main patterns. Isolated atrial amyloidosis and isolated aortic amyloidosis are local forms of senile amyloidosis, while senile systemic amyloidosis involves predominantly the heart with amyloid also deposited in other organs to a much lesser extent. Pathologic deposition of amyloid in the heart, in the vast majority of cases, is due to the presence of two main proteins, monoclonal immunoglobulin light chains and transthyretin.

Localized Amyloidoses

Isolated Atrial Amyloidosis

Isolated atrial amyloidosis (IAA) is an organ-limited senile type of amyloidosis. The incidence

C.D. Tan, MD (✉) • E.R. Rodriguez, MD
Department of Pathology, Cleveland Clinic Lerner
College of Medicine of Case Western Reserve
University, 9500 Euclid Avenue L25, Cleveland,
OH 44195, USA
e-mail: tanc@ccf.org; rodrigr2@ccf.org

and extent of amyloid deposition increase with age, but its functional significance is uncertain. Diagnosis is made only on histologic examination of resected atrial appendages or at autopsy. Amyloid deposits can be found in the atrium as early as the fourth decade, and its prevalence reported as high as 80 % in patients over 80 years [1–4]. The major precursor protein is derived from α (alpha)-atrial natriuretic peptide (ANP) synthesized by atrial cardiac myocytes.

Most studies show a higher incidence of IAA in women. The left atrium is more commonly affected than the right [3, 4]. IAA is most commonly present in the subendocardial myocardium in a patchy distribution. It appears as fine strands and streaks of interstitial deposits around myocytes and less commonly as interstitial small nodular deposits (Fig. 29.1). Amyloid deposits can also be seen within the endocardium and occasionally in the walls of small veins and arterioles. Investigators have reported reactivity with both mature carboxy terminal peptide α-ANP and amino terminal precursor fragment proANP as well as brain natriuretic peptide in the amyloid fibrils by immunoelectron microscopy [5].

The clinical significance of IAA, in particular, a causative relation to atrial tachyarrhythmias, remains controversial [3, 6, 7]. Conditions that lead to increased synthesis and secretion of ANP resulting in a high local concentration of the precursor protein have been postulated to accelerate amyloidogenesis. Accordingly, in some patients

© Springer International Publishing Switzerland 2015
M.M. Picken et al. (eds.), *Amyloid and Related Disorders*, Current Clinical Pathology,
DOI 10.1007/978-3-319-19294-9_29

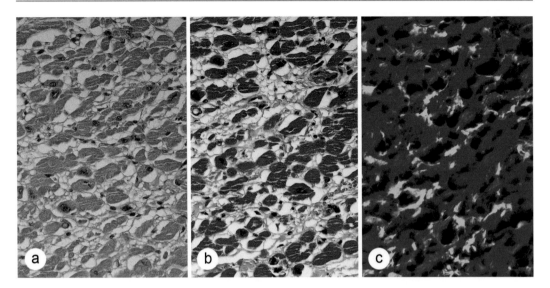

Fig. 29.1 Isolated atrial amyloid. Autopsy examination showed slight rigidity of the left atrial wall. (**a**) The cardiac myocytes show hypertrophy but no distinct eosinophilic infiltrate in the interstitial space (H&E ×400). (**b**) Movat stain shows extracellular material stained *orange red* with *very faint green* strands in the interstitium (Movat stain ×400). (**c**) Examination of the thioflavin S stain under UV light microscopy shows irregular aggregates and strands of amyloid (*light blue* fluorescence) corresponding to the areas of *orange-red* and *green* staining on Movat (thioflavin S ×400)

left atrial dilatation and chronic atrial fibrillation have been associated with increased serum ANP levels and severity of amyloid deposits found in the atrium. Serum ANP is also elevated in the elderly population, probably related to increased incidence of cardiac conditions that stimulate ANP secretion.

Senile Aortic Amyloid

Amyloid deposited in the aorta is believed to be the most common of the age-related amyloidoses, being detectable in 97 % of persons aged 50 or older [8]. Purification and amino acid sequence analysis of aortic amyloid revealed the major fibril protein to be an internal fragment of lactadherin called medin [9]. The precursor protein lactadherin is synthesized locally by vascular smooth muscle cells.

This type of amyloid is seen in the middle part of the media as small irregular aggregates or linear streaks parallel to the elastic lamellae that cause minimal distortion of the medial architecture. The amount of amyloid deposits is found to

be greater in the thoracic aorta than in the abdominal aorta. Amyloid has also been detected in the media of basilar arteries and around the internal elastic lamina of temporal arteries [10].

There are no known consequences of aortic amyloid although one study has shown that oligomeric medin exerts toxic effect to smooth muscle cells in culture [11]. Medin also induces the production of matrix metalloproteinase 2 which degrades elastic laminae.

Senile aortic amyloid is distinct from that occasionally seen in the intima and adventitia. Amyloid derived from wild-type apolipoprotein A1 can be found within atheromatous plaques in the intima [12]. Amyloid occurring in the adventitia and vasa vasorum is part of senile and other types of systemic amyloidosis.

Valvular Amyloidosis

Cardiac valves are commonly infiltrated in systemic amyloidosis with deposits often grossly visible in mitral and tricuspid valves. Infiltration of the semilunar valves is less conspicuous.

Valvular regurgitation associated with amyloid deposition is generally not clinically significant. On the other hand, localized small deposits of amyloid are incidental findings of no clinical importance in surgically excised cardiac valves with a reported prevalence ranging from 15.5 to 67 % in different case series [13–16]. The occurrence of this type of amyloid in valves does not correlate with age. Rather, it is strongly correlated with degenerative and postinflammatory fibrosis and calcification. The amyloid deposits are most common in stenotic aortic valves and are not seen in myxomatous degeneration. Amyloid deposits appear as small irregular plaques within areas of dense fibrosis and hyalinization and are also found at the periphery of calcific deposits (Fig. 29.2). The nature of this amyloid is yet to be established as it does not react with antibodies to the common amyloid proteins that affect the heart.

Systemic Amyloidoses

Immunoglobulin Light Chain Amyloidosis

The most common type of amyloid protein deposited in the heart is derived from monoclonal immunoglobulin light chains (AL) secondary to a plasma cell dyscrasia. This type of amyloidosis, termed AL amyloidosis, involves the heart in about half of the patients with plasma cell dyscrasia. Cardiac amyloidosis almost always occurs in the presence of other organ involvement such as the renal and gastrointestinal system. There is a slight male predominance in most studies, although the gender discrepancy is small compared to that seen in transthyretin amyloidosis. The mean age at diagnosis is 60 years. AL amyloidosis is more commonly due to λ (lambda) immunoglobulin light chains in IgG monoclonal gammopathies. A slight predominance of κ (kappa) immunoglobulin light chains is observed among patients with the rare IgM-related AL amyloidosis [17]. Cardiac involvement confers a poor prognosis with median survival of a year from the time of diagnosis if left untreated [18, 19].

Compared to patients with transthyretin amyloidosis, those who have AL amyloidosis have a higher frequency of hemodynamic impairment despite a lesser degree of cardiac infiltration measured by left ventricular wall thickness on echocardiography [20]. A direct cardiotoxic effect of amyloidogenic light chains has been proposed to explain this discordant clinical observation [21].

In approximately 10 % of primary AL amyloidosis, a monoclonal protein is not demonstrated in serum or urine despite a positive identification of AL amyloidosis on tissue. In such cases, a diagnosis of nonsecretory immunoglobulin-derived amyloidosis is made.

Transthyretin Amyloidosis

The precursor fibril protein of senile systemic amyloidosis (SSA) is normal or wild-type transthyretin (TTR), previously known as prealbumin. TTR is synthesized mainly by the liver and acts as transporter protein for thyroxine and retinol. The protein consists of 127 amino acids encoded by 4 exons located in chromosome 18. Analysis of the protein in SSA revealed normal TTR with predominantly C-terminal fragments admixed with intact full-length monomers [22].

Senile Systemic (Transthyretin) Amyloidosis

The heart is the predominant site of amyloid deposition in SSA; thus, this condition was previously referred to as senile cardiac amyloidosis before it was demonstrated that the amyloid deposit found in other organs is the same as that in the heart. The amyloid deposits are microscopic and patchy in distribution. In the heart, senile amyloid deposits occur in intramural coronary arteries with smaller amounts focally present in the interstitium of the atrial and ventricular myocardium. In organs other than the heart, amyloid is confined mainly in the wall of arteries and sometimes veins [23].

The true incidence of SSA is difficult to determine as a number of autopsy studies predate accurate typing of amyloid. SSA appears to have minimal associated clinical disease manifestations

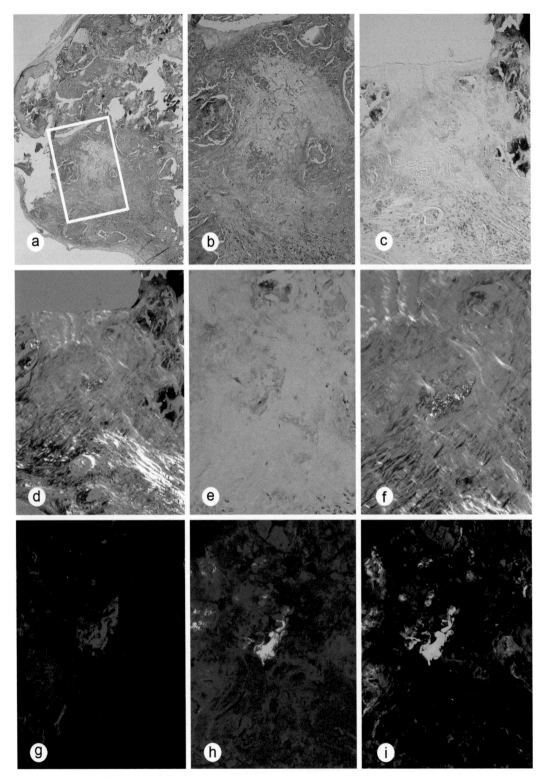

Fig. 29.2 Incidental amyloid in a calcified aortic valve. (**a**) Light micrograph of an aortic valve with marked calcification. There is abundant fibrosis and several cores of basophilic deposits corresponding to areas of calcified extracellular matrix. At this low magnification, there is no overt "amorphous" amyloid deposition identified (H&E ×100). (**b**) The rectangular highlighted portion of the valve in (**a**) shows a close-up of the extracellular matrix and calcium deposits but no overt amyloid deposits (H&E ×300). (**c**) The same area of the valve is shown as a bright field micrograph

and thus it is usually not suspected during life. For unknown reasons, some patients suffer from massive deposition of wild-type TTR that clinically manifest as congestive heart failure or arrhythmias starting in the seventh decade [24]. Interestingly, symptomatic SSA occurs almost exclusively in men.

Transthyretin-Associated Familial Amyloidosis

Single point mutations are thought to destabilize the TTR native structure and cause dissociation, misfolding, and aggregation to form amyloid deposits in tissues. When variant forms of TTR are deposited, it is predominantly found in peripheral nerves and heart causing familial amyloidotic polyneuropathy and familial amyloidotic cardiomyopathy, respectively. To date, there are more than 100 TTR variants reported. The majority of patients are male heterozygous carriers.

Hereditary TTR amyloidosis is autosomal dominant with variable penetrance regarding age of onset and organ involvement. One of the most common variant, Val122Ile, is present in approximately 4 % of the African Americans and is a known cause of late-onset cardiac amyloidosis in this population. In Sweden, Portugal, and Japan, there are endemic foci of Val30Met mutation associated with familial amyloidotic polyneuropathy. In this latter group of patients, cardiomyopathy is a late event and occurs in less than a quarter of patients [25]. The prevalence of other rare mutations varies according to geographical origin and appears to be associated with more pronounced cardiomyopathy rather than polyneuropathy. Patients typically present about a decade earlier than those affected by SSA.

Analysis of extracted amyloid in familial TTR amyloidosis shows both mutant and wild-type TTR. Moreover, fibril composition may be associated with the timing of disease onset and degree of cardiac involvement. In a study of Val30Met mutation carriers, the fibril composition was a mixture of full-length and fragmented forms in patients who manifest late while early disease onset was associated with deposition of only full-length TTR and lesser amount of cardiac deposits [26].

Other Systemic Amyloidoses Affecting the Heart

Amyloid A Protein

Cardiac amyloidosis secondary to deposition of acute-phase reactant serum amyloid A protein (AA) is a rare complication of chronic inflammatory and infectious diseases and malignancy. When it involves the heart, it is usually an incidental finding discovered on autopsy without clinical cardiac dysfunction. Amyloid is distributed mainly in small arteries and arterioles and to a much lesser extent in the myocardial interstitium [27]. In a large series of patients with AA amyloidosis, heart failure was noted in only 1 of 374 patients and cardiac infiltration was detected on echocardiography in 2 of 224 patients [28].

β2-Microglobulin

Patients on long-term dialysis treatment are at risk of developing systemic amyloidosis of β2-microglobulin type with predilection for osteoarticular interstitial deposition. Amyloid deposition within blood vessel wall of visceral

---

Fig. 29.2 (continued) stained with *Congo red*. A small focus of the matrix is stained *red* ("congophilic"). The calcium deposits are basophilic (*Congo red* ×300). (**d**) Examination of the same field under polarized light microscopy shows the extracellular collagen as a birefringent white matrix. In contrast, the small area of congophilic material shows *apple green* birefringence under the polarized visible light (*Congo red* ×300). (**e**) At higher magnification, the congophilic area of the extracellular matrix of the valve stands out in bright field microscopy (*Congo red* ×900). (**f**) Polarized light microscopy shows distinct *apple green* birefringence of the congophilic deposits (*Congo red* ×900). (**g**) Ultraviolet light microscopy of the *Congo red-positive* deposit in the valve is autofluorescent when analyzed with a tetramethylrhodamine isothiocyanate (TRITC) filter (*Congo red* ×900). (**h**) Thioflavin S stain of the same valve shows the amyloid deposition as *bright blue* fluorescence with the 4′,6-diamidino-2-phenylindole (DAPI) filter (thioflavin S ×900). (**i**) The amyloid deposit in the same thioflavin S-stained slide appears *bright green* with the fluorescein isothiocyanate (FITC) filter (thioflavin S ×900)

organs is mainly seen in patients who had been on dialysis for more than 10 years [29]. Small amounts of amyloid are almost always present in the small vessels of the heart and gastrointestinal tract in autopsy series [30]. Amyloid is also seen in the endocardium and cardiac valves. Symptomatic disease is limited to destructive osteoarthropathy and carpal tunnel syndrome. Systemic manifestations are rare with only anecdotal reports of cardiac compromise and death.

Apolipoprotein AI

Aside from transthyretin-associated amyloidosis, the other forms of hereditary autosomal dominant systemic amyloidosis are rare but have been reported to involve the heart in some cases. Apolipoprotein AI is a major component of high-density lipoprotein and is synthesized by the liver and small intestine. The wild-type full-length protein forms amyloid deposits in atherosclerotic plaques. A hereditary systemic amyloidosis associated with mutations in the N-terminal segment of the apolipoprotein AI gene shows preferential involvement of the kidney and liver. However, those mutations occurring in the carboxyl terminal portion of the protein tend to be associated with cutaneous, laryngeal, and slowly progressive cardiac amyloidosis [31].

Fibrinogen

Mutations in the fibrinogen α-chain gene are a common cause of hereditary renal amyloidosis. Cardiovascular amyloid deposition in patients with fibrinogen amyloidosis is noted in the myocardium, in atheromatous plaques, and in arteries and veins of explanted livers [32].

Clinical Features of Cardiac Amyloidosis

Amyloid deposition in the extracellular matrix of the heart alters myocyte contractility and electrical conduction. Only the systemic forms of amyloidosis produce clinically significant heart disease, and there are no distinguishing clinical features for the different molecular types of systemic amyloidosis involving the heart. Symptomatic patients show signs and symptoms of congestive heart failure with or without arrhythmias. The disease can also manifest with acute coronary syndrome or sudden cardiac death [33]. The clinical presentation of cardiac amyloidosis can mimic hypertrophic cardiomyopathy and constrictive pericardial disease.

The serum cardiac biomarkers troponin T or I, B-type natriuretic peptide (BNP), and N-terminal pro-B-type natriuretic peptide (NT-proBNP) are sensitive markers of myocardial dysfunction. Higher levels of these biomarkers are predictive of early mortality in patients with AL amyloidosis [34]. Electrocardiogram shows low voltage in the limb leads and a pseudoinfarction pattern (i.e., the presence of a QS wave pattern in the absence of myocardial infarction).

Imaging will show cardiomegaly with biatrial dilatation and normal or mildly dilated left ventricle. Characteristic echocardiographic findings are suggestive of an infiltrative process with increased ventricular wall thickness in the absence of hypertension, restrictive filling pattern, and sparkling appearance of the interventricular septum. The atrial septum and atrioventricular valves may also be thickened. Pericardial effusion may be present. There is early manifestation of diastolic dysfunction. Ejection fraction is preserved until late in the disease. The presence of accompanying right ventricular hypertrophy and right-sided heart failure is a useful diagnostic clue.

Magnetic resonance imaging of the heart may show late enhancement with gadolinium in a diffuse subendocardial distribution. Technetium-99m pyrophosphate and technetium-99m 3,3-diphosphono-1,2-propanodicarboxylic acid are used as scintigraphic tracers for the visualization of TTR amyloid myocardial infiltration [35]. The use of positron emission tomography (PET) tracer Pittsburgh compound B, ^{11}C-PIB, and ^{18}F-florbetapir has shown promising preliminary results for early detection of cardiac involvement in both AL and ATTR amyloidosis [36, 37].

Clinical Diagnosis

There is no single clinical test that is sufficiently reliable for the diagnosis of cardiac amyloidosis. A tissue biopsy remains the gold standard for diagnosis of amyloidosis. Biopsy of various sites such as abdominal fat and gastrointestinal tract is commonly performed to establish a diagnosis of systemic amyloidosis. A negative biopsy of an extracardiac site, however, does not necessarily rule out cardiac amyloidosis. Moreover, biopsy of a clinically affected organ, such as performing an endomyocardial biopsy in a patient with unexplained heart failure, will have the greatest diagnostic yield. In other instances, the predominant clinical manifestation is that of congestive heart failure or hypertrophic cardiomyopathy; thus, these patients are initially evaluated by cardiologists. Not uncommonly, the diagnosis of a systemic amyloidosis is first made on an endomyocardial biopsy.

Once a tissue diagnosis is made, it is imperative to identify the precursor protein. The typing method used varies by centers and by pathologist experience and preference. In the heart, the clinically relevant forms of amyloidosis are those caused by immunoglobulin light chains and transthyretin. Together, they account for more than 95 % of cardiac amyloidosis that the pathologist is expected to encounter in practice.

A diagnosis of AL amyloidosis is supported by the presence of monoclonal gammopathy as demonstrated in serum or urine immunofixation, serum free light chain assay, and bone marrow biopsy. The criteria for evaluation of organ involvement and treatment response in AL amyloidosis have been standardized by a consensus panel [38]. If TTR staining of diagnostic tissue is positive, DNA testing from blood or tissue must be performed to rule out mutations in the TTR gene. SSA is a diagnosis of exclusion that requires the absence of plasma cell dyscrasia and mutation in the TTR gene. The absence of extracardiac manifestations such as heavy proteinuria and macroglossia is also consistent with a diagnosis of SSA [19]. The heart is occasionally affected in hereditary amyloidosis with predominant renal involvement and sequencing of apolipoprotein AI, AII, gelsolin, and fibrinogen α-chain may be warranted on rare occasions [39, 40].

Gross Morphology of Cardiac Amyloidosis

The localized forms of amyloidosis (isolated atrial or aortic) are practically imperceptible on gross examination. In contrast, examination of hearts from patients with severe amyloid deposition causing cardiac dysfunction often reveals typical gross findings that are diagnostic of amyloidosis. The heart often shows cardiomegaly that can range from mild to severe (Fig. 29.3). The heaviest hearts of up to 1,000 g are observed in TTR amyloidosis. The walls of the atria and ventricles appear rigid and do not easily collapse even in the fresh state upon opening the heart. Both atria are commonly dilated to a moderate degree (Fig. 29.4). Grossly, amyloid can be seen in the mural and valvular endocardium as fine

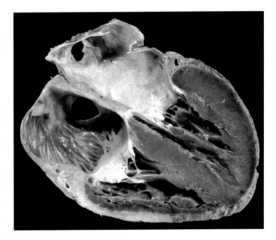

Fig. 29.3 Four-chamber view of a heart infiltrated by amyloid deposits. This image shows a formalin-fixed heart in which the atria are stiff and do not collapse as the atria of a normal heart after fixation. The endocardium of the left atrium is as usual distinctly white because of the normal multiple elastic lamellae present in this chamber but with conspicuous *yellow-ochre* discolored plaques. These *yellow-ochre* plaques represent subendocardial and endocardial amyloid deposits. In addition, the left ventricle shows faint plaques of *paler brown* material towards the subendocardium also representing amyloid deposits

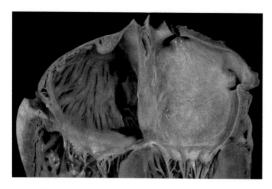

Fig. 29.4 Atrial involvement in transthyretin amyloidosis. Four-chamber view with close-up of the atria in a case of transthyretin-type amyloidosis. There is a fine granularity (resembling wet sandpaper) of the endocardium over the pectinate muscles and crista terminalis of the right atrium as well as the endocardium of the tricuspid valve. The left atrium shows the more conspicuous lesions of *yellow-ochre* plaques throughout the white atrial endocardium. These plaques are also present on the posterior leaflet of the mitral valve

translucent to yellow-tan granularity (Fig. 29.5a). This is most conspicuous in the left atrium and mitral valve. The atrioventricular valves are more commonly affected than the semilunar valves (Fig. 29.5b, c). In about half of patients, all four valves show amyloid deposits. Ventricular dilatation of a moderate degree is uncommon. The myocardium is firm and rubbery in consistency. The right and left ventricles are uniformly increased in wall thickness. The left ventricular hypertrophy is concentric with more or less equal thickness of the free wall and interventricular septum. Some patients will have asymmetric septal hypertrophy that may mimic hypertrophic cardiomyopathy (Fig. 29.5d). Intracardiac thrombi, mostly in the atria, are sometimes present (Fig. 29.5b).

Amyloid can be observed in the endocardium, in the interstitium of the atrial and ventricular myocardium, and in subendocardial adipose tissue (Fig. 29.6). The major epicardial coronary arteries do not show amyloid deposits [41], but amyloid is often demonstrable in the subepicardial adipose tissue and nerves on microscopy. Intramural coronary arteries and arterioles as well as coronary veins are variably involved, but sometimes can be diffuse and severe enough to

cause myocardial ischemia (Fig. 29.7). Amyloid deposition is also found in the conduction system in a minority of cases.

Endomyocardial Biopsy Evaluation

Endomyocardial biopsy is performed first to establish the diagnosis and second to determine the type of amyloid. An adequate specimen should consist of at least 4–6 pieces for routine histologic processing and light microscopy evaluation. A separate piece can be fixed in glutaraldehyde for possible electron microscopy. Histochemical stains used to identify amyloid deposits include Congo red, thioflavin S or T, methyl violet, and modified sulfated Alcian blue. The choice of stain depends on the preference and interpretation experience of the pathologist. It is also recommended to routinely stain all biopsies with trichrome which will be very useful to differentiate amyloid from collagen in the interstitium.

Amyloid is conspicuous on routine hematoxylin and eosin-stained slide as pale eosinophilic material. It is usually described as "amorphous," but it is rather homogeneous and lacks the fibrillary structure of collagen strands in fibrous tissue. It widens the interstitial space causing distortion and separation of myocytes. It can also be seen in any other structure within the biopsy including endocardium, vasculature, and adipose tissue. The pattern of amyloid deposition can be interstitial, endocardial, or vascular. The interstitial pattern can be further described as predominantly pericellular or nodular. In the interstitial pericellular pattern, the amyloid diffusely and completely encircles individual myocytes. The entrapped myocytes commonly undergo atrophy. In the interstitial nodular pattern, the amyloid appears as eosinophilic nodules that expand the interstitium and displace the myocytes. In cases of marked amyloid deposition, a mixed pattern is usually observed. The arterioles are more commonly involved than the small veins. The vessel wall appears thickened with or without significant compromise of the lumen. It should be noted

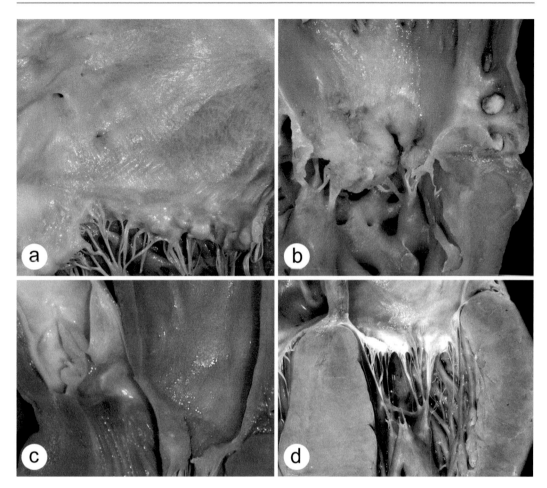

Fig. 29.5 Gross pathology of valvular and septal involvement in amyloidosis. (**a**) Left atrium and mitral valve show distinct plaques of *yellow-ochre* material that bulge on the endocardial surface of these two structures. These deposits have also been described as "glassy" or "waxy." Some thebesian veins opening into the atrium are distinctly visible in *left side* of the image. (**b**) Anterior leaflet of the tricuspid valve is thickened by coarse plaques protruding above its atrial surface. They may resemble organizing vegetations, but on microscopic examination they are composed of amyloid deposits and not of organizing fibrin deposits or fibrous tissue. Note the tan-white, nodular fibrin thrombi lodged in the trabecular portion of the atrial pectinate muscles on the *right side* of the image. (**c**) Long axis view of the left atrium, mitral valve, and aortic valve. The amyloid plaques and small nodules are easily identified over the endocardium of the atrium and the left ventricular outflow tract. Coarser deposits are present on the anterior and posterior leaflets of the mitral valve as well as the posterior and right cusps of the aortic valve. (**d**) This four-chamber view of a heart weighing more than 1,000 g shows distinct asymmetric septal hypertrophy. Note the faint discoloration of the subendocardial myocardium in both the interventricular septum and the left ventricular free wall. In addition, there is fine granularity of the atrial endocardium

that in some biopsies, vascular infiltration is more prominent than interstitial deposition. The ventricular endocardial deposits are usually minimal.

In endomyocardial biopsies, as also observed in autopsy hearts, the pattern of amyloid deposition often provides a clue as to the type of amyloid present (Table 29.1). Interstitial pericellular pattern is often the predominant morphologic feature and is more extensive in distribution in AL amyloidosis, while it is focal with a "chicken wire" appearance in TTR amyloidosis (Fig. 29.8a–e). Vascular amyloid can be seen in both types, but is more readily observed in AL amyloidosis (Fig. 29.8f, g) and rarely seen in

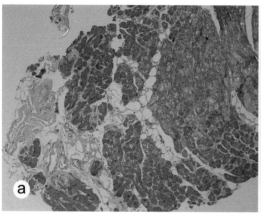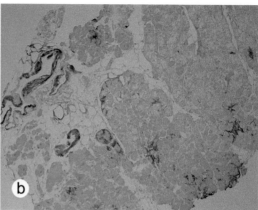

Fig. 29.6 Right ventricular endomyocardial biopsy showing involvement of venules, adipose tissue, and myocardial interstitium. (**a**) Tortuous eosinophilic "amorphous" aggregates are visible towards the *left side* of the micrograph, as well as interspersed within the adipose tissue (H&E ×50). (**b**) Immunohistochemical stain-ing for transthyretin shows that the tortuous material is amyloid present in small collapsed veins, arterioles, and adipose tissue. The stain further highlights the focal amyloid deposits in the myocardial interstitial space which are not very conspicuous on H&E (TTR immuno-histochemistry ×50)

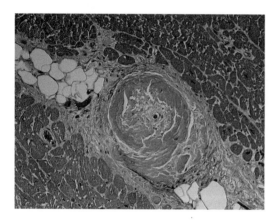

Fig. 29.7 Intramural coronary artery amyloidosis. A pre-dominant involvement of intramural coronary arteries with only mild interstitial amyloid deposition was found in an elderly patient who died suddenly. The patient had a history of angina pectoris with no significant stenosis of the epicardial coronary arteries. The amyloid deposits replace the media and intima, encroaching upon the lumen of this artery (H&E ×400)

TTR amyloidosis on a biopsy. The interstitial nodular pattern is more commonly seen in TTR amyloidosis (Fig. 29.9). Endocardial deposits (Fig. 29.10) are seen in cases with severe amyloid infiltration and are not particularly predominant in one type over the other. Although these differ-ences in the usual pattern of amyloid deposition in the heart exist, these observations do not allow for a reliable means to distinguish between the different types of cardiac amyloidosis based on morphologic features alone.

Amyloid is confirmed by histochemical stain-ing with Congo red (Fig. 29.11) to obtain a dichroic "apple green" birefringence upon polar-ization. However, we find thioflavin stains (S or T) to provide a sensitive and less ambiguous alternative to detect amyloid deposits (Fig. 29.8c, g). Some investigators have reported a difference in Congo red staining in TTR cardiac amyloid [42]. A relatively weak affinity for Congo red and

Table 29.1 Histologic patterns of amyloid deposition in the heart

Pattern of amyloid deposition				
	Interstitial perimyocytic	Interstitial nodular	Vascular	Endocardial
AL amyloidosis	+++	+	++	+/−
TTR amyloidosis	++	+++	+/−	+/−

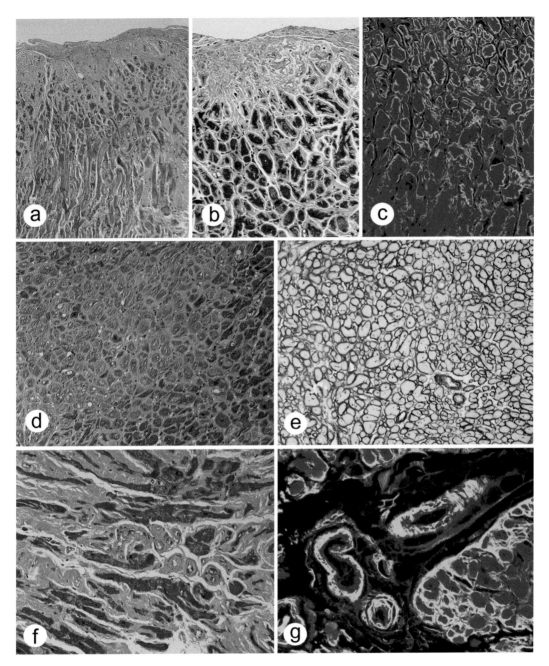

Fig. 29.8 Perimyocytic and arteriolar amyloid deposits.
(**a**) Amyloid deposits are present in perimyocytic location surrounding individual myocytes and also involving the endocardium (H&E ×50). (**b**) Other stains that highlight the interstitial connective tissue can also show the presence of amyloid. In this micrograph, the myocardium is stained with Masson trichrome. The amyloid deposits appear as *dull*, *pale*, *blue-gray* material surrounding individual myocytes in contrast to the typical brighter crisp *blue* of collagen fibers (Masson trichrome ×100). (**c**) Thioflavin S highlights the perimyocytic deposits of amyloid as *bright lighter blue* fluorescence compared to the *darker blue* background fluorescence of the myocytes under ultraviolet light microscopy (thioflavin S ×100).

(**d**) Amyloid deposits follow the contours of the myocytes without forming nodules or producing atrophy of the myocytes (H&E ×100). (**e**) Immunohistochemistry of the case shown in **d** is positive for kappa light chains and shows the exact same pattern of perimyocytic deposition. In addition, two small arterioles are present and also show amyloid deposition (immunohistochemical stain for kappa light chains ×100). (**f**) Diffuse interstitial and arteriolar deposits of amyloid in an endomyocardial biopsy (H&E ×400) with lambda light chain amyloidosis. (**g**) The same case shows bright amyloid deposits in arteriolar as well as interstitial location in this thioflavin S stain examined under ultraviolet light microscopy (thioflavin S ×400)

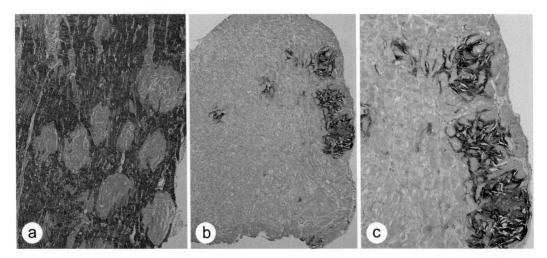

Fig. 29.9 Nodular pattern of myocardial amyloid infiltration. (**a**) Low-magnification view shows the "amorphous" eosinophilic material forming distinct nodules within the myocardium. In contrast to the perimyocytic pattern, the amyloid deposits here have completely obliterated and replaced the myocytes. The collapse of the myocytes allows the amyloid deposits to coalesce and form "nodules" (H&E ×50). (**b**) This endomyocardial biopsy shows distinct TTR-type amyloid nodules (immunohistochemistry for transthyretin ×25). (**c**) This image clearly shows how the encroachment of amyloid and atrophy of myocytes produces the nodular appearance (immunohistochemistry for transthyretin ×100)

weak birefringence is seen in amyloid composed predominantly of TTR fragments, while a stronger reaction and more brilliant birefringence is observed in full-length TTR. A weaker intensity of staining is also seen in localized senile aortic amyloidosis, while AL amyloidosis shows variable intensity [43]. A false-negative result is most commonly due to a small amount of amyloid present.

If histochemical staining is negative, electron microscopy can be performed to rule out amyloidosis in selected cases. Transmission electron microscopic evaluation of amyloid deposits in the heart is in general a straightforward process. The amyloid deposits are readily identifiable in toluidine blue semi-thin sections (Fig. 29.12). The various types of amyloid exhibit similar ultrastructure. The perimyocytic amyloid deposits are electron dense on lead–uranyl-stained thin sections. The amyloid fibrils are straight, or only slightly bent, threadlike filaments which are 10 nm thick. These filaments are commonly seen forming a mesh, and less frequently they can be seen in parallel arrays (Fig. 29.13). Alternation of the bundles of parallel filaments with longitudinal bundles may show as a "checkerboard" pattern at low magnification (i.e., 4,000×) (Fig. 29.14). The myocytes surrounded by amyloid often show degenerative changes. In the arterioles, amyloid fibrils also surround smooth muscle cells.

Amyloid Typing

Immunohistochemical staining, either with immunoperoxidase or immunofluorescence techniques, is widely used to classify the amyloid type in clinical practice. A panel of antibodies is necessary to correctly type the cardiac amyloid present. The choice of antibodies is guided by the prevalence of the different types of systemic amyloidosis that produce clinical heart disease. Localized types of amyloidosis are, in general, incidental findings in the autopsy as they are not associated with significant clinical disease. Of the systemic amyloidosis, only AL and TTR commonly cause symptomatic disease and are likely to be encountered in surgical specimens.

Similar to published large series, our experience with immunohistochemical typing utilizing immunoperoxidase on formalin-fixed paraffin-embedded

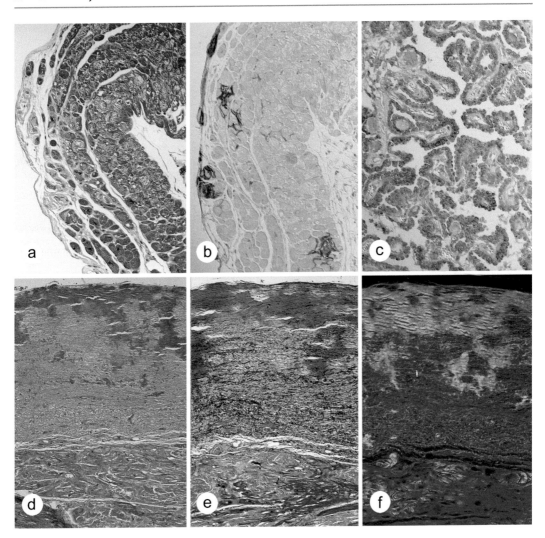

Fig. 29.10 Endocardial amyloid deposits. (**a**) Right ventricular endomyocardial biopsy shows subtle deposition of amyloid in the endocardium as well as around small clusters of cardiac myocytes (H&E ×50). (**b**) Adjacent section to the one shown in A demonstrates positive transthyretin deposits in the endocardium and around small foci of subjacent myocytes (immunohistochemistry for transthyretin ×50). (**c**) Choroid plexus is a useful control for transthyretin immunohistochemistry, as this protein is normally found in the cuboidal epithelium of the choroid plexus (immunohistochemistry for transthyretin ×200). (**d**) Left atrial endocardium showing the microscopic equivalent of the extensive *yellow-ochre* plaques seen on gross examination at autopsy. The amyloid deposits are present as extensive eosinophilic plaques within the endocardium as well as in the subjacent myocardium (H&E ×50). (**e**) The amyloid plaques are distinct from the fibrous tissue (*yellow*) or the elastic tissue (*black*) that normally form the left atrial endocardium. In this stain, the amyloid plaques appear *orange red* (Movat pentachrome ×50). (**f**) Examination under ultraviolet light shows the amyloid plaques in the endocardium and smaller deposits in the subjacent myocardium, analogous to the images in **d** and **e** (thioflavin S ×50)

biopsy material shows AL amyloidosis as the most frequent diagnosis followed by TTR amyloidosis of senile and then familial type [44, 45]. AL amyloidosis of λ light chain origin is at least three times more common than those derived from κ light chains. While we also routinely stain for amyloid A protein, we have not made a diagnosis of AA amyloidosis in a series of at least 100 endomyocardial biopsies. Therefore, the minimum panel of immunostains should always

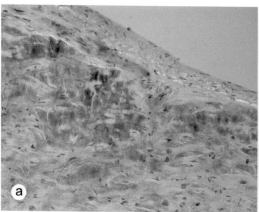 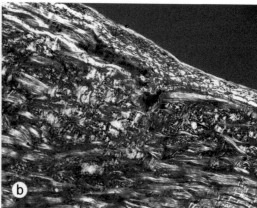

Fig. 29.11 *Congo red* birefringence of cardiac amyloid. (**a**) *Congo red* stain shows "congophilic" deposits upon bright field light microscopy (*Congo red* ×100). (**b**) Examination of the same section under polarized light microscopy shows birefringent collagen in *white* and *apple green* birefringent amyloid deposits corresponding to the congophilic material in A (*Congo red*, polarized light, ×100)

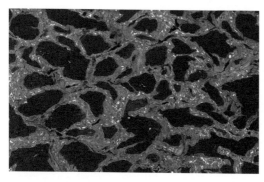

Fig. 29.12 Perimyocytic amyloid deposition in semi-thin plastic-embedded myocardium. This micrograph illustrates perimyocytic amyloid deposits (*pale purple blue*) surrounding and distorting individual myocytes (*dark purple blue*) (toluidine *blue* stain ×800)

include, but are not limited to, antibodies to TTR and immunoglobulin lambda and kappa light chains in the workup of an endomyocardial biopsy. Staining with only one antibody based on the most likely clinical diagnosis is not acceptable.

Despite adequate experience in the interpretation of amyloid immunostains and optimized staining protocol with appropriate controls, the surgical pathologist will encounter challenging cases in amyloid typing because immunohistochemistry has its limitations. In high volume centers, cardiac amyloid typing by immunoperoxidase

staining using commercially available antibodies will be inconclusive in 5–10 % of endomyocardial biopsies. In a much smaller series of cardiac amyloidosis, immunofluorescence staining using fresh frozen tissue was employed for amyloid typing and was successful in 82 % of cases [46]. Amyloid may be unclassifiable by immunostaining due to several reasons. Most common cited reasons are weak, uneven or absent staining, high background staining, and reactivity with more than one antibody. Commercial antibody against TTR (Dako) may react only with full-length TTR and not, or only very weakly, with TTR fragments as shown on Western blotting [26]. Focal or spotty staining of commercial antibodies against light chains in AL amyloidosis due to limited reactivity is also described [47]. In some cases, staining with both anti-λ and anti-κ antibodies is seen and is interpreted as contamination of amyloid by serum proteins.

If immunohistochemical staining as the first step in amyloid typing yields inconclusive results, one should then consider evaluation by other techniques that are more specific and can test for the less common types of hereditary amyloidosis. Classification of amyloid can be performed by immunoelectron microscopy using gold particles for labeling [48]. This technique is both sensitive and highly specific but costly and not widely

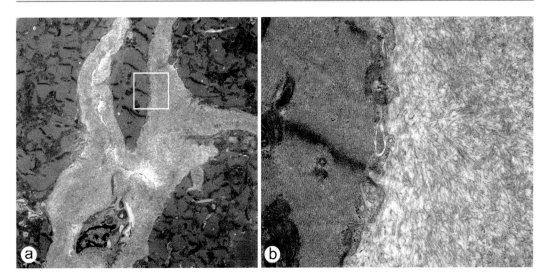

Fig. 29.13 Transmission electron microscopy of amyloid fibrils in the myocardium. (**a**) Myocardium showing segments of sarcoplasm of four myocytes (*left*, *top*, and *right borders*). The myocytes are sectioned in oblique planes and show sarcomeres, Z bands, and multiple mitochondria in the sarcoplasm. The basal laminae are not easily identified at this magnification. An endothelial cell with pinocytic vesicles is present in the lower mid portion of the image. The myocytes and endothelial cells are surrounded by amyloid fibrils (lead citrate and uranyl acetate stain ×4,000). (**b**) Higher magnification of the area shown in the *white square* in **a**. The myocyte sarcomeres show

distinct thick and thin filaments with M and H bands. The more electron-dense material represents the Z bands. Some mitochondria and rare sarcoplasmic glycogen particles are noted. Pinocytic vesicles are present underneath the sarcolemma. The basal lamina of the myocytes is visible as a somewhat uniform electron-dense structure that follows the contour of the sarcolemma. Threadlike amyloid filaments measuring 10 nm in thickness are present in a woven mesh-like arrangement and occupy most of the *right portion* of the micrograph (lead citrate and uranyl acetate stain ×20,000)

available as only a few facilities perform this procedure for diagnostic purposes.

Alternative methods previously employed to make a definitive diagnosis of amyloid type involve extraction of the amyloid fibrils from endomyocardial biopsy tissue and subsequent Western blot analysis or amino acid sequencing [49, 50], but these are rather impractical in evaluating endomyocardial biopsies. More recently, laser microdissection and tandem mass spectrometry-based proteomic analysis has proven to be useful for accurately typing problematic cases [51]. One major advantage of this technique is that formalin-fixed paraffin-embedded tissue can be used for these studies. It is also expected to be able to identify rare cases of hereditary amyloidosis for which antibodies are not readily available. However, a major challenge in using this technique is the need for an adequate amount of amyloid in the biopsy tissue.

To improve clinical outcome, there will be a need for early recognition of organ involvement in systemic amyloidosis. Mass spectrometry might not be feasible if the amyloid deposits in the biopsy are scanty [52].

Differential Diagnosis

The main differential diagnosis of an expanded interstitium in the heart is fibrosis of both interstitial and replacement types. Interstitial fibrosis is commonly associated with cardiac hypertrophy of various etiologies including systemic arterial hypertension and the cardiomyopathies. Replacement fibrosis is associated with myocyte loss or dropout as a result of ischemia. False-positive staining of thick dense collagen may result in green birefringence on Congo red; therefore, one should pay attention to the presence

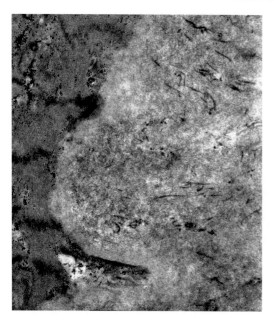

Fig. 29.14 Amyloid and collagen fibrils. As shown in light microscopic sections (Fig. 29.7b), as amyloid fibrils accumulate, they infiltrate and spread apart the normal extracellular matrix. This image shows the edge of a myocyte. The basal lamina is indistinct as its electron density is similar to the 10-nm-thick amyloid fibrils. However, the darker (more electron-dense) collagen fibers are distinctly visible mixed in with the amyloid deposits. They should not pose a diagnostic dilemma for the pathologist (lead citrate and uranyl acetate stain ×20,000)

of typical periodic banding pattern of collagen and to the loss of the green birefringence on rotation of the microscope stage in the horizontal plane during polarization. In addition, Masson trichrome stain provides a clear contrast of the blue collagen fibers against amyloid deposits which appear gray blue in color.

Amyloid deposits may occasionally elicit a giant cell response in the myocardium (Fig. 29.15) and in arteries (Fig. 29.16). This should not be misdiagnosed as giant cell myocarditis or granulomatous vasculitis.

Endocardial fibrosis and fibroelastosis will be seen as thickening of the endocardium. Endocardial fibrosis and fibroelastosis are nonspecific findings but can explain the presence of a restrictive physiology. A trichrome and elastic stain or a Movat pentachrome stain will demonstrate fibrosis with or without elastosis in these cases.

Small vessel disease of intramural coronary arteries is a nonspecific process that results in thickening of the vessel wall with variable luminal narrowing. This can be seen in diverse clinical settings including advanced age, hypertension, diabetes mellitus, hypertrophic cardiomyopathy, collagen vascular diseases, and radiation-induced injury. The pathologic altera-

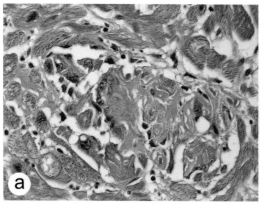 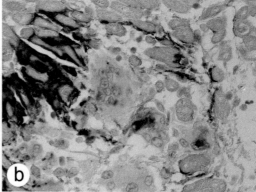

Fig. 29.15 Foreign body giant cell reaction to amyloid deposits in the heart. (**a**) Myocardial amyloid deposits are seen in the center of the field as well as some multinucleated giant cells and histiocytes. It is difficult to see amyloid deposits inside the giant cells (H&E ×400). (**b**) Immunohistochemical staining for transthyretin on a

deeper section of the field shown in **a** distinctly shows a multinucleated giant cell with transthyretin-positive material in its cytoplasm. The extracellular amyloid is also clearly positive for transthyretin (transthyretin immunohistochemistry ×400)

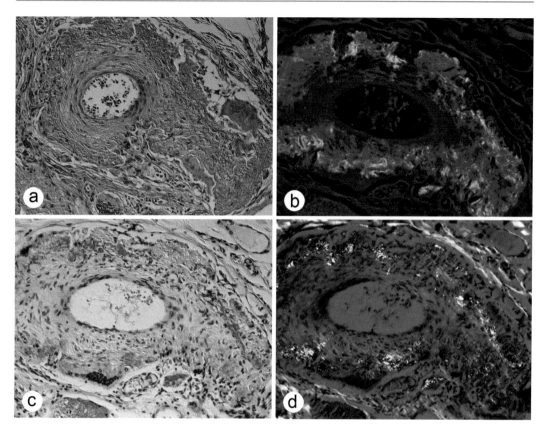

Fig. 29.16 Vascular amyloid with multinucleated giant cells. (**a**) A small artery is shown with expansion of the media by amyloid deposits and prominent giant cell reaction (right side of the artery) in a case of AL amyloidosis of kappa light chain type (H&E ×400). (**b**) Corresponding thioflavin S-stained section examined under fluorescence microscopy reveals a readily identifiable and more exten- sive amyloid deposition in the media (thioflavin S ×400). (**c**) A *Congo red* stain shows mild *red* staining of the eosinophilic extracellular matrix (*Congo red* ×400). (**d**) Upon examination under polarized light, the "congophilic" deposits show "*apple green*" birefringence (*Congo red* ×400)

tions can be due to hyalinization, medial hyperplasia, and medial fibrosis. Hyalin will appear bright magenta on periodic acid–Schiff stain and will be negative on Congo red. A trichrome stain will delineate smooth muscle cells and fibrosis in the media.

On ultrastructural evaluation, it is important to distinguish amyloid fibrils from connective tissue microfibrils which measure 13 nm in thickness and are usually present next to the basal lamina. These are conspicuous in hearts with ongoing fibrosis. Thus, the electron microscopic diagnosis of cardiac amyloidosis should be made carefully considering the information obtained from both light and electron microscopy, particularly in cases where there is no evidence of amyloid deposits in light microscopy, but interstitial fibrosis is present.

Diagnostic Pitfalls

In some patients with plasma cell dyscrasia, monotypic light chain deposition without the formation of amyloid in the myocardium is responsible for heart failure [53]. Light chain deposition disease (LCDD) has a reported incidence of 5 % in patients with multiple myeloma. Symptoms occurring late in the course of the disease and echocardiographic findings are similar to those with cardiac AL amyloidosis. Pathologic examination shows a widened interstitial space in the myocardium that is negative for amyloid on Congo red and thioflavin stains; thus, the diagnosis can be missed unless immunohistochemical staining or electron microscopy is performed. Immunofluorescence staining reveals monotypic light chain deposits in a diffuse perimyocytic and focal vascular pattern. Immunoglobulin typing shows a predominance of κ over λ light chains in LCDD. Electron microscopy reveals discrete granular electron-dense deposits around myocytes and smooth muscle cells of arteries. Occasionally, both fibrillar and nonfibrillar forms of deposition in different organs are observed in the same patient [54].

In the workup of patients with presumed cardiac amyloidosis, the following considerations should be kept in mind. The presence of monoclonal protein in the serum or urine cannot be used to assume a diagnosis of AL amyloidosis without tissue confirmation [55]. This is particularly important in the evaluation of elderly patients because of the following reasons. The incidence of monoclonal gammopathy of undetermined significance rises with age, and it is more common in men and African Americans. A hereditary TTR amyloidosis can also be missed if gene testing is not performed because of absence of a positive family history [56]. Likewise, identification of a gene mutation in the TTR gene from blood samples can be a confounding factor and does not necessarily prove that the cardiac amyloidosis is of TTR type [57]. Bona fide cases of AL amyloidosis do occur in carriers of genetic mutations in one of the amyloidogenic protein genes. An endomyocardial biopsy to establish the diagnosis and ascertain the type of amyloid is essential to avoid misdiagnosis and inappropriate therapy.

Amyloidosis is characteristically derived from one type of precursor protein. However, the possibility of co-deposition of two different types of amyloid fibrils in the same organ has been raised when there is equally strong staining with more than one antibody in the biopsy. A single case of the occurrence of wild-type TTR with mutant apolipoprotein A-I in the skin and larynx of a

patient with cardiac amyloidosis has been reported [58].

A commonly encountered problem in less specialized laboratories is when there appears to be positive staining with antibodies directed to both immunoglobulin light chains and TTR in the same area of amyloid deposition. This scenario is mostly a technical problem than a real condition. On the other hand, an optimized immunohistochemical staining protocol allows for the identification of both immunoglobulin light chains and TTR as distinct amyloid deposits in the same biopsy as shown in Fig. 29.17.

Therapy

Cardiac amyloidosis is still an under-recognized cause of heart failure. Most patients are diagnosed in the advanced stages. Conventional medical therapy for heart failure is of limited benefit in these patients.

Distinction between immunoglobulin-derived amyloidosis from TTR is important because therapy differs for these two forms of amyloidosis. Treatment of AL amyloidosis requires chemotherapy with or without autologous stem cell transplantation. Cardiac dysfunction has an adverse impact on the feasibility to offer patients potentially curative chemotherapy due to a high treatment-related mortality. Chemotherapeutic agents used for AL amyloidosis include corticosteroids combined with alkylating agents (melphalan or cyclophosphamide), immunomodulatory drugs (thalidomide or lenalidomide), and proteasome inhibitors (bortezomib). Selected patients with AL amyloidosis have undergone sequential heart transplantation followed by high-dose myeloablative chemotherapy and autologous stem cell transplantation.

Orthotopic liver transplantation has been performed in familial TTR amyloidosis with the goal of eliminating the major source of the mutant protein and arresting the progression of neurological disease. Heart transplantation alone has been used as a form of therapy for TTR amyloid cardiomyopathy. A combined heart and liver

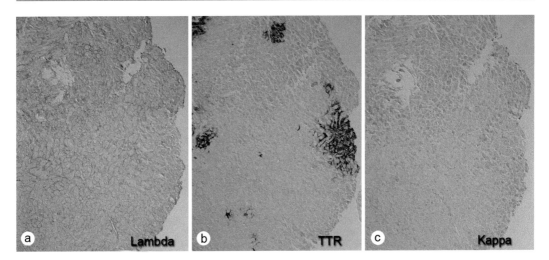

Fig. 29.17 Detection of two types of amyloidosis in an endomyocardial biopsy by immunohistochemistry. This biopsy is from a 90-year-old woman with plasma cell neoplasm and recent onset of heart failure. (**a**) Immunohistochemical staining for lambda light chains shows a somewhat pale but diffuse linear pattern of deposition around individual myocytes throughout this biopsy sample (×100). This has the same pattern as seen in Fig. 29.8. (**b**) The same biopsy shows *darker brown* nodular and coarse perimyocytic deposition of transthyretin similar to that shown in Fig. 29.9b, c (×100). (**c**) Immunohistochemical stain for kappa light chains shows complete absence of staining (×100)

transplantation is a controversial approach to treat familial TTR amyloidosis.

Emerging therapies for TTR amyloidosis aim to slow down or even reverse the amyloid deposition by means of the following strategies: (1) reduction of TTR synthesis in the liver (small interfering RNAs and anti-sense oligonucleotides); (2) stabilization of the TTR tetramer through binding on the thyroxine binding site (diflunisal, tafamidis); and (3) promotion of TTR amyloid fibril clearance (doxycycline, tauroursodeoxycholic acid, epigallocatechin-3-gallate, anti-serum amyloid P component antibodies) [59]. Randomized clinical trials are yet to be completed in the United States to evaluate the efficacy of these novel drug therapies.

Prognosis

Cardiac involvement is the leading cause of death in systemic amyloidosis. Patients usually die of progressive heart failure, but they are also at risk of sudden cardiac death presumed to be due to electromechanical dissociation. The median survival time of AL amyloidosis is approximately 6 months in patients who manifest with heart failure compared to 60 months in SSA [60]. Among the three most frequent systemic amyloidosis affecting the heart, AL amyloidosis is associated with the worse prognosis. Amyloidosis of transthyretin type, whether of the wild-type or mutant protein, is generally a favorable predictor of survival [20]. The median survival of patients with SSA is 5–7 years from the onset of heart failure while those with hereditary TTR amyloidosis is about 2 years [19, 61].

References

1. Steiner I. The prevalence of isolated atrial amyloid. J Pathol. 1987;153:395–8.
2. Cornwell 3rd GG, Murdoch WL, Kyle RA, et al. Frequency and distribution of senile cardiovascular amyloid. A clinicopathologic correlation. Am J Med. 1983;75:618–23.
3. Steiner I, Hajkova P. Patterns of isolated atrial amyloid: a study of 100 hearts on autopsy. Cardiovasc Pathol. 2006;15:287–90.
4. Kawamura S, Takahashi M, Ishihara T, et al. Incidence and distribution of isolated atrial amyloid: histologic

and immunohistochemical studies of 100 aging hearts. Pathol Int. 1995;45:335–42.

5. Pucci A, Wharton J, Arbustini E, et al. Atrial amyloid deposits in the failing human heart display both atrial and brain natriuretic peptide-like immunoreactivity. J Pathol. 1991;165:235–41.

6. Rocken C, Peters B, Juenemann G, et al. Atrial amyloidosis: an arrhythmogenic substrate for persistent atrial fibrillation. Circulation. 2002;106:2091–7.

7. Leone O, Boriani G, Chiappini B, et al. Amyloid deposition as a cause of atrial remodelling in persistent valvular atrial fibrillation. Eur Heart J. 2004;25: 1237–41.

8. Mucchiano G, Cornwell 3rd GG, Westermark P. Senile aortic amyloid: evidence for two distinct forms of localized deposits. Am J Pathol. 1992;140:871–7.

9. Haggqvist B, Naslund J, Sletten K, et al. Medin: an integral fragment of aortic smooth muscle cell-produced lactadherin forms the most common human amyloid. Proc Natl Acad Sci USA. 1999;96:8669–74.

10. Peng S, Glennert J, Westermark P. Medin-amyloid: a recently characterized age-associated arterial amyloid form affects mainly arteries in the upper part of the body. Amyloid. 2005;12:96–102.

11. Peng S, Larsson A, Wassberg E, et al. Role of aggregated medin in the pathogenesis of thoracic aortic aneurysm and dissection. Lab Invest. 2007;87:1195–205.

12. Mucchiano GI, Haggqvist B, Sletten K, et al. Apolipoprotein A-1-derived amyloid in atherosclerotic plaques of the human aorta. J Pathol. 2001;193:270–5.

13. Goffin Y. Microscopic amyloid deposits in the heart valves: a common local complication of chronic damage and scarring. J Clin Pathol. 1980;33:262–8.

14. Cooper JH. Localized dystrophic amyloidosis of heart valves. Hum Pathol. 1983;14:649–53.

15. Ladefoged C, Rohr N. Amyloid deposits in aortic and mitral valves. A clinicopathological investigation of material from 100 consecutive heart valve operations. Virchows Arch A Pathol Anat Histopathol. 1984;404: 301–12.

16. Kristen AV, Schnabel PA, Winter B, et al. High prevalence of amyloid in 150 surgically removed heart valves—a comparison of histological and clinical data reveals a correlation to atheroinflammatory conditions. Cardiovasc Pathol. 2010;19:228–35.

17. Terrier B, Jaccard A, Harousseau JL, et al. The clinical spectrum of IgM-related amyloidosis: a French nationwide retrospective study of 72 patients. Medicine (Baltimore). 2008;87:99–109.

18. Dubrey SW, Cha K, Anderson J, et al. The clinical features of immunoglobulin light-chain (AL) amyloidosis with heart involvement. QJM. 1998;91:141–57.

19. Ng B, Connors LH, Davidoff R, et al. Senile systemic amyloidosis presenting with heart failure: a comparison with light chain-associated amyloidosis. Arch Intern Med. 2005;165:1425–9.

20. Rapezzi C, Merlini G, Quarta CC, et al. Systemic cardiac amyloidoses: disease profiles and clinical courses of the 3 main types. Circulation. 2009;120:1203–12.

21. Guan J, Mishra S, Shi J, et al. Stanniocalcin1 is a key mediator of amyloidogenic light chain induced cardiotoxicity. Basic Res Cardiol. 2013;108:378.

22. Westermark P, Bergstrom J, Solomon A, et al. Transthyretin-derived senile systemic amyloidosis: clinicopathologic and structural considerations. Amyloid. 2003;10 Suppl 1:48–54.

23. Pitkanen P, Westermark P, Cornwell III GG. Senile systemic amyloidosis. Am J Pathol. 1984;117:391–9.

24. Olson LJ, Gertz MA, Edwards WD, et al. Senile cardiac amyloidosis with myocardial dysfunction. Diagnosis by endomyocardial biopsy and immunohistochemistry. N Engl J Med. 1987;317:738–42.

25. Hattori T, Takei Y, Koyama J, et al. Clinical and pathological studies of cardiac amyloidosis in transthyretin type familial amyloid polyneuropathy. Amyloid. 2003;10:229–39.

26. Ihse E, Ybo A, Suhr O, et al. Amyloid fibril composition is related to the phenotype of hereditary transthyretin V30M amyloidosis. J Pathol. 2008;216:253–61.

27. Strege RJ, Saeger W, Linke RP. Diagnosis and immunohistochemical classification of systemic amyloidoses. Report of 43 cases in an unselected autopsy series. Virchows Arch. 1998;433:19–27.

28. Lachmann HJ, Goodman HJ, Gilbertson JA, et al. Natural history and outcome in systemic AA amyloidosis. N Engl J Med. 2007;356:2361–71.

29. Gal R, Korzets A, Schwartz A, et al. Systemic distribution of beta 2-microglobulin-derived amyloidosis in patients who undergo long-term hemodialysis. Report of seven cases and review of the literature. Arch Pathol Lab Med. 1994;118:718–21.

30. Ohashi K, Takagawa R, Hara M. Visceral organ involvement and extracellular matrix changes in beta 2-microglobulin amyloidosis—a comparative study with systemic AA and AL amyloidosis. Virchows Arch. 1997;430:479–87.

31. Rowczenio D, Dogan A, Theis JD, et al. Amyloidogenicity and clinical phenotype associated with five novel mutations in apolipoprotein A-I. Am J Pathol. 2011;179:1978–87.

32. Stangou AJ, Banner NR, Hendry BM, et al. Hereditary fibrinogen A alpha-chain amyloidosis: phenotypic characterization of a systemic disease and the role of liver transplantation. Blood. 2010;115:2998–3007.

33. Neben-Wittich MA, Wittich CM, Mueller PS, et al. Obstructive intramural coronary amyloidosis and myocardial ischemia are common in primary amyloidosis. Am J Med. 2005;118:1287.

34. Kumar S, Dispenzieri A, Lacy MQ, et al. Revised prognostic staging system for light chain amyloidosis incorporating cardiac biomarkers and serum free light chain measurements. J Clin Oncol. 2012;30: 989–95.

35. Bokhari S, Castaño A, Pozniakoff T, et al. (99m) Tc-pyrophosphate scintigraphy for differentiating light-chain cardiac amyloidosis from the transthyretin-related familial and senile cardiac amyloidosis. Circ Cardiovasc Imaging. 2013;6:195–201.

36. Antoni G, Lubberink M, Estrada S, et al. In vivo visualization of amyloid deposits in the heart with 11CPIB and PET. J Nucl Med. 2013;54:213–20.
37. Dorbala S, Vangala D, Semer J, et al. Imaging cardiac amyloidosis: a pilot study using (18)F-florbetapir positron emission tomography. Eur J Nucl Med Mol Imaging. 2014;41:1652–62.
38. Gertz MA, Comenzo R, Falk RH, et al. Definition of organ involvement and treatment response in immunoglobulin light chain amyloidosis (AL): a consensus opinion from the 10th International Symposium on Amyloid and Amyloidosis, Tours, France, 18–22 April 2004. Am J Hematol. 2005;79:319–28.
39. Yazaki M, Liepnieks JJ, Barats MS, et al. Hereditary systemic amyloidosis associated with a new apolipoprotein AII stop codon mutation Stop78Arg. Kidney Int. 2003;64:11–6.
40. Maury CP. Gelsolin-related amyloidosis. Identification of the amyloid protein in Finnish hereditary amyloidosis as a fragment of variant gelsolin. J Clin Invest. 1991;87:1195–9.
41. Roberts WC, Waller BF. Cardiac amyloidosis causing cardiac dysfunction: analysis of 54 necropsy patients. Am J Cardiol. 1983;52:137–46.
42. Bergstrom J, Gustavsson A, Hellman U, et al. Amyloid deposits in transthyretin-derived amyloidosis: cleaved transthyretin is associated with distinct amyloid morphology. J Pathol. 2005;206:224–32.
43. Westermark GT, Johnson KH, Westermark P. Staining methods for identification of amyloid in tissue. Methods Enzymol. 1999;309:3–25.
44. Crotty TB, Li CY, Edwards WD, et al. Amyloidosis and endomyocardial biopsy: correlation of extent and pattern of deposition with amyloid immunophenotype in 100 cases. Cardiovasc Pathol. 1995;4:39–42.
45. Kieninger B, Eriksson M, Kandolf R, et al. Amyloid in endomyocardial biopsies. Virchows Arch. 2010;456:523–32.
46. Collins AB, Smith RN, Stone JR. Classification of amyloid deposits in diagnostic cardiac specimens by immunofluorescence. Cardiovasc Pathol. 2009;18:205–16.
47. Kebbel A, Rocken C. Immunohistochemical classification of amyloid in surgical pathology revisited. Am J Surg Pathol. 2006;30:673–83.
48. Palladini G, Obici L, Merlini G. Hereditary amyloidosis. N Engl J Med. 2002;347:1206–7.
49. Benson MD, Breall J, Cummings OW, et al. Biochemical characterization of amyloid by endomyocardial biopsy. Amyloid. 2009;16:9–14.
50. Murphy CL, Eulitz M, Hrncic R, et al. Chemical typing of amyloid protein contained in formalin-fixed paraffin-embedded biopsy specimens. Am J Clin Pathol. 2001;116:135–42.
51. Vrana JA, Gamez JD, Madden BJ, et al. Classification of amyloidosis by laser microdissection and mass spectrometry-based proteomic analysis in clinical biopsy specimens. Blood. 2009;114:4957–9.
52. Picken MM. Modern approaches to the treatment of amyloidosis: the critical importance of early detection in surgical pathology. Adv Anat Pathol. 2013;20:424–39.
53. Buxbaum JN, Genega EM, Lazowski P, et al. Infiltrative nonamyloidotic monoclonal immunoglobulin light chain cardiomyopathy: an underappreciated manifestation of plasma cell dyscrasias. Cardiology. 2000;93:220–8.
54. Toor AA, Ramdane BA, Joseph J, et al. Cardiac nonamyloidotic immunoglobulin deposition disease. Mod Pathol. 2006;19:233–7.
55. Maleszewski JJ, Murray DL, Dispenzieri A, Grogan M, Pereira NL, Jenkins SM, Judge DP, Caturegli P, Vrana JA, Theis JD, Dogan A, Halushka MK. Relationship between monoclonal gammopathy and cardiac amyloid type. Cardiovasc Pathol. 2013;22:189–94.
56. Lachmann HJ, Booth DR, Booth SE, et al. Misdiagnosis of hereditary amyloidosis as AL (primary) amyloidosis. N Engl J Med. 2002;346:1786–91.
57. Comenzo RL, Zhou P, Fleisher M, et al. Seeking confidence in the diagnosis of systemic AL (Ig light-chain) amyloidosis: patients can have both monoclonal gammopathies and hereditary amyloid proteins. Blood. 2006;107:3489–91.
58. de Sousa MM, Vital C, Ostler D, et al. Apolipoprotein AI and transthyretin as components of amyloid fibrils in a kindred with apoAI Leu178His amyloidosis. Am J Pathol. 2000;156:1911–7.
59. Hanna M. Novel drugs targeting transthyretin amyloidosis. Curr Heart Fail Rep. 2014;11:50–7.
60. Kyle RA, Spittell PC, Gertz MA, et al. The premortem recognition of systemic senile amyloidosis with cardiac involvement. Am J Med. 1996;101:395–400.
61. Ruberg FL, Maurer MS, JUdge DP, et al. Prospective evaluation of the morbidity and mortality of wild-type and V122I mutant transthyretin amyloid cardiomyopathy: the Transthyretin Amyloidosis Cardiac Study (TRACS). Am Heart J. 2012;164:222–8.

Amyloidosis of the Gastrointestinal Tract and Liver

30

Oscar W. Cummings and Merrill D. Benson

Introduction

Amyloidosis is a localized or systemic disease characterized by congophilic protein deposition in many locations throughout the body. The protein can be derived from a number of sources, immunoglobulin light chains (AL), serum amyloid proteins in systemic chronic inflammatory disease (AA), and multiple, rare mutant proteins usually inherited in an autosomal dominant fashion (Chaps. 2, 3, 5) [1–4]. The localized form of amyloid—"amyloidoma"—is more typically encountered outside the GI tract and liver, although it can occur there [5, 6]. Unfortunately one cannot distinguish the localized disorder from the systemic disease by histomorphology alone. The systemic disease is serious, often progressive, commonly affecting the heart and/or

kidney. When the disease affects these major organs, it comes to early attention because of the dramatic clinical signs and symptoms. The kidney is commonly biopsied to evaluate the clinical dysfunction so renal amyloid is well recognized and studied. However, amyloid affecting the GI tract and liver tends to be relatively asymptomatic and only occasionally presents late in the course of the disease with clinical signs. When a patient is clinically suspected of having amyloid, rectal biopsies are often performed to assess whether or not it is systemic and pathologists are well aware of the histopathology in this setting. However, the primary manifestation of amyloid in the liver and GI tract is uncommon and often is discovered as an incidental finding or in autopsy material. Since the GI tract and liver are not commonly sampled to make a primary diagnosis (the rectal biopsy not withstanding), many pathologists are not well acquainted with the histopathology of amyloidosis in these sites. Some of the unusual patterns of amyloid could be easily overlooked by the unwary. Also there is very little literature regarding the surgical pathology of amyloid in the GI tract and liver. The *American Journal of Surgical Pathology*, one of the most widely read histopathology journals, has published only four articles (one a case report) on amyloid relating to the GI tract or liver over a 30-year time span. The following is an attempt to present the panorama of amyloidosis involving the GI tract and liver employing an atlas-like

O.W. Cummings, MD
Department of Pathology, Indiana University Health,
350 West, 11th Street, Room 4054, Indianapolis,
IN 46202, USA
e-mail: ocumming@iupui.edu

M.D. Benson, MD (✉)
Department of Pathology and Laboratory Medicine,
Indiana University School of Medicine,
Van Nuys Medical Science Building,
635 Barnhill Drive, MS-128, Indianapolis,
IN 46202-5126, USA
e-mail: mdbenson@iupui.edu

© Springer International Publishing Switzerland 2015
M.M. Picken et al. (eds.), *Amyloid and Related Disorders*, Current Clinical Pathology,
DOI 10.1007/978-3-319-19294-9_30

approach. Most of the photo micrographs are H&Es, but all the examples have also been stained with Congo red and examined with other techniques to confirm the presence of amyloid. However, most of these confirmatory studies are not illustrated here in order to avoid redundancy. The different types of amyloid have been discussed in Chap. xx and will not be further reviewed here. Neither will the many modalities—histochemical stains, ultrastructure, immunohistochemistry, immunoflouresence, protein sequencing, etc.—used in diagnosis be discussed here (see Chaps. 2–8). Also the details of clinical diagnosis and treatment are beyond the scope of the chapter (see Chaps. 13–24).

GI Tract

Amyloidosis of the GI tract presents with relatively vague signs and symptoms, but they can occasionally be catastrophic (Table 30.1) [7]. Since light chain deposition (AL) is the most common form of amyloid, it is also the most common type seen in the GI tract—with some geographic variations. Also there does not appear to be any pattern of amyloid deposition that is characteristic of any particular type of amyloid— AL vs. AA vs. hereditary—with certain exceptions that will be discussed. The tongue is the most proximal portion of the GI tract and also the most visible. 10–20 % of AL amyloid patients have tongue involvement. Amyloid in this site typically presents with macroglossia that may result in altered speech, excessive salivation, and difficulty eating [8]. The tongue is markedly swollen, but the dorsal rugal pattern is often preserved. There may be indentations from the teeth in the dorsal surface as well as foci of bruising (Fig. 30.1). Grossly the amyloid appears as yellow, waxy infiltrates in the muscle of the tongue (Fig. 30.2). Histologic sections of the tongue show pink amorphous deposits of amyloid in the lamina propria immediately below the squamous epithelium (Fig. 30.3) as well as infiltrating the skeletal muscle (Fig. 30.4).

The earliest amyloid deposition in the esophagus initially involves small arterioles (Fig. 30.5) of the submucosa but later in the course the lamina propria (Fig. 30.6), muscularis mucosa, submucosa, and muscularis propria may all or individually be involved. These same sites may be involved in any part of the GI tract with basically the same appearance, only the mucosa itself being different. Typically esophageal amyloid is asymptomatic but can be seen in 13–22 % of cases based on radiologic and autopsy studies. Deposition in the submucosa and/or the muscularis propria (Fig. 30.7) may lead to achalasia-like symptoms, which can be difficult to control clinically [9].

Symptomatic gastric involvement is also rare (1 %), but gastric deposits have been noted in up to 12 % of cases of amyloid patients at autopsy. Symptoms include nausea, vomiting, and epigastric pain. Gastric outflow obstruction can be seen in patients with amyloid tumors, polyps, or dense mural involvement in the antrum (Fig. 30.8). Plaque-like deposits of amyloid in the mucosa often produce atrophy and damage to the capillaries producing

Table 30.1 Clinical presentation of GI amyloid

Diarrhea
Hematochezia or hematemesis
Obstipation
Obstruction or pseudo-obstruction
Perforation
Malabsorption

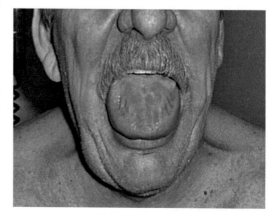

Fig. 30.1 A patient with systemic amyloid and macroglossia. The tongue protrudes at the corners of the mouth and indentation from the teeth can be seen on the ventral surface

Fig. 30.2 Cross section of a tongue from an amyloid patient with macroglossia. The amyloid can be seen as *yellow* plaques within the muscle

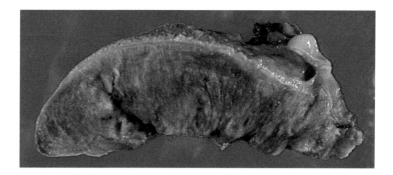

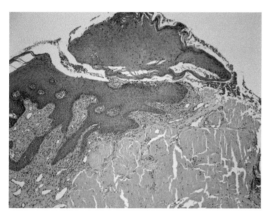

Fig. 30.3 Biopsy from the tongue showing *pink* amorphous material consistent with amyloid deposited in the lamina propria

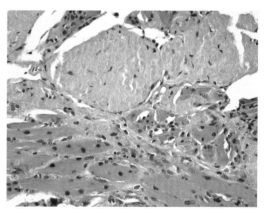

Fig. 30.4 The hyalinized deposits of amyloid are seen dissecting the skeletal muscle of the tongue

a propensity to hemorrhage into the lumen. In the stomach, this can lead to hematemesis that can be quite difficult to control endoscopically (Fig. 30.9) [10, 11]. Emergency resection may be life saving. Involvement of the muscularis mucosae of the tubular gut often produces dysmotility disorders somewhat analogous to achalasia. In the stomach, this lack of involuntary propulsion is often associated with nausea and vomiting which can contribute to systemic wasting. Likewise involvement of the wall of the small intestine may be associated with bacterial overgrowth and malabsorption (Fig. 30.10). Polypoid deposition of amyloid in the stomach, small bowel, and colonic mucosa has been reported [12–14]. In the colon, the impairment of peristalsis may result in constipation and megacolon. Patients with familial amyloidotic polyneuropathy (FAP—mutations in the transthyretin gene) often develop colonic and enteric dysmotility secondary to amyloid deposition. Invariably the muscularis propria is involved when the patients are symptomatic. The intramuscular ganglia do not appear to contain amyloid, but it is unclear whether or not the autonomic fibers are involved Fig. 30.11). It is said by some authors that senile amyloid (wild-type transthyretin) involving the gut can be distinguished from FAP by the lack of involvement of the muscularis propria. Plaque-like involvement of the colonic mucosa can produce life-threatening hematochezia again requiring surgical intervention (Fig. 30.12). The subserosal connective tissue can also be a deposition site for amyloid (Fig. 30.13). It may extend into the adjacent mesentery where it is reminiscent of amyloid seen in abdominal fat pad aspirates (Fig. 30.14) [15–21].

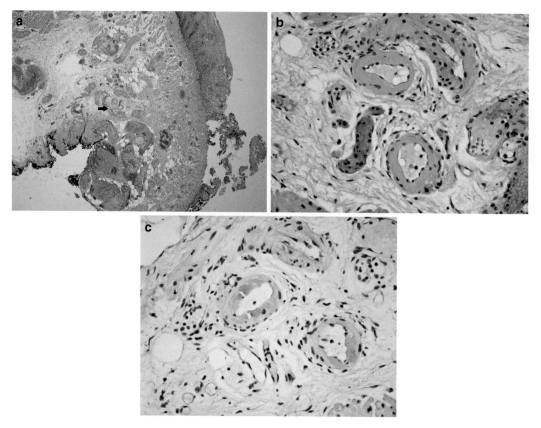

Fig. 30.5 (**a**) Lower power view of an endoscopic mucosa resection from the esophagus. The *arrow* marks the hyalinized vasculature shown better in **b**. This was an incidental finding. (**c**) *Congo red* stain of the same focus as shown in **b**

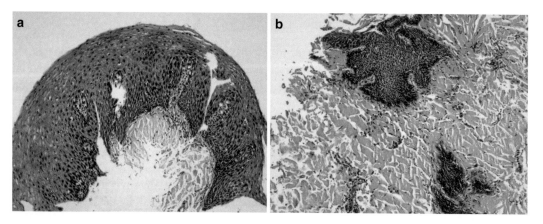

Fig. 30.6 (**a**) An esophageal biopsy showing the amorphous hyalin of amyloid again deposited in the lamina propria. (**b**) A higher magnification showing extensive amyloid deposition in the esophagus with some attenuation of the overlying surface epithelium

Amyloid in the colon may also be deposited in the subepithelial space of the mucosa reminiscent of collagenous colitis (Fig. 30.15). However, this finding is usually not associated with watery diarrhea. Also, unlike collagenous colitis, there is no increase in intraepithelial lymphocytes involving the crypt and surface epithelium and the surface epithelium shows little or no slough-

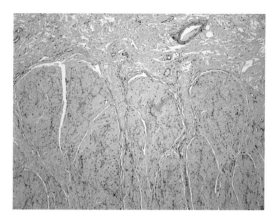 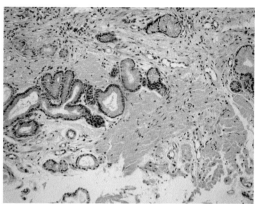

Fig. 30.7 Amyloid dissecting through the muscularis propria of the esophagus. The small arteriole in the overlying submucosa does not appear to be involved. This amount of disease is typically associated with achalasia-type symptoms

Fig. 30.8 Amyloid deposits in the lamina propria of the gastric antrum associated with atrophy of the entrapped glands. This pattern of gastric amyloid can be associated with outlet obstruction or can appear endoscopically as a polyp

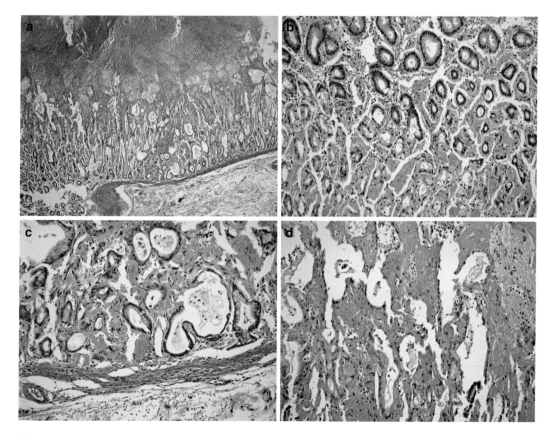

Fig. 30.9 (**a**) Section of stomach showing marked infiltration of amyloid in the lamina propria with overlying erosion and hemorrhage into the lumen. (**b**) Higher magnification of the stomach showing the hyalin material between the gastric glands. In this case, the infiltrate is denser at the muscularis propria. (**c**) In other foci, the amyloid produced is distortion of the usual gastric gland pattern. (**d**) *Congo red* stain of the stomach. The amyloid has an *orange-red* appearance while the fibrin and hemorrhage into the lumen show a *grayish tinge*

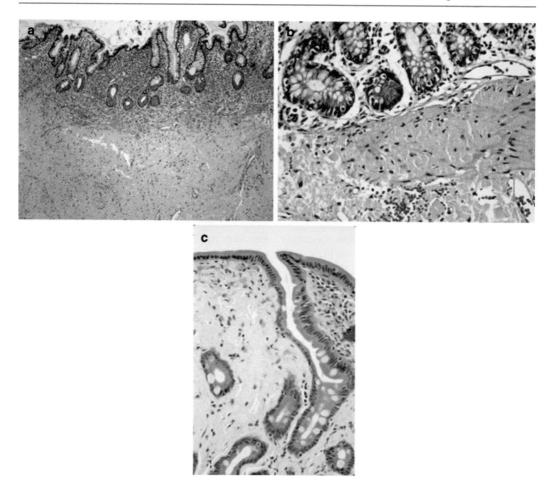

Fig. 30.10 (**a**) A section of small intestine showing dense deposition of amyloid in submucosa that completely spares the mucosa. (**b**) Another section of small intestine showing amyloid infiltrating the muscularis mucosae. The smooth muscle fibers are splayed by the lighter tinged vaguely globular hyalin material. (**c**) This section of small intestine shows infiltration of the lamina propria producing some mild blunting of the villi, a finding that may be associated with malabsorption

ing (Table 30.2). The collagenous colitis pattern of amyloid deposition is usually not present in isolation so amyloid deposition in other parts of the specimen is a clue to the correct interpretation. Special stains will also be useful in distinguishing one from the other [22, 23].

Rarely, mucosal deposition can produce polyps that may be mistaken from more typical colonic polyps by the endoscopist. Histologically, the main differential diagnosis includes the fibromuscular proliferation seen in mucosal prolapse type polyps (MPT) (Fig. 30.16) that may also have an elastic component [24]. These can easily be distinguished by Congo red staining which will be absent in the MPT polyps. Incidental vascular involvement may also be seen in otherwise classic tubular adenoma or hyperplastic polyps (Fig. 30.17). Involvement of the appendix has also been reported [25].

Treatment of GI amyloid is largely supportive—surgery for perforation or bleeding, medication for dysmotility, and antibiotics for bacterial overgrowth. Successful treatment of the underlying etiology of the amyloid may result in significant improvements in the GI symptomatology [26, 27].

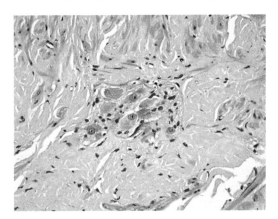

Fig. 30.11 Section of muscularis propria showing amyloid deposition between the inner and outer layers. The amyloid isolates the ganglion neural plexus but does not appear to infiltrate it in this section. This pattern of deposition is typically associated with dysmotility

Liver

The liver is frequently involved in patients with systematic amyloid, up to 90 % in some studies [28]. Signs related to liver involvement can be seen in up to one-half of patients, but symptomatic dysfunction due to amyloid is uncommon and typically a late manifestation of the disease (Table 30.3). Alkaline phosphates' elevation may be detected early, but it is a relatively nonspecific finding with a wide differential diagnosis—amyloidosis being very far down on the list. It is unclear why the hepatic deposition of amyloid results in the elevation of the serum alkaline phosphates. Hepatomegaly is also commonly noted, but the amount of protein deposition may not correlate directly with liver size. Some of the

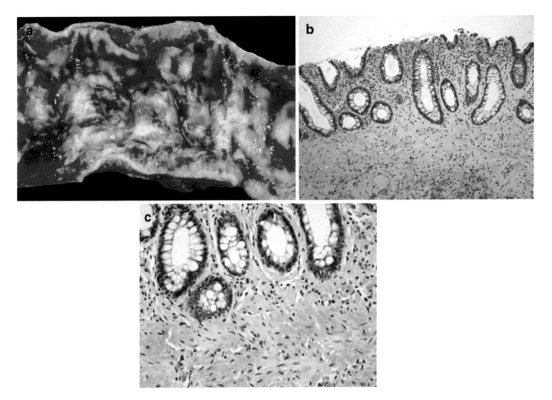

Fig. 30.12 (**a**) A section of colon from a patient with amyloidosis who presented with *bright red* blood per rectum. There are two serpiginous *red* patches of eroded mucosa among the *yellow* amyloid plaques. (**b**) A section of colon showing the amyloid infiltrating the lower portion of the mucosa, the muscularis mucosa, and the submucosa. The submucosa also exhibits acute hemorrhage. (**c**) A *Congo red* stain highlighting the amyloid in the lamina propria and muscularis mucosa

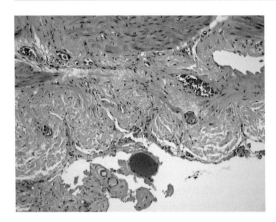

Fig. 30.13 Amyloid deposition in subserosal space that would be visible on the peritoneum

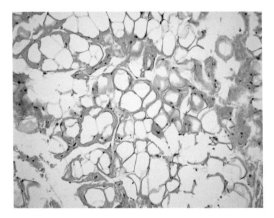

Fig. 30.14 Mesenteric fat with amyloid deposition in the intercellular septum reminiscent of abdominal fat pad biopsies

liver enlargement may be due to passive congestion related to amyloid-induced cardiac failure. As the functioning hepatic parenchyma becomes further compromised by the deposits, jaundice, encephalopathy, and hepatic failure may ensue. Jaundice is a poor sign with most patients succumbing within 6 months of its development.

Fibroscan has been suggested as a noninvasive modality that can be employed to diagnose hepatic amyloid; however, its sensitivity and specificity remain to be determined in everyday clinical use [29]. In the meantime, the liver biopsy remains the gold standard for diagnosis [30–32]. When pathologists think about amyloid deposition in the liver, they typically know about the sinusoidal pattern—by far the most common pattern. The term parenchymal has been used for this pattern by the Japanese; others have called it linear. It is the pattern of amyloid deposition that is present when the patient is symptomatic. However, it is important to remember that there are three other basic patterns of amyloid deposition that can be seen in the liver (Table 30.4). Failure to appreciate these uncommon patterns can greatly complicate the patient's clinical course. Like the GI tract, the type of amyloid in general does not dictate the pattern of deposition with some exceptions that will be noted. In the sinusoidal pattern, hyalinized material is deposited in the space between the sinusoidal lining

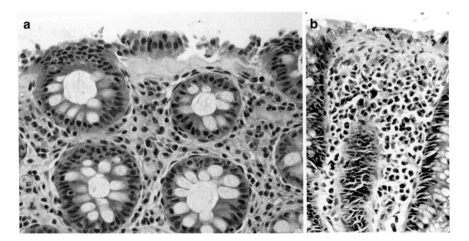

Fig. 30.15 (**a**) Amyloid deposition in the subepithelial reminiscent of collagenous colitis. This is the same patient who is illustrated in Fig. 30.12b, c. (**b**) Collagenous colitis which shows a subepithelial hyalin layer similar to amy-loid but not congophilic. Also note the numerous lymphocytes within the gland and surface epithelium as well as the marked surface epithelial sloughing compared to the amyloid

Table 30.2 Collagenous colitis vs. amyloid

	Subepithelial band	Trichrome	Congo red	IEL	Surface Sl
CC	++	++	–	++	++
Amyloid	++	+	++	–	++

CC collagenous colitis, *IEL* intra-epithelial lymphocytes, *Sl* sloughing

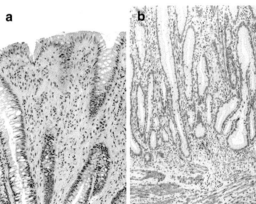
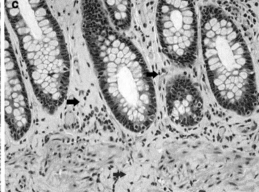

Fig. 30.16 (**a**) Mucosal prolapse polyps are typically seen in the rectum and exhibit fibromuscular hyperplasia involving the lamina propria. The fibromuscular foci have a hyalin appearance and could be confused for amyloid. (**b**) A desmin stain highlighting the fibromuscular hyperplasia and a mucosal type prolapse polyp. (**c**)

Colonic biopsy showing deposition of amyloid in the lamina propria (*arrows*) reminiscent of a mucosal prolapse type polyp. Note that there is infiltration into the submucosa, a finding not always seen; one that would identify the hyalin material is amyloid rather than a mucosal prolapse type polyp

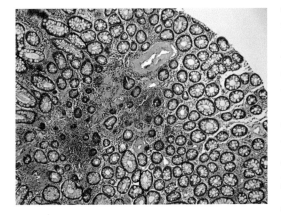

Fig. 30.17 A colonic tubular adenoma (adenomatous portion not shown) showing incidental amyloid involving a vessel

Table 30.3 Clinical presentation of hepatic amyloid

Elevated alkaline phosphatase
Hepatomegaly
Jaundice (late sign)
Portal hypertension
Encephalopathy
Hepatic failure

Table 30.4 Patterns of hepatic amyloid

Sinusoidal
Globular
Arteriolar and/or capsular
Portal

endothelium and the hepatocyte cytoplasm (Fig. 30.18). As with all amyloid depositions it generally has a pinkish tint on H&E stain, but in some preparations it may exhibit a blue-gray tint. This deposition begins in the sinus around the central veins (zone 3) and then spreads throughout the lobule (Fig. 30.19). As the amount of amyloid deposition increases, there is corresponding atrophy of the hepatic plates. In its most extreme form, the underlying liver is almost unrecognizable (Fig. 30.20). Amyloid deposition can also spread into the portal tract. The involvement of the tract can be variable from case to case and also from tract to tract within the same biopsy specimen. Branches of the hepatic artery may also be involved, but again, this is variable (Fig. 30.21). The differential diagnosis includes

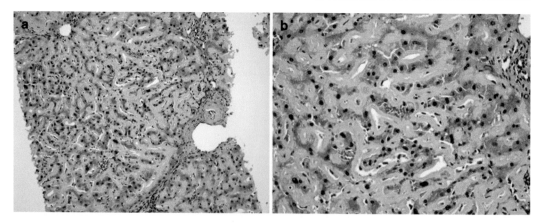

Fig. 30.18 (a) A section of liver showing linear or sinusoidal amyloid deposits in a pan-acinar distribution as well as involving the portal tract. (b) The amyloid is deposited between the sinusoidal lining endothelium and the hepatic plate. There is some atrophy of the hepatocyte cells in the sinusoidal spaces that are difficult to identify

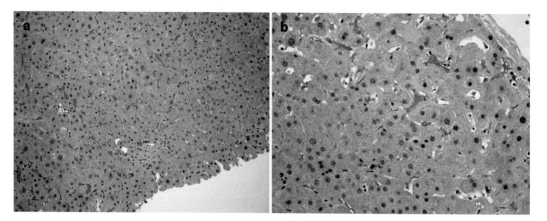

Fig. 30.19 (a) A panoramic view of liver with early sinusoidal amyloid deposition. It is much more difficult to detect than that seen in Fig. 30.18. (b) Higher power view showing a hyalin membrane preferentially lining the sinuses around central vein

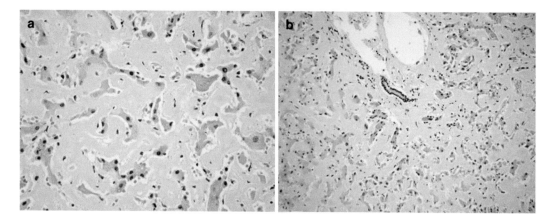

Fig. 30.20 (a) Advanced sinusoidal amyloid deposition almost completely effacing the underlying hepatocytes; (b) even the portal tracts can be difficult to identify in cases with advanced sinusoidal amyloid deposition

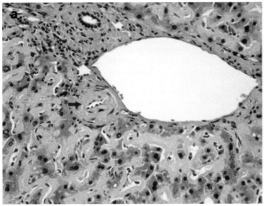
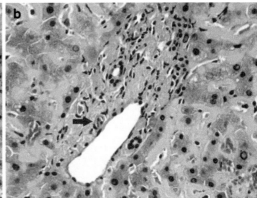

Fig. 30.21 (**a**) Sinusoidal amyloid with involvement of the hepatic artery branch (*arrow*). (**b**) The same liver as seen in part **a** showing no involvement of the hepatic artery in this particular portal tract (*arrow*). The location of amyloid deposits can be somewhat variable from case to case and even in the same organ

Table 30.5 Differential diagnosis of sinusoidal hyaline

Amyloid
Steatohepatitis
Vitamin A toxicity
Venous outflow obstruction
Congenital syphilis
Light chain deposition disease

entities that produce sinusoidal fibrosis including the hepatitis, vitamin A toxicity, venous outflow obstruction, and congenital syphilis as well as light chain deposition disease (Table 30.5). Trichrome stains are a routine part of liver biopsy interpretation and they stain the amyloid in basically the same fashion as fibrosis (Fig. 30.22). This may lead to further confusion if the subtleties of the appearance of amyloid in H&E-stained sections are not appreciated.

The fibrosis in steatohepatitis parallels the sinuses, as one sees in amyloid, but in addition, the lobule exhibits fatty change, "ballooning" hepatocytes, Mallory-Denk bodies, and lobular inflammation which are absent in amyloidosis (Fig. 30.23). Vitamin A toxicity also produces sinusoidal fibrosis as well as prominent finely vacuolated Ito cells. These cells are not visible at the light microscopic level in amyloid deposition disease. With venous outflow obstruction, there is hyalinization of the sinusoidal space as well as atrophy of the hepatic plates (Fig. 30.24).

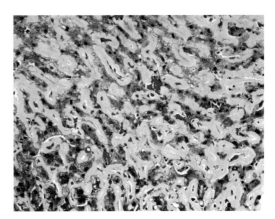

Fig. 30.22 A trichrome stain of sinusoidal amyloid deposits in the liver. Trichrome stain is not helpful in distinguishing amyloid from fibrosis

However, the sinuses are widely dilated and congested in venous outflow obstruction; in amyloid deposition, the sinuses are compressed and difficult to identify. Congenital syphilis can produce a sinusoidal pattern of fibrosis that is also associated with moderate chronic inflammation involving the portal tracts, and chronic venulitis [33]. There is often associated cirrhosis. Light chain deposition disease is very similar to amyloid in that it exhibits amorphous hyalin material in the space of Disse [34, 35]. However, the deposited light chains do not stain with Congo red or component P. The hyalin material is PAS positive and diastase resistant and marks strongly with the

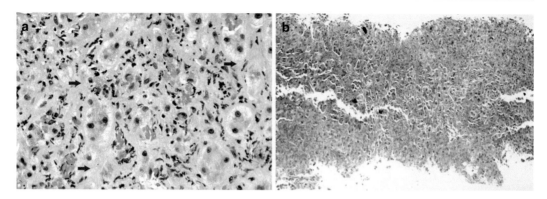

Fig. 30.23 (a) A section of liver showing advanced form of alcoholic steatohepatitis—acute sclerosing hyalin necrosis. There is extensive sinusoidal fibrosis which is somewhat difficult to appreciate because of the inflammatory infiltrate but is highlighted by the *arrows*. This pattern of fibrosis might be confused with sinusoidal amyloid deposition. Note the marked inflammation and numerous Mallory-Denk bodies which would be absent from amyloid cases. (b) The trichrome stain from the same case highlighting the sinusoidal and pericellular nature of the fibrosis

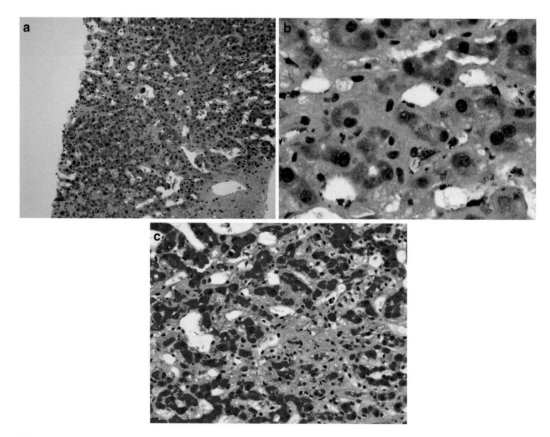

Fig. 30.24 (a) Section of liver showing venous outflow obstruction. There is fibrosis along the sinus which is reminiscent of amyloid deposition. This is more predominant around the central veins, but there is also dilation of the sinusoidal spaces as well as congestion. (b) A higher power view of the fibrosis associated with venous outflow obstruction. (c) The trichrome stain of the same case highlighting the sinusoidal fibrosis

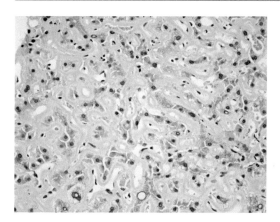

Fig. 30.25 A *Congo red* stain of sinusoidal amyloidosis from a patient with a plasma cell dyscrasia. Note the light staining of the *Congo red* in this instance, possibly leading to confusion with light chain deposition disease. Ultrastructural examination would resolve the dilemma

trichrome stain. It shows a different ultrastructural appearance than classic amyloid fibers. A Congo red stain is very helpful in differentiating light chain deposition disease from amyloid, although some cases of amyloid, usually lambda light chain, often stain weakly with Congo red (Fig. 30.25). Unfortunately, immunoperoxidase staining can be somewhat unreliable so ultrastructural examination can be most helpful in those cases in which the histochemical studies are equivocal [36].

The globular pattern of deposition is not common but has been well described [37, 38]. About 45 cases have been reported, 20 in one series. Men are twice as likely as women to exhibit this pattern of amyloid deposition. The etiology of the amyloid is often not stated, but there is a suggestion that secondary amyloid (AA) is overrepresented in this pattern of liver deposition. However, AL disease has also been noted to produce a globular pattern of amyloid deposits in the liver [39]. This pattern may be confused with other processes because the sinuses lack a hyalin lining and there is no hepatic plate atrophy. Occasionally transitional forms between the globular and sinusoidal pattern have been reported. The globules of amorphous pink amyloid material are distributed in the portal tracts and lobules (Fig. 30.26). The globules can be of various sizes but are generally much larger than

the hepatocytes and should not be confused with intracellular eosinophilic globules such as alpha-1 antitrypsin globules or Lafora bodies (Fig. 30.27). The globules are round and tend to be of similar size to one another, but there is some variability. They tend to cluster together and are often associated with the chronic inflammatory cells. Involvement of vascular structures is commonly encountered. One sub-pattern should be commented on. Leukocyte chemotactic factor 2 (Lect 2) produces a rare amyloid that prominently affects the kidney and the liver [40, 41]. We present three cases of hepatic Lect 2 involvement, all with a globular pattern. The first case was uncomplicated by other liver disease and showed very subtle small eosinophilic globules clustered in the lobule as well as in the portal tracts and around the hepatic artery (Fig. 30.28). The other two are cases that were complicated by cirrhosis, one from ethanol toxicity (Fig. 30.29) and the other from chronic hepatitis C virus infection (Fig. 30.30). In these two latter cases, the globules were somewhat larger than that seen in the first, but smaller than the classically described globular amyloid. These globules were primarily arrayed in the fibrous septa and were especially dense in the remnants of the portal tracts. This finer globular pattern with a predominant involvement of the portal tracts may be relatively specific for Lect 2 amyloid, but further case studies are required to substantiate this impression. There have been suggestions that globular deposits of amyloid may be located within the cytoplasm of hepatocytes. However, we are unaware of any intracellular amyloid deposition outside the central nervous system [42]. The globules are extracellular, but when they occupy the canalicular space they may indent the hepatocyte cytoplasm in such a manner as to give the appearance of an intracytoplasmic location. Also the globules may be associated with macrophages/Kupffer cells leading to the false impression of an intracytoplasmic location of the protein deposit (see Fig. 30.27).

The incidence of the last few patterns of amyloid deposition in the liver is unclear. Most are rare, but the vascular pattern can be quite common in certain subtypes of amyloid such as

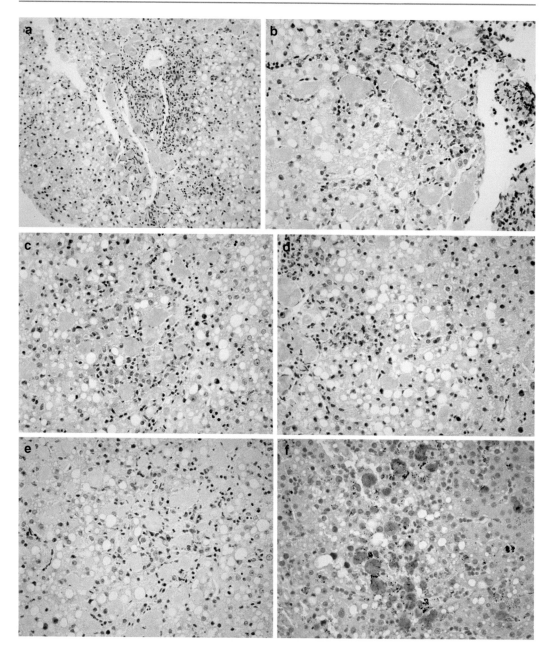

Fig. 30.26 (a) A section of liver with globular amyloid predominantly involving the periportal parenchyma as well as the portal tract. The globules are large and relatively similar in size and shape. There is also involvement of a branch of the artery and mild fatty change. This is a patient with secondary amyloid (AA). (b) Globular amyloid deposition associated with a mild chronic inflammatory cell infiltrate including a few plasma cells. The globules here showed somewhat more variability in size. (c) Globular amyloid deposition in the lobule. (d) Globular amyloid deposition in the lobule began exhibiting some variability in globules size. (e) A *Congo red* stain highlighting the globular amyloid. (f) An immunoperoxidase stain using antibodies directed against serum AA proteins, supporting the secondary nature of the amyloid

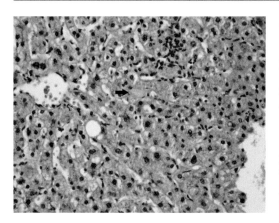

Fig. 30.27 A small fragment of globular amyloid that might be confused for Lafora body, an intracytoplasmic inclusion that can be seen in several diseases. However, amyloid is extracellular except in certain CNS lesions

AA. Some precursors such as transthyretin are primarily manufactured in the liver and do not produce a sinusoidal pattern of deposition there. However, one can see deposition in the fibrous capsule (Fig. 30.31) of the liver with or without deposition in the hepatic arteries (Fig. 30.32) and vice versa. AA and TTR amyloid preferentially involve the arterioles, but the pattern is not specific to those types. AL and AA can also involve the capsule, but generally they also show sinusoidal or arterial involvement as well.

The portal pattern of deposition is also very unusual. Some have referred to this as the stromal pattern. In this setting, large rounded acellular hyalin material almost completely replaces the portal tracts (Fig. 30.33). Occasional vessels may be trapped in the amyloid; the intralobular bile duct and hepatic artery branch are pushed to the periphery and can be difficult to identify. The interface between the lobule is very smooth with broad pushing borders. This pattern is very suggestive of Apolipoprotein A1 deposition [30, 43–46]. On rare occasions one can see AL amyloid replace the portal tracts without significant sinusoidal involvement (Fig. 30.34). These tracts tend to retain a somewhat angular appearance rather than the large bulbous contours seen with Apolipoprotein A1. Rarely, hereditary amyloids may also involve the portal tracts but tend not to obscure the underlying architecture (Fig. 30.35). The differential diagnosis of portal amyloid is

extremely limited. Lipoid proteinosis, an inherited condition associated with mutations in the ECM1 gene, primarily producing muco-cutaneous lesions, can deposit PAS-positive, diastase-resistant, Congo red-negative, hyalin material in the portal tracts [47, 48].

Treatment of hepatic amyloidosis is directed against the underlying etiology of the amyloid protein and symptom relief. Orthotropic liver transplantation is generally contraindicated in AL disease related to plasma cell disorders because of the rapid accumulation of amyloid in the new organ [49]. However, some so-called "domino" transplants have been attempted. Livers from patients with transthyretin (TTR) mutations (the livers are generally morphologically normal) are transplanted into others, while they themselves receive a new liver with wild-type TTR. There have been successes with this approach, but there have also been setbacks [50, 51]. TTR is made not only in the liver but is also secreted from the choroid plexus, so not all donors off TTR mutated livers have had symptomatic improvement and some of the recipients of these mutated livers have become symptomatic with amyloidosis within a few years of the transplant.

Amyloidosis of the gallbladder is most commonly an incidental finding or it is detected at autopsy. The amyloid is deposited primarily in arterials but can also be located in the mucosa, submucosa, or muscularis propria just like the rest of the viscous GI tract (Fig. 30.36). There is a case report describing amyloid involving the mucosa mimicking the clinical appearance of gallbladder carcinoma [52]. There is also a case report of amyloidosis involving the extrahepatic bile ducts [53].

Amyloidosis of the pancreas comes in two main forms. In diabetics, the protein amylin (see Chap. 7) is deposited in the islets and is associated with some atrophy of the beta cells (Fig. 30.37). The deposition appears to be an epiphenomena of the underlying disease rather than a causative factor of the diabetes. Amyloid deposition can also be seen in patients with chronic pancreatitis secondary to cystic fibrosis but is not typically identified in run-of-the-mill chronic pancreatitis. The

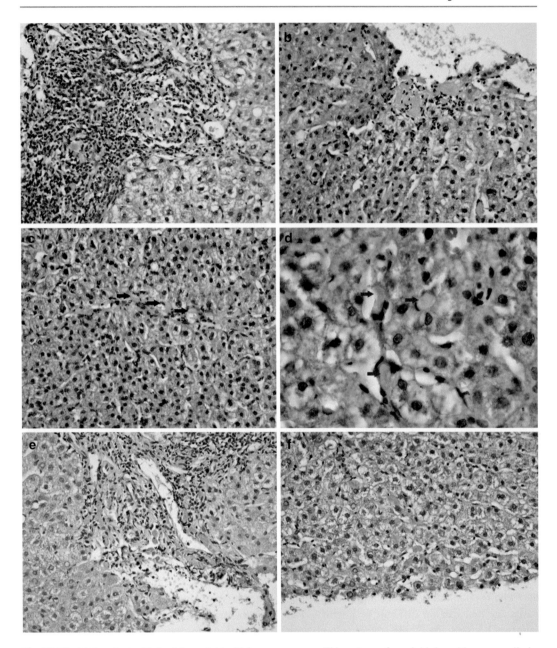

Fig. 30.28 (**a**) A patient with Lect 2 amyloid which can be seen in the portal tracts and lobule fine globules. This section illustrates portal deposition. (**b**) Lect 2 amyloid deposited in the lobule around the central vein. (**c**) Small globular deposits of Lect 2 amyloid highlighted by *arrows*. This pattern of amyloid deposition can easily be missed on casual inspection. (**d**) More of the small globules of Lect 2 amyloid (*arrows*). (**e**) *Congo red* stain highlighting the Lect 2 amyloid in the portal tracts. (**f**) *Congo red* stain highlighting the Lect 2 amyloid in the lobule

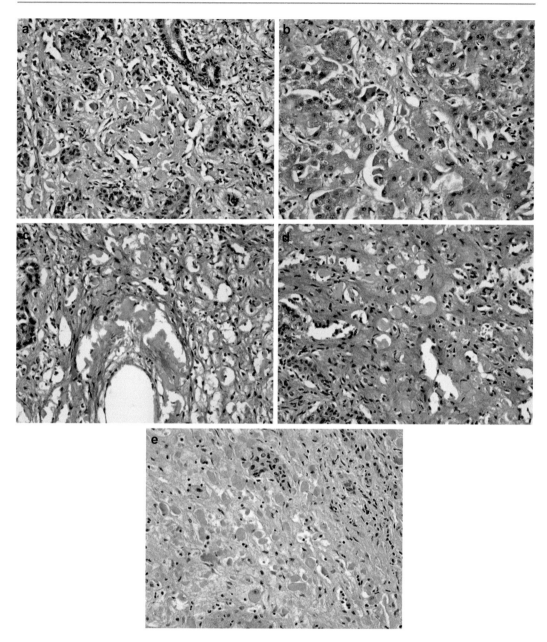

Fig. 30.29 (**a**) A different patient with Lect 2 amyloid and alcohol-induced cirrhosis. Small globules of amyloid are to the primarily in the fibrous septa separating regenerative nodules. (**b**) Several small amyloid globules in regenerating nodule. (**c**) Small globules of Lect 2 amyloid around a vascular structure. (**d**) Fine globules of Lect 2 amyloid and a fibrous band associated with a ductular reaction. (**e**) A *Congo red* stain highlighting small uniform globules of Lect 2 amyloid

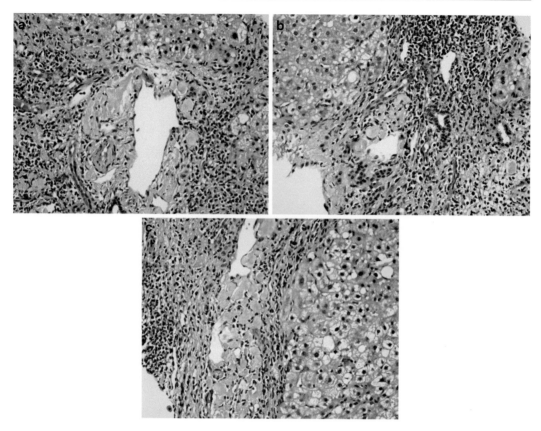

Fig. 30.30 (**a**) A different patient with Lect 2 amyloid and hepatitis C-induced cirrhosis. The fine globules of amyloid were only noted in residual portal tracts and fibrous septa in this case. (**b**) Small Lect 2 amyloid globules in a residual portal structure. (**c**) Coalescent small globules of Lect 2 amyloid

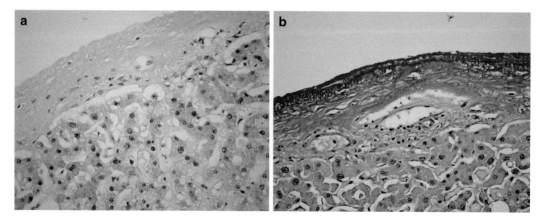

Fig. 30.31 (**a**) Amyloid deposition in the capsule of a resected liver; there was no sinusoidal or vascular involvement in this particular case. (**b**) A *Congo red* stain to highlight the amyloid deposition

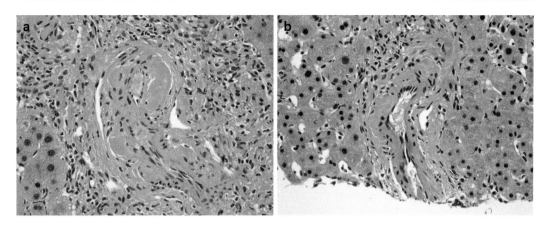

Fig. 30.32 (**a**) The case amyloid deposition only involving the hepatic artery branches; there was no sinusoidal or lobular amyloid noted in this case. The capsule was not available for review. (**b**) Another hepatic arterial in the same patient; confirmation distorted by the amyloid deposition

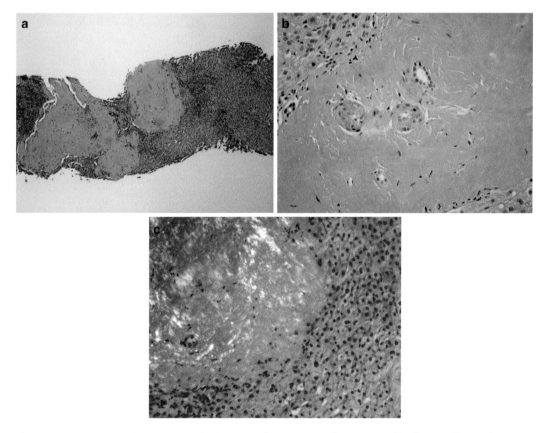

Fig. 30.33 (**a**) Broad bulbous portal deposits of Apolipoprotein A1 amyloid. The sinuses are completely uninvolved in this patient. This large bulbous portal arrangement of the amyloid is relatively characteristic of Apolipoprotein A1 amyloid. (**b**) A *Congo red* stain showing the dense amorphous amyloid deposition entrapping some vascular structures. In other portal tracts, the vascular structures may be pushed to the edge and can be difficult to identify. (**c**) A *Congo red* stain viewed under polarized light showing the classic *apple green* birefringence in Apolipoprotein A1 amyloid

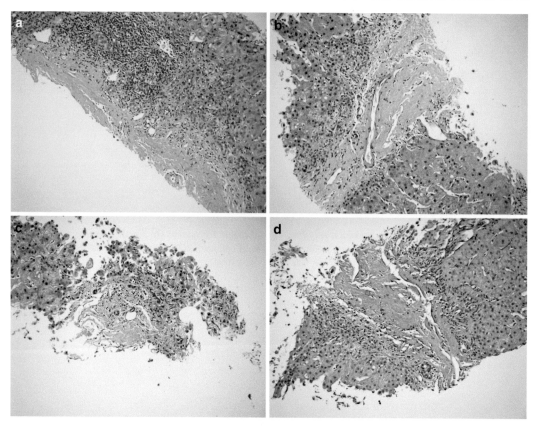

Fig. 30.34 (**a**) An unusual case of systemic AL amyloid involving only the portal tracts. Unlike the Apolipoprotein A1 amyloid, these deposits tend to retain the angular shape of the normal portal tract and can easily be overlooked. There is also moderate chronic inflammatory cell infiltrate and an extensive ductular reaction. Patient was moderately jaundiced. (**b**) Another portal tract with the amyloid tracking along the hepatic artery branch. (**c**) Smaller portal tract involved with amyloid. (**d**) A *Congo red* stain highlighting the portal amyloid deposition. Note the lack of sinusoidal involvement

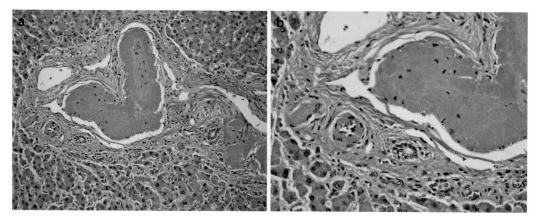

Fig. 30.35 (**a**) An unusual case of transthyretin (TTR) mutation-type amyloid with only involvement of the portal tract. The deposition appears to largely track along the arterioles, but some attached globular component can be appreciated. (**b**) A higher power view of TTR amyloid in the portal tract

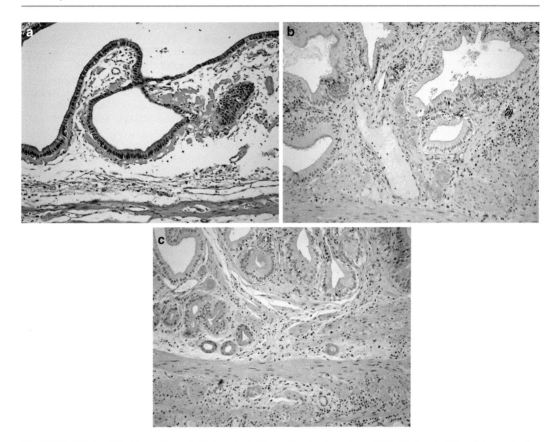

Fig. 30.36 (**a**) A gallbladder with amyloid deposits in the lamina propria producing distortion of the normal architecture. (**b**) A different case again with the lamina propria distribution of amyloid. (**c**) Amyloid involving only the small arterioles of a gallbladder

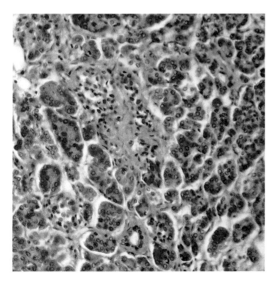

Fig. 30.37 Amyloid involving the pancreatic islets in a diabetic

second form of the disease is the systemic involvement of the pancreas in patients with primary and secondary amyloid. In this instance, the amyloid is deposited in arterials and fibrous septa. Amyloid deposition in the pancreas does not produce clinical manifestations and is either an incidental or autopsy finding [54, 55].

References

1. Pettersson T, Konttinen YT. Amyloidosis-recent developments. Semin Arthritis Rheum. 2010;39: 356–68.
2. Picken MM. Amyloidosis-where are we now and where are we heading? Arch Pathol Lab Med. 2010; 134:545–51.
3. Rocken C, Schwotzer EB, Linke RP, Saeger W. The classification of amyloid deposits in clinicopathological practice. Histopathology. 1996;29:325–35.

4. Hirschfield GM. Amyloidosis: a clinico-pathophysiological synopsis. Semin Cell Dev Biol. 2004;15:39–44.

5. Kyle RA, Gertz MA, Lacy MQ, Dispenzieri A. Localized AL amyloidosis of the colon: an unrecognized entity. Amyloid. 2003;10:36–41.

6. Paccalin M, Hachulla E, Cazalet C, Tricot L, Carreiro M, Rubi M, Grateau G, et al. Localized amyloidosis: a survey of 35 French cases. Amyloid. 2005;12:239–45.

7. Ebert EC, Nagar M. Gastrointestinal manifestations of amyloidosis. Am J Gastroenterol. 2008;103:776–87.

8. Angiero F, Seramondi R, Magistro S, Crippa R, Benedicenti S, Rizzardi C, Cattoretti G. Amyloid deposition in the tongue: clinical and histopathological profile. Anticancer Res. 2010;30:3009–14.

9. Estrada CA, Lewandowski C, Schubert TT, Dorman PJ. Esophageal involvement in secondary amyloidosis mimicking achalasia. J Clin Gastroenterol. 1990;12: 447–50.

10. Iijima-Dohi N, Shinji A, Shimizu T, Ishikawa SZ, Mukawa K, Nakamura T, Maruyama K, et al. Recurrent gastric hemorrhaging with large submucosal hematomas in a patient with primary AL systemic amyloidosis: endoscopic and histopathological findings. Intern Med. 2004;43:468–72.

11. Reddy MB, Poppers DM, Uram-Tuculescu C, Reddy MB, Poppers DM, Uram-Tuculescu C. Recurrent obscure gastrointestinal bleeding in a patient with gastric amyloid. Clin Gastroenterol Hepatol. 2009;7:e1–2.

12. Greaney TV, Nolan N, Malone DE. Multiple gastric polyps in familial amyloid polyneuropathy. Abdom Imaging. 1999;24:220–2.

13. Hemmer PR, Topazian MD, Gertz MA, Abraham SC. Globular amyloid deposits isolated to the small bowel: a rare association with AL amyloidosis. Am J Surg Pathol. 2007;31:141–5.

14. Jensen K, Raynor S, Rose SG, Bailey ST, Schenken JR. Amyloid tumors of the gastrointestinal tract: a report of two cases and review of the literature. Am J Gastroenterol. 1985;80:784–6.

15. Araki H, Muramoto H, Oda K, Koni I, Mabuchi H, Mizukami Y, Nonomura A. Severe gastrointestinal complications of dialysis-related amyloidosis in two patients on long-term hemodialysis. Am J Nephrol. 1996;16:149–53.

16. Borczuk A, Mannion C, Dickson D, Alt E. Intestinal pseudo-obstruction and ischemia secondary to both beta 2-microglobulin and serum A amyloid deposition. Mod Pathol. 1995;8:577–82.

17. Choi HS, Heller D, Picken MM, Sidhu GS, Kahn T. Infarction of intestine with massive amyloid deposition in two patients on long-term hemodialysis. Gastroenterology. 1989;96:230–4.

18. Gono T, Matsuda M, Dohi N, Sekijima Y, Tada T, Sakashita K, Koike K, et al. Gastroduodenal lesions in primary AL amyloidosis. Gastrointest Endosc. 2002; 56:563.

19. Petre S, Shah IA, Gilani N. Review article: gastrointestinal amyloidosis—clinical features, diagnosis and therapy. Aliment Pharmacol Ther. 2008;27:1006–16.

20. Rocken C, Saeger W, Linke RP. Gastrointestinal amyloid deposits in old age. Report on 110 consecutive autopsical patients and 98 retrospective bioptic specimens. Pathol Res Pract. 1994;190:641–9.

21. Yamada M, Hatakeyama S, Tsukagoshi H. Gastrointestinal amyloid deposition in AL (primary or myeloma-associated) and AA (secondary) amyloidosis: diagnostic value of gastric biopsy. Hum Pathol. 1985;16:1206–11.

22. Garcia-Gonzalez R, Fernandez FA, Garijo MF, Fernando Val-Bernal J. Amyloidosis of the rectum mimicking collagenous colitis. Pathol Res Pract. 1998;194:731–5.

23. Groisman GM, Lachter J, Vlodavsky E. Amyloid colitis mimicking collagenous colitis. Histopathology. 1997;31:201–2.

24. Goldblum JR, Beals T, Weiss SW. Elastofibromatous change of the rectum. A lesion mimicking amyloidosis. Am J Surg Pathol. 1992;16:793–5.

25. Ranaldi R, Goteri G, Santinelli A, Rezai B, Pileri S, Poggi S, Bearzi I. Centrocytic-like lymphoma associated with localized amyloidosis of the large intestine. Virchows Arch. 1994;425:327–30.

26. Edwards P, Cooper DA, Turner J, O'Connor TJ, Byrnes DJ. Resolution of amyloidosis (AA type) complicating chronic ulcerative colitis. Gastroenterology. 1988;95:810–5.

27. Katoh N, Matsuda M, Tsuchiya-Suzuki A, Ikeda S. Regression of gastroduodenal amyloid deposition in systemic AL amyloidosis after intensive chemotherapies. Br J Haematol. 2011;153:535–8.

28. Gertz MA, Kyle RA. Hepatic amyloidosis: clinical appraisal in 77 patients. Hepatology. 1997;25:118–21.

29. Loustaud-Ratti VR, Cypierre A, Rousseau A, Yagoubi F, Abraham J, Fauchais AL, Carrier P, et al. Non-invasive detection of hepatic amyloidosis: FibroScan, a new tool. Amyloid. 2011;18:19–24.

30. Booth DR, Tan SY, Booth SE, Tennent GA, Hutchinson WL, Hsuan JJ, Totty NF, et al. Hereditary hepatic and systemic amyloidosis caused by a new deletion/insertion mutation in the apolipoprotein AI gene. J Clin Invest. 1996;97:2714–21.

31. Buck FS, Koss MN. Hepatic amyloidosis: morphologic differences between systemic AL and AA types. Hum Pathol. 1991;22:904–7.

32. Iwata T, Hoshii Y, Kawano H, Gondo T, Takahashi M, Ishihara T, Yokota T, et al. Hepatic amyloidosis in Japan: histological and morphometric analysis based on amyloid proteins. Hum Pathol. 1995; 26:1148–53.

33. Brooks SEH, Audretsch JJ. Hepatic ultrastructure in congenital syphilis. Arch Pathol Lab Med. 1978;102: 502–5.

34. Croitoru AG, Hytiroglou P, Schwartz ME, Saxena R. Liver transplantation for liver rupture due to light chain deposition disease: a case report. Semin Liver Dis. 2006;26:298–303.

35. Randall RE, Williamson WC, Mullinax F, Tung MY, Still WJ. Manifestations of systemic light chain deposition. Am J Med. 1976;60:293–9.

36. Benson MD, Breall J, Cummings OW, Liepnieks JJ. Biochemical characterisation of amyloid by endomyocardial biopsy. Amyloid. 2009;16:9–14.
37. Kanel GC, Uchida T, Peters RL. Globular hepatic amyloid—an unusual morphologic presentation. Hepatology. 1981;1:647–52.
38. Makhlouf HR, Goodman ZD. Globular hepatic amyloid: an early stage in the pathway of amyloid formation: a study of 20 new cases. Am J Surg Pathol. 2007;31:1615–21.
39. Agaram N, Shia J, Klimstra DS, Lau N, Lin O, Erlandson RA, Filippa DA, et al. Globular hepatic amyloid: a diagnostic peculiarity that bears clinical significance. Hum Pathol. 2005;36:845–9.
40. Benson MD, James S, Scott K, Liepnieks JJ, Kluve-Beckerman B. Leukocyte chemotactic factor 2: a novel renal amyloid protein. Kidney Int. 2008;74:218–22.
41. Mereuta OM, Theis JD, Vrana JA, et al. Leukocyte cell-derived chemotaxin 2 (LECT2)-associated amyloidosis is a frequent cause of hepatic amyloidosis in the United States. Blood. 2014;123(10):1479–82.
42. Westermark P, Benson MD, Buxbaum JN, Cohen AS, Frangione B, Ikeda S, Masters CL, et al. A primer of amyloid nomenclature. Amyloid. 2007;14:179–83.
43. Caballeria J, Bruguera M, Sole M, Campistol JM, Rodes J. Hepatic familial amyloidosis caused by a new mutation in the apolipoprotein AI gene: clinical and pathological features. Am J Gastroenterol. 2001;96:1872–6.
44. Coriu D, Dispenzieri A, Stevens FJ, Murphy CL, Wang S, Weiss DT, Solomon A, et al. Hepatic amyloidosis resulting from deposition of the apolipoprotein A-I variant Leu75Pro. Amyloid. 2003;10:215–23.
45. Eriksson M, Schonland S, Yu S, Hegenbart U, von Hutten H, Gioeva Z, Lohse P, et al. Hereditary apolipoprotein AI-associated amyloidosis in surgical pathology specimens: identification of three novel mutations in the APOA1 gene. J Mol Diagn. 2009;11:257–62.
46. Obici L, Palladini G, Giorgetti S, Bellotti V, Gregorini G, Arbustini E, Verga L, et al. Liver biopsy discloses a new apolipoprotein A-I hereditary amyloidosis in several unrelated Italian families. Gastroenterology. 2004;126:1416–22.
47. Burt AD. Liver pathology associated with diseases of other organs or systems. In: Burt AD, Portman BC, Ferrell LD, editors. MacSween's pathology of the liver. 5th ed. Philadelphia, PA: Churchill Livingstone Elsevier; 2007. p. 917.
48. Ien C, Lu L, Hamada T, Sethuraman G, McGrath JA. The molecular basis of lipoid proteinosis: mutations in extracellular matrix protein 1. Exp Dermatol. 2007;16:881–90.
49. Sattianayagam PT, Gibbs SD, Pinney JH, Wechalekar AD, Lachmann HJ, Whelan CJ, Gilbertson JA, et al. Solid organ transplantation in AL amyloidosis. Am J Transplant. 2010;10:2124–31.
50. Liepnieks JJ, Zhang LQ, Benson MD. Progression of transthyretin amyloid neuropathy after liver transplantation. Neurology. 2010;75:324–7.
51. Llado L, Baliellas C, Casasnovas C, Ferrer I, Fabregat J, Ramos E, Castellote J, et al. Risk of transmission of systemic transthyretin amyloidosis after domino liver transplantation. Liver Transpl. 2010;16:1386–92.
52. Kwon A-H, Tsuji K, Yamada H, Okazaki K, Sakaida N. Amyloidosis of the gall bladder mimicking gallbladder cancer. J Gastroenterol. 2007;42:261–4.
53. Sasaki M, Nakanuma Y, Terada T, Hoso M, Saito K, Hayashi M, Kurumaya H. Amyloid deposition in intrahepatic large bile ducts and peribiliary glands in systemic amyloidosis. Hepatology. 1990;12:743–6.
54. Kapurniotu A. Amyloidogenicity and cytototoxicity of islet amyloid polypeptid. Biopolymers (Pept Sci). 2001;60:438–59.
55. Ozdemir D, Dagdelen S, Erbas T. Endocrine involvement in systemic amyloidosis. Endocr Pract. 2010;16:1056–63.

Peripheral Nerve Amyloidosis

31

Adam J. Loavenbruck, JaNean K. Engelstad, and Christopher J. Klein

Introduction

Provided is an overview of the pathology, clinically defining features, and subcategorization of peripheral nerve amyloidosis. This condition is pathologically hallmarked by infiltrative amyloid deposition in varied peripheral neural tissue localizations with associated clinical manifestations. Peripheral nerve involvement is a frequent presenting feature of systemic amyloidosis [1]. As with other organ systems, the diagnosis of amyloid involvement of peripheral nerve is often delayed because the clinical features may mimic many varieties of peripheral neuropathy. Therefore, pathologic discovery of unsuspected amyloidosis is common. The particular amyloid protein can determine the clinical course and preferred treatment modality, as well as potentially alert patients to familial predisposition. Advances in laboratory technology, including most notably mass spectrophotometric evaluation of nerve,

continue to improve the accuracy and sensitivity of amyloid subtyping [2–4]. Appropriate directed peripheral neural biopsy can therefore be instrumental in identifying the diagnosis providing the specific amyloid type, informing prognosis, and directing care in each case.

Historical Pathologic Observations of Nerve Amyloid

In 1938 De Navasquez and Treble demonstrated amorphous material in dorsal roots around small blood vessels, displacing nerve fibers in the endoneurium, and lining epineurial fat deposits [5]. They reviewed the nerve biopsy described in the 1929 paper by De Bruyn and Stern as "hypertrophic polyneuritis", and identified the described "plasmatic bodies" as amyloid deposits [6]. They also noted amyloid in the sympathetic ganglia, where it was thought to compress ganglion cells. Krücke et al. later described similar changes, and demonstrated prominent dorsal root ganglia changes, outlining their findings in two major pathologic reviews in 1959 and 1963 [7, 8]. A large Portuguese family demonstrating inherited peripheral nerve amyloidosis was described by Andrade in 1952 [9] and Horta and Trincao in 1963 [10]. In 1969, Dyck and Lambert outlined ultrastructural findings in sural nerve biopsies taken from cases of dominantly inherited amyloid neuropathy, showing marked loss

A.J. Loavenbruck, MD, MS (✉)
Kennedy Laboratory, Department of Neurology,
University of Minnesota, Diehl Hall J108,
505 Essex St. SE, Minneapolis, MN 55455, USA
e-mail: loave001@umn.edu

J.K. Engelstad, MS • C.J. Klein, MD
Peripheral Nerve Laboratory, Mayo Clinic,
200 1st Street SW, Rochester, MN 55905, USA
e-mail: engelstad.janean@mayo.edu;
klein.christopher@mayo.edu

© Springer International Publishing Switzerland 2015
M.M. Picken et al. (eds.), *Amyloid and Related Disorders*, Current Clinical Pathology,
DOI 10.1007/978-3-319-19294-9_31

of small unmyelinated fibers, and association of endoneurial extracellular amyloid fibrils with collagen replacement [11]. Cohen and Calkins first noted in 1959 that the deposits in various types of amyloidosis appeared essentially similar when viewed by electron microscopy (EM), demonstrating a non-branching, fibrillar structure [12]. In time, fibrils have been shown to measure 70–120 Å in diameter with indeterminate length [13]. We utilize EM rarely in nerve for clinical practice because of the relative sensitivity of tinctorial amyloid staining with Congo red and methyl violet, taken together with the nonspecific EM appearance of the various amyloid types.

Clinical Overview Important in Nerve Amyloid Pathologic Discovery

Amyloidosis is a relatively rare cause of peripheral neuropathy. Rajani et al. reported 13 of 1098 sural nerve biopsies with amyloid deposition [14]. In our own tertiary service-based peripheral nerve laboratory we diagnosed amyloid neuropathy in 62 of 2011 nerve biopsy cases from January 1st 2007 to March 22nd of 2011. Primary amyloidosis (AL) is more common than the other major subset of peripheral nerve amyloidosis, familial amyloid polyneuropathies (FAPs). Both AL (κ-kappa, λ-lambda) and FAPs (TTR-transthyretin, GEL-Gelsolin, APOA1-apo-A1) are subcategorized based on their major amyloid component protein. The familial amyloid varieties have germline nuclear DNA mutations that alter amino acid sequence leading to amyloidogenic potential. In contrast to other forms of amyloidosis, secondary amyloidosis, which can occur in the context of chronic systemic inflammatory conditions such as rheumatoid arthritis, is not known to involve peripheral nerve tissues [2].

The AL and FAP amyloid forms clinically affect the peripheral small nerve fibers or their ganglia early in the course of the disease (aδ fibers conveying cold sensation; c fibers conveying pain and diverse autonomic functions) resulting in a clinical presentation dominated by acral extremity pain and autonomic features of hypohi-

drosis, gastrointestinal dysmotility, orthostasis and impotence [1, 11, 14]. There is typical sparing of Schwann cell function compared to the myelin ensheathed axons, as evidenced by axonal electrophysiologic findings (absence of conduction velocity slowing) and sural nerve pathologic review [11]. Affected persons at the time of presenting to medical attention typically also have clinical involvements of large myelinated fibers (Aβ fibers subserving vibration, gross sensation, and power), causing prominent distal lower extremity weakness and sensory ataxia [15]. Instances of amyloid neuropathy straying from this clinical archetype do occur—most commonly in AL amyloidosis, in which mononeuropathies, plexopathy, asymmetric motor or sensory polyradiculopathy, or selective small-fiber involvement with insensitivity to pain can be seen [16–24]; and in gelsolin amyloidosis, characteristically presenting with insidious facial-onset weakness with corneal lattice dystrophy [25–27]. Rare examples have been reported in TTR amyloid including length-dependent neuropathy with hearing loss or leptomeningeal spread [28, 29]. This variable selective involvement of only certain regions is not understood, but seems important in future discovery for potential strategies to treatment to limit scope of systemic amyloidosis.

Biopsy Sites in Peripheral Nervous System Amyloidosis

In such a clinically heterogeneous condition, the differential diagnosis can be especially broad and proper biopsy location is emphasized to increase yield and limit patient injury (Figs. 31.1 and 31.2). Attempts at evaluating other remote clinically asymptomatic tissues in determination of a person's remote amyloid neuropathy have been generally unsuccessful. By example fat aspiration is commonly attempted in evaluation of neuropathy in question of amyloid but with low yield, i.e., only 6 % of persons with clinical features consistent with amyloid neuropathy [30]. In our own experience, persons with neuropathy and positive fat aspiration for amyloid often have

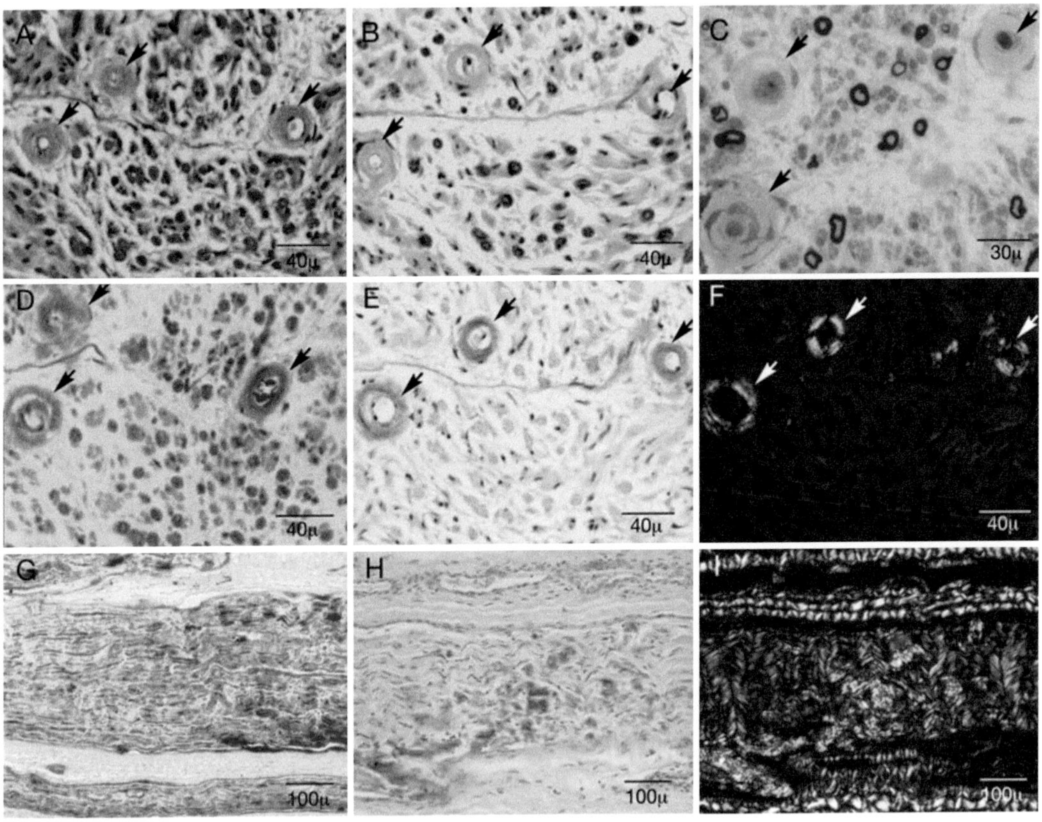

Fig. 31.1 Shown are the characteristic features of amyloid deposition in peripheral sural nerve biopsy tissue studied by light microscopy. Paraffin-stained sections show an acellular and homogenous proteinaceous material on light microscopy on different preparations (**a–f**) and diffuse endoneurial infiltration of amyloid (**g–i**) in a 35-year-old man with primary AL amyloidosis. Vessel walls (*arrows*) are seen to be thickened and acellular on hematoxylin and eosin (**a**), Masson trichrome (**b**), and epoxy-embedded methylene blue-stained sections (**c**). Semithin sections also demonstrate decreased myelinated fiber density with relatively greater loss of small myelinated fibers (**c**). Amyloidal deposits demonstrate magenta metachromasia on methyl violet preparation (**d, g**) and *Congo red* positivity (**e, h**). Demonstrated is the "Maltese cross" appearance under polarized light (**f**)

found alternative non-amyloid neuropathy as cause, i.e., false-positive results. Therefore, currently fat aspiration is insensitive and nonspecific in evaluation of amyloid neuropathy. The implications for a false-positive test are grave with potential application of chemotherapeutic, transplant, and other interventions. Most persons tolerate well different nerve biopsy localizations in amyloid as their pre-biopsy deficits are generally severe, limiting post-procedure new numbness or pain. Since amyloid neuropathy most commonly presents as a distal, sensory and motor neuropathy, whole sural nerve biopsy is most often an appropriate choice for site. Specifically, a 3 cm portion of whole sural nerve is harvested 8 cm above the lateral malleolus. On average 5–13 fascicles are seen. Because the saphenous vein runs juxtaposed to the sural nerve, care in avoiding harvesting this mimic of nerve is emphasized. Helpful in distinction is that the venous branches slope downward (30–60°) in contrast to the sural nerve where its branches arise at right angles (90°) from the main nerve segment. When harvested at the described site the sural nerve typically has 5–13 fascicles allowing for adequate tissue to see amyloid deposits. This sensory nerve provides sensation for the lateral foot, and therefore is consented to be lost post-procedure.

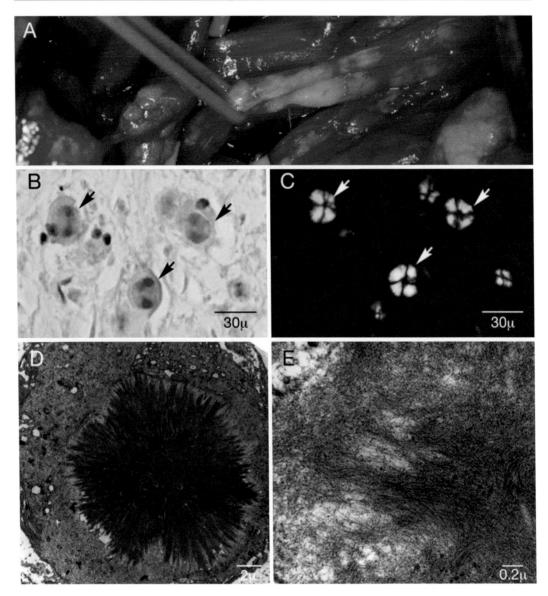

Fig. 31.2 Targeted fascicular biopsy in a 45-year-old man with infiltrative amyloidosis of the lumbosacral roots and sciatic nerve without serum monoclonal protein. Enlarged segments of the peroneal and tibial divisions of the sciatic nerve are seen just distal to the sciatic notch during a fascicular biopsy of the tibial division, with two selected fiber groups held in place with a *red* band (**a**). The biopsied material showed frequent round intracellular inclusions (*arrows*) scattered throughout the endoneurium with congophilia (**b**) and displayed Maltese crosses with polarized light (**c**) (*arrows*). Electron microscopy revealed starburst-shaped inclusions (**d**) with crisscrossing fibril formations typical of amyloid (**e**). Preoperatively he was felt to have a hypertrophic inflammatory neuropathy

Among rare cases, focal or regional amyloid (amyloidoma), reviewed below, has required targeted fascicular biopsy of proximal nerves, roots, plexus, and cranial nerves or their ganglia. In these cases, pre-biopsy suspicion for amyloid is uncommon, despite typical knowledge of circulating monoclonal proteins, with nerve sheath primary tumors or infiltrative neoplasm most commonly suspected by imaging and insidious progressive typically painful course.

Pathogenesis and Histopathologic Findings

The mechanism of tissue destruction in amyloidosis of nerve, as in other organs, is not known. Each amyloidogenic protein (immunoglobulin light chains, or mutated-TTR, GEL, APOA1) is not expressed in the perikaryon or soma of small and large myelinated and unmyelienated fibers nor in Schwann cells. We do not see within the neural tube at or beneath basement membranes or within Schwann cell cytoplasms deposition of amyloid. Rather each fibril forming protein has humoral circulation with deposition in the interstitium of affected nerve fascicles. Endoneurial microvessels most commonly have amyloid deposition with associated apparent spread of amorphous acellular amyloid (Fig. 31.1). There is typically axonal degeneration at the level of the amyloid deposition but also often remotely to the discovered protein. It has been postulated that, due to its tendency to involve blood vessel walls, amyloids' effects might be ischemic, as was initially put forth by Kernohan and Woltman in 1942 [31]. A compressive or structural effect has been suggested by pathologic studies demonstrating physical distortion of nerve fibers by endoneu-

rial amyloid deposits, such as was described by Dyck and Lambert in 1969 [11]. Although rare patients are seen with massive amyloid deposition [19] and poor neurologic course, there seems to be little correlation with extent of deposition and neuropathy severity. This lends credence to the potential for a distal neural apoptotic effect of amyloid fibrils or their precursor proteins and/or its associated pathologic protein microenvironment [32, 33].

Amyloid infiltration of nerve is associated with primary axonal degeneration. Rare examples of demyelination are known to have occurred, though in at least one case demyelination may have been the result of a paraneoplastic effect of an IgM monoclonal gammopathy in association with antibodies to myelin-associated glycoproteins [34] (Fig. 31.3). An increased rate of axonal degeneration and an increased number of empty fibers are the most common abnormalities seen on teased fiber preparation (Fig. 31.4). Additionally, frequently seen in teased fibers is a flocculent deposition at various portions of the nerve fibers (Fig. 31.3).

Depending on chronicity of disease, either active axonal degeneration or resultant fiber loss may be relatively prominent. Semithin sections

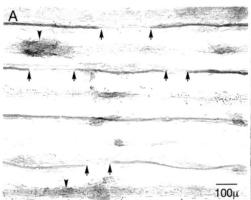
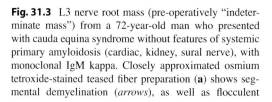
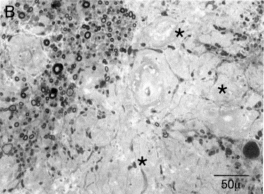

Fig. 31.3 L3 nerve root mass (pre-operatively "indeterminate mass") from a 72-year-old man who presented with cauda equina syndrome without features of systemic primary amyloidosis (cardiac, kidney, sural nerve), with monoclonal IgM kappa. Closely approximated osmium tetroxide-stained teased fiber preparation (**a**) shows segmental demyelination (*arrows*), as well as flocculent material (*arrowheads*) adhering to empty strands, normal fibers, and fibers demonstrating segmental demyelination. An epoxy-embedded methylene *blue*-stained semithin section preparation (**b**) reveals large acellular endoneurial deposits (*asterisks*) with multifocal fiber loss, and fibers with abnormally thin myelin

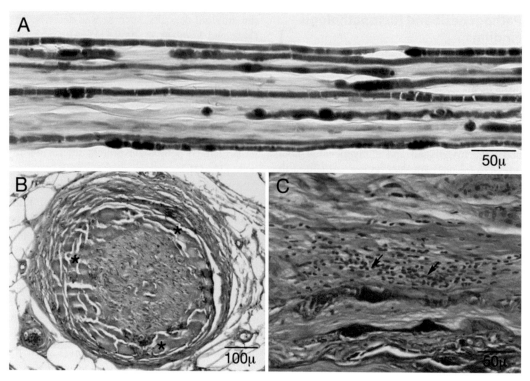

Fig. 31.4 Nerve biopsy from a 76-year-old woman with systemic amyloidosis. Teased fiber preparation (**a**) shows fibers demonstrating axonal degeneration with myelin wrinkling and empty nerve strands. *Congo red* preparation (**b**) shows extensive endoneurial deposition of amy-loid, most prominent subperineurially (*asterisks*). Luxol fast blue–periodic acid Schiff preparation (**c**) demonstrates a moderate size collection of mononuclear cells (*arrows*) adjacent to a small epineurial blood vessel

stained with methylene blue typically show decreased myelinated fiber density (Fig. 31.1). Amyloid infiltrates connective tissues and aggregates in blood vessel walls, more frequently in the endoneurium (Fig. 31.1), though rarely deposits can be seen in nerve arterioles in the epineurium. The amorphous, acellular deposits of amyloid are relatively eosinophillic and PAS positive. Congo red preparations demonstrate congophilia and apple-green birefringence of deposits, and metachromasia can be seen with methyl violet preparations (Fig. 31.1). The absence of congophilia or metachromasia in amorphous, acellular deposits argues strongly against the presence of amyloid, and can be suggestive of amyloid mimicking conditions such as non-amyloidal monoclonal immunoglobulin deposition disease [35], see below section, (Fig. 31.5), or thickening of the basement membrane of endoneurial blood vessels, as can be seen in chronic diabetes [1]. Due to directionality of beta-pleated sheets, cross sections of spherical or tubular deposits of amyloid can demonstrate alternating areas of apple-green birefringence, in some cases manifesting as a Maltese cross appearance of deposits under polarized light (Figs. 31.1 and 31.2) [36]. The examination of Congo red stained slides by fluorescence microscopy using a TRITC (tetramethylrhodamine isothiocyanate) filter shows marked hyperluminescence in areas of amyloid deposits (see Fig. 17.3c, Chap. 17). Collections of perivascular inflammatory cells may be seen in the epineurium and endoneurium, though the frequency and etiologic significance of this finding have not been described (Fig. 31.4).

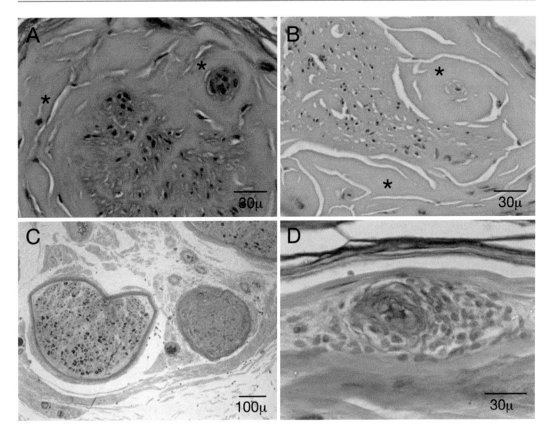

Fig. 31.5 IgM deposition disease (amyloid mimic) in sural nerve biopsy of a 69-year-old man with IgM monoclonal gammopathy. H&E (**a**) and *Congo red* (**b**) preparations show extensive endoneurial infiltration by acellular material involving endoneurial blood vessels (*asterisks*), which was not congophilic. Epoxy-embedded methylene blue-stained semithin sections (**c**) show multifocal myelinated fiber loss with relatively greater loss of small myelinated fibers. (**d**) Luxol fast blue–periodic acid Schiff preparation demon-strates a moderate sized perivascular collection of mononuclear cells in the epineurium, which disrupts the vessel's walls. Mass spectrometry of microdissected deposits detected IgM lambda pentameric macroglobulin with immunoglobulin mu heavy chain constant region, immunoglobulin lambda-light chain constant region, and immunoglobulin J chain, with no evidence of amyloid-associated proteins, serum amyloid protein (SAP), and ApoE, confirming a diagnosis of amyloid-like IgM neuropathy

Regional or Focal Peripheral Nervous System Amyloidosis (Amyloidomas)

Amyloidomas are focal, macroscopic aggregate of amyloid, and an uncommon manifestation of amyloidosis in general. Cases affecting peripheral nerve are exceedingly rare. In several reported cases, nerve roots are affected by amyloidomas arising from vertebral bodies [18, 22, 37]. Only very few cases of amyloidoma arising primarily from peripheral nerve have been reported, involving the lumbosacral plexus (Fig. 31.2), lumbar nerve root (Fig. 31.3), Gasserian ganglion, sciatic nerve, cervical root, brachial plexus, and infraorbital nerve [16, 17, 19–21, 38, 39].

Mass Spectrophotometric Evaluation of Amyloid in Peripheral Nerve Tissues

None of the above described approaches distinguish type of amyloid. One of the most difficult issues arising after the discovery of histologic amyloid in nerves is the correct typing of the specific amyloid proteins. Historically, immuno-histochemical staining (anti-TTR, -lambda-light chain, and kappa-light chain) is performed but is challenging. The difficulties in immunocharacter-ization have been highlighted also in other tissues where misdiagnosis of amyloid type was common and for complex reasons [40, 41]. Contributing to the difficulty in immunocharacterization is the following: (1) antigenic epitopes may be lost by formalin cross-linking in amyloid; (2) circulating contaminant TTR and AL-light chain proteins may produce false-positive results; (3) comparing staining intensities between the different amyloid antibody stains may be unreliable; (4) Pathologic consideration based on clinical, family history and monoclonal serum positivity may be mislead-ing in pathologic interpretation.

We have recently validated application in nerve the use of liquid chromatography tandem mass spectrometry (LC-MS/MS) with laser microdissection (LMD) of amyloid deposits from formalin-fixed, paraffin-embedded sections [4]. This approach eliminates the described problems with immunophenotyping and can be done inde-pendent of often misleading clinical information. Our initial validated studies showed that 21 per-sons with either sural nerve biopsies or proximal root biopsy with amyloid were able to have defined AL, TTR, or GEL cause, whereas earlier attempts at immunophenotyping had failed. Included in the important result was that not only can the predominant amyloid protein be defined, but the specific TTR mutation is determined. This is important as TTR is a normal circulating protein and frequently older persons have circu-lating incidental circulating monoclonal proteins. The approach has had immediate clinical appli-cation in routine practice with large potential for future research with the proteomic microenviron-ment defined by the approach. Based on our experience we have streamlined interpretation away from immunophenotyping.

AL Primary Amyloidosis

Among systemic acquired amyloidoses, only immunoglobulin light chain amyloidosis (AL) has been thought to cause neuropathy. This dogma will require further review with the prolif-eration of proteomic analysis of amyloid by mass spectrophotometry [4, 42]. Lambda-light chains are more commonly involved than kappa-light chains, roughly by twofold [1, 43]. Monoclonal gammopathy, in amyloidosis as in other condi-tions, develops in the setting of plasma cell dys-crasia, multiple myeloma, or MGUS-associated lymphoma including Waldenströms [44, 45]. When monoclonal proteins are identified by serum or urine analysis in patients with amyloi-dosis, AL variety is often given major consider-ation. However, studies have emphasized that the presence of monoclonal protein, particularly in older patients, may be incidental [41, 46]. Therefore, caution should be used in assuming the causality of circulating monoclonal proteins when amyloid is found in peripheral nerves. Conversely, circulating monoclonal proteins may be small, and their detection dependent on the sensitivity of the laboratory methods utilized. The inclusion of serum light chain ratio and 24-h urine analysis provides increased sensitivity beyond that of serum protein electrophoresis and immunofixation [44, 47].

The variability of peripheral nervous sys-tem involvements in AL amyloid is most dra-matic compared to familial forms of systemic amyloidosis affecting nerve. Asymmetric and variable combinations of motor, sensory, and autonomic nerves, roots, and plexus can be involved. However, most commonly, AL causes polyneuropathy involving in length-dependent severity (distal worse than proximal) small nerve fibers, often earlier or more apparently than large nerve fibers, and lower limbs earlier than upper limbs, manifesting in neurologic deficits distally more than proximally (i.e., length dependent). However, isolated mononeuropathy, plexopathy, and radiculopathy are possible, i.e., amyloidoma [16, 17, 19–21, 38, 39] (Figs. 31.2 and 31.3). Involvement of autonomic ganglia and peripheral c fibers are common, and dysautonomic features may include gastrointestinal dysmotility with intractable diarrhea, orthostatic hypotension, urinary incontinence, and erectile dysfunction. Simultaneously, multiple organ systems may be involved, including cardiovascular, renal, hepatic, gastrointestinal, and skin [1, 2, 24, 38, 48–50].

Occasionally, isolated peripheral nervous system amyloidosis may precede spread to other organ systems by years. Presentation with somatic (sensory loss and weakness) non-autonomic peripheral neuropathy in amyloidosis portends on the whole better prognosis. Heart failure and gastrointestinal bleeding being the most common causes of death in systemic AL amyloidosis, though early involvement of autonomic nerves (orthostasis, cardioadrenergic) may also contribute specifically to poorer prognosis [45, 51, 52].

Immunoglobulin Nerve Deposition a Pathologic Mimicker of Amyloid

It is important to be aware of a very rare pathologic mimicker of amyloidosis having intraneural deposition of most commonly IgM macroglobulin in patients with IgM paraproteinemic neuropathy, occurring in monoclonal gammopathy of undetermined significance and Waldenstrom's macroglobulinemia. Few cases are reported in the literature [53–55]. Described patients have presented with asymmetric onset sensory, distal large- and small-fiber deficits with painful dysesthesias which evolve to length-dependent involvements. Notably, there may be relative absence of dysautonomia and systemic organ involvement until very late in the disease course, distinguishing the condition clinically from most cases of peripheral nerve amyloidosis. The mechanism of nerve damage as in amyloidosis remains unexplained—compressive, microvascular, inflammatory, and immune-mediated mechanisms have been considered.

Histopathologically, deposits are seen like amyloid to involve endoneurial blood vessels, with infiltration throughout the endoneurium, often tracking subperineurially (Fig. 31.5). Deposits are eosinophilic, PAS positive, and very similar morphologically to amyloid, though lacking the tinctorial qualities of amyloid on methyl violet and Congo red preparations (Fig. 31.5). Epineurial perivascular mononuclear cell collections may be prominent, suggesting an inflammatory or immune-mediated process. Teased fiber preparation often shows increased numbers of empty nerve strands, floccular aggregates adhering to fibers, and segmental demyelination. Mass spectroscopy of laser microdissected deposits demonstrates that amyloid-like material is composed of μ-heavy chain, λ-light chain, and J-joining chain without serum amyloid protein (SAP) and ApoE, suggesting deposition of IgM pentameric molecules in the absence of amyloid-associated proteins [56]. Deposits show a granulofibrillar structure on electron microscopy, which is slightly distinct from the crisscrossing fibrillar structure of amyloid (Fig. 31.5).

Familial Amyloid Polyneuropathy

FAPs have been subcategorized by the three variant proteins associated with amyloid neuropathy: transthyretin, gelsolin, and apolipoprotein A1 (apo A1). Beta2-microglobulin amyloid deposition, most commonly in the context of chronic hemodialysis, is frequently associated with carpal tunnel syndrome with compressive median neuropathy at the wrist. However, this is known to be due to extraneural deposition within the carpal tunnel and is not as such considered an amyloid neuropathy. More recently, a single family with an apparent, hereditary, systemic amyloidosis, derived from a variant of Beta2-microglobulin, was reported with autonomic and subsequent symmetric sensorimotor axonal polyneuropathy [57].

Transthyretin

Missense point mutation resulting in a valine for methionine substitution at position 30 of TTR among first described by the work of Andrade et al. [9] in Portugal remains the most common alteration associated with inherited amyloid neuropathy. The mutation is inherited in autosomal dominant fashion and has generally high penetrance.

The normal transthyretin protein is a 55 kDa homotetramer of 127-residue monomers, with dimer–dimer formation. The protein has large subregions forming beta-pleated sheets. It is synthesized largely in the liver, choroid plexus, and retina, and its physiologic function is as a transporter of thyroxine and retinol in the serum and cerebrospinal fluid [3, 56, 57]. The protein is encoded by the roughly 7 kbp TTR gene located at 18q12.1. Over 100 mutations of the gene have been reported and found to be amyloidogenic. Generally, mutations lead to destabilization of the homotetrameric formation of the protein, with a greater tendency toward dimerization and subsequently amyloid fibrils. Wild-type transthyretin is known to make up amyloid deposits in Senile Systemic Amyloidosis (SSA), where predominant cardiac involvement occurs, but with primary peripheral nerve involvement not demonstrated [50, 58–60]. However, a case of multifocal spinal column involvement in SSA with resulting compression of adjacent nerve roots and spinal cord has been described [61]. Progression of cardiac amyloidosis after liver transplantation for treatment of TTR amyloidosis has been shown to be attributable to continued deposition of wild-type TTR with a gradually increasing proportion of the wild-type molecules [3, 62–64]. The published ratios of variant to wild-type TTR in tissues were similar to those described by Liepnieks et al. for posttransplant patients with TTR amyloid neuropathy [65].

Though overall epidemiologic studies suggest better survival from the time of symptom onset than in AL amyloidosis [1] TTR amyloid neuropathy cannot be distinguished from primary amyloidosis based on clinical features alone, without the aid of laboratory or histopathologic studies. Like in AL amyloidosis, patients present most commonly with progressive, length-dependent, axonal-predominant polyneuropathy. There is prominent autonomic and small-fiber involvement, manifesting in painful acral paresthesias, thermanesthesia, erectile dysfunction, and gastrointestinal dysmotility. Malabsorption with watery diarrhea may be intractable. Variations exist in presentation, including (1) motor predominant, (2) isolated pain and insensitivity, and (3) isolated dysautonomia. Initially, genotype–phenotype correlations of specific neurologic presentations such as carpal tunnel syndrome were thought possible [66, 67]; however, with subsequent larger case series, these associations are less clear, and substantial phenotypic overlap is recognized between genotypes [68–70]. While the presence of family history of neuropathy or amyloidosis can be helpful in identifying TTR amyloidosis, its absence cannot exclude the diagnosis [69, 71].

Gelsolin

Much less common among FAPs is gelsolin amyloidosis, which causes early and prominent corneal lattice dystrophy, predominant seventh cranial neuropathy, and cutis laxa, and later in the course of the disease a distal polyneuropathy [25, 72]. Gelsolin amyloidosis follows a benign course with relatively late onset, slow progression, and limited morbidity. Inheritance is autosomal dominant. An asparagine for aspartate substitution at position 187 (D187N) of the gelsolin protein has been found, resulting from a missense point mutation in the gelsolin gene. A tyrosine for asparagine substitution at the same position (D187Y) is also known to cause a similar phenotype. The gelsolin protein acts as an actin-modulator and D187N and D187Y mutations make the protein subject to cleavage by the protease molecule furin, by reduced Ca2+ binding at this mutated domain [73]. This occurs in the Golgi complex producing the amyloidogenic protein precursor which then targets the unique distribution of tissues.

Most known patients have been reported in Finland [72], but cases have been reported in the United States, Denmark, the Netherlands, and Japan [74, 75].

Apolipoprotein A1

Apo A-I, secreted by the liver and intestine, is the main protein in high-density lipoprotein (HDL). It is a cofactor for lecithin cholesterol acyltransferase (LCAT), and plays a prominent role in cholesterol transport. The 267-amino acid prepropeptide undergoes two cleavage steps resulting in a functional 243-amino acid protein. Kidney and liver serve as the major sites of Apo A-I breakdown. Decreased plasma HDL (hypoalphalipoproteinemia), hypertriglyceridemia, and/or defective LCAT activation are associated with defects in the protein. Over eight different missense mutations are reported in Apo A-1, but only an arginine for glycine substitution at position 26 (Gly26Arg) and a histine for leucine substitution at position 174 (Leu174His) have been reported to be associated with neuropathy [76–79]. Kidney and heart involvement have been the major causes of clinical presentations.

Apo A-I IOWA was the first Apo A-I variant found to be associated with amyloidosis and peripheral neuropathy, found in an Iowan kindred of British descent 45. The Gly26Arg substitution was seen in Apo A-1 protein making up amyloid fibrils in affected family members. Genetic analysis later discovered heterozygosity for a correlating point mutation of the Apo A-1 gene 43. Variant ApoA1 Gly26Arg was subsequently found in amyloid deposits in two families without neuropathy, including a Massachusetts family of Scandinavian descent and a Canadian family of British descent. Eight additional ApoA1 variants have since been found to be associated with amyloidosis. Chronologically the next two variants to be described were Leu60Arg in a British family and Trp50Arg in an Ashkenazi family, both found to have renal and visceral involvement with variant Apo A-1 amyloid deposits, without neuropathy [80, 81]. Apo A-1 amyloidosis with a 12-residue deletion and Val–Thr insertion was found in a Spanish family [82] in which affected members had both cardiac and renal involvement without neuropathy. An Arg173Pro substitution was found to be associated with cardiac, larynx, and cutaneous involvement [83]. Variant Apo A-1 Leu178His amyloid deposits involving heart, skin, and larynx were found in a small French kindred [76]. One affected member was found to have clinical and neurophysiologic evidence of distal polyneuropathy, though this was not biopsy confirmed. Interestingly, amyloid deposits were found to be composed of both variant ApoA1 and wild-type transthyretin protein.

Treatment of Pathologic Peripheral Nerve Amyloidosis

Symptomatic management of neuropathic pain, orthostasis, weakness, and gastrointestinal complications are important in neurologic management and have been reviewed in detail elsewhere [1]. For pathogenic interventions, the treatment modality is primarily determined by the specific amyloidogenic protein found. The primary goal is to reduce the circulating fibril forming proteins. Therapy for AL-type amyloidosis can be directed at an underlying plasma cell dyscrasia using chemotherapy and stem cell transplantation. Their survival is shown to be improved [84, 85]. Treatment for TTR amyloidosis with liver transplantation has been thought to be helpful in reducing precursor mutant *TTR*. The 5-year survival rate after liver transplantation has varied results reported between 77 and 92 % [86, 87]. However, objective quantitative study of neuropathy is lacking posttransplant, and clinical neurologic progression does occur in a significant portion of treated patients from possibly extrahepatic production of transthyretin. Molecular investigations show deposition of TTR amyloid (wild-type and mutant form) does occur despite liver transplantation [65].

Most recently, pharmacologic attempts at stabilizing fibril forming TTR dimers into their more stable homotetramer state have been demonstrated to be useful in clinical application [88, 89]. The analgesic and anti-inflammatory drug diflunisal, used previously in inflammatory arthropathy, was shown to promote the homotetrameric form of transthyretin in prevention of amyloid fibrils [90, 91]. In a randomized, controlled clinical trial, over 2 years compared to placebo, diflunisal reduced the rate of progression of neurologic impairment and preserved quality of life [92]. Tafamidis was designed specifically to achieve a structure which stabilizes the tetrameric form of transthyretin [93]. In a randomized, controlled clinical trial, tafamadis was well tolerated and delayed impairment associated with peripheral neuropathy in an efficacy evaluable population, but failed to meet primary endpoints in an intention to treat analysis [94]. ISIS-TTR Rx is an antisense oligonucleotide which leads to degradation of transthyretin mRNA thereby silencing expression, and has shown to reduce TTR levels by 80 % in a transgenic mouse model [95]. A phase 2/3 randomized, double-blind, controlled clinical trial began in 2013 [89].

In the case of Gelsolin, molecular therapies have been less clear, and the risk of experimental approaches has generally not been acceptable given the relatively benign course compared to AL and TTR forms. Lubrication of the eyes in prevention of further corneal injury and facial reconstructive surgery are employed in symptomatic management of Gelsolin amyloidosis. Utilization of furin inhibitors or "chemical chaperoning" to stabilize the mutant molecule has been discussed [96].

References

 1. Kyle A, Kelly JJ, Dyck PJ. Amyloidosis and neuropathy. In: Dyck P, editor. Peripheral neuropathies. Philadelphia, PA: Saunders; 2005. p. 2427–51.
 2. Adams D. Hereditary and acquired amyloid neuropathies. J Neurol. 2001;248(8):647–57.
 3. Benson MD, Kincaid JC. The molecular biology and clinical features of amyloid neuropathy. Muscle Nerve. 2007;36(4):411–23.
 4. Klein CJ, et al. Mass spectrometric-based proteomic analysis of amyloid neuropathy type in nerve tissue. Arch Neurol. 2011;68(2):195–9.
 5. De Navasquez S, Treble HA. A case of primary generalized amyloid disease with involvement of the nerves. Brain. 1938;61:12.
 6. De Bruyn RS, Stern RO. A case of the progressive hypertrophic polyneuritis of Dejerine and Sottas, with pathological examination. Brain. 1929;52(1):23.
 7. Krucke W. Histopathologie der Polyneuritis und Polyneuropathie. Dtsch Z Nervenheilkd. 1959;180: 1–39.
 8. Krucke W. Zur pathologischen Anatomie der Paramyloidose. Acta Neuropathol (Berl). 1963;Suppl. II:74–93.
 9. Andrade C. A peculiar form of peripheral neuropathy; familiar atypical generalized amyloidosis with special involvement of the peripheral nerves. Brain. 1952;75(3):408–27.
10. Horta JS, Trincao R. Anatomie pathologique de la paramyloidose de "type Portugais". Acta Neuropathol (Berl). 1963;Suppl. II:54–65.
11. Dyck PJ, Lambert EH. Dissociated sensation in amyloidosis. Compound action potential, quantitative histologic and teased-fiber, and electron microscopic studies of sural nerve biopsies. Arch Neurol. 1969; 20(5):490–507.
12. Cohen AS, Calkins E. Electron microscopic observations on a fibrous component in amyloid of diverse origins. Nature. 1959;183(4669):1202–3.
13. Cohen AS, Shirahama T, Skinner M. Electron microscopy of amyloid. In: Harris I, editor. Electron microscopy of protein. London: Academic; 1982. p. 165–205.
14. Rajani B, Rajani V, Prayson RA. Peripheral nerve amyloidosis in sural nerve biopsies: a clinicopathologic analysis of 13 cases. Arch Pathol Lab Med. 2000;124(1):114–8.
15. Kelly JJ. Neurologic complications of primary systemic amyloidosis. Rev Neurol Dis. 2006;3(4):173–81.
16. Consales A, et al. Amyloidoma of the brachial plexus. Surg Neurol. 2003;59(5):418–23. Discussion 423.
17. Gabet JY, et al. [Amyloid pseudotumor of the sciatic nerve]. Rev Neurol. 1989;145(12):872–6.
18. Haridas A, et al. Primary isolated amyloidoma of the lumbar spine causing neurological compromise: case report and literature review. Neurosurgery. 2005; 57(1):E196. Discussion E196.
19. Ladha SS, et al. Isolated amyloidosis presenting with lumbosacral radiculoplexopathy: description of two cases and pathogenic review. J Peripher Nerv Syst. 2006;11(4):346–52.
20. Laeng RH, et al. Amyloidomas of the nervous system: a monoclonal B-cell disorder with monotypic amyloid light chain lambda amyloid production. Cancer. 1998;82(2):362–74.
21. Pizov G, Soffer D. Amyloid tumor (amyloidoma) of a peripheral nerve. Arch Pathol Lab Med. 1986;110(10): 969–70.
22. Porchet F, Sonntag VK, Vrodos N. Cervical amyloidoma of C2. Case report and review of the literature. Spine. 1998;23(1):133–8.
23. Unal F, et al. Skull base amyloidoma. Case report. J Neurosurg. 1992;76(2):303–6.
24. Wang AK, et al. Patterns of neuropathy and autonomic failure in patients with amyloidosis. Mayo Clin Proc. 2008;83(11):1226–30.
25. Meretoja J. Genetic aspects of familial amyloidosis with corneal lattice dystrophy and cranial neuropathy. Clin Genet. 1973;4(3):173–85.
26. Luttmann RJ, et al. Hereditary amyloidosis of the Finnish type in a German family: clinical and electrophysiological presentation. Muscle Nerve. 2010;41(5):679–84.
27. Tracy JK, Klein CJ. Corneal lattice dystrophy, facial weakness and sensorimotor polyneuropathy-gelsolin amyloidosis. In: Dyck PJ, Amrani K, Klein CJ, Dyck PJB, Low PA, Engelstad J, Spinner RJ editors. Companion to peripheral neuropathy: illustrated cases and new developments. Philadelphia, PA: Saunders; 2011, p. 155–8.
28. Brett M, et al. Transthyretin Leu12Pro is associated with systemic, neuropathic and leptomeningeal amyloidosis. Brain. 1999;122(Pt 2):183–90.
29. Klein CJ, et al. Transthyretin amyloidosis (serine 44) with headache, hearing loss, and peripheral neuropathy. Neurology. 1998;51(5):1462–4.

30. Andrews TR, et al. Utility of subcutaneous fat aspiration for diagnosing amyloidosis in patients with isolated peripheral neuropathy. Mayo Clin Proc. 2002;77(12):1287–90.

31. Kernohan JW, Woltman HW. Amyloid neuritis. Arch Neurol Psychiatr. 1942;47:132–40.

32. Lorenzo A, Yankner BA. Beta-amyloid neurotoxicity requires fibril formation and is inhibited by congo red. Proc Natl Acad Sci U S A. 1994;91(25):12243–7.

33. Simmons LK, et al. Secondary structure of amyloid beta peptide correlates with neurotoxic activity in vitro. Mol Pharmacol. 1994;45(3):373–9.

34. Garces-Sanchez M, et al. Antibodies to myelin-associated glycoprotein (anti-Mag) in IgM amyloidosis may influence expression of neuropathy in rare patients. Muscle Nerve. 2008;37(4):490–5.

35. Buxbaum J, Gallo G. Nonamyloidotic monoclonal immunoglobulin deposition disease. Light-chain, heavy-chain, and light- and heavy-chain deposition diseases. Hematol Oncol Clin North Am. 1999; 13(6):1235–48.

36. Krebs MR, et al. The formation of spherulites by amyloid fibrils of bovine insulin. Proc Natl Acad Sci U S A. 2004;101(40):14420–4.

37. Unal A, Sutlap PN, Kyyyk M. Primary solitary amyloidoma of thoracic spine: a case report and review of the literature. Clin Neurol Neurosurg. 2003;105(3): 167–9.

38. Kyle RA, Bayrd ED. Amyloidosis: review of 236 cases. Medicine (Baltimore). 1975;54(4):271–99.

39. Krishnan J, et al. Tumoral presentation of amyloidosis (amyloidomas) in soft tissues. A report of 14 cases. Am J Clin Pathol. 1993;100(2):135–44.

40. Solomon A, Murphy CL, Westermark P. Unreliability of immunohistochemistry for typing amyloid deposits. Arch Pathol Lab Med. 2008;132(1):14. Author reply 14–5.

41. Lachmann HJ, et al. Misdiagnosis of hereditary amyloidosis as AL (primary) amyloidosis. N Engl J Med. 2002;346(23):1786–91.

42. Vrana JA, et al. Classification of amyloidosis by laser microdissection and mass spectrometry-based proteomic analysis in clinical biopsy specimens. Blood. 2009;114(24):4957–9.

43. Solomon A, Kyle A, Frangione B. Light chain variable region subgroups of monoclonal immunoglobulins in amyloidosis-AL. In: Glenner GG, Osserman EF, Benditt EP, editors. Amyloidosis. New York: Plenum; 1986.

44. Gertz MA. Immunoglobulin light chain amyloidosis: 2011 update on diagnosis, risk-stratification, and management. Am J Hematol. 2011;86(2):180–6.

45. Gertz MA, Kyle RA. Primary systemic amyloidosis— a diagnostic primer. Mayo Clin Proc. 1989;64(12): 1505–19.

46. Kyle RA, et al. Prevalence of monoclonal gammopathy of undetermined significance. N Engl J Med. 2006;354(13):1362–9.

47. Davids MS, Murali MR, Kuter DJ. Serum free light chain analysis. Am J Hematol. 2010;85(10):787–90.

48. Rajkumar SV, Gertz MA, Kyle RA. Prognosis of patients with primary systemic amyloidosis who present with dominant neuropathy. Am J Med. 1998; 104(3):232–7.

49. Kyle RA, Gertz MA. Systemic amyloidosis. Crit Rev Oncol Hematol. 1990;10(1):49–87.

50. Buxbaum JN. The systemic amyloidoses. Curr Opin Rheumatol. 2004;16(1):67–75.

51. Duston MA, et al. Peripheral neuropathy as an early marker of AL amyloidosis. Arch Intern Med. 1989;149(2):358–60.

52. Kyle RA, Greipp PR, O'Fallon WM. Primary systemic amyloidosis: multivariate analysis for prognostic factors in 168 cases. Blood. 1986;68(1):220–4.

53. Vallat JM, et al. Intranervous immunoglobulin deposits: an underestimated mechanism of neuropathy. Muscle Nerve. 2008;38(1):904–11.

54. Moorhouse DF, Fox RI, Powell HC. Immunotactoid-like endoneurial deposits in a patient with monoclonal gammopathy of undetermined significance and neuropathy. Acta Neuropathol. 1992;84(5):484–94.

55. Lamarca J, Casquero P, Pou A. Mononeuritis multiplex in Waldenstrom's macroglobulinemia. Ann Neurol. 1987;22(2):268–72.

56. Figueroa JJ, et al. Amyloid-like IgM deposition neuropathy: a distinct clinico-pathologic and proteomic profiled disorder. J Peripher Nerv Syst. 2012;17(2):182–90.

57. Valleix S, et al. Hereditary systemic amyloidosis due to Asp76Asn variant beta2-microglobulin. N Engl J Med. 2012;366(24):2276–83.

58. Kang GH, et al. A case of a senile systemic amyloidosis patient presenting with angina pectoris and dilated cardiomyopathy. Korean Circ J. 2011;41(4):209–12.

59. Pitkanen P, Westermark P, Cornwell 3rd GG. Senile systemic amyloidosis. Am J Pathol. 1984;117(3):391–9.

60. Kyle RA, et al. The premortem recognition of systemic senile amyloidosis with cardiac involvement. Am J Med. 1996;101(4):395–400.

61. Sueyoshi T, et al. Spinal multifocal amyloidosis derived from wild-type transthyretin. Amyloid. 2011; 18(3):165–8.

62. Stangou AJ, et al. Progressive cardiac amyloidosis following liver transplantation for familial amyloid polyneuropathy: implications for amyloid fibrillogenesis. Transplantation. 1998;66(2):229–33.

63. Olofsson BO, et al. Progression of cardiomyopathy after liver transplantation in patients with familial amyloidotic polyneuropathy, Portuguese type. Transplantation. 2002;73(5):745–51.

64. Dubrey SW, et al. Progression of ventricular wall thickening after liver transplantation for familial amyloidosis. Transplantation. 1997;64(1):74–80.

65. Liepnieks JJ, Zhang LQ, Benson MD. Progression of transthyretin amyloid neuropathy after liver transplantation. Neurology. 2010;75(4):324–7.

66. Thomas PK. Genetic factors in amyloidosis. J Med Genet. 1975;12(4):317–26.

67. Varga J, Wohlgethan JR. The clinical and biochemical spectrum of hereditary amyloidosis. Semin Arthritis Rheum. 1988;18(1):14–28.

68. Ikeda K, et al. Diagnostic pitfalls in sporadic transthyretin familial amyloid polyneuropathy (TTR-FAP). Neurology. 2008;70(17):1576. Author reply 1576–7.

69. Plante-Bordeneuve V, et al. Diagnostic pitfalls in sporadic transthyretin familial amyloid polyneuropathy (TTR-FAP). Neurology. 2007;69(7):693–8.

70. Cappellari M, et al. Variable presentations of TTR-related familial amyloid polyneuropathy in seventeen patients. J Peripher Nerv Syst. 2011;16(2):119–29.

71. Misu K, et al. Late-onset familial amyloid polyneuropathy type I (transthyretin Met30-associated familial amyloid polyneuropathy) unrelated to endemic focus in Japan. Clinicopathological and genetic features. Brain. 1999;122(Pt 10):1951–62.

72. Meretoja J, Teppo L. Histopathological findings of familial amyloidosis with cranial neuropathy as principal manifestation. Report on three cases. Acta Pathol Microbiol Scand A. 1971;79(5):432–40.

73. Chen CD, et al. Furin initiates gelsolin familial amyloidosis in the Golgi through a defect in Ca(2+) stabilization. EMBO J. 2001;20(22):6277–87.

74. Kiuru-Enari S, et al. Neuromuscular pathology in hereditary gelsolin amyloidosis. J Neuropathol Exp Neurol. 2002;61(6):565–71.

75. Kiuru S. Gelsolin-related familial amyloidosis, Finnish type (FAF), and its variants found worldwide. Amyloid. 1998;5(1):55–66.

76. de Sousa MM, et al. Apolipoprotein AI and transthyretin as components of amyloid fibrils in a kindred with apoAI Leu178His amyloidosis. Am J Pathol. 2000;156(6):1911–7.

77. Joy T, et al. APOA1 related amyloidosis: a case report and literature review. Clin Biochem. 2003;36(8):641–5.

78. Nichols WC, et al. A mutation in apolipoprotein A-I in the Iowa type of familial amyloidotic polyneuropathy. Genomics. 1990;8(2):318–23.

79. Van Allen MW, Frohlich JA, Davis JR. Inherited predisposition to generalized amyloidosis. Clinical and pathological study of a family with neuropathy, nephropathy, and peptic ulcer. Neurology. 1969;19(1):10–25.

80. Booth DR, et al. A new apolipoprotein AI variant, Trp50Arg, causes hereditary amyloidosis. QJM. 1995;88(10):695–702.

81. Soutar AK, et al. Apolipoprotein AI mutation Arg-60 causes autosomal dominant amyloidosis. Proc Natl Acad Sci U S A. 1992;89(16):7389–93.

82. Persey MR, et al. Hereditary nephropathic systemic amyloidosis caused by a novel variant apolipoprotein A-I. Kidney Int. 1998;53(2):276–81.

83. Hamidi Asl K, et al. A novel apolipoprotein A-1 variant, Arg173Pro, associated with cardiac and cutaneous amyloidosis. Biochem Biophys Res Commun. 1999;257(2):584–8.

84. Kumar SK, et al. Recent improvements in survival in primary systemic amyloidosis and the importance of an early mortality risk score. Mayo Clin Proc. 2011;86(1):12–8.

85. Dispenzieri A, et al. Superior survival in primary systemic amyloidosis patients undergoing peripheral blood stem cell transplantation: a case-control study. Blood. 2004;103(10):3960–3.

86. Takei Y, et al. Ten years of experience with liver transplantation for familial amyloid polyneuropathy in Japan: outcomes of living donor liver transplantations. Intern Med. 2005;44(11):1151–6.

87. Yamamoto S, et al. Liver transplantation for familial amyloidotic polyneuropathy (FAP): a single-center experience over 16 years. Am J Transplant. 2007;7(11):2597–604.

88. Jono H, et al. Cyclodextrin, a novel therapeutic tool for suppressing amyloidogenic transthyretin misfolding in transthyretin-related amyloidosis. Biochem J. 2011;437(1):35–42.

89. Adams D, et al. FAP neuropathy and emerging treatments. Curr Neurol Neurosci Rep. 2014;14(3):435.

90. Tojo K, et al. Diflunisal stabilizes familial amyloid polyneuropathy-associated transthyretin variant tetramers in serum against dissociation required for amyloidogenesis. Neurosci Res. 2006;56(4):441–9.

91. Sekijima Y, Dendle MA, Kelly JW. Orally administered diflunisal stabilizes transthyretin against dissociation required for amyloidogenesis. Amyloid. 2006;13(4):236–49.

92. Berk JL, et al. Repurposing diflunisal for familial amyloid polyneuropathy: a randomized clinical trial. JAMA. 2013;310(24):2658–67.

93. Bulawa CE, et al. Tafamidis, a potent and selective transthyretin kinetic stabilizer that inhibits the amyloid cascade. Proc Natl Acad Sci U S A. 2012;109(24):9629–34.

94. Coelho T, et al. Tafamidis for transthyretin familial amyloid polyneuropathy: a randomized, controlled trial. Neurology. 2012;79(8):785–92.

95. Benson MD, et al. Targeted suppression of an amyloidogenic transthyretin with antisense oligonucleotides. Muscle Nerve. 2006;33(5):609–18.

96. Sacchettini JC, Kelly JW. Therapeutic strategies for human amyloid diseases. Nat Rev Drug Discov. 2002;1(4):267–75.

Amyloidosis of the Lymph Nodes and the Spleen

32

Filiz Sen and Ahmet Dogan

Introduction

In systemic amyloidosis, involvement of vital organs such as the heart or the kidneys is common. Additionally lymphoid organs such as the peripheral lymph nodes and the spleen may be involved. Clinical features of lymph node and/or spleen involvement can be detected in 10 % of patients with advanced systemic amyloidosis [1]. Additionally the lymph node enlargement and, rarely, the spleen involvement can be the presenting feature in a small number of cases. Given the distinct pathological features of lymph node and spleen amyloidosis, we will discuss these two presentations separately.

F. Sen, MD
Department of Pathology, Memorial Sloan Kettering Cancer Center, 1275 York Avenue, New York, NY 10065, USA
e-mail: senf@mskcc.org

A. Dogan, MD, PhD (✉)
Departments of Pathology and Laboratory Medicine, Memorial Sloan Kettering Cancer Center, 1275 York Avenue, New York, NY 10065, USA
e-mail: dogana@mskcc.org

Amyloidosis Involving Lymph Nodes

Virtually all reported cases of lymph node amyloidosis represent AL amyloidosis [2–31]. In advanced systemic AL amyloidosis, lymph node enlargement can be detected by physical examination up to 10 % of the patients, and can be the sole manifestation at presentation [1]. Rarely lymph node AL amyloidosis may be limited to the lymph nodes without systemic involvement [9, 11, 19, 26, 31, 32]. Lymph node AL amyloidosis is most frequently caused by an underlying systemic plasma cell neoplasm often associated with paraproteinemia and bone marrow involvement [30, 31]. However, in a significant minority of the cases, AL amyloidosis is associated with B-cell lymphoproliferative disorders such as lymphoplasmacytic lymphoma/Waldenstrom's macroglobulinemia or extranodal marginal zone lymphoma [16, 31, 33–36]. These B-cell neoplasms have distinct organ distribution and tendency to involve lymph nodes more frequently than pure plasma cell neoplasms such as plasma cell myeloma.

It is very likely that the lymph nodes are also involved during the course of other systemic amyloidoses such as AA amyloidosis [8], beta-2-microglobulin (B2M) amyloidosis, age-related, or hereditary ATTR amyloidosis. The lymph node biopsies are rarely performed in this context, and reported cases most likely represent incidental

© Springer International Publishing Switzerland 2015
M.M. Picken et al. (eds.), *Amyloid and Related Disorders*, Current Clinical Pathology,
DOI 10.1007/978-3-319-19294-9_32

findings in lymph nodes removed for other pathologies. Other rare causes of lymph node amyloidosis include hereditary systemic amyloidosis causes by Apolipoprotein A1 deposition [37] and extensive localized lymph node amyloidosis associated with metastatic neoplasms producing amyloidogenic proteins such as thyroid medullary carcinoma producing calcitonin.

Histopathology of Lymph Node Amyloidosis

In AL amyloidosis, the affected lymph nodes are often enlarged and firm, and have a waxy appearance on cut surface (Fig. 32.1). Microscopically, the architecture is partially effaced, with occasional well-preserved areas at the periphery of the lymph node. Acellular, amorphous, and faintly eosinophilic material replaces most of the node (Fig. 32.2). The deposits may be surrounded by histiocytes and multinucleated giant cells and are associated with a variable lymphoplasmacytic infiltrate. Misdiagnosis as granuloma with a necrotic "caseous" center should be avoided (Fig. 32.2b). Few residual atrophic follicles may be present within the amorphous deposits. Lymphoid cells, mostly small mature lymphocytes, and plasma cells persist at the periphery or are sprinkled throughout the amorphous deposits

(Fig. 32.2c). Using metachromatic stains such as crystal violet and toluidine blue, amyloid deposits appear red purple. In bright light, Congo red stains deposits of amyloid rose pink, and under polarized light, the deposits show anomalous colors, most typically apple-green birefringence (Fig. 32.2d). PAS stain with and without diastase may be helpful differentiating amyloid from other proteinaceous deposits. While amyloid deposits are typically only weakly PAS positive, the mass-forming non-amyloidotic deposits of light chain deposition disease ("aggregomas"), or other glycoprotein-rich deposits, are strongly PAS positive [38]. Architecturally, diffuse or nodular parenchymal involvement is characteristic of AL amyloidosis, whereas other non-AL systemic amyloidoses predominantly affect medium and large sized vessels in and around the lymph node but spare the parenchyma.

As clinical management depends on the type of amyloid, characterization of amyloid deposits is required in every specimen. This can be achieved by immunohistochemistry [39], and with higher specificity and sensitivity, with mass spectrometry-based proteomics [30, 40]. It is also important to investigate the lymphoid component for evidence of an underlying B-cell or plasma cells proliferative disorder. Flow cytometry-based immunophenotyping is often challenging, especially in lymph nodes extensively

Fig. 32.1 Gross appearances of lymph node involvement in AL amyloidosis. Cut surface of the lymph node involved by AL amyloidosis shows replacement of the parenchyma with a waxy appearing substance consistent with amyloid

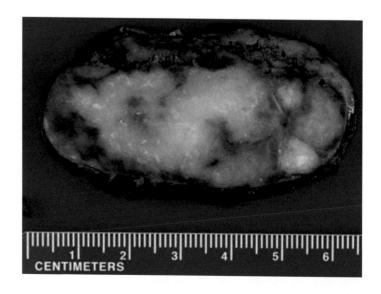

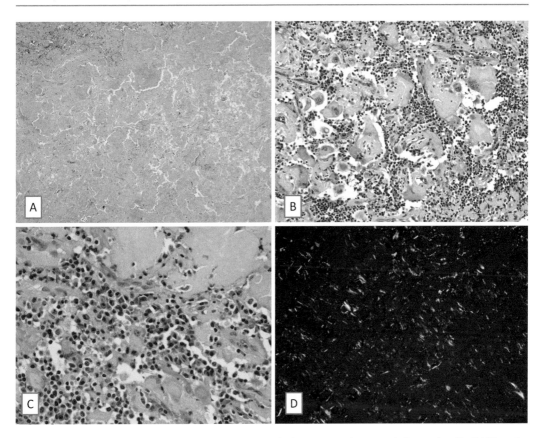

Fig. 32.2 Lymph node involvement in AL amyloidosis. In low-power view, the lymph node architecture is effaced by extensive extracellular eosinophilic amorphous material deposition consistent with amyloidosis (**a**, H&E). In areas, the amyloid deposits are associated with foreign body-type granulomatous inflammation (**b**, H&E), and a lymphoid infiltrate rich in plasma cells (**c**, H&E). *Congo red* stain viewed under polarized light source shows appropriate color change (*apple-green* birefringence) in amyloid deposits (**d**, *Congo red*)

replaced by amyloid deposits. Therefore, immunohistochemistry to detect neoplastic B-cells and/or plasma cells is recommended. Immunohistochemistry tests should include standard workup for low-grade B-cell lymphomas including staining for cytoplasmic immunoglobulin kappa and lambda light chains, and staining for additional markers such as CD56, Cyclin D1, and CD117 often aberrantly expressed by systemic plasma cell disorders. Using such a comprehensive approach, the presence of a clonal B-cell or plasma cell population can be demonstrated in most cases of AL amyloidosis involving the lymph nodes (Fig. 32.3). However, in some cases the neoplastic infiltrate can be very subtle and can only be detected by careful examination or only by molecular techniques. Significantly

higher proportion of AL amyloidosis of lymph nodes are associated with IgM paraproteinemia (2–4 % of systemic AL amyloidosis compared to 20–30 % in lymph node amyloidosis) [30, 31]. Consistent with this, the underlying B-cell neoplasm is more frequently diagnosed as a lymphoplasmacytic lymphoma rather than a pure plasma cell neoplasm.

By mass spectrometry-based proteomics, the exact constitution of amyloid deposits can be identified. Mass spectrometry not only identifies the type of amyloid but also provides detailed information regarding the light chain variable usage and the presence or absence of an immunoglobulin heavy chain component [30]. Interestingly, most cases of AL amyloidosis involving the lymph nodes appear to be composed

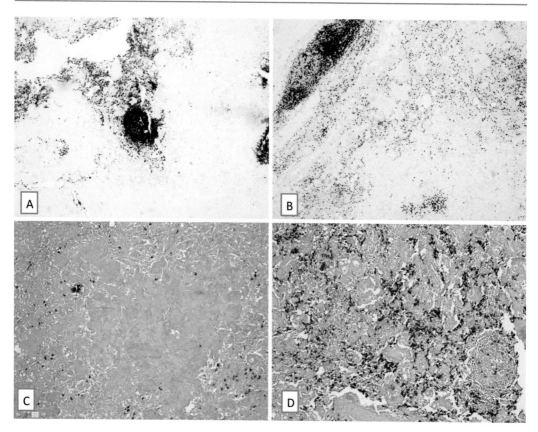

Fig. 32.3 Immunophenotypic features of lymph node involvement in AL amyloidosis. Immunohistochemistry for CD20 (**a**, immunoperoxidase) and CD3 (**b**, immunoperoxidase) highlight B-cell and T-cell areas at the periph- ery. In situ hybridization for kappa and lambda (**c** and **d**, ISH) show that the plasma cell component of the infiltrate is lambda light chain restricted consistent with involvement by a neoplastic process

of both heavy and light chain components. In contrast, amyloid deposits in other organs frequently involved by systemic AL amyloidosis such as the heart or the kidneys are primarily composed of light chains without a heavy chain component. Although the reasons for this difference remain unclear, it is likely that the heavy chain component which has a larger molecular size can be deposited locally in the extracellular environment where it is produced, whereas only the smaller size light chain component can be transported to distant sites.

Amyloidosis Involving the Spleen

Spleen is frequently involved in systemic amyloidosis. By physical examination splenomegaly can be detected in 10 % of patients with systemic

AL or AA amyloidosis [1]. Using special imaging techniques, such as serum amyloid P (SAP) scintigraphy, most patients with systemic amyloidosis show evidence of splenic amyloid deposition [41]. Clinically, splenic amyloidosis may lead to hyposplenism [42–46], and occasionally to splenic rupture [47–58].

Histopathology of Splenic Amyloidosis

Morphological features of splenic amyloidosis have been described in the context of autopsy series and as part of case reports of splenic rupture due to splenomegaly caused by amyloid deposition. Two distinct morphological patterns are reported:

Fig. 32.4 Gross appearances of splenic involvement in AL amyloidosis. A massively enlarged spleen (2500 g) with extensive involvement by systemic AL amyloidosis. Cut surface showed replacement of the parenchyma with a waxy appearing substance consistent with "lardaceous" spleen

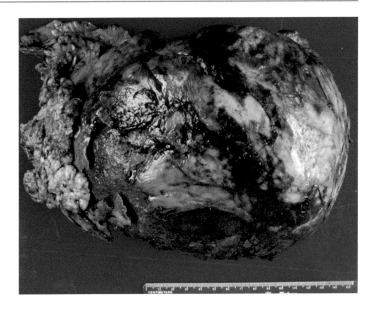

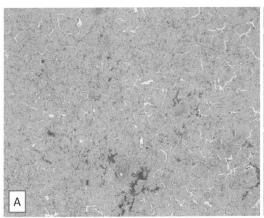
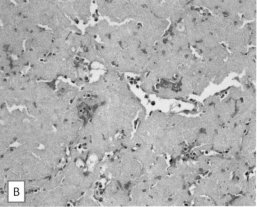

Fig. 32.5 Spleen involvement in AL amyloidosis. In low-power view, the spleen architecture is effaced by extensive extracellular eosinophilic amorphous material deposition consistent with amyloid (**a**, H&E). In high power, the amyloid deposits extensively replace the *red* pulp cord compressing the sinusoids (**b**, H&E)

1. Sago spleen: Amyloid deposits primarily involve the splenic white pulp producing tapioca like granules on gross inspection.
2. Lardaceous spleen: Amyloid deposits primarily involve the red pulp and connective tissue giving a diffuse waxy appearance (Fig. 32.4).

Lardaceous spleen is typical of AL amyloidosis, whereas sago spleen is more frequently associated with AA amyloidosis. Histologically, the amyloid deposits are seen replacing the normal architecture of the spleen. Initially, red pulp cords, connective tissue, and vessels are involved. Eventually the parenchyma is replaced by amyloid deposits (Fig. 32.5). As described for lymph nodes, amyloid deposition can be confirmed by Congo red staining. In splenectomy specimens performed for splenomegaly or splenic rupture amyloid typing is required to establish the nature of the amyloidogenic proteins. In systemic AL amyloidosis, the spleen specimen may contain the neoplastic plasma cell clone in the background of normal lymphoid

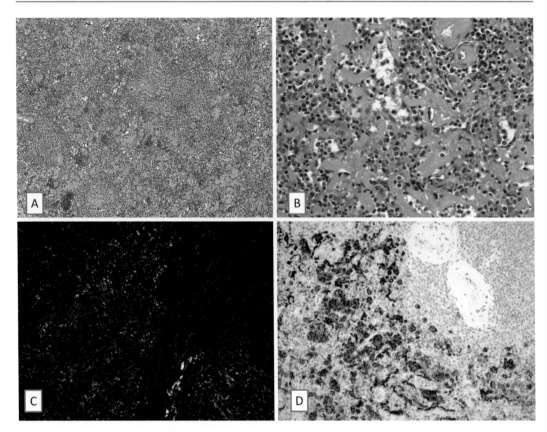

Fig. 32.6 Spleen involvement in ALECT2 amyloidosis. In low-power view, the overall spleen architecture is preserved, but there is patchy extracellular eosinophilic amorphous material deposition consistent with amyloidosis (**a**, H&E). In high power, the amyloid deposits replace the *red* pulp cords, but the sinusoids are patent and func-tional (**b**, H&E). *Congo red* stain viewed under polarized light source shows appropriate color change (*apple-green* birefringence) in amyloid deposits (**c**, *Congo red*). The amyloid deposits are composed of LECT2 protein by immunohistochemistry consistent with ALECT2 amyloidosis (**d**; immunoperoxidase)

population of the spleen [59]. Immunohistochemistry for immunoglobulin light chains may be helpful to identify such clones. The most common causes of splenic amyloidosis include AL amyloidosis and AA amyloidosis, and in patients of Hispanic origin ALECT2 amyloidosis [60] (Fig. 32.6) (see Chap. 4 for ALECT2 amyloidosis).

References

1. Kyle RA, Bayrd ED. Amyloidosis: review of 236 cases. Medicine (Baltimore). 1975;54:271–99.
2. Atkinson AJ. Primary amyloidosis of liver, spleen, kidneys, suprarenals, bone marrow, pancreas, lymph nodes, and blood vessels in lungs. Gastroenterology. 1946;7:477–82.
3. Bauer W, Jones CM, et al. Primary systemic amyloidosis, involving myocardium, cardiac valves, lungs, spleen, lymph nodes and blood vessels. N Engl J Med. 1949;240:572–7.
4. Pilon VA, Gomez LG, Butler JJ. Systemic amyloidosis associated with a benign mesenteric lymphoid mass. Am J Clin Pathol. 1982;78:112–6.
5. Newland JR, Linke RP, Kleinsasser O, Lennert K. Lymph node enlargement due to amyloid. Virchows Arch A Pathol Anat Histopathol. 1983;399:233–6.
6. Melato M, Antonutto G, Falconieri G, Manconi R. Massive amyloidosis of mediastinal lymph nodes in a patient with multiple myeloma. Thorax. 1983;38:151–2.
7. Naschitz JE, Yeshurun D, Pick AI. Intrathoracic amyloid lymphadenopathy. Respiration. 1986;49:73–6.
8. Newland JR, Linke RP, Lennert K. Amyloid deposits in lymph nodes: a morphologic and immunohisto-chemical study. Hum Pathol. 1986;17:1245–9.
9. Kahn H, Strauchen JA, Gilbert HS, Fuchs A. Immunoglobulin-related amyloidosis presenting as

recurrent isolated lymph node involvement. Arch Pathol Lab Med. 1991;115:948–50.

10. Dalton HR, Featherstone T, Athanasou N. Organ limited amyloidosis with lymphadenopathy. Postgrad Med J. 1992;68:47–50.

11. Boss JH. Immunoglobulin-related amyloidosis presenting as recurrent isolated lymph node involvement. Arch Pathol Lab Med. 1993;117:870.

12. Lanzafame S, Magro G, Buffone N, Emmanuele C, Cirino E. Localized primary amyloidosis of axillary lymph nodes. Histopathology. 1996;28:369–71.

13. Spitale LS, Jimenez DB, Montenegro RB. Localised primary amyloidosis of inguinal lymph node with superimposed bone metaplasia. Pathology. 1998;30:321–2.

14. Magro G, Manusia M, Grasso S. Recurrent isolated amyloid lymphadenopathy due to primary plasmacytoma of lymph nodes. Histopathology. 1999;35:581–2.

15. Shi Q, Fan K, Chen H. Localized amyloidosis of cervical lymph nodes. Chin Med J (Engl). 2000; 113:184–5.

16. Meeus G, Ponette J, Delabie J, Verschakelen J, Blockmans D. Immunoglobulin related amyloidosis presenting as isolated lymph node and pulmonary involvement. Leuk Lymphoma. 2000;38:423–7.

17. Mohanty SK, Arora R, Kakkar N, Varma N, Panda N. Amyloidoma of lymph node. Am J Hematol. 2002;70:177–9.

18. Kutlay S, Hasan T, Keven K, Nergizoglu G, Ates K, Karatan O. Primary amyloidosis presenting with massive generalized lymphadenopathy. Leuk Lymphoma. 2002;43:1501–3.

19. Bielsa S, Jover A, Porcel JM. Isolated lymph node amyloidosis. Eur J Intern Med. 2005;16:619.

20. Biewend ML, Menke DM, Calamia KT. The spectrum of localized amyloidosis: a case series of 20 patients and review of the literature. Amyloid. 2006;13: 135–42.

21. Yong HS, Woo OH, Lee JW, Suh SI, Oh YW, Kang EY. Primary localized amyloidosis manifested as supraclavicular and mediastinal lymphadenopathy. Br J Radiol. 2007;80:e131–3.

22. Leiro V, Fernandez-Villar A, Bandres R, Gonzalez A, Represas C, Barros JC, et al. Primary amyloidosis involving mediastinal lymph nodes: diagnosis by transbronchial needle aspiration. Respiration. 2008; 76:218–20.

23. Terrier B, Jaccard A, Harousseau JL, Delarue R, Tournilhac O, Hunault-Berger M, et al. The clinical spectrum of IgM-related amyloidosis: a French nationwide retrospective study of 72 patients. Medicine (Baltimore). 2008;87:99–109.

24. Wechalekar AD, Lachmann HJ, Goodman HJ, Bradwell A, Hawkins PN, Gillmore JD. AL amyloidosis associated with IgM paraproteinemia: clinical profile and treatment outcome. Blood. 2008;112:4009–16.

25. Matsuda M, Gono T, Shimojima Y, Yoshida T, Katoh N, Hoshii Y, et al. AL amyloidosis manifesting as systemic lymphadenopathy. Amyloid. 2008;15:117–24.

26. Sharma S, Kotru M, Gupta R. Isolated amyloidosis of cervical lymph nodes. Acta Cytol. 2010;54:1078–80.

27. Seccia V, Dallan I, Cervetti G, Lenzi R, Marchetti M, Casani AP, et al. A rare case of primary systemic amyloidosis of the neck with massive cervical lymph node involvement: a case report and review of the literature. Leuk Res. 2010;34:e100–3.

28. Matsuda M, Katoh N, Tazawa K, Shimojima Y, Mishima Y, Sano K, et al. Surgical removal of amyloid-laden lymph nodes: a possible therapeutic approach in a primary systemic AL amyloidosis patient with focal lymphadenopathy. Amyloid. 2011;18:79–82.

29. Chan T, Mak HK, Kwong YL. Generalized lymph node immunoglobulin G amyloidoma. Ann Hematol. 2012;91:1503–4.

30. D'Souza A, Theis J, Quint P, Kyle R, Gertz M, Zeldenrust S, et al. Exploring the amyloid proteome in immunoglobulin-derived lymph node amyloidosis using laser microdissection/tandem mass spectrometry. Am J Hematol. 2013;88:577–80.

31. Fu J, Seldin DC, Berk JL, Sun F, O'Hara C, Cui H, et al. Lymphadenopathy as a manifestation of amyloidosis: a case series. Amyloid. 2014;21:256–60.

32. Bhavsar T, Vincent G, Durra H, Khurana JS, Huang Y. Primary amyloidosis involving mesenteric lymph nodes: diagnosis by fine-needle aspiration cytology. Acta Cytol. 2011;55:296–301.

33. Telio D, Bailey D, Chen C, Crump M, Reece D, Kukreti V. Two distinct syndromes of lymphoma associated AL amyloidosis: a case series and review of the literature. Am J Hematol. 2010;85:805–8.

34. Simmonds PD, Cottrell BJ, Mead GM, Wright DH, Whitehouse JMA. Lymphadenopathy due to amyloid deposition in non-Hodgkin's lymphoma. Ann Oncol. 1997;8:267–70.

35. Cohen AD, Zhou P, Xiao Q, Fleisher M, Kalakonda N, Akhurst T, et al. Systemic AL amyloidosis due to non-Hodgkin's lymphoma: an unusual clinicopathologic association. Br J Haematol. 2004;124:309–14.

36. Palladini G, Russo P, Bosoni T, Sarais G, Lavatelli F, Foli A, et al. AL amyloidosis associated with IgM monoclonal protein: a distinct clinical entity. Clin Lymphoma Myeloma. 2009;9:80–3.

37. Eriksson M, Schonland S, Yumlu S, Hegenbart U, von Hutten H, Gioeva Z, et al. Hereditary apolipoprotein AI-associated amyloidosis in surgical pathology specimens: identification of three novel mutations in the APOA1 gene. J Mol Diagn. 2009;11:257–62.

38. Rostagno A, Frizzera G, Ylagan L, Kumar A, Ghiso J, Gallo G. Tumoral non-amyloidotic monoclonal immunoglobulin light chain deposits ('aggregoma'): presenting feature of B-cell dyscrasia in three cases with immunohistochemical and biochemical analyses. Br J Haematol. 2002;119:62–9.

39. Schonland SO, Hegenbart U, Bochtler T, Mangatter A, Hansberg M, Ho AD, et al. Immunohistochemistry in the classification of systemic forms of amyloidosis: a systematic investigation of 117 patients. Blood. 2012;119:488–93.

40. Vrana JA, Gamez JD, Madden BJ, Theis JD, Bergen III HR, Dogan A. Classification of amyloidosis by

laser microdissection and mass spectrometry-based proteomic analysis in clinical biopsy specimens. Blood. 2009;114:4957–9.

41. Hawkins PN, Lavender JP, Pepys MB. Evaluation of systemic amyloidosis by scintigraphy with 123I-labeled serum amyloid P component. N Engl J Med. 1990;323:508–13.

42. Stone MJ. Functional hyposplenism and amyloidosis. Am J Clin Pathol. 1982;78:570.

43. Boyko WJ, Pratt R, Wass H. Functional hyposplenism, a diagnostic clue in amyloidosis. Report of six cases. Am J Clin Pathol. 1982;77:745–8.

44. Gertz MA, Kyle RA, Greipp PR. Hyposplenism in primary systemic amyloidosis. Ann Intern Med. 1983; 98:475–7.

45. Selby CD, Sprott VM, Toghill PJ. Impaired splenic function in systemic amyloidosis. Postgrad Med J. 1987;63:357–60.

46. Powsner RA, Simms RW, Chudnovsky A, Lee VW, Skinner M. Scintigraphic functional hyposplenism in amyloidosis. J Nucl Med. 1998;39:221–3.

47. King FH, Oppenheimer GD. Rupture of amyloid spleen. Ann Intern Med. 1948;29:374–8.

48. Wiley AT, Teeter RR, Schnabel Sr TG. Rupture of the spleen in primary amyloidosis; report of a case. Med Clin North Am. 1951;35:1841–7.

49. Drapiewski JF, Sternlieb SB, Jones R. Primary amyloidosis with spontaneous rupture of the spleen and sudden death. Ann Intern Med. 1955;43:406–12.

50. Wilson H, Yawn DH. Rupture of the spleen in amyloidosis. JAMA. 1979;241:790–1.

51. Cubo T, Ramia JM, Pardo R, Martin J, Padilla D, Hernandez-Calvo J. Spontaneous rupture of the spleen in amyloidosis. Am J Emerg Med. 1997;15:443–4.

52. Gupta R, Singh G, Bose SM, Vaiphei K, Radotra B. Spontaneous rupture of the amyloid spleen: a report of two cases. J Clin Gastroenterol. 1998;26:161.

53. Oran B, Wright DG, Seldin DC, McAneny D, Skinner M, Sanchorawala V. Spontaneous rupture of the spleen in AL amyloidosis. Am J Hematol. 2003;74: 131–5.

54. Aydinli B, Ozturk G, Balik AA, Aslan S, Erdogan F. Spontaneous rupture of the spleen in secondary amyloidosis: a patient with rheumatoid arthritis. Amyloid. 2006;13:160–3.

55. Chau EM, Chan AC, Chan WK. Spontaneous atraumatic rupture of a normal-sized spleen due to AL amyloid angiopathy. Amyloid. 2008;15:213–5.

56. Skok P, Knehtl M, Ceranic D, Glumbic I. Splenic rupture in systemic amyloidosis—case presentation and review of the literature. Z Gastroenterol. 2009;47: 292–5.

57. Baez-Garcia Jde J, Martinez-Hernandez Magro P, Iriarte-Gallego G, Baez-Avina JA. Spontaneous rupture of the spleen secondary to amyloidosis. Cir Cir. 2010;78:533–7.

58. Shobeiri H, Einakchi M, Khajeh M, Motie MR. Spontaneous rupture of the spleen secondary to amyloidosis. J Coll Physicians Surg Pak. 2013;23: 427–9.

59. Solomon A, Macy SD, Wooliver C, Weiss DT, Westermark P. Splenic plasma cells can serve as a source of amyloidogenic light chains. Blood. 2009; 113:1501–3.

60. Dogan A, Theis JD, Vrana JA, Jimenez-Zepeda VH, Lacy MQ, Leung N, et al. Clinical and pathological phenotype of leukocyte cell-derived chemotaxin-2 (LECT2) amyloidosis (ALECT2). Amyloid. 2010;17:69–70.

Amyloidosis of the Lung

33

Karen L. Grogg, Oana Madalina Mereuta,
and Ahmet Dogan

Introduction

The lung is frequently involved in systemic amyloidosis, representing the fifth most common biopsy site that reveals this diagnosis. In about 80 % of these cases, amyloid in the lung represents deposition of abnormal immunoglobulin (Ig) proteins (AL type) followed by secondary amyloidosis (AA type), β2 microglobulin-derived amyloidosis, and familial and senile amyloidosis due to transthyretin (ATTR type) [1]. It usually manifests as a combination of diffuse fine interstitial, vascular, and rarely by nodular deposits [2].

K.L. Grogg, MD
Department of Laboratory Medicine and Pathology,
Mayo Clinic, 200 First Street SW, Rochester,
MN 55905, USA
e-mail: grogg.karen@mayo.edu

O.M. Mereuta, MD, PhD
Department of Pathology, Memorial Sloan Kettering
Cancer Center, 1275 York Avenue, New York, NY
10065, USA
e-mail: mereutao@mskcc.org

A. Dogan, MD, PhD (✉)
Departments of Pathology and Laboratory Medicine,
Memorial Sloan Kettering Cancer Center, 1275 York
Avenue, New York, NY 10065, USA
e-mail: dogana@mskcc.org

In comparison, localized pulmonary amyloidosis is a relatively rare condition. A Mayo Clinic series encompassing a 14-year period reported that only 17 of 55 amyloidosis cases involving the lung were localized [3]. AL type is the most frequently diagnosed type of amyloidosis localized in the lower respiratory tract [1, 2]. Despite the common etiology, the clinical presentation and histologic pattern of amyloid deposition allow distinction into different clinicopathological categories including nodular pulmonary amyloidosis and tracheobronchial amyloidosis. Rare cases of pleural amyloidosis manifesting either as solitary nodules or pleural effusions have also been reported as localized pulmonary AL amyloidosis [3, 4].

Pulmonary Presentation of Systemic Amyloidosis

Diffuse pulmonary interstitial infiltration with amyloid or diffuse alveolar septal amyloidosis has been generally associated with systemic amyloidosis, mostly AL type, and less frequently ATTR type. More rare types include AA and AApoAIV (apolipoprotein AIV) amyloidosis. In less than 10 % of the cases in the literature, interstitial pulmonary involvement was the major manifestation of the disease presenting as dyspnea, cough, or hemoptysis [3, 5–7]. In the series reported by Utz et al. [3], long-term survival was poor in all cases with a median survival of 16 months.

© Springer International Publishing Switzerland 2015
M.M. Picken et al. (eds.), *Amyloid and Related Disorders*, Current Clinical Pathology,
DOI 10.1007/978-3-319-19294-9_33

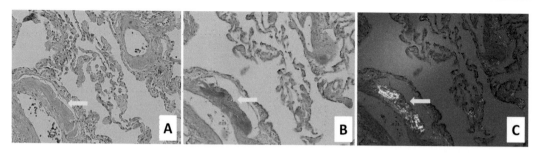

Fig. 33.1 Systemic ATTR amyloidosis involving the lung. Eosinophilic amorphous material consistent with vascular amyloid deposition in the lung (**a**, H&E, *arrow*) stained with *Congo red* (**b**, *arrow*). *Congo red* stain viewed under polarized light (**c**, *Congo red, arrow*)

In this histological pattern, the amyloid deposits are linear and located within the interstitium of the alveolar septae, and are often accompanied by involvement of vessels walls. There is generally no associated lymphoid or plasma cell infiltrate in the lung (Fig. 33.1).

Radiologically, the amyloid deposits appear as nonspecific diffuse interstitial or alveolar opacities, with or without calcification [8]. The differential diagnosis may include idiopathic pulmonary fibrosis, scleroderma, and rheumatoid lung disease.

In the Mayo Clinic study [3], only 1 of 55 cases of pulmonary amyloidosis was found to be of systemic familial ATTR type. In another study over 90-year period, three cases of familial amyloidosis were identified, two of which had pulmonary involvement [9]. In an autopsy study of 19 patients with heterozygotic familial amyloidotic polyneuropathy, all lung samples showed involvement of bronchial/bronchiolar walls, pulmonary artery, and vein walls at various degrees [10].

In contrast, a Swedish autopsy study on 33 individuals with senile ATTR amyloidosis reported the lung as the second most involved site after the heart. The pulmonary amyloid deposits were described as interstitial distribution in a "drop-like" manner [11]. In a similar study, 2 of 21 patients had a diffuse parenchymal involvement of the lung by senile amyloidosis as an incidental finding at the time of autopsy [12]. In a single autopsy case of senile amyloidosis reported

by Ueda et al. [10], the lung tissue revealed scattered patchy amyloid deposits in the pulmonary parenchyma and pulmonary vein. A unique case of confluent nodular senile amyloidosis of the lung associated with scattered lymphoplasmacytic infiltrates composed of polytypic plasma cells and a mixture of small B- and T-lymphocytes has been documented. The radiologic aspect suggested a localized nodular amyloidosis, but immunohistochemistry (IHC), mass spectrometry, and genetic analysis (i.e., to exclude a *TTR* gene mutation) confirmed the senile ATTR type [4]. Patients with pulmonary involvement by senile ATTR amyloidosis are usually asymptomatic and follow a benign course [12].

The autopsy study of Bergstrom et al. [13] revealed codeposition of AApoAIV and TTR in senile systemic ATTR amyloidosis involving the heart. Moreover, in one case was further shown by IHC that the two proteins presented anatomically distinct patterns of distribution within the heart and other organs. For example, in the heart, ApoAIV amyloid deposits presented as small patchy intracellular, interstitial, or larger nodular deposits with bright birefringence on Congo red stain, whereas TTR-positive deposits occurred as interstitial or larger deposits with weak birefringence on Congo red stain. In contrast, in the lung, ApoAIV amyloid was identified in vessel walls, whereas TTR-derived amyloid appeared as small deposits in the alveolar septa [14].

Cases of isolated pulmonary interstitial infiltration have been rarely described [12, 15].

As in other organs, proteomic analysis of lung specimens involved by systemic AL amyloidosis using laser microdissection and liquid chromatography/tandem mass spectrometry (LMD/MS) reveals a fairly pure composition of Ig light chain peptides, without admixed Ig heavy chains [16]. The systemic amyloid distribution should be confirmed with clinical studies and assessment of other organs, in particular the heart and kidney. It is also important to perform serum protein studies and bone marrow biopsy in order to evaluate the presence of an underlying plasma cell neoplasm or systemic B-cell lymphoma.

Clinicopathological Classification of Localized Pulmonary Amyloidosis

Nodular Pulmonary Amyloidosis

Nodular pulmonary amyloidosis (NPA) is often asymptomatic representing an incidental finding on imaging studies (Fig. 33.2a). Patients with autoimmune diseases, in particular Sjogren syndrome, have an increased incidence of NPA [17–21]. The nodules are often multifocal and found in peripheral and subpleural areas. The radiologic appearance of the nodules shows

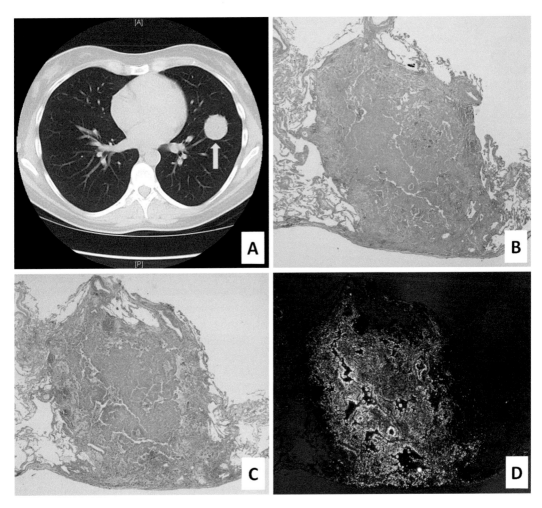

Fig. 33.2 Nodular pulmonary amyloidosis. Nodular amyloid deposition presenting as an isolated nodule in the left lung parenchyma (**a**, CT image, *arrow*). The biopsy shows eosinophilic extracellular deposit (**b**, H&E) stained with *Congo red* (**c**) and showing appropriate color change under polarized light (**d**, *Congo red*)

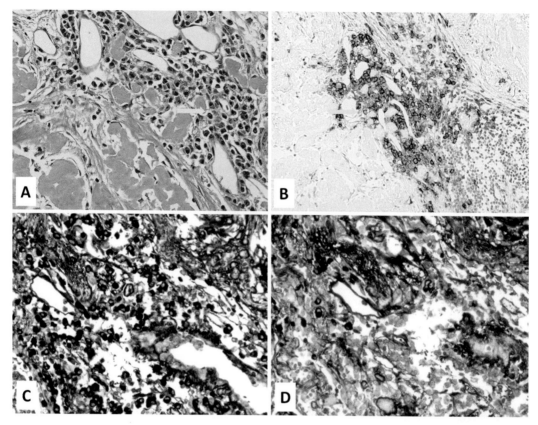

Fig. 33.3 Nodular pulmonary AL kappa amyloidosis involving the lung. Eosinophilic amyloid deposits in the lung and surrounding predominantly plasmacytic infiltrate (**a**, H&E, *arrow*). Immunohistochemistry shows plasma cells expressing CD138 (**b**, immunoperoxidase, *arrow*) and immunoglobulin kappa light chains (**c**, immunoperoxidase for kappa) but not immunoglobulin lambda light chains (**d**, immunoperoxidase for lambda)

discrete borders with frequent calcification, often central or in an irregular pattern within the nodule which may raise concern for a metastatic disease [8, 22, 23].

Histologically, extensive amyloid involvement dominates the lesions of NPA (Fig. 33.2b–d), with aggregates of lymphocytes and plasma cells present within and at the periphery of the nodules (Fig. 33.3a, b). The degree of lymphoplasmacytic infiltrate is quite variable, but generally is scant and may include reactive lymphoid follicles as well as monocytoid small lymphocytes and plasma cells with occasional atypical cytology (Dutcher bodies, Mott cells). The infiltrate may extend beyond the nodule following a lymphangitic distribution. There is often a foreign body giant cell reaction to the amyloid deposits [24].

The chronicity of the process may be reflected by the presence of calcification within the nodule, or even metaplastic ossification [8, 23].

Although NPA derives from Ig proteins, it demonstrates distinct clinicopathological features compared to systemic AL amyloidosis. A recent series of NPA cases analyzed by LMD/MS confirmed the etiology and provided further characterization of the deposits [24]. First of all, NPA was more often related to Ig kappa (k) light chains rather than lambda (λ) Ig light chains, with a ratio of approximately 3:1, in contrast to the λ predominance in systemic AL amyloidosis. Furthermore, the majority of cases (two-thirds) incorporated a mixture of heavy and light chain Ig, designated as Ig-associated amyloidosis (AL/AH type), which is a rare finding in systemic amyloidosis. Before this study, AL/AH amyloidosis has been reported in a single case of localized pulmonary amyloid associated with a lymphoplasmacytoid lymphoma [25]. This characteristic feature may reflect the localized source of the abnormal proteins at the site of amyloid deposition, allowing the entire mixture of proteins to be more readily incorporated into the matrix. In most cases, a clonal population of B cells and/or plasma cells can be identified in close proximity to the amyloid nodules (Fig. 33.3b–d) which differentiates NPA from the usual presentation of primary systemic amyloidosis [24]. Moreover, CD19 expression in monotypic plasma cells has been associated with lymphoplasmacytic neoplasms, only rarely occurring in plasma cell neoplasms that are primary to the bone marrow [26].

Based on these findings, NPA has been considered as a form of extranodal marginal-zone B-cell lymphoma of mucosa-associated lymphoid tissue (MALT) type [27–31]. This concept was further supported by the association of NPA with a connective tissue disorder, in particular Sjogren syndrome [17–21], as well as by the association of Sjogren syndrome and localized amyloid deposition in other anatomic sites that are characteristically involved by MALT lymphoma such as skin, salivary gland, and breast [24, 32]. Therefore, autoimmunity may represent a risk factor for NPA [33].

It is worthwhile to mention that although several *MALT1* gene translocations involving gene locus at 18q21 were reported in 40–60 % of pulmonary MALT lymphomas [34, 35], no translocation was found in NPA cases [24]. Nevertheless, gene expression profiling studies have identified distinct molecular subsets of pulmonary MALT lymphoma, one of these showing increased plasma cells and a predominant plasma cell gene signature but no *MALT1* translocations [36]. Therefore, it has been suggested that NPA may correspond to this particular subset of pulmonary MALT lymphoma [24].

As a localized form, NPA is not associated with a clonal Ig serum protein. The coincident NPA and monoclonal gammopathy of undetermined significance (MGUS) should not be considered evidence of systemic amyloidosis, as this would incorrectly imply a very poor prognosis. In careful study of several patients reported to have both conditions, Ig proteins within the amyloid deposits were found to be unrelated to the clonal serum proteins [24].

In conclusion, NPA represents a lymphoplasmacytic neoplasm in the spectrum of MALT lymphoma. Because of its localized nature, organ dysfunction should not be expected. The clinical course is characterized by indolent behavior and late recurrences either in the lung or other sites. Similar lymphoma recurrence rates (i.e., 33 % and 37 %, respectively) within a median time of 48 months were reported in two series of MALT lymphoma patients [24, 37]. However, the cystic degeneration of the surrounding alveolar parenchyma may occur in a subset of cases, but the underlying pathogenesis of this condition is unknown [38–40].

Tracheobronchial Amyloidosis

Tracheobronchial amyloidosis affects the respiratory tract anywhere along the trachea, bronchi, and bronchioles. It generally presents with symptoms of airway obstruction, such as dyspnea or cough, atelectasis, hemoptysis, and recurrent pneumonia [2, 3]. There also may be vocal changes due to laryngeal involvement. Although rare, patients may present with acute respiratory failure due to subglottic stenosis [2]. Imaging studies show nodular and irregular narrowing of the tracheal lumen, airway wall thickening (Fig. 33.4), and calcification [41]. The amyloid is deposited just underneath the respiratory epithelium, in diffuse deposits or forming nodules, which may appear polypoid on endoscopy. Histologically, the deposits are acellular or may be associated with a very scant lymphoplasmacytic infiltrate [3].

Similar to NPA, tracheobronchial amyloid deposits are comprised of Ig proteins. There is no association with systemic amyloidosis or involvement of other organs. However, the pathogenesis of this disease remains elusive. Previous studies

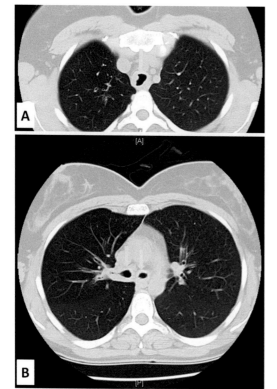

Fig. 33.4 Tracheobronchial amyloidosis. Amyloid deposition in the respiratory tract causing thickening of the tracheal wall and irregular narrowing of the tracheal lumen (**a**, CT image, *arrow*). The same features are identified in the main bronchi (**b**, CT image, *arrows*)

Other "Non-amyloidogenic" Related Conditions Involving the Lung

The lung may also be involved in other Ig deposition syndromes including light chain deposition disease (LCDD) and crystal storing histiocytosis (CSH). These conditions are described more fully in other chapters and will only be briefly addressed here.

Light Chain Deposition Disease

LCDD is a multivisceral disorder presenting with a constant renal involvement. Heart and liver may be frequently involved [44, 45]. Lung involvement is asymptomatic and usually represents an incidental radiological finding. Nodular LCDD restricted to the lung occurs in a similar clinical setting to NPA, with increased frequency in patients with autoimmune disease, especially Sjogren syndrome. Therefore, it is postulated to represent abnormal Ig deposition deriving from an underlying low-grade MALT lymphoma [46]. Multifocal lesions representing nodular LCDD of the lung have been identified concurrently in a patient with Sjogren syndrome. The lesions contained clonally distinct Ig light chains [47]. LCDD may lead to cystic change and a new form of LCDD (i.e., cystic lung LCDD) has been recently described [48–50].

have failed to link this condition with a clonal B-cell or plasma cell population, either residing in the bone marrow or at the site of the amyloid deposits. The lymphoplasmacytic infiltrate, if present, has phenotypic characteristics more consistent with chronic inflammation rather than a lymphoid neoplasm. The peptide composition of the amyloid may show predominance of either k or λ light chains but often a polytypic mixture of k and λ light chains, and sometimes heavy chains as well were identified [15].

Tracheobronchial amyloidosis shows a chronic course that can be complicated by airway obstruction and post-obstructive pneumonia [2]. The lesions are managed with endobronchial laser therapy or cryotherapy with good long-term results [3, 42, 43].

Crystal-Storing Histiocytosis

CSH is a rare disease in which crystalline material accumulates in the cytoplasm of histiocytes. The crystals are most often of Ig k light chain origin without a consistent association of any specific heavy chain [51]. Approximately 90 cases of CSH have been reported so far [52, 53]. In most patients, CSH is a manifestation of an underlying lymphoproliferative disorder, such as multiple myeloma, lymphoplasmacytic lymphoma, and MGUS [53]. The association of CSH and marginal-zone lymphoma has been also reported affecting different anatomic locations,

including the lung and pleura [54–57]. The exact
mechanism of crystal formation in CSH is not
completely understood. It has been proposed that
the aggregated histiocytes in the lung have
engulfed the abnormal Ig proteins produced at
the remote site. An abnormality of the Ig sequence
may prevent normal proteolysis within the lysosomes of the histiocytes, allowing crystal formation to occur [54].

Conclusions

The amyloidosis of the lung remains a challenging
diagnosis which implies accurate differentiation
between localized and systemic forms based on
distinct clinicopathological features. Moreover,
the treatment and prognosis are specific for each
condition and require critical management decisions. Precise typing of the amyloid deposits by
proteomic analysis correlated with IHC findings
as well as molecular studies (i.e., gene expression profiling for MALT lymphoma) provides
new insights into pathogenesis of the localized
amyloidosis involving the lung and underlying
pulmonary lymphoplasmacytic neoplasm.

References

1. Buxbaum JN. The amyloidoses. In: Goldman L,
   Ausiello D, editors. Cecil medicine. 23rd ed.
   Philadelphia, PA: Saunders Elsevier; 2008. p. 2083–7.
2. Howard ME, Ireton J, Daniels F, et al. Pulmonary
   presentations of amyloidosis. Respirology. 2001;6:
   61–4.
3. Utz JP, Swensen SJ, Gertz MA. Pulmonary amyloidosis. The Mayo Clinic experience from 1980 to 1993.
   Ann Intern Med. 1996;124:407–13.
4. Roden AC, Aubry MC, Zhang K, et al. Nodular senile
   pulmonary amyloidosis: a unique case confirmed by
   immunohistochemistry, mass spectrometry, and
   genetic study. Hum Pathol. 2010;41:1040–5.
5. Sumiya M, Ohya N, Shinoura H, et al. Diffuse interstitial pulmonary amyloidosis in rheumatoid arthritis.
   J Rheumatol. 1996;23:933–6.
6. Poh SC, Tija TS, Seah HC. Primary diffuse alveolar
   septal amyloidosis. Thorax. 1975;30:186–91.
7. Celli BR, Rubinow A, Cohen AS, Brody JS. Patterns
   of pulmonary involvement in systemic amyloidosis.
   Chest. 1978;74:543–7.
8. Chan ED, Morales DV, Welsh CH, et al. Calcium
   deposition with or without bone formation in the lung.
   Am J Respir Crit Care Med. 2002;165:1654–69.
9. Smith RR, Hutchins GM, Moore GW, et al. Type and
   distribution of pulmonary parenchymal and vascular
   amyloid. Correlation with cardiac amyloid. Am J
   Med. 1979;66:96–104.
10. Ueda M, Ando Y, Haraoka K, et al. Aging and
    transthyretin-related amyloidosis: pathologic exami-
    nations in pulmonary amyloidosis. Amyloid. 2006;13:
    24–30.
11. Westermark P, Bergström J, Solomon A, et al.
    Transthyretin-derived senile systemic amyloidosis:
    clinicopathologic and structural considerations.
    Amyloid. 2003;10 Suppl 1:48–54.
12. Cordier JF, Loire R, Brune J. Amyloidosis of the
    lower respiratory tract. Clinical and pathologic
    features in a series of 21 patients. Chest. 1986;90:
    827–31.
13. Bergström J, Murphy C, Eulitz M, et al. Codeposition
    of apolipoprotein A-IV and transthyretin in senile sys-
    temic (ATTR) amyloidosis. Biochem Biophys Res
    Commun. 2001;285:903–8.
14. Bergström J, Murphy CL, Weiss DT, et al. Two differ-
    ent types of amyloid deposits-apolipoprotein A-IV
    and transthyretin-in a patient with systemic amyloido-
    sis. Lab Invest. 2004;84:981–9888.
15. Hui AN, Koss MN, Hochholzer I, Wehunt WD.
    Amyloidosis presenting in the lower respiratory tract.
    Clinicopathologic, radiologic, immunohistochemical
    and histochemical studies on 48 cases. Arch Pathol
    Lab Med. 1986;110:212–8.
16. Vrana JA, Gamez JD, Madden BJ, et al. Classification
    of amyloidosis by laser microdissection and mass
    spectrometry-based proteomic analysis in clinical
    biopsy specimens. Blood. 2009;114:4957–9.
17. Ahamed MF, Giampitri EA, Al Shamy A. Pulmonary
    amyloidosis in a patient with lymphocytic interstitial
    pneumonia. Ann Saudi Med. 2007;27:40–4.
18. Adzic TN, Stojsic JM, Radosavljevic-Asic GD, et al.
    Multinodular pulmonary amyloidosis in primary
    Sjogren's syndrome. Eur J Intern Med. 2008;19:
    e97–8.
19. Rodriguez K, Neves F, Stoeterau K, et al. Pulmonary
    amyloidosis in Sjogren's syndrome: a rare diagnosis
    for nodular lung lesions. Int J Rheum Dis. 2009;12:
    358–60.
20. Kawashiri SY, Tamai M, Yamasaki S, et al. A case of
    Sjogren syndrome with pulmonary amyloidosis com-
    plicating microscopic polyangiitis. Mod Rheumatol.
    2011;21:646–50.
21. Beer TW, Edwards CW. Pulmonary nodules due to
    reactive systemic amyloidosis (AA) in Crohn's dis-
    ease. Thorax. 1993;48:1287–8.
22. Gordonson JS, Sargent EN, Jacobson G, et al.
    Roentgenographic manifestations of pulmonary amy-
    loidosis (classification and case illustrations). J Can
    Assoc Radiol. 1972;23:269–72.
23. Ayuso MC, Gilabert R, Bombi JA, et al. CT appear-
    ance of localized pulmonary amyloidosis. J Comput
    Assist Tomogr. 1987;11:197–9.
24. Grogg KL, Aubry MC, Vrana JA, et al. Nodular pul-
    monary amyloidosis is characterized by localized
    immunoglobulin deposition and is frequently associ-

ated with an indolent B-cell lymphoproliferative disorder. Am J Surg Pathol. 2013;37:406–12.

25. Kaplan B, Martin BM, Boykov O, et al. Co-deposition of amyloidogenic immunoglobulin light and heavy chains in localized pulmonary amyloidosis. Virchows Arch. 2005;447:756–61.

26. Morice WG, Chen D, Kurtin PJ, et al. Novel immunophenotypic features of marrow lymphoplasmacytic lymphoma and correlation with Waldenstrom's macroglobulinemia. Mod Pathol. 2009;22:807–16.

27. Dacic S, Colby TV, Yousem SA. Nodular amyloidoma and primary pulmonary lymphoma with amyloid production: a differential diagnostic problem. Mod Pathol. 2000;13:934–40.

28. Moriyama E, Yokose T, Kodama T, et al. Low-grade B-cell lymphoma of mucosa-associated lymphoid tissue in the thymus of a patient with pulmonary amyloid nodules. Jpn J Clin Oncol. 2000;30:349–53.

29. Kurtin PJ, Myers JL, Adlakha H, et al. Pathologic and clinical features of primary pulmonary extranodal marginal zone B-cell lymphoma of MALT type. Am J Surg Pathol. 2001;25:997–1008.

30. Lim JK, Lacy MQ, Kurtin PJ, et al. Pulmonary marginal zone lymphoma of MALT type as a cause of localized pulmonary amyloidosis. J Clin Pathol. 2001;54:642–6.

31. Hourseau M, Virally J, Habib E, et al. Nodular amyloidoma associated with primary pulmonary Malt lymphoma. Rev Mal Respir. 2008;25:1123–6.

32. Wey S-J, Chen Y-M, Lai P-J, et al. Primary Sjogren syndrome manifested as localized cutaneous nodular amyloidosis. J Clin Rheumatol. 2011;17:368–70.

33. Wohrer S, Troch M, Streubel B, et al. MALT lymphoma in patients with autoimmune diseases: a comparative analysis of characteristics and clinical course. Leukemia. 2007;21:1812–8.

34. Streubel B, Huber D, Wohrer S, et al. Frequency of chromosomal aberrations involving MALT1 in mucosa-associated lymphoid tissue lymphoma in patients with Sjogren's syndrome. Clin Cancer Res. 2004;10:476–80.

35. Remstein ED, Dogan A, Einerson RR, et al. The incidence and anatomic site specificity of chromosomal translocations in primary extranodal marginal zone B-cell lymphoma of mucosa-associated lymphoid tissue (MALT lymphoma) in North America. Am J Surg Pathol. 2006;30:1546–53.

36. Chng WJ, Remstein ED, Fonseca R, et al. Gene expression profiling of pulmonary mucosa-associated lymphoid tissue lymphoma identifies new biologic insights with potential diagnostic and therapeutic applications. Blood. 2009;113:635–45.

37. Raderer M, Streubel B, Woehrer S, et al. High relapse rate in patients with MALT lymphoma warrants lifelong follow-up. Clin Cancer Res. 2005;11:3349–52.

38. Sakai M, Yamaoka M, Kawaguchi M, et al. Multiple cystic pulmonary amyloidosis. Ann Thorac Surg. 2011;92:e109.

39. Baqir M, Kluka EM, Aubry MC, et al. Amyloid-associated cystic lung disease in primary Sjogren's syndrome. Respir Med. 2013;107:616–21.

40. Chew KM, Clarke MJ, Dubey N, et al. Nodular pulmonary amyloidosis with unusual, widespread lung cysts. Singapore Med J. 2013;54:e97–9.

41. Kirchner J, Jacobi V, Kardos P, et al. CT findings in extensive tracheobronchial amyloidosis. Eur Radiol. 1998;8:352–4.

42. Thompson PJ, Ryan G, Laurence BH. Laser photoradiation therapy for tracheobronchial amyloid. Aust N Z J Med. 1986;16:229–30.

43. Woo KS, van Hasselt CA, Waldron J. Laser resection of localized subglottic amyloidosis. J Otolaryngol. 1990;19:337–8.

44. Buxbaum J, Gallo G. Nonamyloidotic monoclonal immunoglobulin deposition disease. Light-chain, heavy-chain, and light- and heavy-chain deposition diseases. Hematol Oncol Clin North Am. 1999;13:1235–48.

45. Lin J, Markowitz GS, Valeri AM, et al. Renal monoclonal immunoglobulin deposition disease: the disease spectrum. J Am Soc Nephrol. 2001;12:1482–92.

46. Khoor A, Myers JL, Tazelaar HD, Kurtin PJ. Amyloid-like pulmonary nodules, including localized light-chain deposition: clinicopathologic analysis of three cases. Am J Clin Pathol. 2004;121:200–4.

47. Bhargava P, Rushin JM, Rusnock EJ, et al. Pulmonary light chain deposition disease: report of five cases and review of the literature. Am J Surg Pathol. 2007;31:267–76.

48. Colombat M, Stern M, Groussard O, et al. Pulmonary cystic disorder related to light chain deposition disease. Am J Respir Crit Care Med. 2006;173:777–80.

49. Colombat M, Mal H, Copie-Bergman C, et al. Primary cystic lung light chain deposition disease: a clinicopathologic entity derived from unmutated B cells with a stereotyped IGHV4-34/IGKV1 receptor. Blood. 2008;112:2004–12.

50. Colombat M, Caudroy S, Lagonotte E, et al. Pathomechanisms of cyst formation in pulmonary light chain deposition disease. Eur Respir J. 2008;32:1399–403.

51. Jones D, Bhatia VK, Krausz T, Pinkus GS. Crystal-storing histiocytosis: a disorder occurring in plasmacytic tumors expressing immunoglobulin kappa light chain. Hum Pathol. 1999;30:1441–8.

52. Dogan S, Barnes L, Cruz-Vetrano WP. Crystal-storing histiocytosis: report of a case, review of the literature (80 cases) and a proposed classification. Head Neck Pathol. 2012;6:111–20.

53. Lebeau A, Zeindl-Eberhart E, Muller E-C, et al. Generalized crystal-storing histiocytosis associated with monoclonal gammopathy: molecular analysis of a disorder with rapid clinical course and review of literature. Blood. 2002;100:1817–27.

54. Tahara K, Miyajima K, Ono M, et al. Crystal-storing histiocytosis associated with marginal-zone lymphoma. Jpn J Radiol. 2014;32(5):296–301.

55. Rossi G, Morandi U, Nannini N, et al. Crystal-storing histiocytosis presenting with pleural disease. Histopathology. 2010;56(3):403–5.

56. Rossi G, De Rosa N, Cavazza A, et al. Localized pleuropulmonary crystal-storing histiocytosis: 5 cases of a rare histiocytic disorder with variable clinicoradiologic features. Am J Surg Pathol. 2013;37(6): 906–12.

57. Zhang C, Myers JL. Crystal-storing histiocytosis complicating primary pulmonary marginal zone lymphoma of mucosa-associated lymphoid tissue. Arch Pathol Lab Med. 2013;137:1199–204.

Cutaneous Amyloidosis

34

Oana Madalina Mereuta and Ahmet Dogan

Introduction

Skin is a common site of presentation for localized and systemic amyloidosis. The terminology related to cutaneous amyloidosis is complex and sometimes confusing and reflect cutaneous appearances of the deposits as well as underlying pathogenesis. For practical purposes localized cutaneous amyloidosis is frequently secondary to localized inflammatory and neoplastic skin disorders which lead to local production of the amyloidogenic protein. In contrast, cutaneous involvement in systemic amyloidosis is caused by an abnormal and/or excess amyloidogenic protein produced at a non-cutaneous site. The precise etiology of the cutaneous amyloid deposits often requires histological examination and analysis of biochemical composition of the amyloid

plaques for definitive clinicopathological classification and management of this disorder.

Cutaneous Lesions in Systemic Amyloidosis

Cutaneous amyloidosis can be a manifestation of systemic amyloidosis syndromes (Table 34.1). Two most common types of systemic amyloidosis that involve the skin are AL amyloidosis, which is secondary to deposition of clonal immunoglobulin (Ig) kappa or lambda light chains, and AA amyloidosis, which is caused by excess production of acute phase reactant serum amyloid A (SAA) in chronic inflammatory disorders such as familial Mediterranean fever or rheumatoid arthritis. Cutaneous manifestations of AL amyloidosis are common, occurring in 29–40 % of cases but less frequent in AA amyloidosis [1–4]. Skin can also be involved in systemic β2-microglobulin-derived amyloidosis and familial polyneuropathic type of amyloidosis due to transthyretin (ATTR) as well as in other systemic forms of hereditary amyloidoses (gelsolin, cystatin C, and apolipoprotein A1) [5]. Although rare, mixed amyloid deposits (AA and AL, AA plus β2-microglobulin, AL kappa and ATTR, AL lambda, and β2-microglobulin) were found in large series accounting for 2.5 % of the cases [6–8].

In systemic amyloidosis, the deposits are mainly located in the blood vessel walls in the

O.M. Mereuta, MD, PhD
Department of Pathology, Memorial Sloan Kettering Cancer Center, 1275 York Avenue, New York, NY 10065, USA
e-mail: mereutao@mskcc.org

A. Dogan, MD, PhD (✉)
Departments of Pathology and Laboratory Medicine, Memorial Sloan Kettering Cancer Center, 1275 York Avenue, New York, NY 10065, USA
e-mail: dogana@mskcc.org

© Springer International Publishing Switzerland 2015
M.M. Picken et al. (eds.), *Amyloid and Related Disorders*, Current Clinical Pathology,
DOI 10.1007/978-3-319-19294-9_34

Table 34.1 Clinicopathological classification of cutaneous amyloidosis based on the causative protein

Secondary to systemic amyloidosis	
Primary (AL)	Ig kappa or lambda light chains
Secondary (AA)	SAA
Age-related	TTR
Hereditary[a]	TTR
β2-microglobulin-derived amyloidosis	β2-microglobulin
Primary localized cutaneous amyloidosis	
Lichen	Basal CKs (5 and 14)
Macular	Basal CKs (5 and 14)
Biphasic (mixed)	Basal CKs (5 and 14)
Nodular (AL)	Ig kappa or lambda light chains

[a]Skin may be rarely involved also in other systemic forms of hereditary amyloidosis (gelsolin, cystatin C, and ApoAI) or in some inherited syndromes causing systemic AA amyloidosis

dermis causing wall fragility and subsequent bleeding [5]. Deposits have also been described around lymphatic vessels [9, 10]. Therefore, the main clinical sign observed is purpura [11, 12], many times located around the orbits ("racoon eyes") [13, 14]. Petechiae and ecchymoses also appear even after minimal trauma [15]. Due to the alterations in the coagulation cascade of patients with systemic amyloidosis, cases of disseminated intravascular coagulation and hemangiomas with perihemangiomatous hemorrhage in a targetoid shape have been observed [16, 17].

In advanced disease, amyloid can be deposited also in the subepidermis, adipocytes, glands, vessels, and hair follicles [18]. It presents as non-itchy waxy translucent papulonodular masses mainly around the eyes, mouth, and mucocutaneous junctions. Macroglossia is a common sign of systemic amyloidosis [19]. Nevertheless, other cutaneous clinical manifestations have been reported such as alopecia [20–22], cutis laxa [23, 24], or bullae [25–27]. Blisters due to cleavage developing within the amyloid deposits can occur on the tongue or buccal mucosa and many times are hemorrhagic [28, 29]. Rare forms of presentation include extensive cutaneous ulceration [30] or nail dystrophy [31, 32].

In ATTR, amyloid deposits in the vessels and sweat glands may lead to ulcers, atrophic scars, and petechiae [10, 33, 34]. A case of amyloidogenic His 114 variant presenting with cutaneous nodular amyloidosis was also reported [35].

Although β2-microglobulin-derived amyloidosis rarely involves the skin, some cases of lichenoid plaque-type skin eruptions [36, 37], papules on arms and trunk [38], or flaccid plaques have been reported [39]. It can also appear as subcutaneous nodules, mainly on the buttock [40–44] and lingual papules [38].

Gelsolin deposits may occur in the basal lamina of several cutaneous structures, dermal vessels walls, and elastic fibers leading to the fragmentation and loss of elastic fibers. Therefore, patients present with cutis laxa, dry pruritic skin, hypertrichosis, and loss or thinning of frontotemporal hair. Petechiae and ecchymoses are also frequent [45].

Hereditary cerebral hemorrhage caused by cystatin C deposition may be associated with skin deposits which are usually asymptomatic [46], whereas hereditary apolipoprotein A1 amyloidosis commonly presents as yellowish maculopapular lesions and petechiae [47].

Additionally, some inherited syndromes (Muckle–Wells syndrome, Schnitzler syndrome, and familial Mediterranean fever) may lead to systemic AA amyloidosis [48, 49] and the presence of cutaneous lesions which manifest as Schonlein–Henoch purpura, erythematous erysipelas-like lesions of the lower limbs, panniculitis, and recurrent urticaria [50–52].

It is noteworthy to mention that systemic AA amyloidosis can sometimes be the result of certain cutaneous inflammatory or infectious disorders such as leprosy [53–55], cutaneous tuberculosis, psoriasis, discoid lupus erythematosus, hidradenitis suppurativa, dystrophic epidermolysis bullosa, and other dermatosis [56–59].

Localized Cutaneous Amyloidosis

The term "primary localized cutaneous amyloidosis" (PLCA) refers to a group of conditions that show skin-restricted deposition of amyloid without evidence of systemic organ involvement. The "amyloid" in PLCA may be a combination of degenerate keratin filaments, serum amyloid P

(SAP) component, and secondary deposition of Ig [60]. Two forms of PLCA have been described including keratinic primary localized amyloidosis (kPLCA) and nodular localized primary cutaneous amyloidosis (NLPCA). The kPLCA has been classically described in lichen amyloidosis and macular amyloidosis [5, 61]. Moreover, many patients often show both lichen and macular variants coexisting, and thus, biphasic amyloidosis is not unusual [60]. This suggests a common etiology for the two forms of kPLCA [62].

The clinicopathological classification of PLCA is summarized in Table 34.1.

Keratinic Primary Localized Amyloidosis

The skin in kPLCA shows fibrillary degeneration of basal keratinocytes with increased apoptosis, disruption of dermal unmyelinated nerve fibers, and accumulation of melanosomes in dermal macrophages and Schwann cells [63–65].

kPLCA is due to deposition of cytokeratins (CKs), intermediate filaments found in the basal layer keratinocytes, specific to the dermal deposits of amyloid [66]. This form may be secondary to a dermatologic lesion and it has been described in association with tumors (i.e., basal cell carcinoma [67–69]), nevus [70, 71], seborrheic keratosis, actinic keratosis [72], Bowen's disease [73], and mycosis fungoides [74]. Various forms of PLCA have been reported to coexist with autoimmune connective tissue disorders (e.g., systemic lupus erythematosus, Sjogren syndrome, rheumatoid arthritis, systemic sclerosis, scleroderma, primary biliary cirrhosis, and dermatomyositis [75–80]) as well as multiple endocrine neoplasia type 2A [81].

Clinical Features of kPLCA

The kPLCA usually presents with itching and visible changes of skin hyperpigmentation and thickening (lichenification). In particular, the lesions in macular amyloidosis may be due to or exacerbated by persistent rubbing or scrubbing. Therefore, it is also called frictional amyloidosis [82–85]. Nevertheless, pruritus may be absent in up to 20 % of kPLCA cases, especially in lichen amyloidosis [86].

The most common location for macular amyloidosis is the upper back and usually manifests with a reticulate or "rippled" hyperpigmentation. On the other hand, lichen amyloidosis typically involves the shins and thighs [87], although other locations, such as the arms, back, calves, and dorsum of the feet [85], have been described. It commonly presents with small papules that coalesce into scale-like plaques. Unusual locations for kPLCA are the upper lip and nasolabial folds [88] or external auditory canal [89].

Genetic Linkage Studies in Familial PLCA

Most cases of kPLCA are sporadic, but a genetic predisposition may be present in up to 10 % of cases from South America, Southeast Asia, and China, consistent with an autosomal dominant family history [62].

Following the reports of a possible association between PLCA and the *RET* proto-oncogene, initial genetic linkage studies focused on the *RET* locus on chromosome 10, but no linkage was demonstrated in familial PLCA (FPLCA) pedigrees from China [90]. Further studies on Taiwanese FPLCA cases excluded genetic linkage to a locus on chromosome 1, where the *SAP* gene is located [91]. Genome-wide linkage studies were then performed in these and additional Taiwanese pedigrees, and an interval of probable linkage (5p13.1–q11.2) was identified that spanned the centromere of chromosome 5 [92]. Nevertheless, genetic heterogeneity was suspected as not all autosomal dominant pedigrees mapped to this locus.

FPLCA has been subsequently mapped to a locus on 5p13.1–q11.2 in a large Brazilian family and candidate gene analysis was performed by sequencing genomic DNA [60]. Pathogenic heterozygous missense mutations have been identified in the *OSMR* gene which encodes oncostatin M receptor β (OSMRβ), an interleukin (IL)-6 family cytokine receptor, in all the affected individuals of the Brazilian FPLCA family [60]. The same study also identified a further missense mutation in *OSMR* gene in two Caucasian families with PLCA from the United Kingdom and South Africa. The mutations involved heterozygous amino acid substitutions (p.I691T and p.G618A) within specific extracellular regions of OSMRβ, known as fibronectin type III-like repeat domains (FNIII), regions critical for correct spacing and orientation of the receptor domains. Further pathogenic mutations in the *OSMR* gene have been recently described in various FPLCA pedigrees [62, 93–96].

The cytoplasmic domain of the OSMRβ receptor contains motifs relevant to the recruitment of Janus kinase (JAK)-signal transducers and activators of transcription (STAT) and mitogen-activated protein kinase (MAPK). OSMRβ, however, needs to form a heterodimer for ligand binding and signaling to occur. In fact, OSMRβ is a component of two cytokine receptors, the OSM type II receptor and the IL-31 receptor (IL-31R). The ligands for these two receptors are OSM and IL-31, respectively, which are both members of the IL-6 cytokine family. Signaling via the OSM type II receptor and IL-31R involves activation of both JAK/STAT and MAPK pathways [97]. It has been implicated in keratinocyte cell proliferation, differentiation, apoptosis, and inflammation [98]. Abnormalities in OSMRβ signaling (i.e., reduced activation of JAK/STAT and MAPK pathways) after stimulation of cultured FPLCA keratinocytes with OSM and IL-31 were demonstrated, suggesting that *OSMR* gene mutations may have a direct effect in disrupting intramolecular interactions required for the receptor dimerization and function [60]. Furthermore, identification of these mutations provides new insights into pathophysiological mechanisms of pruritus and keratinocyte apoptosis.

Amyloidosis Cutis Dyschromica

Amyloidosis cutis dyschromica (ACD) is a familial disorder of unknown pathogenesis. Environmental factors, in particular excessive sun exposure and a genetic predisposition, have been suggested as the underlying cause. It has been also suggested that genetic factors may lead to slow DNA repair in keratinocytes due to ultraviolet light damage [99]. The association of ACD with systemic sclerosis, systemic lupus erythematosus, and dermatomyositis has been reported [100].

ACD is a rare condition with only 20 cases reported in the literature. It is characterized by dotted, reticular hyperpigmentation with hypopigmented macules distributed extensively, no or little itch, onset before puberty, and focal subepidermal amyloid deposition. The amyloid is considered to derive from keratinocytes [100].

Histological Findings in kPLCA

The localization of amyloid deposits close to the epidermis suggests that epidermal cells may participate in the pathogenesis of lichen and macular amyloidosis. Amyloid formation in kPLCA results from keratin peptides of degenerating epidermal cells dropped into the dermis (Figs. 34.1a–c and 34.2a–c) [101].

Previous studies using antibodies against epidermal and skin appendageal keratins have been highly contributory to characterizing keratin-derived amyloid which is generally confined to the papillary dermis (Figs. 34.1d and 34.2d) [66, 85, 89, 101, 102].

CKs are a family of intermediate filament proteins that are expressed specifically in the cytoplasm of epithelial cells and are composed of many different polypeptides showing varying degrees of biochemical and immunological relationships. They are classified into two subtypes: type I or acidic CKs (CK9–20) and type II or basic CKs (CK1–8) and they are coexpressed in pairs [103].

These proteins are considered important markers of normal and abnormal cell differentiation. In healthy epidermis, the basal keratinocytes proliferate slowly and express CK5 (type II) and CK14 (type I) and the suprabasal keratinocytes related to terminal differentiation express largely CK1 (type II) and CK10 (type I) with smaller amounts of CK2 (type II) and CK9 (type I) in certain body areas [104].

Immunohistochemical (IHC) studies using monoclonal anti-keratin antibodies produced as purified keratin protein or a mixture of various keratin species were performed on formalin-fixed, paraffin-embedded (FFPE) or frozen tissue sections [66, 89, 101]. All of the CKs detected in amyloid deposits were basic type (type II), in particular CK5. The presence of CK14 was less

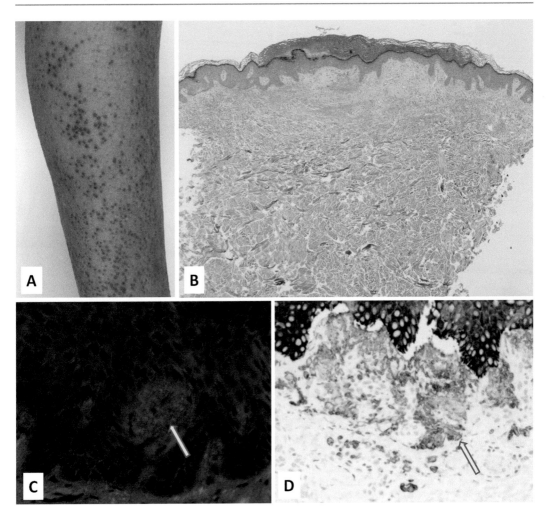

Fig. 34.1 Lichen amyloidosis (**a**). The skin biopsy shows epidermal hyperplasia with hyperkeratosis and accumulation of eosinophilic extracellular material in the papillary dermis (**b**, H&E). The extracellular deposits stain with *Congo red* and show appropriate color change under polarized light (**c**, *Congo red*, *arrow*). Immunohistochemistry shows that the deposits are positive for high molecular weight keratins consistent with a keratinic amyloidosis (**d**, immunoperoxidase)

common suggesting that acidic CKs might be degraded faster than basic types in amyloidogenesis or that FFPE specimens are less sensitive than frozen sections. Moreover, the amyloid deposits were CK14 positive in only 25 % of frozen sections of kPLCA [101]. Therefore, the discrepancy in CK5 and CK14 expression required further investigations. Laser microdissection and proteomic analysis by liquid chromatography/tandem mass spectrometry (LMD/MS) may circumvent many of the pitfalls of IHC demonstrating

that amyloid deposits in kPLCA contain CK5 as well as CK14 (Table 34.1).

Nodular Localized Primary Cutaneous Amyloidosis

Most cases of NLPCA represent AL amyloidosis caused by amyloidogenic light chains produced by a local B-cell/plasma cell disorder [82, 105–107]. Although isolated nodular presentation

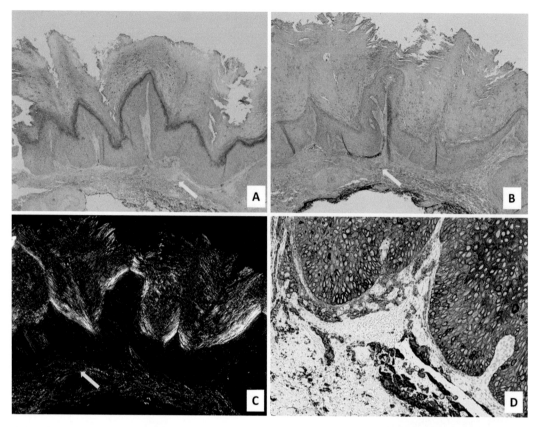

Fig. 34.2 Keratinic cutaneous amyloid deposition associated with squamous carcinoma in situ. There is accumulation of eosinophilic extracellular material in the papillary dermis (**a**, H&E, *arrow*). The extracellular deposits stain with *Congo red* (**b**, *Congo red*, *arrow*) and show appropriate color change under polarized light (**c**, *Congo red*, *arrow*). Immunohistochemistry shows that the deposits are positive for high molecular weight keratins consistent with a keratinic amyloidosis (**d**, immunoperoxidase, *arrow*)

almost always represents localized disease, the possibility of underlying systemic lymphoproliferative disorder with systemic involvement must be excluded [5, 105, 108].

Clinically, NLPCA commonly presents as single or, more rarely, multiple yellowish waxy nodules, and may be located on the extremities, face, trunk, or genitalia, with sizes varying from several millimeters to several centimeters [5, 109]. A bullous variant has been reported [61] as well as the presence of papules and plaques on the nose [110]. NLPCA may be also associated with the CREST (calcinosis, Raynaud phenomenon, esophageal motility disorders, sclerodactyly, and telangiectasia) syndrome, a variant of limited cutaneous systemic sclerosis [111].

Most patients with NLPCA will follow a benign course without development of systemic involvement. However, rare patients may develop systemic AL amyloidosis (i.e., a progression rate of 7–50 % has been reported) or multiple myeloma years later [112, 113]. Nevertheless, local and recurrences of NLPCA are difficult to treat [111].

The histopathology of NLPCA is characterized by primarily dermal deposition of amyloid in a nodular format sometimes involving the local but not distant vessels (Fig. 34.3a–c). The amyloid deposits are frequently associated with a lymphoplasmacytic infiltrate. The infiltrate may be subtle and sometimes can be only detected by IHC. The plasma cells component of the infiltrate

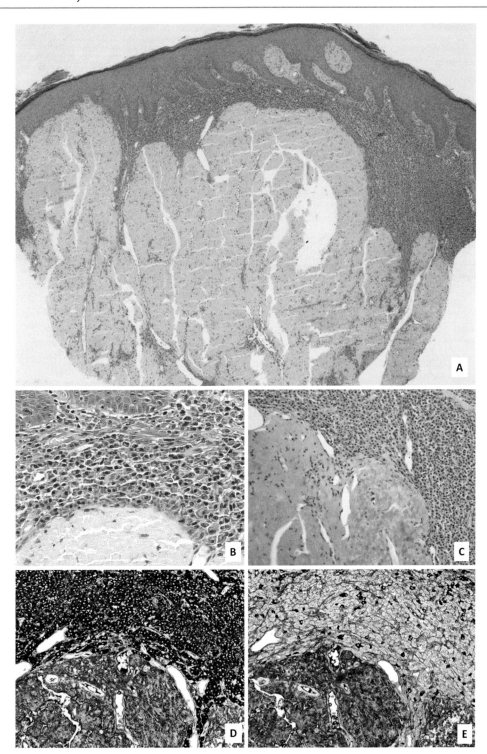

Fig. 34.3 Nodular cutaneous amyloidosis with a large dermal nodule composed of eosinophilic extracellular amorphous material consistent with amyloid (**a**, H&E) and surrounding predominantly plasmacytic infiltrate (**a** and **b**, H&E). The extracellular deposits stain with *Congo red* (**c**, *Congo red*). Immunohistochemistry shows that the plasma cells are positive for immunoglobulin lambda light chains (**d**, immunoperoxidase) but negative for immunoglobulin kappa light chains (**e**, immunoperoxidase) consistent with localized AL (lambda) amyloidosis

Table 34.2 Main clinical features of primary localized cutaneous amyloidosis

Keratinic primary localized amyloidosis	
Lichen	Small papules or scale-like plaques on the shins, thighs, ankles, abdomen, chest, calves, dorsum of the foot Pruritus may be absent
Macular	Reticulate or "rippled" hyperpigmentation on the upper back, extremities, chest, buttocks Pruritus (frictional amyloidosis)
Nodular localized primary cutaneous amyloidosis	
	Single or multiple yellowish waxy nodules on the extremities, face, trunk, genitalia

Table 34.3 Histological features of cutaneous amyloidosis

Histological pattern	Etiology	Localized vs. systemic	Amyloid typing
Subepidermal	Keratin	Localized	IHC
Diffuse dermal	AL	Localized >> systemic	IHC + MS
Vascular	AL, ATTR, AA	Systemic	MS
Subcutaneous	AL, ATTR, AA, Hereditary	Systemic >> localized	MS

is clonal with IHC or molecular testing (Fig. 34.3d, e). In some cases, morphological features of extranodal marginal zone lymphoma with plasmacytic differentiation can be seen.

The clinical presentation and histological findings of kPLCA and NLPCA are summarized in Tables 34.2 and 34.3.

Conclusions

Cutaneous amyloidosis can be localized limited to the skin or manifestation of systemic amyloidosis. The accurate identification of the amyloid type either by immunohistochemical methods or by mass spectrometry-based proteomics is essential for accurate management.

References

1. Schreml S, Szeimies RM, Vogt T, et al. Cutaneous amyloidoses and systemic amyloidoses with cutaneous involvement. Eur J Dermatol. 2010;20:152–60.
2. Brownstein MH, Helwig EB. The cutaneous amyloidoses. II. systemic forms. Arch Dermatol. 1970;102:20–8.
3. Rubinow A, Cohen AS. Skin involvement in generalized amyloidosis: a study of clinically involved and uninvolved skin in 50 patients with primary and secondary amyloidosis. Ann Intern Med. 1978;88:781–5.
4. Barth WF, Willerson JT, Waldmann TA, et al. Primary amyloidosis. Clinical, immunochemical and immunoglobulin metabolism. studies in fifteen patients. Am J Med. 1969;47:259–73.
5. Fernandez-Flores A. Cutaneous amyloidosis: a concept review. Am J Dermatopathol. 2012;34:1–17.
6. Hoshii Y, Takahashi M, Ishihara T, et al. Immunohistochemical classification of 140 autopsy cases with systemic amyloidosis. Pathol Int. 1994;44:352–8.
7. Strege RJ, Saeger W, Linke RP. Diagnosis and immunohistochemical classification of systemic amyloidoses. Report of 43 cases in an unselected autopsy series. Virchows Arch. 1998;433:19–27.
8. Fujimoto N, Yajima M, Ohnishi Y, et al. Advanced glycation end product-modified beta2-microglobulin is a component of amyloid fibrils of primary localized cutaneous nodular amyloidosis. J Invest Dermatol. 2002;118:479–84.
9. Kaiserling E, Krober S. Lymphatic amyloidosis, a previously unrecognized form of amyloid deposition in generalized amyloidosis. Histopathology. 1994;24:215–21.
10. Harkany T, Garzuly F, Csanaky G, et al. Cutaneous lymphatic amyloid deposits in "Hungarian-type" familial transthyretin amyloidosis: a case report. Br J Dermatol. 2002;146:674–9.
11. Rona G. Primary systemic amyloidosis associated with purpura. Can Med Assoc J. 1961;84:1386–9.
12. Kyle RA, Bayrd ED. Amyloidosis: review of 236 cases. Medicine (Baltimore). 1975;54:271–99.
13. Levine N. Bluish discoloration of periorbital area. Eyelid purpura and patient's medical history lead to diagnosis. Geriatrics. 2004;59:20.
14. Lee HJ, Chang SE, Lee MW, et al. Systemic amyloidosis associated with multiple myeloma presenting as periorbital purpura. J Dermatol. 2008;35:371–2.

15. Gamba G, Montani N, Anesi E, et al. Clotting alterations in primary systemic amyloidosis. Haematologica. 2000;85:289–92.
16. Takahashi T, Suzukawa M, Akiyama M, et al. Systemic AL amyloidosis with disseminated intravascular coagulation associated with hyperfibrinolysis. Int J Hematol. 2008;87:371–4.
17. Schmidt CP. Purpuric halos around hemangiomas in systemic amyloidosis. Cutis. 1991;48:141–3.
18. Lee DD, Huang CY, Wong CK. Dermatopathologic findings in 20 cases of systemic amyloidosis. Am J Dermatopathol. 1998;20:438–42.
19. Rigdon RH, Noblin FE. Macroglossia accompanying primary systemic amyloidosis. Ann Otol Rhinol Laryngol. 1949;58:470–8.
20. Wheeler GE, Barrows GH. Alopecia universalis. A manifestation of occult amyloidosis and multiple myeloma. Arch Dermatol. 1981;117:815–6.
21. Hunt SJ, Caserio RJ, Abell E. Primary systemic amyloidosis causing diffuse alopecia by telogen arrest. Arch Dermatol. 1991;127:1067–8.
22. Lutz ME, Pittelkow MR. Progressive generalized alopecia due to systemic amyloidosis. J Am Acad Dermatol. 2002;46:434–6.
23. Yoneda K, Kanoh T, Nomura S, et al. Elastolytic cutaneous lesions in myeloma-associated amyloidosis. Arch Dermatol. 1990;126:657–60.
24. Dicker TJ, Morton J, Williamson RM, et al. Myeloma-associated systemic amyloidosis presenting with acquired digital cutis laxa-like changes. Australas J Dermatol. 2002;43:144–6.
25. Johnson TM, Rapini RP, Hebert AA, et al. Bullous amyloidosis. Cutis. 1989;43:346–52.
26. Robert C, Aractingi S, Prost C, et al. Bullous amyloidosis. Report of 3 cases and review of the literature. Medicine (Baltimore). 1993;72:38–44.
27. Grundmann JU, Bonnekoh B, Gollnick H. Extensive haemorrhagic bullous skin manifestation of systemic AA-amyloidosis associated with IgGlambdamyeloma. Eur J Dermatol. 2000;10:139–42.
28. Stoopler ET, Alawi F, Laudenbach JM, et al. Bullous amyloidosis of the oral cavity: a rare clinical presentation and review. Oral Surg Oral Med Oral Pathol Oral Radiol Endod. 2006;101:734–40.
29. Wang XD, Shen H, Liu ZH. Diffuse haemorrhagic bullous amyloidosis with multiple myeloma. Clin Exp Dermatol. 2008;33:94–6.
30. Alhaddab M, Srolovitz H, Rosen N. Primary systemic amyloidosis presenting as extensive cutaneous ulceration. J Cutan Med Surg. 2006;10:253–6.
31. Mancuso G, Fanti PA, Berdondini RM. Nail changes as the only skin abnormality in myeloma-associated systemic amyloidosis. Br J Dermatol. 1997;137:471–2.
32. Fujita Y, Tsuji-Abe Y, Sato-Matsumura KC, et al. Nail dystrophy and blisters as sole manifestations in myeloma-associated amyloidosis. J Am Acad Dermatol. 2006;54:712–4.
33. Magy N, Liepnieks JJ, Gil H, et al. A transthyretin mutation (Tyr78Phe) associated with peripheral neuropathy, carpal tunnel syndrome and skin amyloidosis. Amyloid. 2003;10:29–33.
34. Ohnishi A, Yamamoto T, Murai Y, et al. Denervation of eccrine glands in patients with familial amyloidotic polyneuropathy type I. Neurology. 1998;51:714–21.
35. Mochizuki H, Kamakura K, Masaki T, et al. Nodular cutaneous amyloidosis and carpal tunnel syndrome due to the amyloidogenic transthyretin His 114 variant. Amyloid. 2001;8:105–10.
36. Miyata T, Nakano T, Masuzawa M, et al. Beta2-microglobulin-induced cutaneous amyloidosis in a patient with long-term hemodialysis. J Dermatol. 2005;32:410–2.
37. Sato KC, Kumakiri M, Koizumi H, et al. Lichenoid skin lesions as a sign of beta 2-microglobulin-induced amyloidosis in a long-term haemodialysis patient. Br J Dermatol. 1993;128:686–9.
38. Ucnotsuchi T, Imafuku S, Nagata M, et al. Cutaneous and lingual papules as a sign of beta 2 microglobulin-derived amyloidosis in a longterm hemodialysis patient. Eur J Dermatol. 2003;13:393–5.
39. Albers SE, Fenske NA, Glass LF, et al. Atypical beta 2-microglobulin amyloidosis following short-term hemodialysis. Am J Dermatopathol. 1994;16:179–84.
40. Sethi D, Hutchison AJ, Cary NR, et al. Macroglossia and amyloidoma of the buttock: evidence of systemic involvement in dialysis amyloid. Nephron. 1990;55:312–5.
41. Fernandez-Alonso J, Rios-Camacho C, Valenzuela-Castano A, et al. Pseudotumoral amyloidosis of beta 2-microglobulin origin in the buttock of a patient receiving long term haemodialysis. J Clin Pathol. 1993;46:771–2.
42. Tom Y, Htwe M, Chandra R, et al. Bilateral beta 2-microglobulin amyloidomas of the buttocks in a long-term hemodialysis patient. Arch Pathol Lab Med. 1994;118:651–3.
43. Lipner HI, Minkowitz S, Neiderman G, et al. Dialysis-related amyloidosis manifested as masses in the buttocks. South Med J. 1995;88:876–8.
44. Shimizu S, Yasui C, Yasukawa K, et al. Subcutaneous nodules on the buttocks as a manifestation of dialysis-related amyloidosis: a clinicopathological entity? Br J Dermatol. 2003;149:400–4.
45. Kiuru-Enari S, Keski-Oja J, Haltia M. Cutis laxa in hereditary gelsolin amyloidosis. Br J Dermatol. 2005;152:250–7.
46. Benedikz E, Blondal H, Gudmundsson G. Skin deposits in hereditary cystatin C amyloidosis. Virchows Arch A Pathol Anat Histopathol. 1990;417:325–31.
47. Hamidi Asl L, Liepnieks JJ, Hamidi Asl K, et al. Hereditary amyloid cardiomyopathy caused by a variant apolipoprotein A1. Am J Pathol. 1999;154:221–7.
48. Haas N, Kuster W, Zuberbier T, et al. Muckle-Wells syndrome: clinical and histological skin findings compatible with cold air urticaria in a large kindred. Br J Dermatol. 2004;151:99–104.

49. Claes K, Bammens B, Delforge M, et al. Another devastating complication of the Schnitzler syndrome: AA amyloidosis. Br J Dermatol. 2008;158:182–4.
50. Barzilai A, Langevitz P, Goldberg I, et al. Erysipelas-like erythema of familial Mediterranean fever: clinicopathologic correlation. J Am Acad Dermatol. 2000;42:791–5.
51. Danar DA, Kwan TH, Stern RS, et al. Panniculitis in familial Mediterranean fever. Case report with histopathologic findings. Am J Med. 1987;82:829–32.
52. Alonso R, Cistero-Bahima A, Enrique E, et al. Recurrent urticaria as a rare manifestation of familial Mediterranean fever. J Investig Allergol Clin Immunol. 2002;12:60–1.
53. Krishnamurthy S, Job CK. Secondary amyloidosis in leprosy. Int J Lepr Other Mycobact Dis. 1966;34:155–8.
54. Anders EM, McAdam KP, Anders RF. Cell-mediated immunity in amyloidosis secondary to lepromatous leprosy. Clin Exp Immunol. 1977;27:111–7.
55. Jayalakshmi P, Looi LM, Lim KJ, et al. Autopsy findings in 35 cases of leprosy in Malaysia. Int J Lepr Other Mycobact Dis. 1987;55:510–4.
56. Anand S, Singh R, Aurora AL, et al. Systemic amyloidosis in psoriasis, lepromatous leprosy & cutaneous tuberculosis. Indian J Dermatol. 1976;21:45–51.
57. Sharma SC, Mortimer G, Kennedy S, et al. Secondary amyloidosis affecting the skin in arthropathic psoriasis. Br J Dermatol. 1983;108:205–10.
58. Powell AM, Albert S, Bhogal B, et al. Discoid lupus erythematosus with secondary amyloidosis. Br J Dermatol. 2005;153:746–9.
59. Yi S, Naito M, Takahashi K, et al. Complicating systemic amyloidosis in dystrophic epidermolysis bullosa, recessive type. Pathology. 1988;20:184–7.
60. Arita K, South AP, Hans-Filho G, et al. Oncostatin M receptor-beta mutations underlie familial primary localized cutaneous amyloidosis. Am J Hum Genet. 2008;82:73–80.
61. LaChance A, Phelps A, Finch J, et al. Nodular localized primary cutaneous amyloidosis: a bullous variant. Clin Exp Dermatol. 2014;39:344–7.
62. Tanaka A, Arita K, Lai-Cheong JE, et al. New insight into mechanisms of pruritus from molecular studies on familial primary localized amyloidosis. Br J Dermatol. 2009;161:1217–24.
63. Kumakiri M, Hashimoto K. Histogenesis of primary localized cutaneous amyloidosis: sequential change of epidermal keratinocytes to amyloid via filamentous degeneration. J Invest Dermatol. 1979;73:150–62.
64. Kobayashi H, Hashimoto K. Amyloidogenesis in organ-limited cutaneous amyloidosis: an antigenic identity between epidermal keratin and skin amyloid. J Invest Dermatol. 1983;80:66–72.
65. Schepis C, Siragusa M, Gagliardi M, et al. Primary macular amyloidosis: an ultrastructural approach to diagnosis. Ultrastruct Pathol. 1999;23:279–84.
66. Apaydin R, Gurbuz Y, Bayramgurler D, et al. Cytokeratin expression in lichen amyloidosus and macular amyloidosis. J Eur Acad Dermatol Venereol. 2004;18:305–9.
67. Hashimoto K, Brownstein MH. Localized amyloidosis in basal cell epitheliomas. Acta Derm Venerel. 1973;53:331–9.
68. Weedon D, Shand E. Amyloid in basal cell carcinomas. Br J Dermatol. 1979;101:141–6.
69. Looi LM. Localized amyloidosis in basal cell carcinoma. A pathologic study. Cancer. 1983;52:1833–6.
70. Zhuang L, Zhu W. Inflammatory linear verrucose epidermal nevus coexisting with lichen amyloidosus. J Dermatol. 1996;23:415–8.
71. MacDonald DM, Black MM. Secondary localized cutaneous amyloidosis in melanocytic naevi. Br J Dermatol. 1980;103:553–6.
72. Hashimoto K, King Jr LE. Secondary localized cutaneous amyloidosis associated with actinic keratosis. J Invest Dermatol. 1973;61:293–9.
73. Speight EL, Milne DS, Lawrence CM. Secondary localized cutaneous amyloid in Bowen's disease. Clin Exp Dermatol. 1993;18:286–8.
74. Romero LS, Kantor GR, Levin MW, et al. Localized cutaneous amyloidosis associated with mycosis fungoides. J Am Acad Dermatol. 1997;37:124–7.
75. Azon-Masoliver A. Widespread primary localized cutaneous amyloidosis (macular form) associated with systemic sclerosis. Br J Dermatol. 1995;132:163–5.
76. Yoneyama K, Tochigi N, Oikawa A, et al. Primary localized cutaneous nodular amyloidosis in a patient with Sjögren's syndrome: a review of the literature. J Dermatol. 2005;32:120–3.
77. Ogiyama Y, Hayashi Y, Kou C, et al. Cutaneous amyloidosis in patients with progressive systemic sclerosis. Cutis. 1996;57:28–32.
78. Orihara T, Yanase S, Furuya T. A case of sclerodermatomyositis with cutaneous amyloidosis. Br J Dermatol. 1985;112:213–9.
79. Fujiwara K, Kono T, Ishii M, et al. Primary localized cutaneous amyloidosis associated with autoimmune cholangitis. Int J Dermatol. 2000;39:768–71.
80. Naldi L, Marchesi L, Locati F, et al. Unusual manifestations of primary cutaneous amyloidosis in association with Raynaud's phenomenon and livedo reticularis. Clin Exp Dermatol. 1992;17:117–20.
81. Verga U, Fugazzola L, Cambiaghi S, et al. Frequent association between MEN 2A and cutaneous lichen amyloidosis. Clin Endocrinol (Oxf). 2003;59:156–61.
82. Breathnach SM. Amyloid and the amyloidosis of the skin. In: Burns T, Breathnach S, Cox C, Griffiths C, editors. Rook's textbook of dermatology, vol. 3. Oxford: Blackwell; 2004. p. 57.36–51.
83. Venkataram MN, Bhushnurmath SR, Muirhead DE, et al. Frictional amyloidosis: a study of 10 cases. Australas J Dermatol. 2001;42:176–9.
84. Iwasaki K, Mihara M, Nishiura S, et al. Biphasic amyloidosis arising from friction melanosis. J Dermatol. 1991;18:86–91.
85. Salim T, Shenoi SD, Balachandran C, et al. Lichen amyloidosus: a study of clinical, histopathologic and

immunofluorescence findings in 30 cases. Indian J Dermatol Venereol Leprol. 2005;71:166–9.

86. Ramirez-Santos A, Labandiera J, Monteagudo B, et al. Lichen amyloidosus without itching indicates that it is not secondary to chronic scratching. Acta Derm Venereol (Stockh). 2006;86:561–2.

87. Wood AC, Hsu S. Pruritic papules on the shins. Lichen amyloidosis. Postgrad Med. 2000;107:249–50.

88. Jhingan A, Lee JS, Kumarasinghe SP. Lichen amyloidosis in an unusual location. Singapore Med J. 2007;48:E165–7.

89. Wenson SF, Jessup CJ, Johnson MM, et al. Primary cutaneous amyloidosis of the external ear: a clinicopathological and immunohistochemical study of 17 cases. J Cutan Pathol. 2012;39:263–9.

90. Lee DD, Huang JY, Wong CK, et al. Genetic heterogeneity of familial primary cutaneous amyloidosis: lack of evidence for linkage with the chromosome 10 pericentromeric region in Chinese families. J Invest Dermatol. 1996;107:30–3.

91. Lin MW, Lee DD, Lin CH, et al. Suggestive linkage of familial primary cutaneous amyloidosis to a locus on chromosome 1q23. Br J Dermatol. 2005;152:29–36.

92. Lee DD, Lin MW, Chen IC, et al. Genome-wide scan identifies a susceptibility locus for familial primary cutaneous amyloidosis on chromosome 5p13.1–q11.2. Br J Dermatol. 2006;155:1201–8.

93. Saeedi M, Ebrahim-Habibi A, Haghighi A, et al. A novel missense mutation in oncostatin M receptor beta causing primary localized cutaneous amyloidosis. Biomed Res Int. 2014;2014:653724.

94. Wang WH, Li LF, Huang ES, et al. A new c.1845A→T of oncostatin M receptor-β mutation and slightly enhanced oncostatin M receptor-β expression in a Chinese family with primary localized cutaneous amyloidosis. Eur J Dermatol. 2012;22:29–33.

95. Schreml S, Weber BH, Schroder J, et al. Familial primary localized cutaneous amyloidosis with an oncostatin M receptor-β mutation, Pro694Leu. Clin Exp Dermatol. 2013;38:932–5.

96. Arita K, Abe R, Baba K, et al. A novel OSMR mutation in familial primary localized cutaneous amyloidosis in a Japanese family. J Dermatol Sci. 2009;55:64–5.

97. Heinrich PC, Behrmann I, Haan S, et al. Principles of interleukin (IL)-6-type cytokine signalling and its regulation. Biochem J. 2003;374:1–20.

98. Chattopadhyay S, Tracy E, Liang P, et al. Interleukin-31 and oncostatin-M mediate distinct signaling reactions and response patterns in lung epithelial cells. J Biol Chem. 2007;282:3014–26.

99. Moriwaki S, Nishigori C, Horiguchi Y, et al. Amyloidosis cutis dyschromica: DNA repair reduction in the cellular response to UV light. Arch Dermatol. 1992;128:966–70.

100. Garg T, Chander R, Jabeen M, et al. Amyloidosis cutis dyschromica: a rare pigmentary disorder. J Cutan Pathol. 2011;38:823–6.

101. Chang YT, Liu HN, Wang WJ, et al. A study of cytokeratin profiles in localized cutaneous amyloids. Arch Dermatol Res. 2004;296:83–8.

102. Borowicz J, Gillespie M, Miller R. Cutaneous amyloidosis. Skinmed. 2011;9:96–100.

103. Irvine AD, McLean WHI. Human keratin diseases: the increasing spectrum of disease and subtlety of the phenotype-genotype correlation. Br J Dermatol. 1999;140:815–28.

104. Steinert PM. Structure, function, and dynamics of keratin intermediate filaments. J Invest Dermatol. 1993;100:729–34.

105. Borowicz J, Shama L, Miller R. Nodular cutaneous amyloidosis. Skinmed. 2011;9:316–8.

106. Hagari Y, Mihara M, Hagari S. Nodular localized cutaneous amyloidosis: detection of monoclonality of infiltrating plasma cells by polymerase chain reaction. Br J Dermatol. 1996;135:630–3.

107. Hagari Y, Mihara M, Konohana I, et al. Nodular localized cutaneous amyloidosis: further demonstration of monoclonality of infiltrating plasma cells in four additional Japanese patients. Br J Dermatol. 1998;138:652–4.

108. Moon AO, Calamia KT, Walsh JS. Nodular amyloidosis: review and long-term follow-up of 16 cases. Arch Dermatol. 2003;139:1157–9.

109. Santos-Juanes J, Galache C, Curto JR, et al. Nodular primary cutaneous amyloidosis. J Eur Acad Dermatol Venereol. 2004;18:224–6.

110. Evers M, Baron E, Zaim MT, et al. Papules and plaques on the nose. Nodular localized primary cutaneous amyloidosis. Arch Dermatol. 2007;143:535–40.

111. Summers EM, Kendrick CG. Primary localized cutaneous nodular amyloidosis and CREST syndrome: a case report and review of the literature. Cutis. 2008;82:55–9.

112. Brownstein MH, Helwig EB. The cutaneous amyloidoses. I. localized forms. Arch Dermatol. 1970;102:8–19.

113. Woollons A, Black MM. Nodular localized primary cutaneous amyloidosis: a long-term follow-up study. Br J Dermatol. 2001;145:105–9.

Iatrogenic Pharmaceutical Amyloidosis Associated with Insulin and Enfuvirtide Administration

35

Ahmet Dogan and Oana Madalina Mereuta

Iatrogenic systemic amyloidosis has been documented among patients on long-term dialysis and the recipients of "domino" (sequential) liver transplants, who developed amyloid derived from β2microglobulin and acquired familial amyloid polyneuropathy, respectively; also, iatrogenic cerebral amyloidosis (iatrogenic Creutzfeldt–Jakob disease) has been reported in patients exposed to the infectious prions via corneal transplantation, stereotactic EEG, neurosurgery, dura-mater graft, growth hormone, gonadotropin, and blood transfusions. In recent years, another form of iatrogenic amyloidosis has emerged, which is related to the subcutaneous injection of medications ("pharmaceutical"), and thus represents a form of localized amyloidosis directly derived from the administered drug. Peptides and poly-peptides have been used as drugs since the beginning of the twentieth century. Early examples include peptide morphine, cyclic peptide penicil-lin, and the polypeptide insulin; current examples include recombinant peptides specifically designed to block or activate receptors and peptides with antimicrobial or antiviral functions such as enfuvirtide [1, 2]. Some of these drugs are delivered by subcutaneous injection and may require lifelong use in order to control chronic diseases such as diabetes. The intrinsic chemical properties of the drugs vary widely depending on the pharmaceutical target, but at least a subset, such as the insulin polypeptide, are known to have a tendency to form beta-pleated sheets and amyloid-like structures in in vitro systems, under special conditions, especially when present in excess quantities. It is now recognized that at least two peptide drugs, insulin [3] and enfu-virtide (Fuzeon©) [4, 5], can cause localized amyloidosis in vivo at the subcutaneous injection site after prolonged pharmacological use.

A. Dogan, MD, PhD (✉)
Departments of Pathology and Laboratory Medicine, Memorial Sloan Kettering Cancer Center, 1275 York Avenue, New York, NY 10065, USA
e-mail: dogana@mskcc.org

O.M. Mereuta, MD, PhD
Department of Pathology, Memorial Sloan Kettering Cancer Center, 1275 York Avenue, New York, NY 10065, USA
e-mail: mereutao@mskcc.org

Iatrogenic Insulin-Associated Amyloidosis (AIns)

AIns was first described in an animal model and a human subject in 1983 [3]. Since the recognition of the amyloidogenic potential of insulin, the polypeptide has been extensively used in the laboratory as a model for amyloid fibril formation [6]. Insulin can self-assemble to form a crystalline nidus, which then, after a lag time, can assemble into fibrils, central to the amyloidogenic process. These processes are accelerated by an acidic environment and higher concentrations of insulin [7]. The native proinsulin protein, when translated in human pancreas islet beta cells, is a polypeptide composed of a signal peptide and so-called A, B, and C peptides. The signal peptide directs the proinsulin polypeptide to the endoplasmic reticulum, where the functional folding of the polypeptide chain occurs and the signal peptide is cleaved. The proinsulin is then converted into mature insulin protein by cleavage of the C peptide and the resulting molecule is composed of A and B peptides, linked together by disulfide bonds. It is the mature insulin protein that has amyloidogenic potential but not the proinsulin molecule, which includes the C peptide. Pharmacological recombinant preparations of insulin mimic the structure of the mature insulin polypeptide, sometimes with additional minor modifications.

Only a handful of incidents of AIns amyloidosis have been described in the literature [8–11]. However, the condition is likely to be far more prevalent, given the number of insulin users in the general population. AIns amyloidosis appears to occur at injection sites after repeated subcutaneous injections in one area. The most common clinical presentation is the presence of an abdominal subcutaneous mass or masses, either identified by the patient or during physical examination for other reasons [12]. Rarely, the patients may inject at other soft tissue sites, and cases presenting as masses on the leg or arms have been described. Some patients may present with development of insulin resistance due to reduced systemic absorption through the amyloid plaques. If the tissue integrity is disturbed, areas of hemorrhage can be seen.

The diagnosis requires biopsy of the lesion and histological examination. Histologically, there is often marked subcutaneous amyloid deposition replacing normal structures (Fig. 35.1). As expected, the deposits are strongly Congophilic and show all of the appropriate optical qualities of amyloid. If the clinical context is known, the diagnosis is straightforward. However, in many instances, clinical information may not be available to the surgeon or pathologist. This may lead to a mistaken diagnosis of systemic amyloidosis, in particular AL amyloidosis. For this reason, typing of amyloid either by immunohistochemistry for insulin (Fig. 35.1) or by mass spectrometry is required [12].

Clinically, AIns is invariably a localized process, without risk of systemic dissemination. Management includes a change of injection sites and, if necessary, the excision of mass lesions. It is important to keep in mind that, in some cases, the change of injection site may cause hypoglycemia as the insulin dose may have been increased to accommodate for resistance caused by injection into the amyloid deposit.

Iatrogenic Enfuvirtide-Associated Amyloidosis (AEnf)

The viral spike of HIV-1 is composed of three gp120 envelope glycoproteins attached noncovalently to three gp41 transmembrane molecules. Virus entry is initiated by binding of this complex to the CD4 receptor on the cell surface of T-cells and dendritic cells. Enfuvirtide is a synthetic peptide which binds gp41 and blocks the fusion of the virus to the host cell through the CD4 receptor. Enfuvirtide was approved by the FDA in March 2003 for use in adults, and in children aged 6 and older with advanced HIV infection, and is marketed under the brand name Fuzeon©. The drug is administered by subcutaneous injections, and has been associated with a variety of skin reactions occurring in more than 80 % of patients [13, 14]. In rare cases, it has also been associated with subcutaneous localized amyloidosis [4, 5, 12]. Recently, mass spectrometry-based proteomics studies showed that these amyloid deposits were composed of the synthetic peptide of enfuvirtide [12], and enfuvirtide-induced amyloidosis (AEnf) was

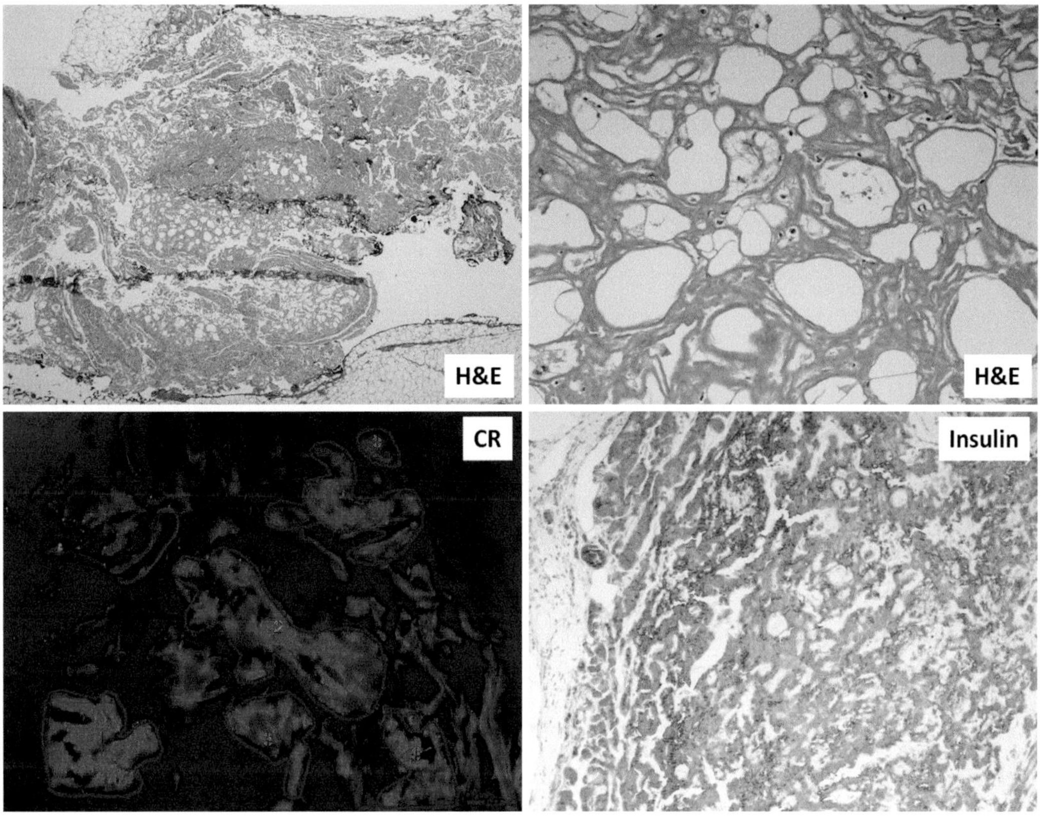

Fig. 35.1 AIns amyloidosis secondary to subcutaneous insulin injection to control diabetes. The incisional subcutaneous biopsy shows extensive deposition of eosinophilic extracellular material in the subcutaneous adipose tissue (low and high power H&E). The deposits are Congophilic and show appropriate optical qualities under fluorescent light (*Congo red*; CR). The deposits are positive for insulin by immunohistochemistry (insulin, immunoperoxidase)

recognized as a novel type of iatrogenic amyloidosis by the Nomenclature Committee of the International Society of Amyloidosis [15].

AEnf amyloidosis presents as hemorrhagic nodules at the site of injections, which may persist after discontinuation of the drug. A biopsy with histological examination is required for diagnosis. The histology shows marked subcutaneous amyloid deposition replacing normal structures. As expected, the deposits are strongly Congophilic and show the appropriate optical qualities of amyloid (Fig. 35.2). If the clinical context is known, the diagnosis is straightforward. If typing is required, mass spectrometry-based proteomics is the only method available, as the peptide is synthetic and no antibody-based immunohistochemical assays are available [12] (Fig. 35.2).

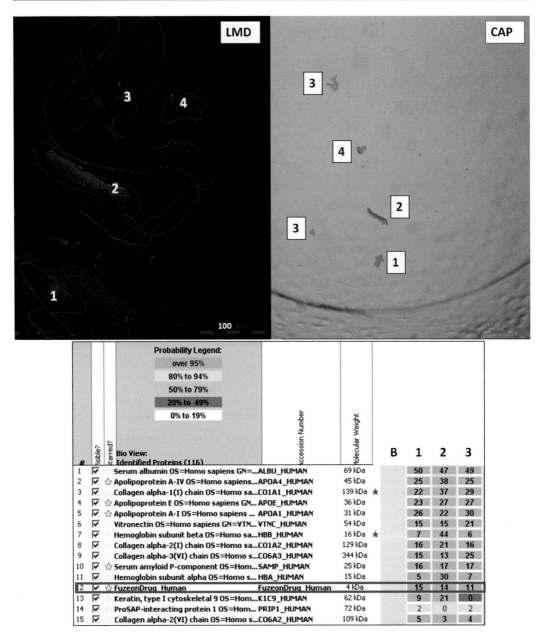

Fig. 35.2 AEnf amyloidosis secondary to subcutaneous enfuvirtide injections to manage advanced HIV infection. The incisional subcutaneous biopsy shows extensive deposition of extracellular material in the subcutaneous adipose tissue. The deposits are Congophilic and show appropriate optical qualities under fluorescent light. They were laser microdissected for mass spectrometry analysis (LMD). These are seen in the cap (CAP). Mass spectrometry-based proteomic analysis was performed in three replicates (1–3), with a blank control (B). Enfuvirtide (referred as Fuzeon© in the figure) was identified as the cause of amyloidosis (*red box*)

References

1. Lazzarin A, Clotet B, Cooper D, Reynes J, Arasteh K, Nelson M, et al. Efficacy of enfuvirtide in patients infected with drug-resistant HIV-1 in Europe and Australia. N Engl J Med. 2003;348:2186–95.
2. Lalezari JP, Henry K, O'Hearn M, Montaner JS, Piliero PJ, Trottier B, et al. Enfuvirtide, an HIV-1 fusion inhibitor, for drug-resistant HIV infection in North and South America. N Engl J Med. 2003;348: 2175–85.
3. Storkel S, Schneider HM, Muntefering H, Kashiwagi S. Iatrogenic, insulin-dependent, local amyloidosis. Lab Invest. 1983;48:108–11.
4. Morilla ME, Kocher J, Harmaty M. Localized amyloidosis at the site of enfuvirtide injection. Ann Intern Med. 2009;151:515–6.
5. Naujokas A, Vidal CI, Mercer SE, Harp J, Kurtin PJ, Fox LP, et al. A novel form of amyloid deposited at the site of enfuvirtide injection. J Cutan Pathol. 2012;39:220–1. Quiz 19.
6. Amdursky N, Gazit E, Rosenman G. Formation of low-dimensional crystalline nucleus region during insulin amyloidogenesis process. Biochem Biophys Res Commun. 2012;419:232–7.
7. Landreh M, Stukenborg JB, Willander H, Soder O, Johansson J, Jornvall H. Proinsulin C-peptide interferes with insulin fibril formation. Biochem Biophys Res Commun. 2012;418:489–93.
8. Westermark P, Eizirik DL, Pipeleers DG, Hellerstrom C, Andersson A. Rapid deposition of amyloid in human islets transplanted into nude mice. Diabetologia. 1995;38:543–9.
9. Swift B, Hawkins PN, Richards C, Gregory R. Examination of insulin injection sites: an unexpected finding of localized amyloidosis. Diabet Med. 2002;19:881–2.
10. Nagase T, Katsura Y, Iwaki Y, Nemoto K, Sekine H, Miwa K, et al. The insulin ball. Lancet. 2009;373:184.
11. D'Souza A, Theis JD, Vrana JA, Buadi F, Dispenzieri A, Dogan A. Localized insulin-derived amyloidosis: a potential pitfall in the diagnosis of systemic amyloidosis by fat aspirate. Am J Hematol. 2012;87:E131–2.
12. D'Souza A, Theis JD, Vrana JA, Dogan A. Pharmaceutical amyloidosis associated with subcutaneous insulin and enfuvirtide administration. Amyloid. 2014;21:71–5.
13. Maggi P, Ladisa N, Cinori E, Altobella A, Pastore G, Filotico R. Cutaneous injection site reactions to long-term therapy with enfuvirtide. J Antimicrob Chemother. 2004;53:678–81.
14. Mirza RA, Turiansky GW. Enfuvirtide and cutaneous injection-site reactions. J Drugs Dermatol. 2012;11: e35–8.
15. Sipe JD, Benson MD, Buxbaum JN, Ikeda S, Merlini G, Saraiva MJ, et al. Nomenclature 2014: amyloid fibril proteins and clinical classification of the amyloidosis. Amyloid. 2014;21:221–4.

Part VI

Clinical Issues and Therapy

Clinical and Pathologic Issues in Patients with Amyloidosis: Summary and Practical Comments Regarding Diagnosis, Therapy, and Solid Organ Transplantation

36

Maria M. Picken and Kevin Barton

Introduction

The care of patients with amyloidosis requires accurate diagnosis, including amyloid typing, staging of disease, therapy, and subsequent reevaluations of response to therapy, relapses, recurrence, and/or development of secondary complications. Diagnosis of amyloidosis and its staging involve critical interactions between clinicians and pathologists. This chapter provides a brief summary of clinical issues in patients with amyloidosis and practical advice to pathologists involved in their care.

Suspicion of Amyloidosis

Diagnosis of amyloidosis should ideally occur at a relatively early stage in the disease process, prior to significant organ dysfunction [1–4].

M.M. Picken, MD, PhD (✉)
Department of Pathology, Loyola University Medical Center, Loyola University Chicago, Building 110, Room 2242, 2160 South First Avenue, Maywood, IL 60153, USA
e-mail: mpicken@luc.edu; MMPicken@aol.com

K. Barton, MD
Division of Hematology/Oncology, Department of Medicine, Loyola University Medical Center, 2160 S. First Avenue, Maywood, IL 60153, USA
e-mail: kbarton@lumc.edu

This, of course, requires consideration of the diagnosis by both clinicians and pathologists. Because of the vague constellation of symptoms, which also mimic more common diseases, clinicians are often delayed in considering a diagnosis of amyloidosis. Weakness, abdominal pain, arthritis, carpal tunnel syndrome, neuropathies, proteinuria, and heart failure rarely have clinicians considering amyloidosis initially. The classic findings of macroglossia or periorbital purpurs are found only in a small minority of patients (14 % and 11 %, respectively, please see Chap. 2, Fig. 2.3). Amyloidosis-associated factor X deficiency and associated bleeding is also an unusual finding. Thus, help from pathologists, with a raised index of suspicion, will often direct the clinician toward a diagnosis that had not previously been considered. Prior biopsies that are reexamined for amyloid deposits are often found to be positive. This indicates not only a delay in diagnosis and early treatment but also potentially increased morbidity to the patient, who continues to undergo unnecessary procedures for his or her symptoms, and a delay in treatment. Amyloidosis should be suspected in any patient with unexplained nephrotic range proteinuria, cardiomyopathy, peripheral neuropathy, hepatomegaly, or symptoms of bowel pseudo-obstruction [1–4]. Amyloidosis should be suspected not only in patients with underlying plasma cell disorders such as MGUS, asymptomatic myeloma, and symptomatic

© Springer International Publishing Switzerland 2015
M.M. Picken et al. (eds.), *Amyloid and Related Disorders*, Current Clinical Pathology,
DOI 10.1007/978-3-319-19294-9_36

multiple myeloma but also in patients with chronic lymphocytic leukemia, Waldenström's macroglobulinemia, extranodal marginal zone lymphoma of mucosa-associated lymphoid tissue (MALT) lymphomas, or any mature B-cell lymphoproliferative disorder where a paraprotein may be produced [1–6]. Laboratory evaluation with serum free light chain assay together with immunofixation of the serum and urine now has a sensitivity of near 100 % for detection of an abnormal light chain in patients with AL-type amyloidosis [7] (please see also Chap. 25). Patients with a detectable paraprotein or abnormal light chain levels will require biopsies for diagnosis of amyloidosis [1–4, 7].

Biopsy Types

The biopsy may be an involved organ or an alternative site [1–4]. Kidney, heart, and/or peripheral nerves are the most commonly involved sites in systemic amyloidoses and pathologists should routinely consider amyloidosis in the differential diagnosis of these biopsies. Hence, it is practical, and strongly recommended, to routinely perform appropriate stains, in particular Congo red stain, on these biopsies. The goal should be an early detection of amyloid, *before* it can be suspected on H&E stain. Other organs may include minor salivary gland biopsy, rectal biopsy, or gastrointestinal biopsies with morphology of collagenous colitis, ischemic changes, and/or ulcers mimicking amyloid deposits. Specimens with features of MALT lymphoma should be also investigated for amyloidosis [5, 6]. Vascular involvement by amyloid can be associated with wall thickening, mimicking hypertensive changes, and even vasculitis (please see also Chap. 9). Among soft tissue sites, skin, muscle (with pseudo-hypertrophy and a shoulder pad sign), peri-articular tissues, and temporal artery may be biopsied. Other sites may include submandibular gland (clinically with swelling) and lymph nodes (with lymphadenopathy); tongue biopsy is only rarely performed. Clinically symptomatic vascular amyloid may be associated with claudication of the limbs and jaw. Thus, pathologic evaluation of these sites should

include stain(s) for amyloid deposits. Importantly, however, localized amyloid deposits, in particular, may mimic malignancy and may come to the pathologist's attention at the time of frozen section examination. Given the differences in management (please see also below), it is critical to consider amyloid and to avoid potentially more extensive surgery.

Alternatively, biopsy of a surrogate site may be considered, such as abdominal fat, minor salivary gland, rectum, or bone marrow (please see Chap. 16; [1]); deep skin punch biopsies, including underlying fat, have also been used. Patients with a high suspicion for systemic amyloidosis should undergo both abdominal fat and bone marrow biopsies, which may need to be periodically repeated. Positive results from these surrogate sites may spare the patient more invasive internal organ biopsies (please see Chaps. 16 and 17). Such biopsies should also be performed if a diagnosis of amyloidosis was suspected but inconclusive in prior specimens due to sample size limitation and/or sample representativity error (please see also Chap. 14). The advantages of using an actual small surgical fat biopsy over fine-needle aspiration biopsy (FNAB) are discussed in Chaps. 16 and 17. Moreover, repeated fat biopsies may be easily performed (please see Chap. 16; [1–4]).

Diagnosis

Generic diagnosis of amyloidosis requires the demonstration in tissue section of deposits that are Congo red positive and birefringent under polarized light [1]. Recently published updated recommendations on amyloid diagnosis and nomenclature, agreed upon at the XIVth Symposium of the International Society of Amyloidosis, include an acknowledgment that, besides apple-green birefringence, other anomalous colors, such as yellow or orange, are also diagnostic of amyloid [8]. This expanded definition of the diagnostic results of Congo red stain birefringence acknowledges that, while pure green can be seen under *ideal optical conditions*, more often than not orange and yellow are also present, caused by strain birefringence, or by uncrossing of the polarizer and analyzer (please see Chap. 17, Figs. 17.1 and 17.2). Other modifications of Congo red and alternative stains, useful for screening purposes, are discussed in Chaps. 13–15 and 17. Congo red stains may show false-positive or false-negative results based on technical issues [1]. It is thus important that the biopsies are processed appropriately and interpreted by experienced pathologists. Pathologic diagnosis of amyloid also involves determination of the amyloid fibril protein type. Historically, patients with a paraprotein and amyloidosis were inferred to have AL-type amyloidosis. While this is often true, confirmation of the specific amyloid protein type in tissue deposits is mandatory before a specific therapy can be considered. This has traditionally been achieved by immunohistochemical studies (performed on paraffin or frozen sections) and, most recently, by mass spectrometry (discussed in Chaps. 18–24; [1, 9, 10]). Correct determination is critical in view of the markedly different treatment options available for these patients and is particularly important in selected patients with hereditary amyloidoses and coincidental monoclonal gammopathy [11, 12]. One should be mindful that the pathology reporting of both the amyloid type is legally binding. Hence, if your investigations are not diagnostic of the amyloid type, you must clearly state so (please see also Chap. 39).

Since amyloidoses are handled rather infrequently by most general surgical pathology laboratories, it is preferable to refer the evaluation of such specimens to specialized laboratories, both for the confirmation of a generic diagnosis and for amyloid-type determination [1]. Thus, the most important, and in fact critical, contribution of general surgical pathologists is sensitive screening for amyloid deposits in general.

Please note that repeated biopsies may be needed in order to establish an initial diagnosis of amyloidosis in patients with known risk factors such as an underlying plasma cell disorder, chronic inflammatory states, or a known potentially amyloidogenic mutation. Moreover, the evaluation of response to treatment or detection of disease recurrence may also be aided by biopsies [13–15]. The definition of organ involvement and response to treatment in AL, which has been established thus far, and which is routinely used by clinicians, also involves pathologic parameters [13, 14]. Therefore, the pathology report should contain the required information. Hence, it is important to specify whether amyloid deposits are limited to the vasculature or are interstitial. To this end, for example, vascular deposits limited to hepatic venules or portal triad vessels are insufficient for the definition of hepatic involvement. Similarly, deposits limited to vessels in the gastrointestinal tract, which are seen in 80 % of patients with AL and are asymptomatic, are not considered evidence of intestinal organ involvement *for the purposes of staging* [13]. In contrast, the presence of interstitial deposits in the liver and the lamina propria of the gastrointestinal tract is usually symptomatic and meets these criteria. In the lungs, nodular and tracheobronchial amyloidosis is often localized, but diffuse interstitial amyloidosis is associated with pulmonary involvement in systemic amyloidosis. Pleural effusions may be caused by direct pleural infiltration with amyloid. In peripheral nerves, amyloidosis affects small unmyelinated fibers. Carpal tunnel syndrome, due to amyloid deposition, does not constitute peripheral neuropathy [13]. With regard to cardiac specimens, it is critical to specify the biopsy site, i.e., ventricular versus atrial. The latter may be involved by localized amyloid deposits and is frequently associated with atrial fibrillation. The definition of organ involvement and response to treatment in non-AL amyloidosis has also been proposed [15]. Unique challenges associated with the follow-up of patients post-liver (including domino liver and other solid organ) transplantation are briefly discussed later in this chapter.

Staging

Localized Amyloidosis

Amyloidosis presenting in the urinary bladder or in the tracheobronchial tree may often be localized [1]. Some other anatomic areas such as the skin, gastrointestinal tract, tonsil, lymph node, and breast may also have localized amyloidosis (please see also Chaps. 7, 28, and 32–34; [1, 5, 6]). These patients often present a challenge and require careful evaluation to exclude systemic disease. Thus, patients with possible localized disease should undergo abdominal fat and bone marrow examinations. Clinical evaluation for possible cardiac involvement, with laboratory studies that include B-type natriuretic peptides (BNP) and troponin, along with echocardiogram and cardiac MRI, may be useful [2–4, 16]. The patient should undergo clinical evaluation for renal involvement, with a 24-h urine collection to assess for proteinuria and paraproteins. If the localized amyloid is of the AL type, without evidence of systemic disease, a search to rule out a plasma cell/B-cell lymphoproliferative process, in particular extranodal marginal zone lymphoma of mucosa-associated lymphoid tissue (MALT) lymphoma as the cause of the local light chain production, should be undertaken [5, 6]. Patients who prove to have localized disease may require local therapy, such as laser, radiation therapy, or surgery, to remove an obstructive tracheobronchial, gastrointestinal, or genitourinary mass (see Chap. 28; [5, 6]). Targeted therapies (Rituximab, Bendamustine + Retuximab) are being tested for the treatment of multifocal disease associated with MALT lymphoma [5, 6]. If paraprotein is present, patients are considered for a lymphoma therapy. These patients should be followed since recurrences with obstruction and/or mass symptoms can occur. Such lesions may also be, at times, bilateral and even multifocal within the tracheobronchial tree or extrarenal genitourinary system. While it is perceived that, once correctly diagnosed, localized amyloid rarely progresses to systemic disease, this possibility, nevertheless, should be kept in mind (please see also Chaps. 7, 28, and 33).

Systemic Amyloidosis

The manifestations of systemic amyloidosis are indeed protean. Many organs may be involved. The heart, however, is clearly the critical target organ with regard to prognosis and with regard to determining which therapies are possible (please see also Chap. 2, Fig. 2.3) [2–4, 16]. The critical distinction is between AL versus other types of systemic amyloidoses. Figure 36.1 presents an algorithm for the evaluation of suspected amyloidosis [2].

Cardiac Staging

Staging for cardiac burden is a critical part of the initial evaluation since the prognosis in AL amyloidosis is a function of the extent of cardiac involvement [2–4, 13, 14, 16]. In the case of hereditary amyloidoses, significant cardiac involvement may require combined liver and cardiac transplantation (please see below) [15]. Serum troponins (I or T) and B-type natriuretic peptides (either BNP or NT-proBNP) are highly sensitive markers for cardiac involvement and normal values exclude clinically significant cardiac amyloid [2–4, 13, 14, 16]. Electrocardiography and echocardiography should be performed to evaluate for arrhythmias and restrictive cardiomyopathy. Consideration should be given to cardiology consultation in cases where any abnormalities are found. Cardiac MRI is also an emerging modality for the evaluation of amyloid infiltration. Cardiac biomarkers are prognostic for survival in AL patients and can also be used to monitor the effect of treatment. Post-therapy, patients with a greater than 30 % reduction and a greater than 300 ng/L decrease in the NT-proBNP level, from baseline, are correlated with improved survival; increases of the same amount are associated with a reduced survival rate [2–4, 13, 14, 16].

Bone Marrow Evaluation

Systemic AL amyloidosis is caused by free light chains produced by clonal plasma cells, or rarely (2 % of the time), by mature B-cell lymphomas (please see Chap. 26; [2–4, 17]). In contrast to multiple myeloma, AL amyloid patients may have significant end organ damage with <10 % plasma cells found on bone marrow examination (please see Chap. 2) [17]. The cytogenetics and FISH studies that have prognostic value in myeloma are not yet well validated for amyloid. Please see also Chaps. 26 and 27.

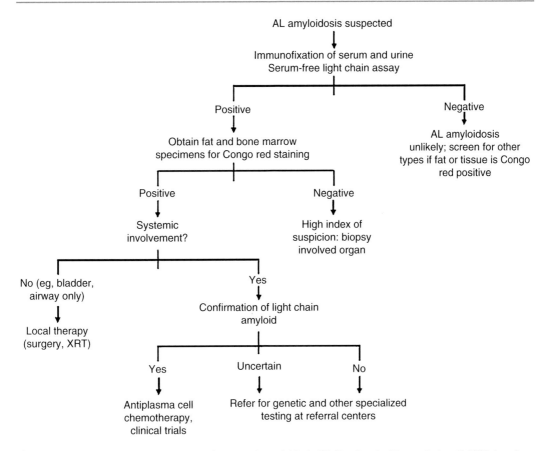

Fig. 36.1 An algorithm for the evaluation of suspected amyloidosis [2]. Reprinted with permission. © 2008 American Society of Clinical Oncology. All rights reserved. Merlini G et al. J Clin Oncol. 2011;29:1924–33 [2]

Therapy

Appropriate treatment for amyloidosis differs based on the amyloid protein type and the staging, highlighting the importance of an accurate diagnosis at presentation [1–4]. Localized disease is generally managed with local treatments or, in select cases, by observation with planned reevaluations. Although localized amyloidosis, if diagnosed correctly, is felt to progress rarely to a systemic process, these patients require periodic reevaluation to exclude recurrences or progression, which may take years to develop (please see Chap. 25). Recurrences may also occur. Various risk-adapted therapies, including personalized targeted therapies, are currently being used for the treatment of multifocal disease associated

with MALT lymphoma [5, 6]. Other amyloidoses, including AA, hereditary, and senile forms, are not responsive to cytotoxic therapies and their management involves evaluation for organ transplantation and/or pharmacologic therapies (see below and Chaps. 37 and 38). The most critical step in the management of patients with a newly diagnosed amyloidosis is distinction between systemic AL versus other amyloidoses [1–4, 10].

Systemic AL Amyloidosis

The goal of therapy in patients with AL amyloidosis is to reduce the production of abnormal free light chains to as low a level as possible, for as long as possible, and as soon as possible [2–5].

Patients with amyloidosis associated with CLL or non-Hodgkin's lymphoma should have their therapy directed against the specific associated disease. It is important to recognize that eliminating the source of the damaging light chains can reverse AL-related organ damage and improve the functional status of these patients [2–5, 7, 16, 17]. Despite improvements in diagnosis and staging, the effective treatment of AL amyloidosis remains a challenge. The median survival from diagnosis is mainly driven by the degree of cardiac involvement [2–4, 16, 17]. Thus, in patients with scores ranging from 0 to 3 median survival ranges from 94.1 to 5.8 months, respectively [3]. Delayed/late diagnosis continues to play a major role in early mortality while undergoing treatment [2–4, 16]. Failure to achieve a 50 % reduction in involved free light chain has been associated with a significantly reduced survival [2–4, 16]. Increasing evidence supports the notion that it is the pre-fibrillar monomers, rather than the actual amyloid fibrils, that are the toxic entity [17]. Hence, a rapid reduction in the level of circulating light chains is an important issue.

A broad range of therapies are available for patients who have plasma cell disorders underlying their amyloidosis. We will briefly summarize some of the most common current and emerging therapies. There is abundant literature pertaining to this subject and a more detailed review is beyond the scope of this chapter. The choice of therapy for an individual patient is dependent on their comorbidities, their overall condition, and, particularly, the cardiac staging, referred to as "risk-adapted" therapies. The most significant independent prognostic determinants are cardiac involvement and response to therapy [2–4, 16, 17].

High-Dose Chemotherapy and Autologous Bone Marrow Transplantation

Autologous bone marrow transplantation allows for the use of otherwise potentially lethal doses of chemotherapy, since it replenishes the ablated bone marrow with the patient's own collected stem cells. The response of amyloidogenic light chains to chemotherapy is dose dependent, and

this method may be the most effective long-term therapy in AL amyloidosis, provided the patient can tolerate the procedure. At one center, 25 % of patients receiving autologous stem cell transplantation (ASCT) were reported to be 10-year survivors and, of those who achieved a complete remission, the 10-year survival rate was 53 % [3, 4, 18]. At diagnosis of systemic AL amyloidosis, clinicians should determine if the patient is an appropriate candidate for autologous transplantation.

Historically, AL amyloid patients have experienced a much higher mortality rate when undergoing autologous stem cell transplantation than that found for other diseases, most probably due to underlying organ dysfunction. Historically, treatment-related mortality rates with autologous stem cell transplantation in AL amyloidosis have been reported to be in excess of 20 % [2–4, 18]. Due to the increased treatment-related mortality risk associated with high-dose therapy and autologous stem cell transplantation in AL amyloid patients, proper patient selection is essential in order to optimize clinical outcomes. Poor performance status, advanced heart failure, elevated cardiac troponins, significant renal dysfunction, and extensive multi-organ involvement represent contraindications to transplantation [3, 4]. With appropriate patient selection and improved supportive care, the treatment-related mortality has decreased to the range of 3–7 % at many experienced centers [3, 4, 18]. Nonetheless, only approximately 20 % of patients are good candidates for high-dose therapy and better options are still needed for those not suitable for this treatment.

Melphalan-Based Therapies

One of the early, landmark, prospective studies in the treatment of AL amyloidosis compared the standard colchicine regimen (which has a known benefit in the treatment of secondary amyloidosis in familial Mediterranean fever) to melphalan (an oral alkylating agent with a known effect against plasma cell neoplasms) with prednisone versus a third group that received all three agents [19]. The results showed a significant overall survival benefit to those receiving melphalan and prednisone (18 months vs. 8.5 months for the colchicine alone group) [19]. This study thus initiated the use of a myeloma-type regimen for the effective treatment of AL amyloidosis. Oral melphalan and dexamethasone have traditionally been one of the standard frontline treatments for systemic AL amyloidosis [18, 19]. The use of high-dose dexamethasone with melphalan led to an improvement in the median time to response (4.5 months) as compared to prednisone with melphalan [18].

High-dose melphalan (HDM) and autologous peripheral blood stem cell transplantation (SCT) can lead to durable remissions and long-term survival in AL amyloidosis [18]. Survival strongly depends on the achievement of a complete hematologic response, and patients treated at earlier stages, with less organ involvement and an absence of cardiac involvement, have a better outcome. While melphalan-based therapies represent an advance in the treatment of AL amyloidosis, it is the emergence of novel agents that has revolutionized the treatment of these diseases.

The Immunomodulatory Derivatives

The Immunomodulatory drugs (IMiDs), thalidomide and its derivatives (lenalidomide and pomalidomide), are oral drugs that have been found to be potent agents in the treatment of multiple myeloma, as well as AL amyloidosis. The exact mechanisms of action are unclear, but it does appear that the use of IMiDs decreases binding of multiple myeloma cells to bone marrow stromal cells, inhibits the production in the bone marrow milieu of cytokines (IL-6, vascular endothelial growth factor [VEGF], TNF-α) that mediate the growth and survival of the myeloma cells, blocks angiogenesis, and stimulates host anti-tumor natural killer cell immunity [2–4, 18, 20]. Recently, Lu et al. [21] and Krönke et al. [22], respectively, reported that thalidomide and derivative compounds have a toxic effect on multiple myeloma by causing the degradation of two transcription factors, Ikaros and Aiolos, which are targets for proteasome inhibitors. This loss halts myeloma growth while simultaneously altering immune cell function.

Major side effects of this class of drugs include significant risk of thromboembolism, which can be reduced by the use of anti-platelet agents and/or anticoagulation.

Thalidomide is an oral agent that was first developed as a drug in the 1950s for its sedating and anti-nausea properties, but which quickly earned a notorious reputation due to its teratogenic effects. A resurgence of interest occurred in the 1990s when its anti-angiogenic properties were demonstrated and it was tested for use in the treatment of multiple myeloma [23–25]. Although thalidomide introduced the class of immunomodulatory agents, it is poorly tolerated in AL amyloidosis due to fatigue, edema, thromboembolism, bradycardia, and neurotoxicity. Newer IMiDs have essentially supplanted it for use in patients with systemic amyloidosis.

Thus, Lenalidomide appears to be largely replacing thalidomide in the treatment of AL amyloidosis. It is administered with or without dexamethasone. Toxicities include fatigue and myelosuppression, which are dose limiting. This drug also carries an increased risk of thromboembolism and, therefore, appropriate anticoagulation measures should be taken in all patients [2–4]. A notable confounding aspect of IMiD therapy is a rise in cardiac biomarkers, which does not appear to correlate with worsening cardiac status or hematologic progression. The third-generation immunomodulatory drug, Pomalidomide, is an oral agent, with structural similarities to both lenalidomide and thalidomide, that was formulated to maintain efficacy but avoid the neurotoxicity of thalidomide and the myelosuppression associated with lenalidomide [26]. Pomalidomide is promising in combination with Dexamethasone (Pom/dex) [26]. Further investigation of its frontline use is being explored.

Proteasome Inhibitors

The proteasome is found in both the nucleus and the cytoplasm of cells and acts to degrade unneeded or damaged proteins by proteolysis. Inhibiting the function of the proteasome in sensitive cells may lead to an overwhelming load for

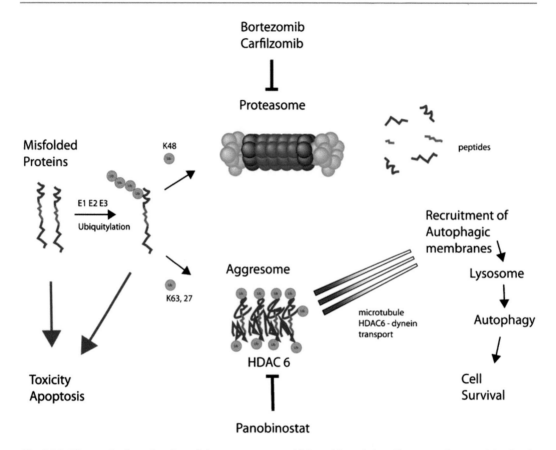

Fig. 36.2 The mechanism of action of the proteasome inhibitors bortezomib (PS-341) and carfilzomib (PR-171) along with the pan-HDAC inhibitor panobinostat (LBH589) [25, 27, 28]. The combined inhibition of both the proteasome and aggresome pathways may result in the accumulation of unfolded and misfolded amyloid protein, which could result in cell stress and cytotoxicity for the plasma cells producing the abnormal light chains. Abbreviations: *E1* ubiquitin-activating enzyme, *E2* ubiquitin-conjugating enzyme, *E3* ubiquitin ligases, *Ub* poly-ubiquitin chain, K27, 48, 63 lysine residues, *HDAC6* histone deacetylase-6

the endoplasmic reticulum and ultimate apoptosis by disrupting the regulated degradation of pro-growth cell cycle proteins (Fig. 36.2; [27–32]). Clonal plasma cell disorders, including those associated with AL amyloidosis, appear to be exquisitely sensitive to proteasome inhibition, making it an attractive target for treatment. Bortezomib is the first-in-class proteasome inhibitor and appears to be one of the most active agents in the treatment of AL amyloidosis [29–32]. Cyclophosphamide, bortezomib, and dexamethasone (CyBorD) treatment continues to be a commonly used active therapy for AL amyloidosis; subcutaneous delivery of bortezomib has improved the prior dose-limiting neurotoxicity

[29–32]. Bortezomib has minimal myelosuppression (when compared to other agents), making it an attractive option for patients in whom ASCT is a consideration. Due to an increased risk of viral infections, including shingles and disseminated herpes, prophylactic antivirals are indicated with the use of bortezomib.

Carfilzomib is an irreversible proteasome inhibitor that was developed to address the limiting neurotoxicity of bortezomib. Carfilzomib is approved for multiple myeloma and is being studied in AL amyloidosis. Ixazomib is expected to be the first oral proteasome inhibitor and will probably be available in the near future [33, 34].

Aggresome Inhibition

It is speculated that the aggresome can act as a secondary mechanism to the proteasome in the disposal of cellular contents and, therefore, is an attractive alternative target of inhibition (Fig. 36.2). There is some optimism that dual inhibition of both the proteasome and the aggresome may offer synergistic effects, or may be useful in those who become refractory to proteasome inhibition alone. The drug panobinostat[1] is a histone deacetylase (HDAC) inhibitor that also functions to inhibit the aggresome. This drug is being studied as a single agent and in combination with proteasome inhibitors.

Monoclonal Antibodies

Several monoclonal antibodies show promising activity in multiple myeloma and amyloidosis. However, none have been, as of this writing (February 2015), approved by the FDA for use in human subjects [35–37]. These include Daratumumab anti-CD38 and Elotuzumab anti-CS1. Anti-amyloid monoclonal antibody NEOD001 is currently in phase III clinical trials.

Other Systemic Amyloidoses

Not all systemic amyloidoses are, at present, treatable, but new possibilities are emerging. Modern therapies for AA amyloidosis and emerging therapies for other amyloidoses are discussed in Chaps. 37 and 38. The role of solid organ transplantation in the management of patients with various systemic amyloidoses, hereditary as well as non-hereditary, is also increasing [38–46].

For several hereditary amyloidoses, the liver is the predominant (transthyretin), exclusive (fibrinogen), or partial (apolipoprotein AI) source of abnormal protein. Based on this, liver transplantation was offered to affected patients as

a form of "surgical" gene therapy, where replacement of the variant gene with a normal gene is achieved by replacement of the liver [38]. Thus, in the early 1990s, the first patients with familial amyloid polyneuropathy (FAP) due to a mutation in the ATTR gene were treated by liver transplantation and there is now a worldwide registry of such transplantations (please see www.fapwtr.org; [38]). Currently, liver transplantation is an acceptable treatment option, halting progress of the disease; however, long-term outcomes are variable. The results appear to be better in younger patients who are affected by the most prevalent variant of transthyretin (Met30), and who are at the early stages of the disease, with mild symptoms [40, 42, 43]. Thus, regression of visceral amyloid deposits has been reported, as well as improvements in autonomic and, to a lesser extent, peripheral nerve function. Unexpectedly, however, some patients, who were affected by certain mutations, experienced a rapid progression of cardiac amyloidosis after liver transplantation, even though the deposits elsewhere had stabilized or regressed [43, 44]. It is proposed that this is due to enhanced deposition of wild-type TTR on a template of amyloid derived from the variant TTR [38, 44]. This phenomenon appears to be mutation dependent. In sum, it appears that the outcome of liver transplantation in patients with FAP depends on many variables, including the type of mutation, severity of neuropathy and the degree of cardiac amyloid involvement, as well as nutritional status and age; thus, early diagnosis and transplantation is critical. Unfortunately, given the variability of penetrance and the late onset of disease in many mutations, a family history is often missing. De novo mutations are also possible. For these reasons, the diagnosis is often delayed.

With the exception of being a source of abnormal protein, which causes systemic disease, livers from patients with ATTR are otherwise structurally and functionally normal. Usually, the livers contain only microscopic amyloid deposits in hilar vessels and nerves and are otherwise uninvolved [44, 47]. Thus, given the shortage of livers available for transplantation, since 1995, such explanted livers have been used

---

[1] Please note that Panobinostat has not been, as of this writing (February 2015), approved by the FDA for use in human subjects.

sequentially as donor grafts for recipients with liver malignancies or conditions that make them unacceptable (or low priority) candidates for conventional cadaveric liver transplantation ("marginal recipients"). This type of dual, sequential transplantation has been named "domino" liver transplantation [47–53]. The domino surgery has not been found to add additional risk to the FAP-liver donor or recipient. However, importantly, domino surgery increases the organ pool, allowing the transplantation of marginal recipients who would not otherwise be eligible to receive a deceased donor liver [48, 51–53].

Since the penetrance of the disease varies substantially and amyloid deposition and symptoms occur in affected persons only in adulthood, it was considered that the danger of de novo disease in the recipient was minimal. Indeed, hundreds of patients have benefited from domino transplants. However, with longer survival times post-domino liver transplantation, rare patients were found to develop polyneuropathy. The first such reported case was a patient who developed polyneuropathy associated with ATTR amyloid deposits, in his peripheral nerves, 8 years post-domino liver transplantation [54]. More recent reports suggest that overt polyneuropathy may be preceded by subclinical gastrointestinal transthyretin amyloid deposits [55, 56]. Thus, it appears that polyneuropathy symptoms may appear 3 or 4 years after the histological demonstration of amyloid deposition elsewhere in the body. Even earlier, non-fibrillar deposits of transthyretin may also be detected in the skin [55]. Hence, at the present time, long-term monitoring of domino FAP recipients, using annual abdominal fat or gastro-duodenal mucosal biopsies, is recommended in order to detect amyloid deposits at an early stage of disease. Nerve biopsy is required to diagnose de novo amyloid polyneuropathy and to consider retransplantation. Pharmacologic therapies, some of which are currently in clinical trials, are also becoming available [57, 58]. Further, nonsteroidal anti-inflammatory drugs have been shown to stabilize the native tetramer of TTR molecules, to inhibit transthyretin amyloidogenesis, and to

reduce the risk of posttransplant amyloid polyneuropathy [39].

In individuals with a TTR gene mutation, it takes >20 years before the onset of amyloid deposition in their organs and several more years before FAP symptoms develop. While it is difficult to explain why some recipients of FAP livers develop TTR amyloidosis within a much shorter incubation period (in comparison with genetically determined FAP patients), the age factor may play a role. In this regard, recipients of domino livers have typically been older and, hence, subject to age-related amyloidogenesis. The TTR molecule, being composed largely of beta-sheet structure, is inherently amyloidogenic. In older individuals, even the wild-type molecule may promote amyloidogenesis, in particular affecting the heart (please see also Chaps. 5 and 7). Thus, in older patients, who are recipients of domino livers, amyloidogenesis may be accelerated due to older age [54–56]. The Familial Amyloidotic Polyneuropathy World Transplant Registry also collects data on domino liver transplants (The Domino Liver World Transplant Registry at: http://www.fapwtr.org/ram1.htm; [47]).

Variants of fibrinogen A alpha-chain (AFib) cause the most common type of hereditary renal amyloidosis in Europe and possibly also in the United States [59, 60]. This type of hereditary amyloidosis appears to target primarily the kidney, leading to the development of nephrotic syndrome, hypertension, and kidney failure as the main clinical manifestations. Initially, kidney transplantation was offered to affected patients, but solitary renal allografts were found to fail within 1–7 years as a consequence of recurrent amyloidosis. Since the variant fibrinogen is solely produced in the liver, currently, a combined liver and kidney transplantation is performed. Moreover, data published recently by Stangou et al. [59] even encourage the consideration of a *preemptive solitary* liver transplantation, early in the course of amyloid nephropathy, in order to obviate the need for subsequent hemodialysis and kidney transplantation. These authors also propose that early solitary liver transplantation

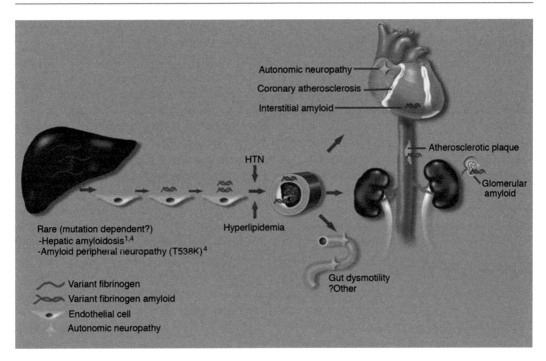

Fig. 36.3 Proposed pathogenesis of fibrinogen amyloidosis [60]. Reprinted with permission from Picken MM. Blood. 2010;115:2985 [60]

may also prevent significant cardiovascular amyloidosis. This is based on their evidence that AFib is a systemic and serious disorder, affecting more organs than just the kidneys, and that, therefore, renal transplantation can be compromised by ongoing damage to other tissues and to the new renal graft (Fig. 36.3; [59, 60]).

Thus, similar to FAP, patients affected by AFib are considered for transplantation at the earlier stages of the disease. However, issues associated with the clinical management of asymptomatic carriers of a potentially amyloidogenic mutation are still largely unresolved [59]. In general, due to variable penetrance, aggressive treatments are delayed until onset of the disease is clinically apparent, a situation that may occur quite late in some patients. This may change, however, in view of the data presented by Stangou et al. suggesting that, even in clinically healthy carriers of a mutation, damage to the systemic vasculature may already have occurred (Fig. 36.3; [59, 60]). The development of pharmacologic gene therapy should alleviate some of the issues

associated with transplantation in hereditary amyloidoses. Conventional pharmacologic therapies for overt ATTR disease are also in clinical trials (please see also Chap. 37).

Apolipoprotein AI (AApoAI), which can cause hereditary amyloidosis, is secreted by the liver and intestine [61]. Here, amyloid disease progression may be very slow and the natural history of the condition can be favorably altered in patients who receive a liver transplant. Moreover, it has been advocated that, in hereditary AApoAI amyloidosis, failing organs should be replaced, since graft survival is excellent and transplantation confers substantial survival benefit [61]. In Apolipoprotein AII (AApoAII) hereditary amyloidosis, the major morbidity is associated with renal failure. Hence, kidney dialysis and renal transplantation are, presently, the only two therapeutic options. Renal transplantation is an effective therapy for apolipoprotein AII amyloidosis, since recurrence of amyloid in the graft and progression of other organ involvement may be very slow [62].

Transplantation in the Management of Patients with Non-hereditary Systemic Amyloidoses

Because of delays in diagnosis, vital organ failure is not uncommon in AL. Indeed, organ failure may, in turn, delay or even prevent the aggressive therapy that is needed. However, solid organ transplantation, to overcome organ failure, is controversial because of the multisystem nature of this disease and the risk of disease recurrence in the graft; for these reasons, transplantation has rarely been performed in AL amyloidosis. Nonetheless, available data demonstrate the feasibility of the concept and support a potential role for this procedure in selected patients [63–70]. Alternative strategies might also involve solid organ transplantation before treatment, in order to permit high-dose chemotherapy and ASCT or, after successful treatment, during remission [65, 66, 68]. In AL, the kidney is the most frequently affected organ. Patients with end-stage kidney disease due to amyloidosis have a poor prognosis, tolerate dialysis poorly, have increased episodes of hypotension, and have issues with vascular access. Kidney transplantation can be successfully performed in AL patients who have a complete hematologic response and meet the usual kidney transplantation selection criteria. Outcomes appear similar to those found in other recipients, regardless of whether the hematologic response was achieved with ASCT or by nonmyeloablative therapy [66]. Apart from the kidney, other organ transplants have also been performed while in hematologic remission after ASCT, including the liver [65]. Patients with renal failure caused by AA amyloidosis are also eligible for renal transplantation but require careful management of both cardiovascular and infectious complications in order to reduce the high risk of mortality [71, 72]. Recurrent AA amyloidosis in a kidney transplant is rare, especially when the underlying inflammatory condition is controlled, but it has been reported [72]. In the case of ALECT2, kidney transplantation is associated with recurrent amyloidosis [73]. However, since the major morbidity is associated with renal failure and, currently, no specific therapies are available for patients affected by ALECT2, kidney transplantation remains a reasonable option [10].

Examples of Patients with Different Types of Systemic Amyloidosis, Illustrating the Different Evaluation and Treatment Options

1. A 54-year-old African American male who presented to his primary care provider with complaints of increasing lower extremity edema, shortness of breath, and an unintentional 20-lb. weight loss. He had a history of chronic back pain, peripheral neuropathies, carpal tunnel syndrome, sleep apnea, and chronic diarrhea. Echocardiography showed a restrictive cardiomyopathy with a thickened interventricular septum. Family history was significant for a father who died at age 69 of heart failure. Following cardiac catheterization a myocardial biopsy was performed which showed amyloidosis derived from transthyretin. Subsequent studies demonstrated a mutation (V122I) and the patient was diagnosed with hereditary (familial) ATTR. His family was referred for genetic counseling. With progressing symptoms, he underwent orthotopic liver and heart transplantation 1 year later.

2. A male in his 70s presented with progressive restrictive cardiomyopathy. One year prior, he had a cholecystectomy for recurring abdominal pain with constipation; pathology did not reveal any diagnostic abnormalities in his gallbladder and he has not noted any change in his pain since surgery. He subsequently developed chronic renal insufficiency, gastroparesis, and fatigue. Echocardiography revealed an enlarged heart and endomyocardial biopsy demonstrated amyloid derived from transthyretin (ATTR). No mutation in the transthyretin gene was detected by molecular studies and a diagnosis of wild-type ("senile") ATTR was made. The patient received supportive care and nonsteroidal

anti-inflammatory drugs; with worsening renal function he was subsequently placed on dialysis. His clinical course continued to deteriorate and he passed away of multi-organ failure 6 years after diagnosis of amyloidosis by endomyocardial biopsy. Autopsy revealed massive amyloid deposits in the heart and moderately abundant amyloid in his lungs and systemic vasculature. Amyloid deposits were also present in the kidneys and in the gastrointestinal tract. There was also a mild hepatomegaly with congestion and fibrosis, but without evidence of amyloidosis in the parenchyma.

3. A 67-year-old male with a history of progressive, unintentional, 25 lb. weight loss and loose stools over the past year, who presented to the emergency room with severe abdominal pain and fatigue. His primary care doctor had recently noted that he had a mild macrocytic anemia with a severely low vitamin B12 level and started him on supplementation. Mild chronic peripheral neuropathy was also attributed to his B12 deficiency. He was found to have a partial small bowel obstruction and required volume resuscitation and pain control. CT scans showed irregularities throughout his colon. Colonoscopy demonstrated patches of inflammatory changes, most prominent at the terminal ileum. He was empirically started on high-dose steroids for presumed Crohn's disease. Pathology demonstrated amorphous deposits and Congo red staining was positive for amyloid, subsequently typed as AL-lambda. Serum and urine electrophoresis confirmed a monoclonal protein; free lambda light chain was also increased. Bone marrow exam demonstrated 12 % monoclonal lambda light chain-restricted plasma cells without evidence of amyloid. Twenty-four-hour urine protein revealed nephrotic range proteinuria at over 4 g/day. Echocardiography revealed a normal ejection fraction without evidence of cardiac involvement. NT-BNP and cardiac troponins were normal. Once stabilized, he was initiated on treatment with bortezomib and dexamethasone with an immediate improvement by light chain assay evaluation. He went on to receive high-dose melphalan-based chemotherapy and ASCT with an excellent response to treatment.

Reevaluation

As an incurable disease, surveillance for progression remains essential in the management of systemic amyloidosis. In patients with disease associated with light chain, monitoring with serum free light chain assays is mandatory. Careful attention should be paid to the follow-up monitoring of patients diagnosed with localized amyloidosis, since there remains a risk of progression to systemic disease, which, although generally small, can be difficult to reliably predict in an individual patient. However, in patients with MALT lymphoma and localized amyloidosis recurrences do occur. In AL amyloidosis, the serum free light chain assay is used to monitor the burden of light chains and correlates well with progression of the disease and its response to treatment. Therapy should be aimed at preventing the progression of cardiac biomarkers (NT-proBNP and troponins) since cardiac disease remains the ultimate cause of death in the majority of these patients.

The Future

Although systemic amyloidosis remains an incurable condition, both the diagnosis and the treatment of amyloidosis have recently undergone major advances. Essential to this progress is an active awareness, by clinicians and pathologists, of amyloid diseases and their potential presentations. In this, an appropriate interaction between clinician and pathologist, the use of newer tests that have increased the accuracy of diagnosis of the disease, and the use of appropriate treatment algorithms, including evaluation by an experienced bone marrow transplantation center, are important adjuncts. Please see also Chaps. 2, 37 and 38. For hereditary amyloidoses, solid organ transplantation will remain the treatment of choice until effective gene therapy becomes available. Currently, several pharmacologic therapies are in clinical trials. The availability of pharmacologic therapies will allow us to address, at a much earlier stage, issues of management that pertain to carriers of potentially amyloidogenic mutations. Additionally, a better insight into the relationship between hereditary amyloidosis and aging will help our understanding of aging in general and may also, perhaps, aid us in devising age-deferring strategies.

Acknowledgments We would like to acknowledge the help of Brad Daleiden-Brugman with the drawing of Fig. 36.2 and JS Dalal for his contribution to this chapter in the prior edition.

References

1. Picken MM. Modern approaches to the treatment of amyloidosis—the critical importance of early detection in surgical pathology. Adv Anat Pathol. 2013; 20(6):424–39.
2. Merlini G, Seldin DC, Gertz MA. Amyloidosis: pathogenesis and new therapeutic options. J Clin Oncol. 2011;29:1924–33.
3. Gertz MA. Immunoglobulin light chain amyloidosis: 2014 update on diagnosis, prognosis, and treatment. Am J Hematol. 2014;89:1133–40.
4. Mahmood S, Palladini G, Sanchorawala V, Wechalekar A. Update on treatment of light chain amyloidosis. Haematologica. 2014;99:209–21. doi:10.3324/haematol.2013.087619.
5. Ryan RJH, Sloan JM, Collins AB, Mansouri J, Raje NS, Zukerberg LR, Ferry JA. Extranodal marginal zone lymphoma of mucosa-associated lymphoid tissue with amyloid deposition: a clinicopathologic case series. Am J Clin Pathol. 2012;137:51–64.
6. Said SM, Reynolds C, Jimenez RE, Chen B, Vrana JA, Theis JD, Dogan A, Shah SS. Amyloidosis of the breast: predominantly AL type and over half have concurrent breast hematologic disorders. Mod Pathol. 2013;26:232–8. Published online 28 September 2012.
7. Kaufman GP, Dispenzieri A, Gertz MA, Lacy MQ, Buadi FK, Hayman SR, Leung N, Dingli D, Lust JA, Lin Y, Kapoor P, Go RS, Zeldenrust SR, Kyle RA, Rajkumar SV, Kumar SK. Kinetics of organ response and survival following normalization of the serum free light chain ratio in AL amyloidosis. Am J Hematol. 2015;90(3):181–6. doi:10.1002/ajh.23898 [Epub ahead of print].
8. Sipe JD, Benson MD, Buxbaum JN, Ikeda S, Merlini G, Saraiva MJ, Westermark P. Nomenclature 2014:

amyloid fibril proteins and clinical classification of the amyloidosis. Amyloid. 2014;21(4):221–4. Epub 2014 Sep 29.
9. Vrana JA, et al. Classification of amyloidosis by laser microdissection and mass spectrometry-based proteomic analysis in clinical biopsy specimens. Blood. 2009;114:4957–9.
10. Picken MM. Alect2 amyloidosis: primum non nocere (first, do no harm). Kidney Int. 2014;86(2):229–32. doi:10.1038/ki.2014.45.
11. Lachmann HJ, Booth DR, Booth SE, Bybee A, Gillbertson JA, Gillmore JD, Pepys MB, Hawkins PN. Misdiagnosis of hereditary amyloidosis as AL (primary) amyloidosis. N Engl J Med. 2002;346(23): 1786–91.
12. Comenzo RL, Zhou P, Fleisher M, Clark B, Teruya-Feldstein J. Seeking confidence in the diagnosis of systemic AL (Ig light-chain) amyloidosis: patients can have both monoclonal gammopathies and hereditary amyloid proteins. Blood. 2006;107(9):3489–91. Epub 26 Jan 2006.
13. Gertz MA, Comenzo R, Falk RH, Fermand JP, Hazenberg BP, Hawkins PN, Merlini G, Moreau P, Ronco P, Sanchorawala V, Sezer O, Solomon A, Grateau G. Definition of organ involvement and treatment response in immunoglobulin light chain amyloidosis (AL): a consensus opinion from the 10th International Symposium on Amyloid and Amyloidosis, Tours, France, 18–22 April 2004. Am J Hematol. 2005;79(4):319–28.
14. Gertz MA, Wechalekar A, Palladini G. Looking for consensus: organ involvement and response criteria in AL. In: Hazenberg BPC, Bijzet J, editors. The proceedings of the XIIIth international symposium on amyloidosis, 6–10 May 2012, Groningen, The Netherlands. GUARD (Groningen Unit for Amyloidosis Research and Development); 2013. p. 466–9.
15. Merkies ISJ, Obici L, Suhr OB. Organ involvement and response criteria in non-AL amyloidosis: special attention to peripheral neuropathies and cardiomyopathy in ATTR amyloidosis. In: Hazenberg BPC, Bijzet J, editors. The proceedings of the XIIIth international symposium on amyloidosis, 6–10 May 2012, Groningen, The Netherlands. GUARD (Groningen Unit for Amyloidosis Research and Development); 2013. p. 470–4.
16. Merlini G, Palladini G. Light chain amyloidosis: the heart of the problem. Haematologica. 2013;98(10): 1492–5.
17. Merlini G, et al. Dangerous small B-cell clones. Blood. 2006;108:2520–30.
18. Sanchorawala V. High dose melphalan and autologous peripheral blood stem cell transplantation in AL amyloidosis. Hematol Oncol Clin North Am. 2014;28:1131–44.
19. Kyle RA, Gertz MA, Greipp PR, Witzig TE, Lust JA, Lacy MQ, Therneau TM. A trial of three regimens for primary amyloidosis: colchicine alone, melphalan and prednisone, and melphalan, prednisone, and colchicine. N Engl J Med. 1997;336:1202–7.

20. Wechalekar AD, Gillmore JD, Bird J, Cavenagh J, Hawkins S, Kazmi M, Lachmann HJ, Hawkins PN, Pratt G, on behalf of the BCSH Committee. Guidelines on the management of AL amyloidosis. Br J Haematol. 2015;168(2):186–206. doi:10.1111/bjh.13155. http://www.bcshguidelines.com/index.html.
21. Lu G, Middleton RE, Sun H, Naniong M, Ott CJ, Mitsiades CS, Wong KK, Bradner JE, Kaelin Jr WG. The myeloma drug lenalidomide promotes the cereblon-dependent destruction of Ikaros proteins. Science. 2014;343(6168):305–9. doi:10.1126/science.1244917. Epub 2013 Nov 29.
22. Krönke J, Udeshi ND, Narla A, Grauman P, Hurst SN, McConkey M, Svinkina T, Heckl D, Comer E, Li X, Ciarlo C, Hartman E, Munshi N, Schenone M, Schreiber SL, Carr SA, Ebert BL. Lenalidomide causes selective degradation of IKZF1 and IKZF3 in multiple myeloma cells. Science. 2014;343(6168):301–5. doi:10.1126/science.1244851.
23. Singhal S, Mehta J, Desikan R, Ayers D, Roberson P, Eddlemon P, Munshi N, Anaissie E, Wilson C, Dhodapkar M, Zeddis J, Barlogie B. Antitumor activity of thalidomide in refractory multiple myeloma. N Engl J Med. 1999;341(21):1565–71.
24. Van Rhee F, Dhodapkar M, Shaughnessy JD, et al. First thalidomide clinical trial in multiple myeloma: a decade. Blood. 2008;112(4):1035–8.
25. Stewart AK. How thalidomide works against cancer. Science. 2014;343(6168):256–7. doi:10.1126/science.1249543.
26. Dispenzieri A, et al. Activity of pomalidomide in patients with immunoglobulin light-chain amyloidosis. Blood. 2012;119(23):5397–404.
27. Hideshima T, Bradner JE, Wong J, Chauhan D, Richardson P, Schreiber SL, Anderson KC. Small-molecule inhibition of proteasome and aggresome function induces synergistic antitumor activity in multiple myeloma. Proc Natl Acad Sci U S A. 2005;102(24):8567–72.
28. McConkey D. Proteasome and HDAC: who's zooming who? Blood. 2010;116(3):308–9.
29. Jaccard A, Comenzo RL, Hari P, Hawkins PN, Roussel M, Morel P, Macro M, Pellegrin JL, Lazaro E, Mohty D, Mercie P, Decaux O, Gillmore J, Lavergne D, Bridoux F, Wechalekar AD, Venner CP. Efficacy of bortezomib, cyclophosphamide and dexamethasone in treatment-naïve patients with high-risk cardiac AL amyloidosis (Mayo Clinic stage III). Haematologica. 2014;99(9):1479–85. doi:10.3324/haematol.2014.104109. ©2014 Ferrata Storti Foundation. This is an open-access paper.
30. Palladini G, et al. Melphalan and dexamethasone with or without bortezomib in newly diagnosed AL amyloidosis: a matched case–control study on 174 patients. Leukemia. 2014;28:2311–6.
31. Kastritis E, Roussou M, Gavriatopoulou M, Migkou M, Kalapanida D, Pamboucas C, Kaldara E, Ntalianis A, Psimenou E, Toumanidis S, Tasidou A, Terpos E, Dimopoulos MA. Long term outcomes of primary systemic light chain (AL) amyloidosis in patients treated upfront with bortezomib or lenalidomide and the importance of risk adapted strategies. Am J Hematol. 2015;90(4):E60–5. doi:10.1002/ajh.23936 [Epub ahead of print].
32. San-Miguel JF, et al. Panobinostat plus bortezomib and dexamethasone versus placebo plus bortezomib and dexamethasone in patients with relapsed or relapsed and refractory multiple myeloma: a multicentre, randomised, double-blind phase 3 trial. Lancet Oncol. 2014;15:1195–206.
33. Kumar SK, Berdeja JG, Niesvizky R, Lonial S, Laubach JP, Hamadani M, Stewart AK, Hari P, Roy V, Vescio R, Kaufman JL, Berg D, Liao E, Di Bacco A, Estevam J, Gupta N, Hui AM, Rajkumar V, Richardson PG. Safety and tolerability of ixazomib, an oral proteasome inhibitor, in combination with lenalidomide and dexamethasone in patients with previously untreated multiple myeloma: an open-label phase 1/2 study. Lancet Oncol. 2014;15(13):1503–12. www.thelancet.com/oncology.
34. Kumar SK, Bensinger WI, Zimmerman TM, et al. Phase 1 study of weekly dosing with the investigational oral proteasome inhibitor ixazomib in relapsed/refractory multiple myeloma. Blood. 2014;124(7):1047–55.
35. Laubach JP, Tai YT, Richardson PG, Anderson KC. Daratumumab granted breakthrough drug status. Expert Opin Investig Drugs. 2014;23(4):445–52. doi:10.1517/13543784.2014.889681. Epub 2014 Feb 20.
36. Lonial S, Kaufman J, Laubach J, Richardson P. Elotuzumab: a novel anti-CS1 monoclonal antibody for the treatment of multiple myeloma. Expert Opin Biol Ther. 2013;13(12):1731–40. doi:10.1517/14712598.2013.847919. Epub 2013 Oct 23. Review.
37. Wall JS, Kennel SJ, Williams A, Richey T, Stuckey A, Huang Y, Macy S, Donnell R, Barbour R, Seubert P, Schenk D. AL amyloid imaging and therapy with a monoclonal antibody to a cryptic epitope on amyloid fibrils. PLoS One. 2012;7(12), e52686.
38. Ericzon BG, Wilczek HE, Larsson M, Wijayatunga P, Stangou A, Rodrigues Pena J, Furtado E, Barroso E, Danie J, Samuel D, Adam R, Karam V, Poterucha J, Lewis D, Ferraz-Neto BH, Waddington Cruz M, Munar-Ques M, Fabregat J, Ikeda S, Ando Y, Heaton N, Otto G, Suhr O. Liver transplantation for hereditary transthyretin amyloidosis: after 20 years still the best therapeutic alternative? Transplantation 2015;doi:10.1097/TP.0000000000000574.
39. Ueda M, Ando Y. Recent advances in transthyretin amyloidosis therapy. Transl Neurodegener. 2014;3:19. http://www.translationalneurodegeneration.com/content/3/1/19.
40. Holmgren G, Ericzon BG, Groth CG, et al. Clinical improvement and amyloid regression after liver transplantation in hereditary transthyretin amyloidosis. Lancet. 1993;341:1113–6.
41. Obici L, Merlini G. An overview of drugs currently under investigation for the treatment of transthyretin-related hereditary amyloidosis. Expert Opin Investig Drugs. 2014;23(9):1239–51. doi:10.1517/13543784.2014.922541. Epub 2014 Jul 8.

42. Stangou AJ, Hawkins PN. Liver transplantation in transthyretin-related familial amyloid polyneuropathy. Curr Opin Neurol. 2004;17(5):615–20.

43. Ohya Y, Okamoto S, Tasaki M, Ueda M, Jono H, Obayashi K, Takeda K, Okajima H, Asonuma K, Hara R, Tanihara H, Ando Y, Inomata Y. Manifestations of transthyretin-related familial amyloidotic polyneuropathy: long-term follow-up of Japanese patients after liver transplantation. Surg Today. 2011;41(9): 1211–8. Epub 2011 Aug 26.

44. Stangou AJ, Hawkins PN, Heaton ND, Rela M, Monaghan M, Nihoyannopoulos P, O'Grady J, Pepys MB, Williams R. Progressive cardiac amyloidosis following liver transplantation for familial amyloid polyneuropathy: implications for amyloid fibrillogenesis. Transplantation. 1998;66(2):229–33.

45. Davis MK, Kale P, Liedtke M, Schrier S, Arai S, Wheeler M, Lafayette R, Coakley T, Witteles RM. Outcomes after heart transplantation for amyloid cardiomyopathy in the modern era. Am J Transplant. 2015;15(3):650–8. doi:10.1111/ajt.13025 [Epub ahead of print].

46. Barreiros AP, Post F, Hoppe-Lotichius M, Linke RP, Vahl CF, Schäfers HJ, Galle PR, Otto G. Liver transplantation and combined liver-heart transplantation in patients with familial amyloid polyneuropathy: a single-center experience. Liver Transpl. 2010;16(3):314–23.

47. Wilczek HE, Larsson M, Yamamoto S, Ericzon BG. Domino liver transplantation. J Hepatobiliary Pancreat Surg. 2008;15(2):139–48.

48. Kitchens WH. Domino liver transplantation: indications, techniques, and outcomes. Transplant Rev (Orlando). 2011;25(4):167–77.

49. Mazzaferro V, Regalia E, Doci R, et al. Liver transplantation for the treatment of small hepatocellular carcinomas in patients with cirrhosis. N Engl J Med. 1996;334:693–700.

50. Stangou AJ, Heaton ND, Rela M, Pepys MB, Hawkins PN, Williams R. Domino hepatic transplantation using the liver from a patient with familial amyloidotic polyneuropathy. Transplantation. 1998;65:1496–8.

51. Ericzon BG, Larsson M, Wilczek HE. Domino liver transplantation: risks and benefits. Transplant Proc. 2008;40(4):1130–1. doi:10.1016/j.transproceed. 2008.03.020.

52. Tincani G, Hoti E, Andreani P, Ricca L, Pittau G, Vitale V, Blandin F, Adam R, Castaing D, Azoulay D. Operative risks of domino liver transplantation for the familial amyloid polyneuropathy liver donor and recipient: a double analysis. Am J Transplant. 2011; 11(4):759–66.

53. Yamamoto S, Ericzon BG. Domino liver transplantation as a valuable option. Transpl Int. 2014;27(4):e27–8. doi:10.1111/tri.12235. Epub 2013 Nov 29.

54. Stangou AJ, Heaton ND, Hawkins PN. Transmission of systemic transthyretin amyloidosis by means of domino liver transplantation. N Engl J Med. 2005; 352(22):2356.

55. Sousa MM, Ferrao J, Fernandes R, et al. Deposition and passage of transthyretin through the blood-nerve barrier in recipients of familial amyloidotic polyneuropathy livers. Lab Invest. 2004;84:865–73.

56. Adams D, Lacroix C, Antonini T, Lozeron P, Denier C, Kreib AM, Epelbaum S, Blandin F, Karam V, Azoulay D, Adam R, Castaing D, Samuel D. Symptomatic and proven de novo amyloid polyneuropathy in familial amyloid polyneuropathy domino liver recipients. Amyloid. 2011;18 Suppl 1:169–72.

57. Coelho T, Maia LF, da Silva AM, Cruz MW, Planté-Bordeneuve V, Suhr OB, Conceiçao I, Schmidt HH, Trigo P, Kelly JW, Labaudinière R, Chan J, Packman J, Grogan DR. Long-term effects of tafamidis for the treatment of transthyretin familial amyloid polyneuropathy. J Neurol. 2013;260:2802–14.

58. Ando Y, Coelho T, Berk JL, Waddington Cruz M, Ericzon BG, Ikeda S, Lewis WD, Obici L, Planté-Bordeneuve V, Rapezzi C, Said G, Salvi F. Guideline of transthyretin-related hereditary amyloidosis for clinicians. Orphanet J Rare Dis. 2013;8:31. http://www.ojrd.com/content/8/1/31.

59. Stangou AJ, Banner NR, Hendry BM, Rela M, Portmann B, Wendon J, Monaghan M, Maccarthy P, Buxton-Thomas M, Mathias CJ, Liepnieks JJ, O'Grady J, Heaton ND, Benson MD. Hereditary fibrinogen A alpha-chain amyloidosis: phenotypic characterization of a systemic disease and the role of liver transplantation. Blood. 2010;115(15):2998–3007.

60. Picken MM. Fibrinogen amyloidosis: the clot thickens! Blood. 2010;115(15):2985–6.

61. Gillmore JD, Stangou AJ, Lachmann HJ, Goodman HJ, Wechalekar AD, Acheson J, Tennent GA, Bybee A, Gilbertson J, Rowczenio D, O'Grady J, Heaton ND, Pepys MB, Hawkins PN. Organ transplantation in hereditary apolipoprotein AI amyloidosis. Am J Transplant. 2006;6(10):2342–7.

62. Magy N, Liepnieks JJ, Yazaki M, Kluve-Beckerman B, Benson MD. Renal transplantation for apolipoprotein AII amyloidosis. Amyloid. 2003;10(4):224–8.

63. Sattianayagam PT, Gibbs SD, Pinney JH, Wechalekar AD, Lachmann HJ, Whelan CJ, Gilbertson JA, Hawkins PN, Gillmore JD. Solid organ transplantation in AL amyloidosis. Am J Transplant. 2010;10(9):2124–31.

64. Gibbs SD, Sattianayagam PT, Hawkins PN, Gillmore JD. Cardiac transplantation should be considered in selected patients with either AL or hereditary forms of amyloidosis: the UK National Amyloidosis Centre experience. Intern Med J. 2009;39(11):786–7.

65. Binotto G, Cillo U, Trentin L, Piazza F, Zaninotto M, Semenzato G, Adami F. Double autologous bone marrow transplantation and orthotopic liver transplantation in a patient with primary light chain (AL) amyloidosis. Amyloid. 2011;18 Suppl 1:127–9.

66. Herrmann SM, Gertz MA, Stegall MD, Dispenzieri A, Cosio FC, Kumar S, Lacy MQ, Dean PG, Prieto M, Zeldenrust SR, Buadi FK, Russell SJ, Nyberg SL, Hayman SR, Dingli D, Fervenza FC, Leung N. Long-term outcomes of patients with light chain amyloidosis (AL) after renal transplantation with or without stem cell transplantation. Nephrol Dial Transplant. 2011;26(6):2032–6.

67. Bridoux F, Ronco P, Gillmore J, Fermand JP. Editorial Comment Renal transplantation in light chain amyloidosis: coming out of the cupboard. Nephrol Dial Transplant. 2011;26(6):1766–8. doi:10.1093/ndt/gfr191. Epub 2011 Apr 12.

68. Pinney JH, Lachmann HJ, Bansi L, Wechalekar AD, Gilbertson JA, Rowczenio D, Sattianayagam PT, Gibbs SDJ, Orlandi E, Wassef NL, Bradwell AR, Hawkins PN, Julian D, Gillmore JD. Outcome in renal AL amyloidosis after chemotherapy. J Clin Oncol. 2011;29(6):674–81. doi:10.1200/JCO.2010.30.5235JCO. 2011 by American Society of Clinical Oncology. Published online before print January 10, 2011.

69. Gursu M, Yelken B, Caliskan Y, Kazancioglu R, Yazici H, Kilicaslan I, Turkmen A, Sever MS. Outcome of patients with amyloidosis after renal transplantation: a single-center experience. Int J Artif Organs. 2012;35(6):444–9. doi:10.5301/ijao.5000091.

70. Gilstrap LG, Niehaus E, Malhotra R, Ton VK, Watts J, Seldin DC, Madsen JC, Semigran MJ. End stage cardiac amyloidosis: predictors of survival to cardiac transplantation and long term outcomes. J Heart Lung Transplant. 2014;33(2):149–56. doi:10.1016/j.healun.2013.09.004.

71. Kofman T, Grimbert P, Canouï-Poitrine F, Zuber J, Garrigue V, Mousson C, Frimat L, Kamar N, Couvrat G, Bouvier N, Albano L, Le Thuaut A, Pillebout E, Choukroun G, Couzi L, Peltier J, Mariat C, Delahousse M, Buchler M, Le Pogamp P, Bridoux F, Pouteil-Noble C, Lang P, Audard V. Renal transplantation in patients with AA amyloidosis nephropathy: results from a French multicenter study. Am J Transplant. 2011;11(11):2423–31 [Epub ahead of print].

72. Sethi S, El Ters M, Vootukuru S, Qian Q. Recurrent AA amyloidosis in a kidney transplant. Am J Kidney Dis. 2011;57(6):941–4.

73. Said SM, Sethi S, Valeri AM, Chang A, Nast CC, Krahl L, Molloy P, Barry M, Fidler ME, Cornell LD, Leung N, Vrana JA, Theis JD, Dogan A, Nasr SH. Characterization and outcomes of renal leukocyte chemotactic factor 2-associated amyloidosis. Kidney Int. 2014;86:370–7. doi:10.1038/ki.2013.558. Published online 22 January 2014.

Emerging Therapies for Amyloidosis

37

Merrill D. Benson

Once upon a time, the diagnosis of amyloidosis was considered a medical death sentence. This, of course, was the perception of immunoglobulin light chain (primary) amyloidosis for which there was a 15–18-month median survival after diagnosis. Indeed, the median survival did not change after the institution of treatment with oral melphalan and low-dose prednisone, although a minority of patients did have favorable response to this drug regimen. Now there are a number of therapeutic agents used alone or in combination which show significant efficacy in the treatment of AL amyloidosis. Table 37.1 lists some of these agents, commonly used regimens, and side effects. Development of effective therapy for AL amyloidosis (the most common type of amyloidosis) has been of great benefit to many patients but has had serious adverse effects for a number of patients who have other forms of amyloidosis. There are at least 26 proteins which can give amyloidosis in humans, and 11 of these are associated with systemic forms of amyloidosis which can be easily mistaken for the clinical features of AL amyloidosis [1]. This is particularly true for AA (secondary, reactive) amyloidosis and several

of the systemic types of hereditary (familial) amyloidosis. When there was no specific therapy for any form of systemic amyloidosis, there was less concern about making a correct diagnosis as to the specific type of amyloidosis. Now, with the development of many specific therapies for different types of amyloidosis, it is imperative that the correct type of amyloidosis be made expeditiously. All too many patients with familial forms of amyloidosis have been treated with chemotherapeutic agents as a result of an incorrect diagnosis as the more common AL amyloidosis.

So, what are the specific therapies we have at the present time for the different forms of systemic amyloidosis? We have already alluded to the chemotherapy treatment of AL (primary) amyloidosis, its effectiveness, and that it continues to evolve with new drugs and new regimens. We will, however, leave further discussion of treatment of systemic AL amyloidosis to others and only emphasize that it is not considered the best medicine to treat other forms of amyloidosis with chemotherapeutic drugs as a result of less than rigorous pathologic diagnosis.

AA (reactive) amyloidosis appears to be much less common than it was when there was less effective therapy for the inflammatory diseases (rheumatoid arthritis, Crohn's disease, psoriatic arthritis) or infectious diseases (osteomyelitis, tuberculosis). Even so, there continue to be occasional patients who present with renal or hepatic amyloidosis on biopsy, and clinically,

M.D. Benson, MD (✉)
Department of Pathology and Laboratory Medicine,
Indiana University School of Medicine, Van Nuys Medical
Science Building, 635 Barnhill Drive, Room A128,
Indianapolis, IN 46202-5126, USA
e-mail: mdbenson@iupui.edu

© Springer International Publishing Switzerland 2015
M.M. Picken et al. (eds.), *Amyloid and Related Disorders*, Current Clinical Pathology,
DOI 10.1007/978-3-319-19294-9_37

Table 37.1 Chemotherapy agents for AL amyloidosis and toxicities: why diagnosis of AL should be confirmed before treatment

Drug	Toxicity
Melphalan (Alkeran) (oral)	Bone marrow suppression Myelodysplastic syndrome
Melphalan (IV with stem-cell rescue)	Bone marrow suppression Infection
Bortezomib (Velcade)	Neuropathy
Lenalidomide (Revlimid)	Thrombocytopenia GI dysmotility Deep venous thrombosis Bone marrow suppression
Dexamethasone (Decadron)	Electrolyte imbalance, hypoglycemia Psychological changes
Vincristine (Oncovin)	Neuropathy GI dysmotility
Doxorubicin (Adriamycin)	Cardiotoxicity, bone marrow suppression
Cyclophosphamide (Cytoxan)	Bone marrow suppression Cystitis

there is no apparent predisposing inflammatory condition. Some of these patients may have type II familial Mediterranean fever, one of the various TRAPS syndromes, or some as yet unrecognized condition that generates chronic elevated blood levels of serum amyloid A (SAA) [2]. For the pathologist, these patients can be easily identified by immunohistochemistry using specific antibody to amyloid AA protein. These antisera are available commercially and are reliable when used on formalin-fixed and paraffin-embedded biopsy tissues.

Treatment of AA amyloidosis has been non-specific and principally aimed at suppressing the inflammatory condition that predisposed to hepatic synthesis of SAA. With the advent of biologic agents to treat inflammatory arthritis, this form of therapy presents a viable option for AA patients. Recently, a drug (sodium eprodisate) with the clinical name, Kiacta, has been tested for inhibiting AA amyloid formation. This drug is effective in the murine model of induced AA amyloidosis [3]. The initial human trial did not meet the levels of significance required by the FDA [4]. Further clinical trials are being done.

β_2-*Microglobulin amyloidosis* is seen in patients with renal failure who have usually been

on hemodialysis for a number of years. Therapy is aimed at lowering serum levels of β_2-microglobulin, and, with the newer dialysis membranes, the frequency of this form of amyloidosis has dwindled. Diagnosis of this form of amyloidosis is essentially made at the clinical level with the recognition of osseous involvement, although it is important to distinguish it from the bone involvement of AL amyloidosis. Immunohistochemistry may, or may not, be definitive or very helpful.

Transthyretin (TTR) amyloidosis is the most common form of hereditary amyloidosis, and, in addition, increasing numbers of senile systemic or senile cardiac amyloidosis patients are being identified. These patients in the past have been the most common victims of inappropriate treatment with chemotherapeutic agents due to misdiagnosis as AL amyloidosis. While TTR amyloidosis is hereditary, a considerable number of patients do not have an informative family history due to lack of penetrance of the condition or delayed clinical onset until advanced age. Many of these patients have cardiomyopathy which is indistinguishable from the AL cardiac presentation. From the surgical pathology viewpoint, immunohistochemistry with anti-TTR antibodies may be helpful, but this is not 100 % reliable perhaps due to variations in fixation techniques. The only specific treatment for TTR amyloidosis developed so far has been liver transplantation [5, 6]. Plasma TTR is synthesized by the liver, and liver transplantation will eliminate the source of the amyloidogenic variant protein. Approximately 2000 liver transplantations for TTR amyloidosis have been performed since 1990 and reported to the Transplant Registry [7]. It is recognized that an additional number of treated patients may not have been reported to the Transplant Registry. Results have been good but are somewhat variable depending upon the TTR mutation. The Val30Met patients from Portugal, Sweden, and Japan, where neuropathy is the major manifestation of the disease, have shown significant benefit with 5-year survival at 80–85 %. It is now recognized that patients in a more advanced stage of the disease with a modified body mass index (BMI) less than 600 (modified BMI = BMI × serum albumin level expressed in grams per liter) have not fared as well [8]. Hepatic transplant patients who have a non-Val30Met mutation, which includes at least 45 different TTR mutations, have only a 50–55 % 5-year survival. In these patients, there is often progression of amyloid deposition by amyloid fibrils made from wild-type (normal) TTR. This is logical since we already know that senile systemic amyloidosis occurs in elderly individuals (mainly male) without the benefit of any TTR mutation.

The lack of consistent response from liver transplantation has spurred efforts to find medical treatments for TTR amyloidosis. Two drugs shown to stabilize the TTR tetramer in vitro have been studied for slowing the progression of peripheral neuropathy in patients with TTR amyloidosis. Tafamidis (Vyndaqel) has been approved in Europe for treatment of patients with stage 1 peripheral neuropathy and, while not approved in the United States, is the subject of additional studies [9]. Diflunisal (Dolobid) has shown statistically significant results for slowing the progression of peripheral neuropathy in patients with TTR amyloidosis and, while only FDA approved for treatment of arthritis, is available by prescription (off-label) [10]. Another drug available by prescription is doxycycline which has shown some evidence for preventing amyloid fibril formation in vivo. Efficacy in humans has not been proven to date. The same is true for the use of sulfites and other compounds which have been available to patients on a nonprescription basis. Potential treatments aimed at decreasing variant transthyretin synthesis by the liver include gene conversion which has only been reported in an animal model and the use of antisense oligonucleotide (ASO) or siRNA compounds which specifically target TTR mRNA [11, 12]. Both TTR-specific ASO and siRNA have been shown to be effective in suppressing hepatic synthesis of TTR in vivo and are now being evaluated for safety and potential efficacy in humans.

Apolipoprotein A-I (ApoA-I) amyloidosis, whether due to mutations that cause nephropathy or cardiomyopathy, is a form of amyloidosis that can be easily mistaken for AL amyloidosis. ApoA-I mutations associated with laryngeal amyloid may be confused with AL amyloidosis which also has a high frequency of laryngeal involvement. Fortunately, AL laryngeal amyloidosis is usually a localized phenomenon and does not warrant chemotherapy. A number of liver transplants have been done for ApoA-I amyloidosis. Most have been for patients with the Gly26Arg mutation [13]. It is not entirely clear whether this form of specific therapy is beneficial [14]. Some patients have definitely benefited, but others appear to have progression of disease. One problem is that the renal disease has often progressed to a relatively advanced stage before liver transplantation is entertained. At that point, liver and kidney transplantation or liver transplantation followed by the need for renal transplantation has often been the course of events. Some patients with mutations associated with cardiomyopathy have benefited from cardiac transplantation without liver transplantation. Not enough subjects have been studied to know whether affected organ replacement or liver transplantation is the better option. ApoA-I is synthesized by both the liver and small intestine, so liver transplantation does not entirely eliminate circulating variant ApoA-I [13].

Fibrinogen Aα-chain (FibAα-chain) amyloidosis The liver is the sole source for fibrinogen Aα-chain. The fact that only peptides from the variant form of FibAα-chain are incorporated into the amyloid fibrils indicates that liver transplantation would be a cure for this form of amyloidosis [15]. FibAα-chain amyloidosis specifically gives nephropathy. If renal transplantation is done without liver transplantation, amyloid recurs in the renal graph within 1–10 years. The question is as follows: when should a person with the FibAα-chain mutation receive a liver transplant? Fortunately, there appears to be a reduced penetrance of this condition, and many gene carriers will not develop the disease even until advanced age. Therefore, it is obvious that liver transplantation should not be done until the disease manifests itself. Once the renal disease has been detected, it probably is a good idea to consider liver transplantation before the renal disease has progressed to the point of needing dialysis, and perhaps even earlier considering that antirejection drugs taken after liver transplantation are nephrotoxic [16]. In addition, it has become obvious that patients who are maintained on dialysis have a heightened risk for atherosclerotic disease and may not tolerate liver transplantation as well as those with relatively well-maintained renal function. No specific medical therapy for FibAα-chain amyloidosis has been proposed since it would be necessary to target synthesis of only the variant form of the protein. Fibrinogen is an important member of the clotting system.

Lysozyme amyloidoses There is no specific therapy for lysozyme amyloidosis. It may be mistaken for other types of systemic amyloidosis, so a definite diagnosis is important. Hepatic and renal transplants for organ failure have benefitted a number of patients [17]. In some cases, renal function has been adequate as long as two decades after renal transplantation [18].

Apolipoprotein AII (ApoA-II) amyloidosis While there is no specific therapy for this primarily nephropathic form of amyloidosis, patients who received a renal transplant have survived for greater than 10 years without evidence of amyloid in the graft [19]. Cardiac or other organ amyloid deposition may progress after kidney transplant.

Gelsolin amyloidosis There is no specific treatment for this disease. The phenotype is very specific, and there is little reason to mistake this amyloidosis for other types.

Cystatin C amyloidosis There is no specific treatment for this disease. It has been suggested that amyloid fibril formation is enhanced at increased body temperature, so avoidance and early treatment of febrile conditions should be considered [20].

LECT2 amyloidosis It is too soon after discovery of this form of amyloidosis to know if renal transplantation for this disease will give acceptable prolongation of life [21]. Liver transplanta-

tion has been done for one patient with terminal hepatic failure and has survived for greater than 3 years.

In summary, it is important to determine the specific type of the amyloid for each patient to avoid inappropriate treatment, especially chemotherapy for misdiagnosis as AL amyloidosis, and consider specific therapy if available.

References

1. Sipe JD, Benson MD, Buxbaum JN, Ikeda S, Merlini G, Saraiva MJ, Westermark P. Amyloid fibril protein nomenclature: 2010 recommendations from the nomenclature committee of the International Society of Amyloidosis. Amyloid. 2010;17:101–4.
2. Kastner DL, Aksentijevich I. Intermittent and periodic arthritis syndromes. In: Koopman WJ, Moreland LW, editors. Arthritis and allied conditions: a textbook of rheumatology, vol. 2. 15th ed. Philadelphia: Lippincott Williams and Wilkins; 2004. p. 1411–61. Chapter 68.
3. Kisilevsky R, Lemieux LJ, Fraser PE, Kong X, Hultin PG, Szarek WA. Arresting amyloidosis in vivo using small-molecule anionic sulphonates or sulphates: implications for Alzheimer's disease. Nat Med. 1995;1:143–8.
4. Dember LM, Hawkins PN, Hazenberg BP, Gorevic PD, Merlini G, Butrimiene I, Livneh A, Lesnyak O, Puéchal X, Lachmann HJ, Obici L, Balshaw R, Garceau D, Hauck W, Skinner M. Eprodisate for the treatment of renal disease in AA amyloidosis. N Eng J Med. 2007;356:2349–60.
5. Holmgren G, Ericzon BG, Groth CG, Steen L, Suhr O, Andersen O, Wallin BG, Seymour A, Richardson S, Hawkins PN, Pepys MB. Clinical improvement and amyloid regression after liver transplantation in hereditary transthyretin amyloidosis. Lancet. 1993; 341:1113–6.
6. Holmgren G, Steen L, Ekstedt J, Groth CG, Ericzon BG, Eriksson S, Andersen O, Karlberg I, Nordén G, Nakazato M, Hawkins P, Richardson S, Pepys M. Biochemical effect of liver transplantation in two Swedish patients with familial amyloidotic polyneuropathy (FAP-met30). Clin Genet. 1991;40:242–6.
7. Familial World Transplant Registry. http://www.fapwtr.org/ram_fap.htm. Accessed 2 Sept 2011.
8. Suhr O, Danielsson A, Holmgren G, Steen L. Malnutrition and gastrointestinal dysfunction as prognostic factors for survival in familial amyloidotic polyneuropathy. J Intern Med. 1994;235:479–85.
9. Coelho T, Maia L, Martins da Silva A, Waddingtion-Cruz M, Planté-Bordeneuve V, Lozeron P, Suhr OB, Campistol J, Conceiçao IM, Conceiçao H, Schmidt H, Trigo P, Packman J, Grogan DR. Tafamidis (Fx-1006A): a first-in-class disease-modifying

therapy for transthyretin familial amyloid. Amyloid. 2010;17:75–6.

10. Berk JL, Suhr OB, Obici L, Sekijima Y, Zeldenrust SR, Yamashita T, Heneghan MA, Gorevic PD, Litchy WJ, Wiesman JF, Nordh E, Corato M, Lozza A, Cortese A, Robinson-Papp J, Colton T, Rybin DV, Bisbee AB, Ando Y, Ikeda S, Seldin DC, Merline G, Skinner M, Kelly JW, Dyck PJ, Diflunisal Trial Consortium. Repurposing diflunisal for familial amyloid polyneuropathy: a randomized clinical trial. JAMA. 2013;310:2658–67.

11. Nakamura M, Ando Y, Nagahara S, Sano A, Ochiya T, Maeda S, Kawaji T, Ogawa M, Hirata A, Terazaki H, Haraoka K, Tanihara H, Ueda M, Uchino M, Yamamura K. Targeted conversion of the transthyretin gene in vitro and in vivo. Gene Ther. 2004;11: 838–46.

12. Benson MD, Kluve Beckerman B, Zeldenrust SR, Siesky AM, Bodenmiller DM, Showalter AD, Sloop KW. Targeted suppression of an amyloidogenic transthyretin with antisense oligonucleotides. Muscle Nerve. 2006;33:609–18.

13. Gillmore JD, Stangou AJ, Lachmann HJ, Goodman HJ, Wechalekar AD, Acheson J, Tennent GA, Bybee A, Gilbertson J, Rowczenio D, O'Grady J, Heaton ND, Pepys MB, Hawkins PN. Organ transplantation in hereditary apolipoprotein AI amyloidosis. Am J Transplant. 2006;6:2342–7.

14. Gillmore JD, Stangou AJ, Tennent GA, Booth DR, O'Grady J, Rela M, Heaton ND, Wall CA, Keogh JA, Hawkins PN. Clinical and biochemical outcome of hepatorenal transplantation for hereditary systemic

amyloidosis associated with apolipoprotein AI Gly26Arg. Transplantation. 2001;71:986–92.

15. Benson MD, Liepnieks J, Uemichi T, Wheeler G, Correa R. Hereditary renal amyloidosis associated with a mutant fibrinogen α-chain. Nat Genet. 1993; 3:252–5.

16. Stangou AJ, Banner NR, Hendry BM, Rela M, Portmann B, Wendon J, Monaghan M, MacCarthy P, Buxton-Thomas M, Mathias CJ, Liepnieks JJ, O'Grady J, Heaton ND, Benson MD. Hereditary fibrinogen A α-chain amyloidosis: phenotypic characterization of a systemic disease and the role of liver transplantation. Blood. 2010;115:2998–3007.

17. Pepys MB, Hawkins PN, Booth DR, Vigushin DM, Tennent GA, Soutar AK, Totty N, Nguyen O, Blake CCF, Terry CJ, Feest TG, Zalin AM, Hsuan JJ. Human lysozyme gene mutations cause hereditary systemic amyloidosis. Nature. 1993;362:553–7.

18. Yazaki M, Farrell SA, Benson MD. A novel lysozyme mutation Phe57Ile associated with hereditary renal amyloidosis. Kidney Int. 2003;63:1652–7.

19. Magy N, Liepnieks JJ, Yazaki M, Kluve-Beckerman B, Benson MD. Renal transplantation for apolipoprotein AII amyloidosis. Amyloid. 2003;10:224–8.

20. Abrahamson M, Grubb A. Increased body temperature accelerates aggregation of the Leu-68 Gln mutant cystatin C, the amyloid-forming protein in hereditary cystatin C amyloid angiopathy. Proc Natl Acad Sci U S A. 1994;91:1416–20.

21. Benson MD, James S, Scott K, Liepnieks JJ, Kluve-Beckerman B. Leukocyte chemotactic factor 2: a novel renal amyloid protein. Kidney Int. 2008;74:218–22.

Modern Therapies in AA Amyloidosis

Amanda K. Ombrello

The field of rheumatology has experienced major therapeutic developments in the past 25 years. Whereas conditions such as rheumatoid arthritis and ankylosing spondylitis used to tread a progressive course resulting in bone and joint destruction, newer medications can now significantly stanch and in some cases even halt the destruction. Likewise, many of these biologic medications are used to treat the subset of rheumatologic diseases known as the autoinflammatory diseases.

AA amyloidosis is a condition that develops in patients who have long-standing inflammatory conditions. The chronic inflammatory state leads to misfolding of the AA amyloid protein and resultant deposition in tissues. Chronic arthritis conditions such as rheumatoid arthritis (RA), ankylosing spondylitis (AS), and systemic juvenile arthritis (SJIA), inflammatory bowel disease (IBD), as well as autoinflammatory diseases such as familial Mediterranean fever (FMF) and tumor necrosis factor receptor associated periodic syndrome (TRAPS) and the group of diseases known as the cryopyrinopathies comprise a major portion of AA amyloidosis cases both in the United States and in Europe. Currently, there is not any

established therapy for AA amyloidosis and treatment is targeted at reducing the underlying inflammatory condition. As newer therapies have been developed to treat the underlying condition, there is emerging evidence that the annual incidence of AA amyloidosis is decreasing [1, 2].

The class of medications referred to as the anti-tumor necrosis factor (anti-TNF) alpha drugs have been paramount in the management of RA and other autoimmune diseases. Although more are in the process of being developed and approved for therapy, the three most studied anti-TNFs include the soluble p75 TNFR:Fc fusion protein, etanercept, the mouse–human chimeric anti-TNF antibody, infliximab, and the fully human monoclonal antibody, adalimumab. Etanercept is given as a weekly injection, adalimumab is administered subcutaneously every 2 weeks, and infliximab is given via infusion every 4–8 weeks. Not only have these medications been approved for wide use in RA patients, but they are also used in other rheumatologic conditions such as AS, juvenile idiopathic arthritis (JIA), and psoriatic arthritis as well as IBD. Additionally, etanercept has been successfully used to treat patients with TRAPS, but, notably, infliximab and adalimumab have been associated with worsened disease and complications when used in TRAPS patients [3, 4]. In both autoimmune and autoinflammatory conditions with accompanying AA amyloidosis, there are case reports documenting the effectiveness of anti-TNF agents in blunting

A.K. Ombrello, MD (✉)
Inflammatory Disease Section, National Human Genome Research Institute, National Institutes of Health, 10 Center Drive, 4N/208 MSC 1375, Bethesda, MD 20892, USA
e-mail: ombrelloak@mail.nih.gov

© Springer International Publishing Switzerland 2015
M.M. Picken et al. (eds.), *Amyloid and Related Disorders*, Current Clinical Pathology,
DOI 10.1007/978-3-319-19294-9_38

the progression of the amyloidosis [5–11]. There are newer anti-TNF agents such as certolizumab, the human anti-TNF-α (alpha) antibody Fab′ fragment that is chemically linked to polyethylene glycol (approved for use in patients with RA and Crohn's disease), and golimumab, the human IgG1κ (kappa) monoclonal antibody specific for human TNF-α (approved for use in patients with RA and AS) whose efficacy has not yet been reported in patients with AA amyloidosis.

Regarding adverse effects of the anti-TNF medications, reactivation of tuberculosis and hepatitis B are two well-established complications (Table 38.1). Additionally, the development of various antibodies, autoantibodies, as well as autoimmune disease has been noted in patients taking anti-TNF agents. There has been a lot of investigation into a potential risk for malignancies, especially lymphoma, solid tumor, and non-melanoma skin cancer. Although an association with non-melanoma skin cancer has been established, there is no other compelling evidence that supports patients having an increased risk of malignancy on anti-TNF agents. A potential association between these medications and malignancy has been difficult to parse out as the diseases treated by anti-TNF agents, historically, have predisposition for malignancy development [12]. Extreme caution should be used if prescribing anti-TNF agents to patients with a history of congestive heart failure or demyelinating disease, as use can cause exacerbations in their underlying cardiac and neurologic disease.

The interleukin-1 (IL-1) pathway is the target of multiple biologic medications used in autoimmune and autoinflammatory diseases. The three available IL-1 antagonists include anakinra (IL-1 receptor antagonist), rilonacept (soluble IL-1 receptor decoy), and C (long-acting, fully human IgG1 anti-Il-1β (beta) monoclonal antibody). Due to their markedly different half-lives,

anakinra is given as a daily subcutaneous injection, whereas rilonacept is given via weekly subcutaneous injection and canakinumab is given subcutaneously every 8 weeks. Anakinra has been an effective treatment for patients with RA, SJIA, and polyarticular JIA [13, 14]. In patients with periodic fever syndromes, anakinra has been used in patients with FMF who are nonresponders to colchicine as well as patients with TRAPS, the deficiency of IL-1 receptor antagonist (DIRA), and hyper-IgD syndrome (HIDS) and those with one of the cryopyrinopathies [familial cold auto-inflammatory syndrome (FCAS), Muckle–Wells syndrome (MWS), and neonatal onset multisystem autoinflammatory disease/chronic infantile neurologic cutaneous and articular syndrome (NOMID/CINCA)] [15–22]. The longer acting rilonacept and canakinumab have been approved for use in patients with FCAS and MWS and are also being used in NOMID patients [21–26]. Regarding patients with AA amyloidosis, the various IL-1 inhibitors have been successful at slowing the progression of and, in some cases, treatment results in regression of amyloid-associated proteinuria [15, 26–30].

A newer therapy for the treatment of RA and SJIA is tocilizumab, the humanized anti-human IL-6 receptor antibody. Preliminary evidence has shown efficacy in treating both RA- and SJIA-associated AA amyloidosis [31, 32]. Currently ongoing is an international trial using the molecule, eprodisate disodium, in patients with AA amyloidosis-associated nephropathy. By binding the amyloidogenic precursor proteins, eprodisate disodium attempts to prevent the deposition of amyloid in organs, hence preserving renal function. For more information regarding ongoing clinical trials involving these medications for the diseases discussed above, the website: www.clinicaltrials.gov maintains a database of federally and privately supported clinical trials conducted worldwide.

Table 38.1 The anti-TNF medications

Anti-TNF medication	Type	Administered	Diseases treated	AA amyloidosis treatment	Infection risk	Use with caution in patients with	Monitoring	Antibody, autoimmune associations
Etanercept	Soluble p75 TNFR:Fc fusion protein	Subcutaneous	RA AS Psoriatic arthritis TRAPS JIA	Case reports	Tuberculosis Fungal opportunistic hepatitis B reactivation	Congestive heart failure Demyelinating disease Hematologic disorders	Annual PPD Hepatitis B screening prior to therapy	Lupus-like syndrome
Adalimumab	Fully humanized monoclonal antibody	Subcutaneous	RA AS Psoriatic arthritis IBD JIA	Case reports	Tuberculosis Fungal opportunistic hepatitis B reactivation	Congestive heart failure Demyelinating disease Hematologic disorders	Annual PPD Hepatitis B screening prior to therapy	Lupus-like syndrome Human antihuman antibodies
Infliximab	Chimeric antibody (mouse/human)	Intravenous	RA Psoriatic arthritis AS IBD	Case reports	Tuberculosis Fungal infections Opportunistic infections	Congestive heart failure Demyelinating disease Hematologic disorders	Annual PPD Hepatitis B screening prior to therapy	Lupus-like syndrome Human antichimeric antibodies
Certolizumab	Pegylated humanized Fab' fragment	Subcutaneous	RA Crohn's disease AS Psoriatic arthritis	No reports	Tuberculosis Fungal infections Opportunistic infections	Congestive heart failure Demyelinating disease Hematologic disorders	Annual PPD Hepatitis B screening prior to therapy	Lupus-like syndrome
Golimumab	Human IgG1κ (kappa) antibody	Subcutaneous	RA AS Psoriatic arthritis Ulcerative colitis	No reports	Tuberculosis Fungal infections Opportunistic infections	Congestive heart failure Demyelinating disease Hematologic disorders	Annual PPD Hepatitis B screening prior to therapy	Not described

References

1. Immonen K, Savolainen A, Kautiainen H, Hakala M. Longterm outcome of amyloidosis associated with juvenile idiopathic arthritis. J Rheumatol. 2008;35:907–12.
2. Immonen K, Finne P, Gronhagen-Riska C, et al. A marked decline in the incidence of renal replacement therapy for amyloidosis associated with inflammatory rheumatic diseases—data from nationwide registries in Finland. Amyloid. 2011;18:25–8.
3. Drewe E, Powell RJ, McDermott EM. Comment on: failure of anti-TNF therapy in TNF receptor 1-associated periodic syndrome (TRAPS). Rheumatology (Oxford). 2007;46:1865–6.
4. Jacobelli S, Andre M, Alexandra JF, Dode C, Papo T. Failure of anti-TNF therapy in TNF receptor 1-associated periodic syndrome (TRAPS). Rheumatology (Oxford). 2007;46:1211–2.
5. Nakamura T, Higashi S, Tomoda K, Tsukano M, Shono M. Etanercept can induce resolution of renal deterioration in patients with amyloid A amyloidosis secondary to rheumatoid arthritis. Clin Rheumatol. 2010;29:1395–401.
6. Kuroda T, Otaki Y, Sato H, et al. A case of AA amyloidosis associated with rheumatoid arthritis effectively treated with infliximab. Rheumatol Int. 2008;28:1155–9.
7. Kuroda T, Wada Y, Kobayashi D, et al. Effective anti-TNF-alpha therapy can induce rapid resolution and sustained decrease of gastroduodenal mucosal amyloid deposits in reactive amyloidosis associated with rheumatoid arthritis. J Rheumatol. 2009;36:2409–15.
8. Kobak S, Oksel F, Kabasakal Y, Doganavsargil E. Ankylosing spondylitis-related secondary amyloidosis responded well to etanercept: a report of three patients. Clin Rheumatol. 2007;12:2191–4.
9. Iizuka M, Sagara S, Etou T. Efficacy of scheduled infliximab maintenance therapy on systemic amyloidosis associated with Crohn's disease. Inflamm Bowel Dis. 2011;17(7):E67–8.
10. Park YK, Han DS, Eun CS. Systemic amyloidosis with Crohn's disease treated with infliximab. Inflamm Bowel Dis. 2008;14:431–2.
11. Drewe E, Huggins ML, Morgan AG, Cassidy MJ, Powell RJ. Treatment of renal amyloidosis with etanercept in tumour necrosis factor receptor-associated periodic syndrome. Rheumatology (Oxford). 2004;43:1405–8.
12. Le Blay P, Mouterde G, Barnetche T, Morel J, Combe B. Risk of malignancy including non-melanoma skin cancers with anti-tumor necrosis factor therapy in patients with rheumatoid arthritis: meta-analysis of registries and systematic review of long-term extension studies. Clin Exp Rheumatol. 2012;30(5):756–64.
13. Jiang Y, Genant HK, Watt I, et al. A multicenter, double-blind, dose-ranging, randomized, placebo-controlled study of recombinant human interleukin-1 receptor antagonist in patients with rheumatoid arthritis:

radiologic progression and correlation of Genant and Larsen scores. Arthritis Rheum. 2000;43:1001–9.
14. Quartier P, Allantaz F, Cimaz R, et al. A multicentre, randomized, double-blind, placebo-controlled trial with the interleukin-1 receptor antagonist in patients with systemic-onset juvenile idiopathic arthritis (ANAJIS trial). Ann Rheum Dis. 2011;70:747–54.
15. Meinzer U, Quartier P, Alexandra JF, Hentgen V, Retornaz F, Kone-Paut I. Interleukin-1 targeting drugs in familial Mediterranean fever: a case series and a review of the literature. Semin Arthritis Rheum. 2011;41(2):265–71.
16. Gattorno M, Pelagatti MA, Meini A, et al. Persistent efficacy of anakinra in patients with tumor necrosis factor receptor-associated periodic syndrome. Arthritis Rheum. 2008;58(5):1516–20.
17. Aksentijevich I, Masters SL, Ferguson PJ, et al. An autoinflammatory disease with deficiency of the interleukin-1-receptor antagonist. N Engl J Med. 2009;360:2426–37.
18. Hoffman HM, Rosengren S, Boyle DL, et al. Prevention of cold-associated acute inflammation in familial cold autoinflammatory syndrome by interleukin-1 receptor antagonist. Lancet. 2004;364:1779–85.
19. Kuemmerle-Deschner JB, Tyrrell PN, Koetter I, et al. Efficacy and safety of anakinra therapy in pediatric and adult patients with the autoinflammatory Muckle-Wells syndrome. Arthritis Rheum. 2011;63(3):840–9.
20. Goldbach-Mansky R, Daily NJ, Canna SW, et al. Neonatal-onset multisystem inflammatory disease responsive to interleukin-1 beta inhibition. N Engl J Med. 2006;355:581–92.
21. Hoffman HM, Throne ML, Amar NJ, et al. Efficacy and safety of rilonacept (interleukin-1 trap) in patients with cryopyrin-associated periodic syndromes results from two sequential placebo-controlled studies. Arthritis Rheum. 2008;58(8):2443–52.
22. Moll M, Kuemmerle-Deschner JB. Inflammasome and cytokine blocking strategies in autoinflammatory disorders. Clin Immunol. 2013;147(3):242–75.
23. Goldbach-Mansky R, Shroff SD, Wilson M, et al. A pilot study to evaluate the safety and efficacy of the long-acting interleukin-1 inhibitor rilonacept (interleukin-1 trap) in patients with familial cold autoinflammatory syndrome. Arthritis Rheum. 2008;58:2432–42.
24. Kuemmerle-Deschner JB, Ramos E, Blank N, et al. Canakinumab (ACZ885, a fully human IgG1 anti-IL-1β (beta) mAb) induces sustained remission in pediatric patients with cryopyrin-associated periodic syndrome (CAPS). Arthritis Res Ther. 2011;13(1):R34.
25. Lachmann HJ, Kone-Paut I, Kuemmerle-Deschner JB, et al. Use of canakinumab in the cryopyrin-associated periodic syndrome. N Engl J Med. 2009;360:2416–25.
26. Ter Haar N, Lachmann H, Ozen S, et al. Treatment of autoinflammatory diseases: results from the Eurofever Registry and a literature review. Ann Rheum Dis. 2013;72(5):678–85.
27. Obici L, Meini A, Cattlini M, et al. Favourable and sustained response to anakinra in tumour necrosis

factor receptor-associate periodic syndrome (TRAPS) with or without AA amyloidosis. Ann Rheum Dis. 2011;70(8):1511–2.

28. Leslie KS, Lachmann HJ, Bruning E, et al. Phenotype, genotype, and sustained response to anakinra in 22 patients with autoinflammatory disease associated with *CIAS-1/NALP3* mutations. Arch Dermatol. 2006;142:1591–7.

29. Neven B, Marvillet I, Terrada C, et al. Long-term efficacy of the interleukin-1 receptor antagonist anakinra in ten patients with neonatal-onset multisystem inflammatory disease/chronic infantile neurologic, cutaneous, articular syndrome. Arthritis Rheum. 2010;62(1):258–67.

30. Thornton BD, Hoffman HM, Bhat A, Don BR. Successful treatment of renal amyloidosis due to familial cold autoinflammatory syndrome using and interleukin 1 receptor antagonist. Am J Kidney Dis. 2007;49(3):477–81.

31. Inoue D, Arima H, Kawanami C, et al. Excellent therapeutic effect of tocilizumab on intestinal amyloid A deposition secondary to active rheumatoid arthritis. Clin Rheumatol. 2010;29:1195–7.

32. Okuda Y, Takasugi K. Successful use of a humanized anti-interleukin-6 receptor antibody, tocilizumab, to treat amyloid A amyloidosis complicating juvenile idiopathic arthritis. Arthritis Rheum. 2006;54: 2997–3000.

Timothy Craig Allen

Diagnostic and Therapeutic Amyloidosis Advances

Amyloidosis, characterized by the deposition of amyloid protein in an abnormal fibrillar form [1–3], involves a variety of uncommon and complex systemic diseases, the classification of which necessitates the timely identification of the specific molecular type of amyloid protein fibril involved [1]. More than 25 different types of proteins, and many additional variants, may cause amyloidosis [1]. It may occur as systemic, localized, systemic and localized, cerebral, or extracerebral disease [1]. There may be multiple organ involvement, with the kidney most commonly involved. Heart, lung, and liver involvement may also be found [1–3]. Systemic amyloidosis typically occurs as AL amyloidosis, also termed primary amyloidosis, which is derived from an immunoglobulin light chain or a light chain fragment; or may occur as AA amyloidosis, formerly termed secondary amyloidosis, which is associated with chronic inflammatory processes or chronic infections [1]. Hereditary amyloidoses,

thought to be an underdiagnosed amyloidosis, may clinically mimic AL amyloidosis, and include, among others, amyloid derived from fibrinogen A alpha chain (Afib), amyloid derived from transthyretin (ATTR), amyloid derived from a mutant of lysozyme (ALys), and amyloidosis derived from apolipoprotein AI (AApo AI) [1]. More recently amyloidosis derived from leukocyte chemotactic factor-2 (ALect-2) was added to systemic amyloidosis [2]. There has recently been a "formidable evolution" of systemic amyloidoses treatments from one of entirely supportive disease management to one dependent upon the specific molecular type of amyloid protein involved, utilizing "quite diverse, radical, and aggressive treatments," including chemotherapeutic regimens, some with stem cell rescue; stem cell transplantation; liver transplantation; and liver transplantation combined with heart or kidney transplantation [1]. Currently, treatments once only provided to younger patients are showing benefits in older adults, and research is ongoing [1]. These remarkable therapeutic advances for some specific types of amyloidosis depend upon early, specific, and accurate amyloidosis diagnosis in order to best ensure appropriate patient treatment and optimize prognosis [1]. Hence not only late diagnosis but also misdiagnosis of the amyloidosis-type consequently leading to the application of aggressive treatment is dangerous [1, 4].

T.C. Allen, MD, JD (✉)
Department of Pathology, The University of Texas
Medical Branch, 301 University Blvd., Galveston,
TX 77555, USA
e-mail: tcallen@utmb.edu

© Springer International Publishing Switzerland 2015
M.M. Picken et al. (eds.), *Amyloid and Related Disorders*, Current Clinical Pathology,
DOI 10.1007/978-3-319-19294-9_39

Increased Medical-Legal Risk Due to Alleged Diagnostic Delay or Misdiagnosis

Amyloidosis may mimic many other diseases and is frequently difficult to diagnose; patients present with variable and often general symptoms and progress variably in their disease courses [3]. In some cases other diseases mask amyloidosis' sometimes subtle signs and symptoms. Because of these concerns, "it is imperative that the criteria for amyloid-type diagnoses be stringent" [1]. Diagnostic workup may not end with the diagnosis of amyloidosis; for example, kidney biopsy may be used in considering liver transplantation [1].

Pathology workup continues to evolve. Although Congo red stain is still considered the "gold standard" for amyloidosis, some other older methods have been eliminated. For example: "[i]t must be stressed that potassium permanganate stain currently has no role in amyloid typing" [1]. Further, diagnosing AL type and differentiating it from hereditary amyloidosis may be challenging [1]. Although immunohistochemical diagnosis of AA-type amyloidosis remains generally reliable, it may require the use of panels of immunostains, including repeat panels, for accurate diagnosis [1]. Electron microscopy and Western blotting may also need to be employed for diagnosis, as they have been shown to in some cases provide better diagnostic results than immunohistochemical staining [1]. In other cases, tandem mass spectrometry with laser microdissection has been successfully applied to amyloid typing [5]. When therapy was supportive, diagnosis did nothing to alter patient prognosis; however, diagnostic and therapeutic advances increase the potential for diagnostic delay or misdiagnosis, ultimately to the patients' detriment, with consequentially increased physician risk of medical malpractice lawsuits.

Physician responsibility for timely and accurate amyloidosis diagnosis is now correspondingly greater. Delayed diagnosis, failure to diagnose, and misdiagnosis are the typical allegations in medical malpractice lawsuits, and due to the potential for serious injury where there is spe- cific, effective therapy available, would likely be the alleged cause of action in cases of amyloidosis misdiagnosis or diagnostic delay [4, 6–8]. The potential for large damage awards exists, because damage allocation may include the cost of medical care, lost wages and income, loss of spousal companionship, potential permanent disfigurement, and pain and suffering [7].

While lawsuits for failure to diagnose, misdiagnosis, or delayed diagnosis of amyloidosis have not yet emerged in the legal literature, their likelihood is increasing, as discussed below. As such, it behooves physicians, both specialists in amyloidosis and nonspecialists, to better understand the basics of medical malpractice, including possible avenues for plaintiff claims and potential defenses.

Medical Malpractice Basics

Detailed examinations of the medical malpractice system can be found [6]. Briefly, a claim of failure to diagnose or delayed diagnosis is a claim of medical malpractice, which is an alleged tort. A tort is "damage, injury, or a wrongful act done willfully, negligently, or in circumstances involving strict liability, but not involving breach of contract, for which a civil suit can be brought" [9]. Medical malpractice tort allegations generally involve allegations of negligence [6]. Negligence is "[c]onduct which falls below the standard established by law for the protection of others against unreasonable risk of harm; it is a departure from the conduct expectable of a reasonably prudent person under like circumstances" [10]. To be held negligent, a physician must be found to have committed a medical error that rises to the level of a breach of duty of care to the patient, i.e., not met the standard of care required in caring for the patient [6]. Today's "reasonable person" standard is determined by whether a physician "proceed[ed] with such reasonable caution as a prudent man would have exercised under such circumstances" [6, 11]. Unfortunately, what constitutes the medical malpractice standard of care in a courtroom has not been well settled; and currently, there are numerous definitions and explanations of "standard of care" in medical malpractice [6]. The standard of care may not be straightforward or easily determined [6, 12]. As Richard Epstein noted, "Everyone supports a standard of reasonable care, but everyone interprets it just a little bit differently" [6, 13]. Standard of care is frequently determined by the court from the testimony of expert witnesses [14]. The expert has an obligation of candor toward the court; however, "standards of care are routinely interpreted oppositely by expert witnesses…[and] both sides devote considerable effort to screening and disqualifying consultant experts whose views do not represent the 'standard' the attorney needs to make the case. The attorney is doing his or her job" [6, 15]. As such, expert witness shopping for "hired guns" often leads to a confusing "battle of the experts" [6].

The Expansion of the "Loss-of-Chance" Doctrine

Traditional tort theory requires that for a plaintiff to succeed in a medical malpractice lawsuit, a physician's actions must be proved to "more likely than not" have caused the injury [16–18]. In other words, "[i]f the plaintiff had a 51% chance of survival, and the misdiagnosis reduced that chance to zero, the estate is awarded full wrongful death damages, but if the patient had only a 49% chance of survival, and the misdiagnosis reduced it to zero, the plaintiff receives nothing. Thus, whenever the chance of survival is less than even, the 'all or nothing' rule gives a 'blanket release from liability for doctors and hospitals…regardless of how flagrant the negligence'" [17]. Claims of injustice from this "all-or-nothing approach" has led courts, and over the last two decades, to adopt the "loss-of-chance" doctrine, which views a person's prospect for surviving a serious medical condition as something of value, "even if the possibility of recovery was less than even (i.e., less than a 50 % chance) prior to the physician's allegedly tortuous conduct" [17, 19].

Courts are increasingly adopting the "loss-of-chance" doctrine in medical malpractice cases

[20–27]. Courts that accept that a physician's action would "more likely than not" caused a patient's injury can hold physicians liable for patient injury [28]. Courts that accept less of an injury, i.e., a patient's "loss of chance" of any clinical improvement or prolonged survival, can nonetheless impose liability [24]. Currently, "loss-of-chance" liability is accepted by approximately half the states, and the legal trend shows increasing acceptance, with five of seven state supreme courts accepting the doctrine [29]. The doctrine nonetheless is controversial [18, 30–35]. "One of the most debated issues involving the loss of chance is causation" [36]. "A majority of states adopting an exception for loss-of-chance plaintiffs have done so by relaxing the causation standard to less than the normal preponderance-of-the-evidence threshold. In applying a relaxed standard, "freed from its moorings" [21], these states provide a loss-of-chance plaintiff an opportunity to recover damages despite an inability to prove causation by a preponderance of the evidence. This is achieved by allowing the presentation of expert testimony to demonstrate that the plaintiff was either deprived of a 'substantial possibility' of survival or recovery or simply incurred an 'increased risk' of suffering the ultimate injury as a result of the defendant's negligence" [36]. With today's new diagnostic criteria, new diagnostic methods, and new therapies for patients with amyloidosis which are more specific to the exact type of fibril protein causing the amyloidosis, and for which early therapy yields a better prognosis, it is reasonable to imagine that "loss-of-chance" doctrine may be useful for plaintiffs who cannot show that the delayed diagnosis or misdiagnosis was more likely than not the proximate cause of the plaintiff's injury.

Amyloidosis' varied presentations mimicking other diseases, its new specific diagnostic criteria and therapies, its chronic nature, and the prognostic benefit of its early diagnosis all increase the medical-legal risk of its misdiagnosis or delayed diagnosis; and suggest that the "loss-of-chance" doctrine might be an advantageous theory of physician liability [30]. The complexity and difficulty in diagnosing amyloidosis early, and diagnosing the specific type of fibril protein involved accurately, will likely be considered by plaintiffs' attorneys to be part of "routine" medical practice and the "standard of care." As one medical malpractice attorney group makes clear, "Not every patient presents to a physician with 'classic' signs and symptoms. If they did, we would not need skilled physicians. At [our law office] we do not accept the 'the symptoms were atypical' defense when a preventable injury has occurred" [37].

Supporters of the "loss-of-chance" doctrine note that "the loss-of-chance doctrine makes up for all of the traditional all-or-nothing approach's shortcomings. First, where the traditional approach forecloses recovery to those whose injuries do not meet its arbitrary thresholds, the loss-of-chance doctrine provides a theory of causation that allows a jury to award recovery to any plaintiff who can prove a real loss resulting from a physician's negligence. Next, instead of awarding full damages or no damages at all, one of the essential traits of the doctrine is to provide a tailor-made recovery for a prevailing plaintiff that is proportional to the actual harm incurred. Lastly, the loss-of-chance doctrine is an improvement because it deters negligence, in contrast to the traditional rule which fails to hold physicians accountable in their treatment of seriously ill and injured patients. The loss-of-chance doctrine's policy of allowing recovery to all patients who can prove a lost chance, regardless of what their original chance was, provides a mechanism to deter negligent treatment of those patients who can least afford to suffer it" [38].

Critics of the "loss-of-chance" doctrine, "which has been described as 'the most pernicious example of a new tort action resulting in expanded liability,'" consider it "a cause of action unique to medical malpractice litigation [which] permits a patient-turned-plaintiff to recover damages from a doctor-turned-defendant without even needing to establish that the doctor was probably (i.e., more likely than not) responsible for the patient's alleged injury" [39]. The "loss-of-chance" doctrine "seemingly thwarts our civil litigation system's presumption that a defendant should not be held liable unless the plaintiff demonstrates that the defendant more likely than not

caused the plaintiff's injury. To hold a defendant liable in any other instance, opponents of the doctrine argue, is to 'undercut the truth-seeking function of the courts'" [39]. Proponents of the "loss-of-chance" doctrine respond that "pure loss of chance allows for recovery when the plaintiff proves to a preponderance of the evidence that the doctor caused the lost chance. In this light, when the recovery is for the lost chance, the [proximate cause] standard is upheld" [40]. Another common complaint about the "loss- of-chance" doctrine is that calculation of damages is extremely difficult [41]. "Pure loss of chance involves complex statistical analysis and expert testimony that may be confusing for the jury and result in inappropriate decisions" [40]. Indeed, calculation of damages has been called "a 'rabbit-out-of-the-hat' approach" in "loss-of-chance" lawsuits [32]. There are also other issues regarding the use of the "loss-of-chance" doctrine, including when, if ever, a state's statute of limitations precludes a medical malpractice lawsuit utilizing the "loss-of-chance" doctrine; and whether state wrongful death statutes preclude the use of the "loss-of-chance" doctrine [42, 43].

Another concern among critics of the "loss-of-chance" doctrine is that by lowering the standard for which plaintiffs can bring medical malpractice lawsuits that "'we're going to see a barrage…of stand-alone loss of chance cases apart from the wrongful-death medical-malpractice claims that have always been allowed'" [44]. However, proponents of the "loss-of-chance" doctrine disagree, noting that "in cases where the chances of survival were modest, plaintiffs will have little monetary incentive to bring a case to trial because damages would be drastically reduced to account for the preexisting condition" [44]. And, "[a]s a whole, courts in states that have adopted the lost-chance doctrine have shown an ability to confine the doctrine's scope and overall effect on civil litigation. This has been accomplished by expressly limiting the doctrine to medical malpractice cases only, refusing to relax expert testimony requirements, continuing to require valid statistical evidence, and refusing to apply the doctrine in situations where traditional but-for causation is more appropriate. Thus, while opponents of the doctrine may have fears that the lost-chance concept will lead to unwanted consequences, judges have thus far been able to apply the doctrine carefully and appropriately" [45].

Conclusion

Given the complexity inherent in the diagnosis of amyloidosis, as well as the current need for accurate and early diagnosis, "loss-of-chance" doctrine might be employed in determining liability in some amyloidosis-related medical malpractice lawsuits. Even with increased medical malpractice risk in diagnosing amyloidosis, physicians can take proactive steps that help ensure patient care quality and resultantly reduce medical malpractice risk. As with any medical situation, the best protection from an amyloidosis diagnosis-related medical malpractice lawsuit is appropriate physician understanding of amyloidosis, including the complexities of amyloidosis diagnosis and treatment. Further, similar to other medical malpractice situations, clear and careful documentation is essential to explain physician actions and decisions, so providing the best defense in an amyloidosis diagnosis-related medical malpractice lawsuit. Many cases alleging delayed diagnosis "can be defended on the basis of the aggressiveness of the [disease] but only with adequate documentation of clinical findings, clinical impressions and outcomes of tests and biopsies. Because patients' refusal to undergo recommended procedures can independently form the basis of a defense, practitioners also must document these actions" [7].

References

1. Picken MM. New insights into systemic amyloidosis: the importance of diagnosis of specific type. Curr Opin Nephrol Hypertens. 2007;16(3):196–203.
2. Picken MM. Modern approaches to the treatment of amyloidosis: the critical importance of early detection in surgical pathology. Adv Anat Pathol. 2013;20(6):424–39.
3. Rajagopala S, Singh N, Gupta K, Gupta D. Pulmonary amyloidosis in Sjogren's syndrome: a case report and systematic review of the literature. Respirology. 2010;15(5):860–6.
4. Picken MM. Alect2 amyloidosis: primum non nocere (first, do no harm). Kidney Int. 2014;86(2):229–32.
5. Vrana JA, Gamez JD, Madden BJ, Theis JD, Bergen 3rd HR, Dogan A. Classification of amyloidosis by laser microdissection and mass spectrometry-based proteomic analysis in clinical biopsy specimens. Blood. 2009;114(24):4957–9.
6. Allen TC. Medicolegal issues in pathology. Arch Pathol Lab Med. 2008;132(2):186–91.
7. Epstein JB, Sciubba JJ, Banasek TE, Hay LJ. Failure to diagnose and delayed diagnosis of cancer: medicolegal issues. J Am Dent Assoc. 2009;140(12):1494–503.
8. Kern KA. The delayed diagnosis of breast cancer: medicolegal implications and risk prevention for surgeons. Breast Dis. 2001;12:145–58.
9. The American Heritage dictionary of the English language. 4th ed. Boston: Houghton Mifflin; 2000.
10. Black's law dictionary. 6th ed. St. Paul, MN: West; 1991.
11. Vaughan v. Menlove, 132 Eng Rep 490 (CP) 1837.
12. The negligence issue. In: Epstein RA, editor. Cases and materials on torts. Boston, MA: Little Brown; 1995. p. 229.
13. Epstein RA. History, doctrine, and evolution of liability, Mortal peril: our inalienable right to health care? New York: Addison Wesley; 1997. p. 376.
14. Havighurst CC, Hutt PB, McNeil BJ, Miller W. Evidence: its meanings in health care and in law. (Summary of the 10 April 2000 IOM and AHRQ Workshop, "Evidence": its meanings and uses in law, medicine, and health care). J Health Polit Policy Law. 2001;26(2):195–215.
15. Jones JW, McCullough LB, Richman BW. Standard of care: what does it really mean? J Vasc Surg. 2004;40(6):1255–7.
16. Buckler S. Loss of chance: recovery for the lost opportunity of survival—Matsuyama v. Birnbaum, 890 N.E.2d 817 (Mass. 2008). J Health Biomed Law. (2009);5:117–129.
17. Renehan JF. A new frontier: the loss of chance doctrine in medical malpractice cases. BBJ. 2009;53:14, 15.
18. Leslie K, Bramley D, Shulman M, Kennedy E. Loss of chance in medical negligence. Anaesth Intensive Care. 2014;42(3):298–302.
19. Dyer C. Negligence through loss of chance. Br Med J (Clin Res Ed). 1986;293(6561):1560–1.
20. Negligence—Failure to carry out physical examination and biopsy—damages for loss of chance of extended lifespan. Brown v Willington [2001] ACTSC 100. J Law Med. 2002;9:397–8.
21. Garwin MJ. Risk creation, loss of chance, and legal liability. Hematol Oncol Clin North Am. 2002;16(6):1351–63.
22. Faunce T, McEwan A. The High Court's lost chance in medical negligence: Tabet v Gett (2010) 240 CLR 537. J Law Med. 2010;18:275–83.

23. Molinelli A, Bonsignore A, Capecchi M, Calabria G. Loss of chance: a new kind of damage to ophthalmologic patients from Europe to Italy. Eur J Ophthalmol. 2011;21(3):310–4 [Epub ahead of print].
24. Johnson LJ. State laws on loss of chance of survival continue to evolve. Med Econ. 2013;90(1):46–7.
25. Tibballs J. Loss of chance: a new development in medical negligence law. Med J Aust. 2007;187(4): 233–5.
26. Beraldo Ade M, Pereira PM. The theory of loss of chance in medical liability applied within Brazilian jurisprudence. Med Law. 2012;31(2):265–81.
27. Bhatia N, Tibballs J. Legal clarification of "loss of chance of a better outcome" in Australia. Med J Aust. 2012;196(3):167–8.
28. Saver JL. Number needed to treat estimates incorporating effects over the entire range of clinical outcomes: novel derivation method and application to thrombolytic therapy for acute stroke. Arch Neurol. 2004;61(7):1066–70.
29. Dahl D. 'Loss of chance' damages gaining acceptance. *Lawyers USA.* 2008; Aug. 11. http://www.allbusiness.com/legal/trial-procedure-suits-claims/11483848-1.html. Accessed 29 July 2014.
30. Bal BS, Brenner LH. Medicolegal sidebar: the law and social values: loss of chance. Clin Orthop Relat Res. 2014;472(10):2923–6.
31. Jerjes W, Upile T. English law for the surgeon III: loss of chance: Gregg v Scott revisited. Head Neck Oncol. 2012;4:67.
32. Brahams D. Loss of chance of survival. Lancet. 1996;348(9042):1604.
33. Brahams D. Loss of a chance of survival: US and UK compared. Med Leg J. 1996;64(Pt 4):135–6.
34. Bird S. Loss of chance: what loss? Aust Fam Physician. 2006;35(5):351–2.
35. Casacelli B. Losing a chance to survive: an examination of the loss of chance doctrine within the context of a wrongful death action. J Health Biomed Law. 2014;9:521, 552.
36. Warzecha CM. The loss of chance doctrine in Arkansas and the door left open: revisiting Holt ex rel. Holt v. Wagner. Ark Law Rev. 2010;63:785, 803.
37. Chicago brain hemorrhage misdiagnosis lawyers. http://www.cirignani.com/Brain-Injuries/Missed-Brain-Hemorrhage.shtml. Accessed 4/9/11.
38. Warzecha CM. The loss of chance doctrine in Arkansas and the door left open: revisiting Holt ex rel. Holt v. Wagner. Ark Law Rev. 2010;63:785, 802.
39. Koch SR. Whose loss is it anyway? Effects of the "lost-chance" doctrine on civil litigation and medical malpractice insurance. NCL Rev. 2010;88:595, 598–9.
40. Buckler S. Loss of chance: recovery for the lost opportunity of survival—Matsuyama v. Birnbaum, 890 N.E.2d 819 (Mass. 2008). J Health Biomed Law. 2008;5:117, 128.
41. Frasca R. Loss of chance rules and the valuation of loss of chance damages. J Legal Econ. 2009;15:91.
42. Buckler S. Loss of chance: recovery for the lost opportunity of survival—Matsuyama v. Birnbaum, 890 N.E.2d 819 (Mass. 2008). J Health Biomed Law. 2008;5:117, 123.
43. Zarick AL. Damage deferred: determining when a cause of action begins to accrue for a cancer misdiagnosis claim. Univ Toledo Law Rev. 2010;41:445, 460–1.
44. Koch SR. Whose loss is it anyway? Effects of the "lost-chance" doctrine on civil litigation and medical malpractice insurance. NCL Rev. 2010;88:595, 619.
45. Koch SR. Whose loss is it anyway? Effects of the "lost-chance" doctrine on civil litigation and medical malpractice insurance. NCL Rev. 2010;88:595, 635.

Amyloidosis from the Patient's Perspective

Muriel Finkel

The information and views presented in this chapter are derived from e-mail and personal contacts with members of the Amyloidosis Support Groups, Inc.(ASG), a 501(c)(3) charity-based in the United States. Despite its corporate status, this is a not-for-profit entity whose primary purpose is to offer advice and support to patients who, for the first time, are confronted by a diagnosis of amyloidosis. Initial encounters with patients frequently derive from contacts instigated via the group's websites (http://www.amyloidosissupport.org and http://www.amyloidosisonline.com) and typically arise as a result of patients searching for information about amyloidosis on the Internet. The support group currently has over 3000 members in the USA and over 2000 registered with amyloidosisonline.com at Yahoo. In total, since its inception, the support group has advised over 4500 patients worldwide. Being a support advocacy group, we strive to stay current with the latest developments, and to maintain contacts with amyloidosis experts at centers specializing in its treatment. We have a medical advisory board to answer the medical questions that constantly arise from our online group sessions and face-to-face meetings. We also ask our members to share their experiences with their local doctors, in order to enhance grassroots awareness of the disease.

In the vast majority of cases, the patient's first response to a diagnosis of amyloidosis is a total lack of comprehension, never having encountered the term on any previous occasion. The most common concerns are: "Am I going to die? I can't even pronounce it. My doctor had to leave the room and look it up. What "stage" is it? What about my family and how will their lives be disrupted? What organs are involved and can my local doctor, in my small town, take care of them? Why is there no center specializing in the treatment of amyloidosis in my big city? Why me? How did I get this disease?" The list of questions and concerns is as long as it would be for a common disease, plus extra queries for the rare disease.

These questions usually prompt the patient to search for information on the Internet. Of the literally millions of possible "hits" for amyloidosis that are available from the Internet, only a few are accurate, current, and peer-reviewed. Almost invariably, articles informing the patient that death is imminent are the result. Typically, the patient then feels more overwhelmed than after first receiving the diagnosis. For these reasons, the ASG tries to be as prominent as possible among the results of Internet searches, so that patients find and contact us, using our toll-free telephone number, in search of help and guidance.

M. Finkel (✉)
Amyloidosis Support Groups, Inc.,
232 Orchard Drive, Wood Dale, IL 60191, USA
e-mail: muriel@finkelsupply.com;
http://www.amyloidosissupport.org

© Springer International Publishing Switzerland 2015

525

M.M. Picken et al. (eds.), *Amyloid and Related Disorders*, Current Clinical Pathology,
DOI 10.1007/978-3-319-19294-9_40

The ASG then tries to expedite the patient's search for factual information and to guide them towards experienced centers and doctors specializing in amyloidosis treatment. The ASG's strategy is to provide information on a gradual, steadily increasing basis, reserving the more technical articles until the patient (or caregiver) is calmer and more able to absorb information. In a perfect world, the diagnosis would be made, a recommendation to an experienced center specializing in the treatment of amyloidosis would follow, the patient's insurance company would comply with the recommended treatments, and all would be well. This, however, is typically not the case; in addition to fighting the disease, the patient may also be fighting the insurance company and, in some cases, their local doctor, who may be reluctant to transfer the patient into specialist care. Some patients put themselves completely in the hands of their local general practitioner, often for reasons that, when distilled to their essence, amount to little more than pure sentiment. Unfortunately, this doctor frequently does not know how to treat amyloidosis and is often unwilling to contact experts for help. Up to this point in his/her life, the patient may well have thought of doctors as "all-knowing"; the onset of disillusionment invariably fosters a growing sense of frustration with the medical world. Often, patients resent having to know technical details of amyloid diagnosis (such as the importance of a Congo red stain) and/or treatment, when their general practitioner clearly does not. Typically, patients feel that they have the right to a quick and proper diagnosis by doctors and pathologists working in collaboration.

Table 40.1 presents representative results of a questionnaire that was sent to ASG members who had been diagnosed with amyloidosis. While it was not practical to include all replies, short answers from a selected few are presented, and the table comprises a compilation of the results. As can be seen, there were 20 males and 11 females. Their age at diagnosis ranged from <40 to >70 years. Of the two patients who were younger than 40, one had a family history that was positive for amyloidosis. This patient was subsequently confirmed to have familial amyloidosis and was the *only* patient for whom a diag-

nosis of amyloidosis was not unexpected. The other patient was diagnosed with AL at the age of 37. Most patients (>50 % in this group) were 50–60 years old when the diagnosis was made. While, for many patients, it took several months from the onset of symptoms to a definitive diagnosis of amyloidosis, in approximately 50 % of patients this diagnosis was finally made after >1 year and, in some cases, after several years. Amyloid typing was also delayed in many patients. While initial symptoms were nonspecific in many cases, kidney symptoms proved to be the most efficient pathway to a definitive diagnosis, as a consequence of a kidney biopsy being performed. Many patients had more than one type of biopsy (typically in addition to a bone marrow biopsy). Abdominal fat pad biopsy, which is essentially a noninvasive procedure, currently appears to be underutilized; it was performed in only 24 % of *all* ASG members surveyed. Again, these results illustrate that there is a clear need to increase awareness of amyloidosis, and the available treatment options, among clinicians and pathologists. Please note that many ASG members mentioned the need for increased use of the Congo red stain; a frequent question was: "*Why is it that Congo red stain is not used more often by pathologists?*".

Two of the most common symptoms of amyloidosis are shortness of breath and severe fatigue; these are also, unfortunately, very common and nonspecific. Edema is typically associated with kidney and/or heart problems, which may be due to involvement by amyloidosis. Periorbital purpura may be noticed by the patient, but not always by the physician, since it may be transient. One ASG member, a pregnant woman from New York (age 30+), had edema, periorbital purpura, enlarged tongue, fatigue, weight loss, shortness of breath, and tingling and numbness of the extremities. Amyloidosis was finally diagnosed after about 2 months, by kidney biopsy, but treatment had to be delayed until after the pregnancy. A healthy baby was born and the mother received a stem cell transplant. After many additional chemotherapy treatments to maintain her response, she is now about to embark on a second autologous stem cell transplant. Carpal tunnel

Table 40.1 Excerpts from the ASG patient survey

Age and sex at dx	Interval from symptoms to dx	How long did it take to type it	Initial symptoms	What bx was diagnostic, how many?	What was your life after the dx	What message would you like to convey to the pathologists
72 M	5 years	Immediate	SOB, fatigue, back pain, weight/strength loss, food tasting bad	Kidney bx	N/A	Had gallbladder removed and told my back pain was arthritis. Why no one was checking?
50s M	Several years	3 months	Edema, blood clots	Kidney bx	Returned to a less active normal life, foot amputated	Nephrologists should be more aware, advise regarding biopsy options
40s F	2 months	Immediate	N/A	Bone marrow, fat, kidney bx	Shock, disbelief, depression	Diagnosis should be explained
60 M	>Year	10 weeks		Heart	N/A	More awareness
50s M	Delay—insurance issues	6 months	Foamy frothy urine, and edema	Kidney (+), bone marrow ×2 (−)	Bedridden/wheelchair for the first 5 months	Early treatment is best, best treatment options at specialized centers
70s M	Years	2 months	SOB, fatigue, weakness, edema	Bone marrow, heart bx	I was told there was no treatment	The pathologist's analysis of the biopsy was accurate
50s M	3 years	Months	SOB, proteinuria, hypogammaglobulinemia	Kidney biopsy	ASCT, chemotherapy with full response	The pathologist found my amyloidosis on the first try
50s M	1.5 years	Immediate at referral center	Back pain, proteinuria, edema	Kidney, fat pad, bone marrow	Had ASCT	Do Congo red stains more often
50s M	2 months	Patient unsure	Stomach pains, diarrhea, inability to eat or drink	Heart, kidney, adrenals	Did not tolerate chemotherapy well	More awareness
60s M	1 month	2 months	Edema, Irregular heartbeat	Kidney, bone marrow bx	ASCT, chemotherapy ×2	More Congo red stains, routinely on certain organs
50s F	1 month	2 weeks	Slight edema	Kidney and bone marrow bx	Steroids are difficult and feel overwhelmed	My nephrologist knew nothing, the pathologist found it
50s M	1.5 years	Month	Proteinuria, hoarseness, ED, dizzy standing, fatigue, weight loss, PN	Kidney and bone marrow bx	Trying to cope	If someone has multiple organ or system complaints, do a Congo red stain!
50s F	10 months	Immediately	Proteinuria	Kidney, bone marrow, tongue	After SCT had many side effects, now ok	Do a Congo red stain!
70s M	Several days	Several weeks	Fatigue	Heart, fat, bone marrow	Life is good if I avoid stairs	Test early with Congo red. Awareness
61 F	2 years	Month	Fatigue	Kidney	Support group important	

(continued)

Table 40.1 (continued)

Age and sex at dx	Interval from symptoms to dx	How long did it take to type it	Initial symptoms	What bx was diagnostic, how many?	What was your life after the dx	What message would you like to convey to the pathologists
50s M	Few months	1 month	Spots on face	Skin and bone marrow	Seeking knowledge and to find support	More Congo red-stained biopsies
50s M	6 months	Few days, known MM	Weakness, SOB, loss of appetite	Heart bx	Died a few days after bx	Awareness, patients with MM should be monitored for amyloidosis
61 M	11 months	Few days	Protein in urine	Liver and bone marrow	Devastated, felt alone	More Congo red stains, do not delay giving results
60s F	Years	N/A	Fatigue, kidney Failure, carpal tunnel	Bone marrow, fat pad, kidney	I am still not typed	More Congo red stains
56 F	3 weeks	6 weeks	Lump on upper arm	Biopsy of the lump	Many questions	More testing with Congo red
50s F	1 year	Few weeks	Proteinuria	Fat aspirate and bone marrow	Spent a year undergoing treatments	N/A
60s F	<3 years	3 months	SOB, enlarged tongue, black/blue eyes, fatigue, loss of appetite, edema	Fat (+) bone marrow (−)	Symptoms became worse, thought I was going to die	Congo Red stain, more awareness and knowledge among doctors
37 F	2 months	N/A	Edema, black eyes, enlarged tongue, fatigue, weight loss, PN, SOB	Kidney	Have not been able to return to work	More Congo red stains!
40s F	2 years	1 week	Pea size nodule on the leg that grew	Mass on leg	Scared	More Congo red stains
30S M	2 weeks Dx was expected	Immediate— familial	Cough, fatigue, diarrhea, weight loss	Fat and colonoscopy	Difficult maintaining normal activities	N/A
50s M	2 years	Months	PN, carpal tunnel	Nerve and fat	Still overwhelmed and scared	N/A
50s M	2 years	Immediate	Proteinuria	Kidney	Shock, frightened	More Congo red staining
60s F	3 years	6 months	Proteinuria	Kidney and bone marrow	None	More Congo red staining
70s M	9 months	Immediate	Pleural effusion, SOB, fainting, edema	Bone marrow	No pain, some PN	More Congo red staining
50s M	6 months	1 month	PN, fatigue, arrhythmia	Kidney	Partial response, now 6 years post dx	More Congo red staining
50s M	3 weeks	Immediate	Proteinuria	Kidney and bone marrow	Anxiety and uncertainty	More Congo red staining

syndrome is also frequently mentioned by ASG members. This highlights the contention between doctors and amyloidosis patients over the issue of whether all carpal tunnel syndrome patients should be investigated by biopsy, with analysis by Congo red stain? Doctors say no. Patients say yes. Enlarged tongue (macroglossia), when present, should raise a suspicion of amyloidosis. Nevertheless, one ASG member with multiple myeloma (which is also a risk factor for amyloidosis) had her tongue biopsied, with the resultant diagnosis: "nonspecific mucositis." In this case, a Congo red stain was not performed. Skin changes and easy bruising are two other symptoms of amyloidosis that can mimic many other diseases. An ASG member had what looked like "blood spots" on his face. A dermatologist had the spots biopsied and a diagnosis of amyloidosis was made. After several bone marrow biopsies, the patient was diagnosed with AL amyloidosis and multiple myeloma. After an autologous stem cell transplant, performed over 2 years ago, the patient continues to feel well and is being closely followed. He is, however, deeply concerned about the future. He worries about the return of his disease with symptoms that may be worse than simply "spots on his face."

The possibility of false-positive or false-negative results and/or incorrect typing by less-experienced doctors are also issues that need to be addressed. Thus, one ASG member commented on the questionnaire: "*If they work with a lab that is not familiar with amyloidosis, they should at least tell the patient, and have the sample(s) sent elsewhere.*" The need for consultation with specialized laboratories and amyloidosis treatment centers cannot be over-emphasized. It is critical to obtain proper therapy and to obtain it in a timely fashion. Too often, the ASG sees a considerable delay in contacting centers with experience in treating amyloidosis.

Another ASG member commented: "*When I had 'all' the procedures and tests completed by my gastroenterologist, and nothing was positive, and perhaps they thought I was crazy, why didn't they conduct a fat pad or rectal biopsy? Amyloidosis never entered the doctor's mind even though, put together, all my symptoms pointed to it, and it was not in my imagination.*" This patient was finally diagnosed with familial amyloidosis, had a liver transplant, and is currently doing well.

Amyloidosis is a rare disease, and, therefore, not unexpectedly, many physicians may lack extensive firsthand experience of its diagnosis and treatment. In this connection, the majority of the ASG members who were diagnosed with amyloidosis, and are still living, are patients who were treated at specialized amyloidosis treatment centers. It is extremely important to *screen for amyloidosis* in order to detect it at an early stage among the many patients who present with similar symptoms and to identify those who have, or may be suspected of having, the disease. A proactive approach to the diagnosis of amyloidosis is needed from all physicians, general practitioners, specialists, and pathologists, since this is a disease that can indeed be "hiding in plain sight," as stated in a cover article of CAP TODAY, published by the College of American Pathologists in November 2005 [1]. To achieve this, we need to mobilize the awareness and support of the entire medical community, both clinicians and pathologists.

Acknowledgment The author wishes to thank Dr. Maria M. Picken for helpful suggestions and editing.

Reference

1. Titus K. Amyloidosis hiding in plain sight. CAP TODAY, November 2005, cover story. http://www.cap.org

Index

© Springer International Publishing Switzerland 2015

M.M. Picken et al. (eds.), *Amyloid and Related Disorders*, Current Clinical Pathology,
DOI 10.1007/978-3-319-19294-9